ANESTHESIOLOGY
REVIEW

Third Edition

Edited by

Ronald J. Faust, M.D.

Professor
Department of Anesthesiology
Mayo Medical School
Rochester, Minnesota

Associate Editors

Roy F. Cucchiara, M.D.
Professor
Department of Anesthesiology
University of Florida College of Medicine
Gainesville, Florida

Steven H. Rose, M.D.
Assistant Professor
Department of Anesthesiology
Mayo Medical School
Rochester, Minnesota

Thomas N. Spackman, M.D.
Assistant Professor
Department of Anesthesiology
Mayo Medical School
Rochester, Minnesota

Denise J. Wedel, M.D.
Professor
Department of Anesthesiology
Mayo Medical School
Rochester, Minnesota

C. Thomas Wass, M.D.
Assistant Professor
Department of Anesthesiology
Mayo Medical School
Rochester, Minnesota

ANESTHESIOLOGY
REVIEW

Third Edition

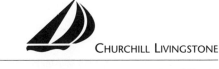

CHURCHILL LIVINGSTONE

An Imprint of Elsevier

CHURCHILL LIVINGSTONE
An Imprint of Elsevier

The Curtis Center
Independence Square West
Philadelphia, Pennsylvania 19106

Library of Congress Cataloging-in-Publication Data

Anesthesiology review / edited by Ronald J. Faust; associate editors, Roy F. Cucchiara . . . [et al.].—3rd ed.

p.   cm.

Includes bibliographical references and index.

ISBN 0–443–06601–9

1. Anesthesiology—Examinations, questions, etc.   I. Faust, Ronald J.   II. Cucchiara, Roy F.

RD82.3.A53 2002   617.9′6′076—dc21

DNLM/DLC   2001017365

Publishing Director, Surgery: Richard Lampert
Senior Acquisitions Editor: Allan Ross
Developmental Editor: Deborah Thorp
Project Manager: Scott Filderman
Senior Production Manager: Natalie Ware
Illustrations Specialist: Walt Verbitski

ANESTHESIOLOGY REVIEW   ISBN 0–443–06601–9

Third Edition © Mayo Foundation 2002
Second Edition © Mayo Foundation 1994
First Edition © Mayo Foundation 1991

Last digit is the print number: 9   8   7   6   5   4

CONTRIBUTORS

Martin D. Abel, M.D.
Associate Professor, Department of Anesthesiology
  Mayo Medical School, Rochester, Minnesota

Roxann D. Barnes, M.D.
Assistant Professor, Department of Anesthesiology
  Mayo Medical School, Rochester, Minnesota

David R. Becker, M.D.
Anesthesiologist, Phoenix, Arizona

Eric A. Bedell, M.D.
Anesthesiologist, University of Texas Medical
  Branch, Galveston, Texas

Richard Belmont, D.O.
Anesthesiologist, Eau Claire, Wisconsin

Keith H. Berge, M.D.
Assistant Professor, Department of Anesthesiology
  Mayo Medical School, Rochester, Minnesota

Ines H. Berger, M.D.
Assistant Professor, Department of Anesthesiology
  Mayo Medical School, Rochester, Minnesota

William G. Binegar, M.D.
Anesthesiologist, Boise, Idaho

Michael L. Bishop, M.D.
Anesthesiologist, Warrenton, Virginia

Susan Black, M.D.
Professor, Department of Anesthesiology
  University of Alabama School of Medicine
  Birmingham, Alabama

Daniel R. Brown, M.D., Ph.D.
Assistant Professor, Department of Anesthesiology
  Mayo Medical School, Rochester, Minnesota

Pamela Jensen-Bundy, M.D.
Anesthesiologist, Port Angeles, Washington

Paul E. Carns, M.D.
Instructor, Department of Anesthesiology
  Mayo Medical School, Rochester, Minnesota

Renee E. Caswell, M.D.
Assistant Professor, Department of Anesthesiology
  Mayo Medical School, Scottsdale, Arizona

Thomas J. Christopherson, M.D.
Instructor, Department of Anesthesiology
  University of South Dakota School of Medicine
  Sioux Falls, South Dakota

David J. Cook, M.D.
Associate Professor, Department of Anesthesiology
  Mayo Medical School, Rochester, Minnesota

Robert M. Craft, M.D.
Assistant Professor, Department of Anesthesiology
  University of Tennessee Graduate School of
  Medicine, Knoxville, Tennessee

Frank D. Crowl, M.D.
Anesthesiologist, Chevy Chase, Maryland

Roy F. Cucchiara, M.D.
Professor, Department of Anesthesiology
  University of Florida College of Medicine
  Gainesville, Florida

David R. Danielson, M.D.
Assistant Professor, Department of Anesthesiology
  Mayo Medical School, Rochester, Minnesota

William J. Davis, M.D.
Anesthesiologist, Victoria, British Columbia

Maria DeCastro, M.D.
Anesthesiologist, Los Angeles, California

Ann E. Decker, J.D.
Legal Department, Mayo Clinic
  Rochester, Minnesota

Martin L. DeRuyter, M.D.
Assistant Professor, Department of Anesthesiology
  Mayo Medical School, Rochester, Minnesota

Niki M. Dietz, M.D.
Associate Professor, Department of Anesthesiology
  Mayo Medical School, Rochester, Minnesota

Jerry A. Dorsch, M.D.
Associate Professor, Department of Anesthesiology
  Mayo Medical School, Jacksonville, Florida

Douglas A. Dubbink, M.D.
Anesthesiologist, St. Paul, Minnesota

Beth A. Elliott, M.D.
Assistant Professor, Department of Anesthesiology
  Mayo Medical School, Rochester, Minnesota

John K. Erie, M.D.
Anesthesiologist, Sioux Falls, South Dakota

Scott A. Eskuri, M.D.
Anesthesiologist, Duluth, Minnesota

Ronald J. Faust, M.D.
Professor, Department of Anesthesiology
  Mayo Medical School, Rochester, Minnesota

Neil G. Feinglass, M.D.
Assistant Professor, Department of Anesthesiology
  Mayo Medical School, Jacksonville, Florida

James Findlay, M.B., Ch.B., F.R.C.A.
Assistant Professor, Department of Anesthesiology
  Mayo Medical School, Rochester, Minnesota

Randall P. Flick, M.D.
Assistant Professor, Department of Anesthesiology
  Mayo Medical School, Rochester, Minnesota

Robert J. Friedhoff, M.D.
Assistant Professor, Department of Anesthesiology
  Mayo Medical School, Rochester, Minnesota

Scott A. Gammel, M.D.
Anesthesiologist, Lafayette, Louisiana

Stephen T. Gott, M.D.
Anesthesiologist, St. Paul, Minnesota

Robert E. Grady, M.D.
Anesthesiologist, Sioux Falls, South Dakota

Brian A. Hall, M.D.
Assistant Professor, Department of Anesthesiology
  Mayo Medical School, Rochester, Minnesota

Jerry A. Hall, M.D.
Assistant Professor, Department of Anesthesiology
  University of Colorado Health Sciences Center
  Denver, Colorado

James D. Hannon, M.D.
Assistant Professor, Department of Anesthesiology
  Mayo Medical School, Rochester, Minnesota

Barry A. Harrison, M.D.
Assistant Professor, Department of Anesthesiology
  Mayo Medical School, Rochester, Minnesota

Roger E. Hofer, M.D.
Assistant Professor, Department of Anesthesiology
  Mayo Medical School, Rochester, Minnesota

Terese T. Horlocker, M.D.
Associate Professor, Department of Anesthesiology
  Mayo Medical School, Rochester, Minnesota

Michael P. Hosking, M.D.
Associate Professor, Department of Anesthesiology
  University of Tennessee Graduate School of
  Medicine, Knoxville, Tennessee

Paul J. Hubbell, M.D.
Anesthesiologist, Metairie, Louisiana

Daniel J. Janik, M.D.
Associate Professor, Department of Anesthesiology
  University of Colorado Health Sciences Center
  Denver, Colorado

Christopher J. Jankowski, M.D.
Assistant Professor, Department of Anesthesiology
  Mayo Medical School, Rochester, Minnesota

Mary B. Jedd, M.D.
Anesthesiologist, Chico, California

Michael E. Johnson, M.D., Ph.D.
Assistant Professor, Department of Anesthesiology
  Mayo Medical School, Rochester, Minnesota

Robert V. Johnson, M.D.
Assistant Professor, Department of Pediatric &
  Adolescent Medicine, Mayo Medical School
  Rochester, Minnesota

Michael J. Joyner, M.D.
Professor, Department of Anesthesiology
  Mayo Medical School, Rochester, Minnesota

Mark T. Keegan, M.D.
Assistant Professor, Department of Anesthesiology
  Mayo Medical School, Rochester, Minnesota

Brian C. Kerr, M.D.
Anesthesiologist, Boise, Idaho

Michelle A. O. Kinney, M.D.
Instructor, Department of Anesthesiology
  Mayo Medical School, Rochester, Minnesota

Tim J. Lamer, M.D.
Assistant Professor, Department of Anesthesiology
Mayo Medical School, Jacksonville, Florida

Theresia L. Lee, M.D.
Anesthesiologist, San Antonio, Texas

Scott A. Lockwood, M.D.
Instructor, Department of Anesthesiology
University of South Dakota School of Medicine
Sioux Falls, South Dakota

Elizabeth Noël Lumpkin, M.D.
Anesthesiologist, Longview, Washington

Robert J. Lunn, M.D.
Anesthesiologist, Sioux Falls, South Dakota

Carlos B. Mantilla, M.D.
Assistant Professor, Department of Anesthesiology
Mayo Medical School, Rochester, Minnesota

David P. Martin, M.D., Ph.D.
Assistant Professor, Department of Anesthesiology
Mayo Medical School, Rochester, Minnesota

Brian P. McGlinch, M.D.
Instructor, Department of Anesthesiology
Mayo Medical School, Rochester, Minnesota

John C. McMichan, M.B.B.S., Ph.D.
Associate Professor, Department of Anesthesiology
Mayo Medical School, Scottsdale, Arizona

K.A. Kelly McQueen, M.D.
Anesthesiologist, Phoenix, Arizona

Pamela A. Mergens, M.D.
Instructor, Department of Anesthesiology
Mayo Medical School, Rochester, Minnesota

Linda K. Miller, M.D.
Instructor, Division of Preventive & Occupational
Medicine, Mayo Medical School
Rochester, Minnesota

David R. Mumme, M.D.
Anesthesiologist, Indianapolis, Indiana

Donald A. Muzzi, M.D.
Anesthesiologist, Duluth, Minnesota

Bradly J. Narr, M.D.
Assistant Professor, Department of Anesthesiology
Mayo Medical School, Rochester, Minnesota

Gregory A. Nuttall, M.D.
Assistant Professor, Department of Anesthesiology
Mayo Medical School, Rochester, Minnesota

Doris B. Ockert, M.D.
Associate Professor, Department of Anesthesiology
University of Wisconsin Medical School, Madison,
Wisconsin

William C. Oliver, Jr., M.D.
Assistant Professor, Department of Anesthesiology
Mayo Medical School, Rochester, Minnesota

Steven G. Peters, M.D.
Associate Professor, Division of Pulmonary &
Critical Care Medicine, Mayo Medical School
Rochester, Minnesota

Susanne D. Pfeffer, M.D.
Resident, Department of Anesthesiology
Mayo Graduate School of Medicine, Rochester,
Minnesota

Christopher Powers, M.D.
Instructor, Department of Anesthesiology
Mayo Medical School, Rochester, Minnesota

Mary M. Rajala, M.D.
Anesthesiologist, Green Bay, Wisconsin

Karen S. Reed, M.D., Ph.D.
Anesthesiologist, Elmira, New York

Guy S. Reeder, M.D.
Professor, Division of Cardiovascular Diseases
Mayo Medical School, Rochester, Minnesota

Kent H. Rehfeldt, M.D.
Instructor, Department of Anesthesiology
Mayo Medical School, Rochester, Minnesota

Edwin H. Rho, M.D.
Instructor, Department of Anesthesiology
Mayo Medical School, Rochester, Minnesota

Richard H. Rho, M.D.
Instructor, Department of Anesthesiology
Mayo Medical School, Rochester, Minnesota

Kevin P. Ronan, M.D.
Anesthesiologist, Sioux Falls, South Dakota

Steven H. Rose, M.D.
Assistant Professor, Department of Anesthesiology
Mayo Medical School, Rochester, Minnesota

Joseph J. Sandor, M.D.
Anesthesiologist, Scottsdale, Arizona

Timothy S. J. Shine, M.D.
Assistant Professor, Department of Anesthesiology
  Mayo Medical School, Jacksonville, Florida

Peter A. Southorn, M.D., F.R.C. Anes.
Professor, Department of Anesthesiology
  Mayo Medical School, Rochester, Minnesota

Thomas N. Spackman, M.D.
Assistant Professor, Department of Anesthesiology
  Mayo Medical School, Rochester, Minnesota

Wolf H. Stapelfeldt, M.D.
Instructor, Department of Anesthesiology
  Mayo Medical School, Jacksonville, Florida

Paul E. Stensrud, M.D.
Assistant Professor, Department of Anesthesiology
  Mayo Medical School, Rochester, Minnesota

Michael D. Taylor, M.D.
Anesthesiologist, Edmond, Oklahoma

Norman E. Torres, M.D.
Assistant Professor, Department of Anesthesiology
  Mayo Medical School, Rochester, Minnesota

Mark F. Trankina, M.D.
Associate Professor, Department of Anesthesiology
  University of Alabama School of Medicine
  Birmingham, Alabama

Terrence L. Trentman, M.D.
Instructor, Department of Anesthesiology
  Mayo Medical School, Scottsdale, Arizona

Claude A. Vachon, M.D.
Resident, Department of Anesthesiology
  Mayo Graduate School of Medicine
  Rochester, Minnesota

Jerald O. Van Beck, M.D.
Anesthesiologist, Des Moines, Iowa

John M. Van Erdewyk, M.D.
Anesthesiologist, Mitchell, South Dakota

G.M.S. Vasdev, M.D., F.R.C. Anes.
Assistant Professor, Department of Anesthesiology
  Mayo Medical School, Rochester, Minnesota

Pamela Vick, M.D.
Assistant Professor, Division of Pain Management
  University of North Carolina School of Medicine
  Chapel Hill, North Carolina

Wayne H. Wallender, D.O.
Anesthesiologist, Rogersville, Missouri

David O. Warner, M.D.
Professor, Department of Anesthesiology
  Mayo Medical School, Rochester, Minnesota

Mark A. Warner, M.D.
Professor, Department of Anesthesiology
  Mayo Medical School, Rochester, Minnesota

Mary Ellen Warner, M.D.
Assistant Professor, Department of Anesthesiology
  Mayo Medical School, Rochester, Minnesota

C. Thomas Wass, M.D.
Assistant Professor, Department of Anesthesiology
  Mayo Medical School, Rochester, Minnesota

Joseph G. Weber, M.D.
Anesthesiologist, Minneapolis, Minnesota

Mary B. Weber, M.D.
Anesthesiologist, Wyoming Medical Center
  Casper, Wyoming

Denise J. Wedel, M.D.
Professor, Department of Anesthesiology
  Mayo Medical School, Rochester, Minnesota

Margaret R. Weglinski, M.D.
Assistant Professor, Department of Anesthesiology
  Mayo Medical School, Rochester, Minnesota

Roger D. White, M.D.
Professor, Department of Anesthesiology
  Mayo Medical School, Rochester, Minnesota

Jack L. Wilson, M.D.
Assistant Professor, Department of Anesthesiology
  Mayo Medical School, Rochester, Minnesota

Lawrence J. Winikur, M.D.
Anesthesiologist, Martinsville, Virginia

Gilbert Y. Wong, M.D.
Assistant Professor, Department of Anesthesiology
  Mayo Medical School, Rochester, Minnesota

Glenn E. Woodworth, M.D.
Anesthesiologist, Phoenix, Arizona

Fernando A. Zepeda, M.D.
Anesthesiologist, Johnson City, Tennessee

Preface to the Third Edition

Just after the second edition of this text was published in 1994, a publishing company executive told me that electronic publishing would largely replace conventional textbooks by 2000. He's in another field now, and business at the local bookshop seems to be as good as ever.

Although we have access to electronic information in ways never dreamed of 5 years ago, computers do not yet match the utility, portability, and popularity of printed books. More important, the printed page seems to better fit the learning style of many students who use underlining, highlighting, and reviewing to enhance learning of important topics. Computer access varies from teaching institution to institution, hospital to hospital, student to student, and country to country. Although the possibilities are theoretically unlimited in the Age of Information, better access, new hardware, and improved computer skills among users are implemented at a slow pace with great variability across the global village.

Readers who used a previous edition might notice a shift in the information presentation in this 3rd edition. Focusing on key word phrases, the first two editions of *Anesthesiology Review* attempted to close the gap in the process through which the American Board of Anesthesiology (ABA)/American Society of Anesthesiology (ASA) Joint Council on In-Training Examinations conducts its annual written examination. That group starts with its Content Outline from which question writers develop questions (see Figure). These questions are carefully edited before inclusion in the ABA/ASA Annual In-Training Examination. After the exam, key word phrases are constructed from each question, and feedback is given to each resident on which phrases were answered incorrectly. The first two editions of *Anesthesiology Review* attempted to give readers an organized way to study as many key word phrases, derived from examinations of recent years, as possible.

A problem with this approach to learning lies in its inconclusiveness. Important topics in our specialty might be missed year after year because they do not readily lend themselves to question writing. Key word phrases might bear little resemblance to the area of the Content Outline from which a question was originally derived. New topics of undeniable importance might not yet have made their way into the examination process.

The Associate Editors and I have taken a new

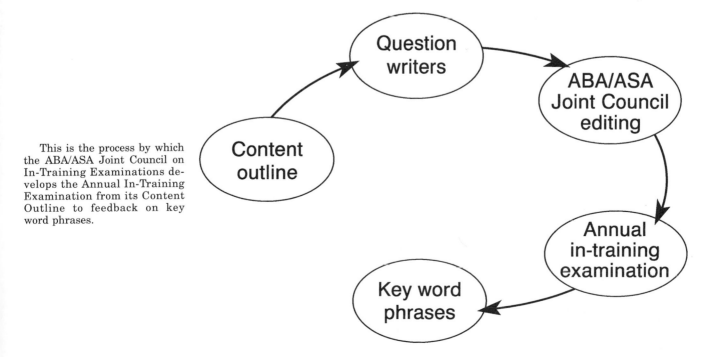

This is the process by which the ABA/ASA Joint Council on In-Training Examinations develops the Annual In-Training Examination from its Content Outline to feedback on key word phrases.

approach in constructing this edition. We tried to concentrate on what we thought was missing or incomplete in the first two editions and chose contributors with special expertise in those areas. Over 60 new or totally revised chapters have been added, although great effort has been taken to delete or combine chapters from the previous editions so that the text would not lose its portability.

The many kind expressions of thanks I have received from readers of the first two editions have been the motivation to create the third. It is hoped that readers will continue to find it useful.

Ronald J. Faust, M.D.

Preface to the First Edition

Although the release of new anesthesia textbooks and monographs in the 1980s paralleled the growth of knowledge in the field, the success rate of candidates applying for certification in the specialty continues to be disappointing. Data from the American Board of Anesthesiology (ABA) reveal that over 15 percent of United States medical school graduates taking their first ABA written examination fail. Only 75 percent of candidates taking their first ABA oral examination were successful in the late 1980s. More than 20 percent of residents who completed training by 1987 and applied to the ABA were still not certified by spring, 1991.

Why is the success rate on ABA examinations not higher? Most would agree that the quality of physicians coming into the specialty has risen over the past 15 years. Has the growth of knowledge in the specialty outstripped the ability of residents to master it? Has the proliferation of new journals in the specialty increased the burden on anesthesiology students by diffusing pertinent new information? Or are the priorities of ABA examiners that much different from those who write the texts used by anesthesiology residents?

Candidates should have an understanding of the process through which the written examination is formulated each year. The American Board of Anesthesiology—American Society of Anesthesiologists Joint Council on In-Training Examinations publishes a 17-page Content Outline, last revised in June, 1987. It is organized into areas on physiologic, physical, and clinical sciences. Each year the Joint Council assigns sections of the Content Outline to experienced anesthesiologists who function as question writers. The Council then carefully edits selected questions before each July examination. Anesthesiology residents take the test annually as an in-training practice. Those who have completed the required training and have been admitted to the certification process by the ABA take a subset of the same examination to qualify for the oral evaluation which must be passed for certification. After each examination, the Joint Council reports a list of key word phrases to program directors. This list contains over 300 items tested with percentage of correct answers for each program and for the nation as a whole. Each resident in training also receives a list of key word phrases that he or she answered incorrectly.

Thus, the Joint Council makes public where the examination originated (the Content Outline) and where it ended (the key word phrase list) each year. In spite of this information, success rates do not improve. This may be attributed to many factors, including difficulty with studying from the Content Outline and the key word phrase lists. These sources may be too inclusive to be researched in depth by one person.

Anesthesiology Review provides a new approach to preparation for this examination. Over 200 key word phrases from the 1986 through 1989 written examinations have been selected and edited for this review. A synopsis has been prepared on each key word based on knowledge that is current in anesthesia journals and texts. The selected key word phrases are grouped into sections on physiologic, physical, and clinical sciences in a manner similar to the organization of the Content Outline, which is included as an appendix. The goal is to concentrate on essential information rather than produce a reference text.

Anesthesiology Review provides students of the specialty with a fresh approach to preparation for ABA examinations. By reducing the available information into an abbreviated format, a conciseness is achieved that also makes the book a manual useful for clinical practice. All key word phrase sections were written by current or former residents in the Department of Anesthesiology at the Mayo Clinic and edited by my capable associate editors.

Ronald J. Faust, M.D.

Contents

PHYSICAL SCIENCES

CLINICAL SCIENCES

Physiologic Sciences

1
Pulmonary Function Test Interpretation

David O. Warner, M.D.

Normal values for pulmonary function tests in normal subjects are shown in Table 1–1, and typical alterations in disease are shown in Table 1–2. The anesthesiologist should be aware that although these tests provide an assessment of the severity of lung disease, no single test or combination of tests is necessarily predictive of perioperative pulmonary complications.[3]

Tests to Measure Lung Volumes

Spirometry. Spirometry measures the volume of gas passing through the airway opening. During spirometry, the patient first breathes normally, then is asked to inhale maximally and exhale maximally (Fig. 1–1). Measurements obtained by spirometry include inspiratory capacity (IC), inspiratory reserve volume (IRV), expiratory reserve volume (ERV), and vital capacity (VC). These measurements are all effort-dependent.

Functional Residual Capacity Measurements. Functional residual capacity (FRC) measures the amount of gas in the lungs at the end of expiration during tidal breathing. Three types of methods are available: (1) **equilibration methods,** in which FRC is calculated from the concentration of a tracer gas (usually helium) in a closed system in equilibrium with the patient's lungs; (2) **washout methods**, in which FRC is calculated from the lung washout of a tracer gas (usually nitrogen); and (3) **plethysmographic methods**, in which the total thoracic gas volume is measured by a technique based on Boyle's law. This method measures the total amount of gas in the thorax, whereas the other two methods measure the amount of gas in communication with the airway opening. When combined with spirometry, FRC measurements allow calculation of total lung capacity (TLC) and residual volume (RV). Decreased TLC and RV is the hallmark of restrictive lung disease.

Tests of Gas Flow

Forced Expiratory Spirography. In this test, the subject exhales as forcefully as possible from a maximal inhalation, and expiratory flow and volume are measured using a spirometer or pneumotachograph (Fig. 1–2). In any individual, after the maximal forced expiratory flow (FEF_{max}), the flow during maximal effort depends only on lung volume and lung characteristics, not on the effort. The most useful parameters obtained from forced expiratory spirography are forced vital capacity (FVC) and forced expiratory volume in 1 second (FEV_1). The

Table 1–1. Normal Values for a 40-Year-Old Male (Height 178 cm) and Female (Height 165 cm)

	Male	Female
VC and FFV (l)	5	3.5
RV (l)	1.8	1.7
TLC (l)	6.8	5.2
FRC (l)	3.4	2.6
FEV_1 (l)	4.1	2.9
$FEV_1\%$	82	83
FEF_{25-75} (l/sec)	4.3	3.3
MVV (L/min)	168	112
DL_{CO} (mL/min/mm Hg)	33	24

See text for definition of abbreviations. (Adapted from Taylor AE Rehder K, Hyatt RE, et al[2].)

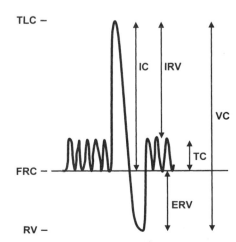

Figure 1–1. Changes in lung volume over time during spirometry. See text for abbreviations. (Adapted from Conrad SA and George RB.[1])

Table 1–2. Patterns of Disease

	Restriction		Obstruction		
	Chest Wall	*Parenchyma*	*Asthma*	*Bronchitis*	*Emphysema*
TLC	↓	↓	↑	− or ↑	↑
VC			− or ↓	− or ↓	− or ↓
RV	− or ↑	↓	↑	↑	↑
FRC	↓	↓	↑	↑	↓
MVV	− or ↓	− or ↓			↓
D_LCO	−	↓	− or ↑	− or ↓	↓
FEV_1	↓	↓			↓
$FEV_1\%$	−	−	↓	↓	↓

↓ = decreased; ↑ = increased; − = normal. See text for definitions of abbreviations. (Adapted from Taylor AE, Rehder K, Hyatt RE, et al.[2])

ratio of FEV_1 to FVC ($FEV_1\%$) normalizes FEV_1 measurements for each individual's lung volume. For example, a patient with restrictive lung disease will have a low FEV_1 because of low lung volume, not airway obstruction. Reduced FEV_1 and $FEV_1\%$ is the hallmark of obstructive lung disease. $FEV_1\%$ values of 60% to 70% indicate mild obstruction; 40% to 60%, moderate obstruction; and less than 40%, severe obstruction. These measurements are not valid if the patient does not perform at maximum effort. Forced expiratory flow from 75% to 25% of VC (FEF_{25-75}) is another spirography measurement that may be less effort-dependent. If maximal inspiratory flows are also measured, then the **flow-volume loop** can be useful in identifying the source of airway obstruction (Fig. 1–3). In patients with obstructive lung disease, forced expiratory spirography may be done before and after the inhalation of a bronchodilator to assess the reversibility of airway obstruction. (A greater than 10% change in FEV_1 indicates reversibility.) Analogously, airway challenge with methacholine is used to diagnose asthma. Patients with asthma will exhibit abnor-

mally decreased flow parameters (a greater than 15% decrease in FEV_1) in response to methacholine.

Maximal Voluntary Ventilation (MVV). In this test, the subject breathes as quickly and deeply as possible through a pneumotachograph for 12 seconds. The exhaled volume is measured and multiplied by 5 to yield the maximal ventilation during 1 minute. Because this test measures patient motivation and effort as well as lung and thorax properties, it may be a particularly useful screening test before surgery.

Tests of Diffusing Capacity

Several methods are available to measure diffusing capacity, all of which measure the diffusion of carbon monoxide across the alveolar-capillary membrane. Diffusing capacity ($D_{L_{CO}}$) decreases with the loss of parenchyma (e.g., in emphysema) or thickening of the alveolar-capillary membrane (e.g., in fibrosis).

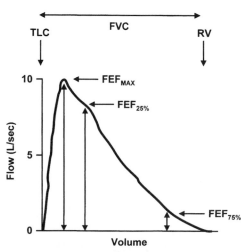

Figure 1–2. Maximal expiratory flow-volume curve. See text for abbreviations. (Adapted from Conrad SA, George RB.[1])

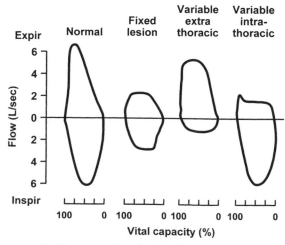

Figure 1–3. Maximal inspiratory and expiratory flow-volume curves used to diagnose airway obstruction. (Adapted from Taylor AE, Rehder K, Hyatt RE, et al.[2])

Selected References

1. Conrad SA, George RB. Clinical pulmonary function testing. In George RB, Light RW, Matthay RA, eds. Chest Medicine. New York: Churchill Livingstone, 1984:161.

2. Taylor AE, Rehder K, Hyatt RE, et al. Clinical Respiratory Physiology. Philadelphia, WB Saunders, 1989.

3. Tisi GM. Preoperative evaluation of pulmonary function. Am Rev Respir Dis 1979;119:293.

2
Factors Affecting Pulmonary Compliance and Airway Resistance

Michael L. Bishop, M.D.

Tissue Elasticity and Compliance

Elasticity is that property of tissue that causes a return to resting shape after deformation by an external force. Perfectly elastic tissues will obey **Hooke's law** such that application of one unit of force will result in one unit of stretch, two units of force will result in two units of stretch, and so on up to the tissue's elastic limit. The slope of the line that results from plotting the change in length (stretch) versus the change in force will indicate the stiffness, or mechanical **compliance,** of the tissues. Compliance of the lungs and thorax is defined as the change in volume for a given change in pressure (dV/dP); the clinical units are L/cm H_2O. This measurement specifically refers to **static pressure–volume** relationships. In contrast, airway **resistance** refers to **dynamic pressure–flow** relationships.

Lung and Thoracic Cage Compliance Relationships

Resting volumes are lower in isolated lungs than in lungs in the intact chest. Resting volumes of the thoracic cage are greater with the lungs removed than with the lungs in situ. Thus, the resting position is a balance between two forces: the force of the thoracic cage attempting to expand outward and the force of the lungs attempting to recoil inward. The volume within the lungs at this balance point is termed the **functional residual capacity** (FRC). Muscular energy is required to both increase and decrease lung volume from this resting position. The compliance of the combined thoracic cage and lung is less than the compliance of either component alone. It is calculated by the following formula:

$$\frac{1}{C_{Total}} = \frac{1}{C_{Lung}} + \frac{1}{C_{Thoracic\ Cage}}$$

Normal values are:
- Lung compliance 0.2 L/cm H_2O.
- Thoracic cage compliance 0.2 L/cm H_2O.
- Total compliance 0.1 L/cm H_2O.

Experiments have demonstrated that compliance varies with lung volume. Thus, compliance measurements must be interpreted with knowledge of lung volume (usually FRC). For example, a lung compliance of 60% of normal does not indicate that the lungs are stiffer than normal unless the lung volume (FRC) is known to be normal. To address this problem, some investigators report **specific compliance** (compliance related to FRC).

Lung Compliance

- The pressure in a bubble (or alveolus) is inversely proportional to the radius (**LaPlace's law**). That is, a small bubble would empty into a larger one.
- Pulmonary surfactant **increases** compliance by altering surface tension relationships in the alveoli; surfactant **decreases** surface tension as alveoli decrease in size. This allows small alveoli to exist at the same pressure as larger alveoli.
- Pulmonary edema **decreases** compliance, perhaps by altering surfactant concentration or changing alveolar geometry.
- When pulmonary surfactant is damaged or removed, increased surface tension in smaller alveoli causes them to collapse. High pressure is needed to re-expand them.
- Ascites, pleural effusion, pericardial effusion, and cardiomegaly all **decrease** compliance by decreasing FRC, among other mechanisms.
- Pleural, interstitial or alveolar fibrosis all **decrease** compliance by decreasing the elastic properties of the lung tissue and decreasing FRC.
- Atelectasis and pneumonia **decrease** compliance secondary to decreased FRC and decreased surfactant.
- Airway occlusion by bronchospasm **decreases** compliance secondary to decreased FRC.
- Poliomyelitis and kyphoscoliosis **decrease** compliance secondary to decreased FRC.
- Pulmonary artery obstruction **decreases** compliance by decreasing FRC and pulmonary surfactant.
- General anesthesia **decreases** compliance by decreasing FRC.

□ Emphysema **increases** compliance secondary to loss of normal elastic recoil of the lungs. (Normal transpulmonary pressure results in an elevated FRC.)

Thoracic Cage Compliance. Kyphoscoliosis, pectus excavatum, arthritic spondylitis, skeletal muscle diseases resulting in rigidity or spasticity, abdominal disorders with marked diaphragmatic elevation, and marked obesity all **decrease** thoracic cage compliance.

Effects of Decreased Compliance

□ Decreased compliance causes **increased work** of breathing, because higher pressures are needed to increase lung volume. Compensatory mechanisms to decrease the work of breathing include increased respiratory rate and decreased tidal volume.

□ Pulmonary compliance is not uniform throughout the lung, and thus alveolar ventilation is also uneven. This results in regional ventilation–perfusion variability.

Airway Resistance

Driving pressure is that pressure necessary to move air through the airways during inspiration and expiration. This equals atmospheric pressure – alveolar pressure during inspiration and alveolar pressure – atmospheric pressure during expiration. Because pressure = flow × resistance (**Ohm's law**), **resistance = driving pressure/flow**. Airway resistance is created by friction between molecules of flowing gas and the airway walls; it is expressed in units of $cmH_2O \cdot L^{-1} \cdot sec^{-1}$.

For **laminar** gas flow, by **Poiseuille's law**, resistance = $8 Nl/\Pi r^4$, where N = viscosity of the gas in poises, l = length of airway, and r = radius of the airway. Thus, resistance to flow is affected most significantly by the radius of the airway. Reducing the radius by 50% increases resistance 16-fold (i.e., 2^4).

Resistance is also dependent on the nature of the gas flow. With **laminar flow**, pressure is proportional to the volume of gas flow times a constant related to gas **viscosity**. However, with **turbulent** flow, pressure is proportional to the volume of the gas flow squared times a constant related to gas **density**. Assuming constant flow, according to Ohm's law, resistance with turbulent flow exceeds that during laminar flow. Turbulence occurs at airway branch points and with irregularities in the walls of the airways (e.g., mucus, exudate, tumor, foreign body, and partial glottic closure). In normal lungs, most airway resistance occurs in the large lobar bronchi and diminishes progressively as gas moves peripherally, because of progressively increased total airway area with resultant decreased flow velocity. Resistance is minimal in peripheral respiratory bronchioles. Thus, large changes can occur in the diameter of peripheral bronchioles before changes occur in measured airway resistance. Normal adult airway resistance is 0.5 to 1.5 $cmH_2O \cdot L^{-1} \cdot sec^{-1}$.

Factors Affecting Airway Resistance

□ Airway resistance **decreases** with increased lung volume as the elastic tissues of the lung increase airway diameter.

□ Bronchospasm and airway secretions associated with asthma result in **increased** airway resistance, thereby facilitating turbulent flow.

□ Emphysema causes **increased** resistance because airways tend to collapse. In addition, as these patients attempt to overcome the increased resistance with forced expiration, the positive intrapleural pressure developed tends to collapse airways further.

□ Airway resistance is **increased** by other causes of decreased airway lumen size including mucosal congestion, edema, inflammation, pneumothorax, presence of exudate or foreign bodies, compression, and fibrosis.

□ Iatrogenic causes of **increased** resistance include long, narrow endotracheal tubes.

Effects of Increased Airway Resistance

□ Increased resistance increases the time needed to complete exhalation. This results in increased FRC if the respiratory rate is kept constant. To compensate, patients may depend on active exhalation, which increases the work of breathing.

□ Increased airway resistance may cause dyspnea, particularly during exhalation.

□ In an attempt to decrease airway resistance, patients may decrease their rate of breathing, to allow decreased flow velocity, and exhale against pursed lips, to decrease the pressure gradient, which tends to collapse the airways.

Suggested References

Comroe JH. Physiology of Respiration. Chicago, Year Book Medical, 1974.

Comroe JH, Forster RE, DuBois AB, et al. The Lung. Chicago, Year Book Medical, 1962.

Lewis WD, Chwals W, Benotti PN, et al. Bedside assessment of the work of breathing. Crit Care Med 1988;16:117–122.

Tobin MJ, Guenther SM, Perez W, et al. Konno–Mead analysis of ribcage-abdominal motion during successful and unsuccessful trials of weaning from mechanical ventilation. Am Rev Respir Dis 1987;135:1320–1328.

3
Effect of Surfactant on Lung Mechanics

Thomas J. Christopherson, M.D.

Surfactant Production and Composition

Surfactant is a saturated phospholipid material that promotes alveolar stability and expansion by **lowering surface tension**.

Production. Surfactant production is under the control of the hypothalamic-pituitary-adrenal axis. This develops late in fetal life; **type II pneumocytes** differentiate at approximately 24 weeks' gestation, and begin to synthesize surfactant at about 34 weeks' gestation. Steroid administration may increase the number of type II alveolar cells and thus stimulate surfactant production.[1]

Surfactant's short half-life (14 to 48 hours) makes it quite sensitive to various influences that affect pulmonary integrity in critically ill patients.[2] Atelectasis, oxygen toxicity, transudate in alveolar spaces, and vascular obstruction with hypoperfusion can all markedly diminish surfactant production.

Composition. Surfactant is composed predominantly of dipalmityl phosphatidylcholine with some phosphatidylglycerol and other saturated phospholipids.[3] Surfactant is confined to a 50-Å layer on the alveolar surface. The fatty acid portion of the molecule is hydrophobic and projects into the alveolar cavity. The other end of the molecule is hydrophilic and lies within the alveolar fluid. During expiration, surfactant molecules become more densely packed as alveolar surface area decreases. This results in decreased alveolar surface tension.

Bovine surfactant (e.g., beractant, calfactant, colfosceril) is available for intratracheal or nebulized administration through an endotracheal tube to infants with neonatal respiratory distress syndrome (RDS). These agents' efficacy in treating chronic pulmonary disease has not been clearly demonstrated, however.

Effect of Surfactant on Alveolar Surface Tension

The effect of surfactant on alveolar surface tension and pressure can be illustrated by **Laplace's law**:

$$P \propto 2T/r$$

As the alveolus grows smaller during expiration, alveolar membrane pressure (P) increases to twice the surface tension (T) divided by the alveolar radius (r). As the alveolar radius decreases, membrane pressure increases, leading to collapse (i.e., atelectasis). By diminishing alveolar surface tension in concert with decreasing alveolar radius, surfactant allows for a small transpulmonic pressure (i.e., 4 to 5 cmH_2O) to maintain alveolar integrity during expiration.

Effect of Surfactant on Foreign Particles

Surfactant has been shown to be protective against certain bacteria and toxic agents. It is **bactericidal** toward some microorganisms, especially gram-positive bacteria present in oral secretions. On the other hand, gram-negative organisms are resistant to surfactant, but may be susceptible to one or more partially defined alveolar fluid peptides.

Surfactant has also been shown to be an opsonic agent that facilitates phagocytosis of *Staphylococcus aureus* by macrophages in vitro. Surfactant may also reduce toxicity of certain inhaled particles (e.g., silica) by coating the particle and altering its composition or charge.[4]

Selected References

1. Murphy BE. Evidence of cortisol deficiency at birth in infants with the respiratory distress syndrome. J Clin Endocrinol Metab 1978;38:158.
2. Morgan TE. Pulmonary surfactant. N Engl J Med 1971;284:1185–1193.
3. Nunn JF. Elastic forces and lung volumes. In Nunn JF, ed. Nunn's Applied Respiratory Physiology. 4th ed. Cambridge: UK, Butterworth-Heinemann, 1995:36–60.
4. Kelley WN. Textbook of Internal Medicine. Philadelphia, JB Lippincott, 1989.

4
Factors Affecting Pulmonary Ventilation and Perfusion

Michael E. Johnson, M.D., Ph.D.

Ventilation ($\dot{V}$)

In an awake, spontaneously breathing patient, in all positions, ventilation per unit lung volume is smallest at the highest portion (e.g., the apex in an upright patient) and increases with vertical distance down the lung. The lung is more compressed in the most dependent portion because gravity creates a gradient in intrapleural pressure. Basal alveoli are one-quarter the volume of apical alveoli at end-expiration. This puts the basal alveolar characteristics on a steeper portion of the pressure-volume (P-V) curve (Fig. 4–1); the basal alveoli are smaller than apical alveoli initially, but expand more during inspiration.

General anesthesia changes the effect of gravity on alveolar ventilation. In the supine patient, anesthesia with paralysis and mechanical ventilation decreases the difference between the ventilation of the dependent and nondependent alveoli, causing more nearly uniform distribution of ventilation throughout the lung. This is attributed to a decreased functional residual capacity (FRC), shifting alveolar characteristics downward on the P-V curve (see Fig. 4–1), and altered respiratory mechanics. In the lateral decubitus position, anesthesia re-verses the distribution of ventilation, so that the nondependent (up) lung receives greater ventilation than the dependent (down) lung. This holds for both spontaneous and mechanical ventilation. This is clinically significant because the dependent lung has greater perfusion (see later), which causes increased ventilation/perfusion ($\dot{V}/\dot{Q}$) mismatch. The change in ventilatory distribution in the lateral decubitus position is attributed to (1) decreased FRC, causing a shift along the P-V curve (which can be partially reversed by positive end-expiratory pressure [PEEP]), (2) greater compression of the dependent lung by the mediastinum and abdominal contents, and (3) increased compliance of the nondependent hemithorax.

Pulmonary Blood Flow ($\dot{Q}$)

The two major determinants of pulmonary blood flow are (1) gravity and (2) hypoxic pulmonary vasoconstriction. Pulmonary artery (PA) pressure decreases by 1.25 mm Hg/cm of vertical distance up the lung. Because the pulmonary circulation is a low-pressure system, this causes significant differences in perfusion pressure between the lower and

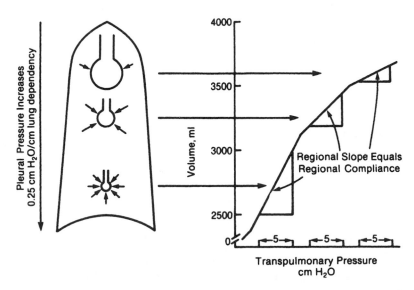

Figure 4–1. Pleural pressure increases 0.25 cm H_2O every centimeter down the lung. The increase in pleural pressure causes a fourfold decrease in alveolar volume. The caliber of the air passages also decreases as lung volume decreases. When regional alveolar volume is translated over to a regional transpulmonary pressure–alveolar volume curve, small alveoli are on a steep (large slope) portion of the curve, and large alveoli are on a flat (small slope) portion of the curve. The regional slope equals regional compliance. Over the normal tidal volume range (2500 to 3000 mL), the pressure-volume relationship is linear. Lung volume values in this diagram relate to the upright position. (From Benumof JL.[1])

The Four Zones of the Lung

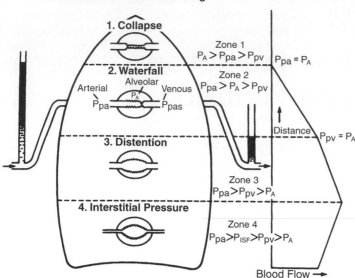

Figure 4-2. Distribution of blood flow in the isolated lung. In zone 1, alveolar pressure (PA) exceeds pulmonary artery pressure (Ppa) and no flow occurs, presumably because collapsible vessels are directly exposed to alveolar pressure. In zone 2, arterial pressure exceeds alveolar pressure, but alveolar pressure exceeds venous pressure (Ppv). Flow in zone 2 is determined by the arterial-alveolar pressure difference, which steadily increases down the zone. In zone 3, pulmonary venous pressure now exceeds alveolar pressure and flow is determined by the arterial-venous pressure difference (Ppa − Ppv), which is constant down the lung. However, the pressure across the walls of the vessels increases down zone 3, so that their caliber increases, as does flow. In zone 4, flow is determined by the arterial interstitial pressure difference (Ppa − PISF), because interstitial pressure exceeds both Ppv and PA. (From Benumof JL.[1])

higher regions of the lung, with greater perfusion going to the lower lung regions. The actual perfusion (Q̇) to an alveolus also depends on the alveolar pressure (PA) which opposes the PA pressure (Ppa) and pulmonary venous pressure (Ppv). This interaction is summarized in Figure 4–2. All these relationships are dynamic, varying throughout the cardiac and respiratory cycles. There are four defined zones of blood flow in the lung. In zone 1, at the apex of an upright lung, PA > Ppa, preventing any blood flow and thereby creating alveolar dead space. Zone 1 is negligible in healthy lungs. In zone 2, Ppa > PA > Ppv, so that Q̇ depends only on Ppa − PA. In zone 3, Ppa > Ppv > PA, and Q̇ is a function of Ppa − Ppv, independent of PA. In general, decreases in Ppa (e.g., hemorrhagic shock) will increase the size of the upper zones (1 and 2) at the expense of the lower zones (2 and 3), whereas increases in Ppa have the opposite effect. Increases in PA (e.g., with PEEP) may recruit alveoli from lower zones into higher zones (i.e., increase the volumes of zones 1 and 2).

Hypoxic pulmonary vasoconstriction (HPV) is a local response of PA smooth muscle to a decreased regional alveolar P_{O_2}. It acts to decrease Q̇ to underventilated regions of lung and maintain normal V̇/Q̇. HPV is effective only when there is a significant section of normally ventilated and oxygenated lung to which flow can be diverted (e.g., one-lung ventilation during thoracic surgery). Intravenous anesthetics do not inhibit HPV, whereas the volatile anesthetics and potent vasodilators do. Therapeutically inhaled nitric oxide is a unique pulmonary-specific vasodilator that does not worsen HPV and often improves oxygenation, because it is delivered only to alveoli that are already being ventilated.

Ventilation/Perfusion Ratio (V̇/Q̇)

Both V̇ and Q̇ increase toward the dependent part of the lung, but at different rates (Fig. 4–3).

Therefore, V̇/Q̇ >1 at the top, V̇/Q̇ = 1.0 at the third rib in upright lungs, and V̇/Q̇ <1 below the third rib. V̇/Q̇ is, of course, also affected by the factors that affect V̇ or Q̇ separately (see earlier).

Dead Space (VD)

VD is that portion of a breath that does not participate in gas exchange. VT is the tidal volume. VD/VT is the fraction of the tidal volume composed of dead-space volume. Anatomic dead space [VD(an)] is that volume of gas that ventilates the conducting airways only. Alveolar dead space [VD(al)] is that

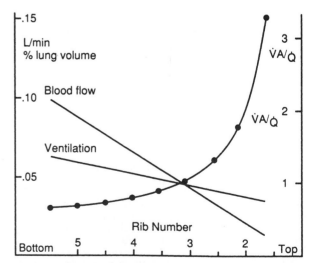

Figure 4–3. Distribution of ventilation and perfusion (left vertical axis) and the ventilation/perfusion ratio (right vertical axis) in normal upright lung. Both ventilation and perfusion are expressed in L/min/percent alveolar volume and have been drawn as smoothed-out linear functions of vertical height. The closed circles mark the ventilation/perfusion ratios of horizontal lung slices. A cardiac output of 6 L/min and a total minute ventilation of 5.1 L/min was assumed. (From West JB.[2])

volume of gas not taking part in effective gas exchange at the alveolar level; i.e., ventilated but unperfused alveoli. Total (or physiologic) $V_D = V_D(an) + V_D(al)$. Normally, the ratio of the physiologic dead space to the tidal volume $(V_D/V_T) = 1/3$, and $V_D(an) = 0.5$ mL/kg body weight. In awake, healthy, supine patients, $V_D(al)$ is negligible. One mechanism contributing to this is a bronchiolar constrictive reflex that constricts airways to alveoli that are unperfused.

V_D/V_T may be measured by Bohr's method, based on the fact that all expired CO_2 comes from perfused alveoli and none from dead space:

$$V_D/V_T = \frac{(\text{alveolar } P_{CO_2} - \text{expired } P_{CO_2})}{\text{alveolar } P_{CO_2}}$$

Clinically, we assume that arterial = alveolar P_{CO_2}. Expired P_{CO_2} is the average P_{CO_2} in an expired gas sample; this is *not* the same as the end-tidal P_{CO_2}.

Factors Affecting V_D and V_D/V_T

V_D and V_D/V_T are affected by $\dot{V}$, $\dot{Q}$, and the anatomy of the conducting airways.

□ *Decreased Ppa* (e.g., hemorrhage, drug effects) causes increased $V_D(al)$ due to an increase in zone 1.

□ *Loss of perfusion* to ventilated alveoli despite normal or high PA pressures causes increased $V_D(al)$. These conditions may result from pulmonary emboli (including venous air embolism), PA thrombosis, surgical manipulation of pulmonary arterial tree, or emphysema with loss of alveolar septa and vasculature.

□ *Increased airway pressure* (e.g., positive-pressure ventilation [PPV]) causes increased $V_D(an)$ from radial traction on conducting airways by surrounding lung parenchyma and increased $V_D(al)$ from increased zone 1.

□ *Extended neck and protruded jaw* cause a twofold increase in $V_D(an)$ compared to a flexed neck and depressed chin.

□ *Erect posture* causes increased $V_D(al)$ compared to supine, because decreased perfusion to uppermost alveoli causes increased volume of zone 1.

□ *The dead space of anesthesia apparatus* increases V_D/V_T ratio from the normal 0.3 to values of 0.4 to 0.5 with endotracheal intubation and Y-piece connectors or 0.64 with face mask.

□ *Tracheostomy or intubation* decreases $V_D(an)$ by roughly half unless the anesthesia apparatus is added to the breathing circuit.

□ *General anesthesia*, with spontaneous or controlled respiration, increases V_D and V_D/V_T. Etiology is multifactorial and incompletely understood; it may be partially due to moderate pulmonary hypotension, loss of skeletal muscle tone, or loss of bronchoconstrictor tone.

□ *Rapid, short inspirations* increase V_D by ventilating a greater fraction of noncompliant and badly perfused alveoli than slower, deeper inspirations.

□ *Increasing age* increases both anatomic and alveolar dead space due to decreased elasticity of lung tissues. Additionally, closing volume and closing capacity increase with aging.

Selected References

1. Benumof JL. Respiratory physiology and respiratory function during anesthesia. In Miller RD, ed. Anesthesia, 5th ed. Philadelphia: Churchill Livingstone, 2000:578–618.
2. West JB. Respiratory Physiology. 2nd ed. Baltimore, Williams & Wilkins, 1970.

Suggested References

Eisenkraft JB, Cohen E, Neustein SM. Anesthesia in thoracic surgery. In Barash PG, Cullen BF, Stoelting RK, eds. Clinical Anesthesia, 3rd ed. Philadelphia: Lippincott-Raven, 1996:769–803.

Prough DS, Mathru M. Acid-base, fluids, and electrolytes. In Barash PG, Cullen BF, Stoelting RK, eds. Clinical Anesthesia. 3rd ed. Philadelphia: Lippincott-Raven, 1996:157–187.

Rehder K, Sessler AD, Marsh HM. General anesthesia and the lung. Ann Rev Resp Dis 1975;112:541.

Stock MC. Respiratory function in anesthesia. In Barash PG, Cullen BF, Stoelting RK, eds. Clinical Anesthesia. 3rd ed. Philadelphia: Lippincott-Raven, 1996:747–768.

Zapol WM. Inhaled nitric oxide. Acta Anaesthiol Scand 1996;109 (Suppl):81–83.

5
Clinical Implications of the Alveolar Gas Equation

Pamela Jensen Bundy, M.D.

The alveolar air equation is used to determine the partial pressure of oxygen in alveoli (PAO_2). Clinically, PAO_2 is important when calculating the alveolar-arterial oxygen tension difference ($A\text{-}aDO_2$). Knowledge of the magnitude of this difference can indicate whether a functional deficit in oxygen exchange exists. These values can be calculated using the following equations:

$$PAO_2 = (PB - PH_2O)(FIO_2) - PaCO_2/R$$

$$A\text{-}aDO_2 = A\text{-}a \text{ gradient} = PAO_2 - PaO_2$$

where PB = barometric pressure (760 mm Hg at sea level); PH_2O = partial pressure of water in alveoli (47 mm Hg at 37°C); FIO_2 = fraction of inspired oxygen; and R = respiratory quotient (i.e., CO_2 production/O_2 consumption, 0.8). Arterial oxygen tension (PaO_2) and arterial carbon dioxide tension ($PaCO_2$) are determined by arterial blood gas analysis. As can be seen from the above equations, reductions in PAO_2 result from decreased PB or FIO_2, or increased $PaCO_2$ (i.e., hypoventilation). Normal PaO_2 decreases with age according to the equation:

$$PaO_2 = 102 - \frac{age\ (yr)}{3}$$

Alveolar-Arterial Oxygen Difference

A gradient between the alveolar and arterial oxygen tensions (i.e., $A\text{-}aDO_2$) normally exists. Such differences are often referred to as A-a gradients. Normal $A\text{-}aDO_2$ is <10 mm Hg in healthy individuals and increases with age. The gradient is due to (1) normal "physiologic" shunting through bronchial and thebesian (coronary) veins that drain deoxygenated blood directly into the left side of the heart, and (2) normal ventilation-perfusion gradients. The clinical usefulness of the A-a gradient is limited because values are dependent on FIO_2. That is, the A-a gradient increases with increasing FIO_2 regardless of normal or abnormal pulmonary physiology. For example, the gradient may increase to 70 mm Hg in normal individuals inspiring an FIO_2 of 100%.

Abnormal A-a Gradients

Increased A-a gradients occur for several reasons:

- **Anatomic shunting**. Shunting may result from congenital heart disease with right-to-left shunting or pulmonary arteriovenous malformations.
- **Diffusion impairment**. If the capillary-alveolar interface is thickened, as in interstitial lung disease, then oxygen delivery to the pulmonary capillary blood may be hindered. There is usually adequate pulmonary transit time. However, in exercise or other high-output states, pulmonary blood flow may be so high that red cells do not remain in alveolar capillaries long enough to become fully oxygenated (usually 0.3 second).
- **Ventilation-perfusion ($\dot{V}/\dot{Q}$) mismatch**. $\dot{V}/\dot{Q}$ may be altered by a change in either ventilation or perfusion.

In **low $\dot{V}/\dot{Q}$ areas**, perfusion exceeds ventilation, resulting in intrapulmonary shunting. General anesthesia reduces functional residual capacity (FRC) by approximately 400 mL, and the supine position decreases FRC by about 800 mL. This decrease may bring the end-expiratory level or even the entire tidal volume range below closing capacity, greatly decreasing regional lung ventilation without changing perfusion. Further complicating matters, volatile anesthetics, aminophylline, nitroprusside, nitroglycerin, and hypocapnia inhibit hypoxic pulmonary vasoconstriction (HPV), a protective physiologic measure causing regional pulmonary vasoconstriction in areas of hypoxia. HPV causes diversion of blood from these underventilated areas, thereby maintaining normal $\dot{V}/\dot{Q}$ relationships. When HPV is blunted or abolished, low $\dot{V}/\dot{Q}$ areas develop. This may severely affect oxygenation, particularly during one-lung ventilation in the lateral position. Additionally, exposure to 100% oxygen can lead to absorption atelectasis. Because hemoglobin from high $\dot{V}/\dot{Q}$ areas is already fully saturated and unable to increase its oxygen content further, local hyperventilation (increased $\dot{V}/\dot{Q}$) cannot compensate for decreased arterial oxygen content resulting from low $\dot{V}/\dot{Q}$ regions.

In **high $\dot{V}/\dot{Q}$ areas**, ventilation exceeds perfusion, resulting in alveolar dead space. High $\dot{V}/\dot{Q}$ areas exist with embolic events due to air, tumor, fat, or thrombi. However, pulmonary emboli also release vasoactive substances that cause regional or widespread vasoconstriction, resulting in increased shunting. Surgical clamping of pulmonary arterial vasculature will also decrease perfusion.

Suggested References

Stoelting RK. Pulmonary gas exchange and blood transport of gases. In Stoelting RK, ed. Pharmacology and Physiology in Anesthesia Practice. 3rd ed. Philadelphia: Lippincott-Raven, 1999:692–701.

Isserles SA, Breen PH. Can changes in end-tidal PCO_2 measure changes in cardiac output? Anesth Analg 1991;73:808–814.

Weinberger SE. Principles of Pulmonary Medicine. 3rd ed. Philadelphia, WB Saunders, 1998.

West JB. Respiratory Physiology: The Essentials. 6th ed. Philadelphia, Lippincott Williams & Wilkins, 2000.

6

Measurement and Implications of $\dot{Q}s/\dot{Q}t$

Gregory A. Nuttall, M.D.

As discussed in Chapter 5, the alveolar-arterial oxygen tension difference (A-a gradient, A-a DO_2) is normally less than 10 mm Hg with fraction of inspired oxygen (FIO_2) = 0.21. However, the magnitude of the A-a gradient is not linear with FIO_2, and at an FIO_2 of 1.0, the normal A-a gradient is less than 100 mm Hg. This has led to other methods of measuring the efficiency of oxygen gas exchange. The a/A ratio is one such method. The a/A ratio is equal to arterial oxygen tension (PaO_2)/alveolar oxygen concentration (PAO_2). A normal a/A ratio is greater than 0.75 regardless of the FIO_2 or PAO_2.

$\dot{V}/\dot{Q}$ Matching

The normal matching of pulmonary ventilation to perfusion ($\dot{V}/\dot{Q}$) is 0.8. A normal lung segment has matched ventilation and perfusion ($\dot{V}/\dot{Q}$ = 1). An absolute shunt is represented by lung segments that are perfused but not ventilated ($\dot{V}/\dot{Q}$ = 0). Deadspace is represented by lung segments that are ventilated but not perfused ($\dot{V}/\dot{Q}$ = infinity). The normal $\dot{V}/\dot{Q}$ ratio may be altered by the distribution of ventilation, the distribution of perfusion, and the relationship of these two distributions. An important concept is that local hyperventilation (increased $\dot{V}/\dot{Q}$) cannot compensate for the decreased PaO_2 secondary to areas of shunting (low $\dot{V}/\dot{Q}$). Hypoxic pulmonary vasoconstriction (HPV) is an intrapulmonary mechanism that attempts to minimize $\dot{V}/\dot{Q}$.

Shunt (Venous Admixture)

Some pulmonary capillary blood normally bypasses ventilated alveoli so that venous blood is added to arteriolized blood. An estimated 2% to 5% of cardiac output is normally shunted through these pulmonary shunts, which accounts for the normal A-a gradient. There are thought to be three types of shunts:

□ Physiologic (capillary) shunts are the most common and are secondary to atelectasis or consolidation of alveoli.

□ Postpulmonary shunts are secondary to bronchial, mediastinal, pleural, and thebesian veins.
□ Pathoanatomic shunts are secondary to congenital or traumatic anomalies and intrapulmonary tumors. The absolute shunt is equal to the sum of the anatomic and physiologic shunting.

Calculation of Shunt Fraction ($\dot{Q}s/\dot{Q}t$)

The fraction of cardiac output that passes through a shunt is expressed as the shunt fraction ($\dot{Q}s/\dot{Q}t$):

$$\dot{Q}s/\dot{Q}t = \frac{(Cc - Ca)}{(Cc - Cv)}$$

where Cc = oxygen content of end-pulmonary capillary blood, Ca = oxygen content of arterial blood, and Cv = oxygen content of mixed venous blood.

$$Ca = (1.39)(Hb)(\% \ sat) + (0.003)(PaO_2)$$

where Hb = hemoglobin concentration (g/dL), % sat = percent oxygen saturation, and PaO_2 = arterial blood oxygen concentration.

When cardiac output is normal and PaO_2 is greater than 175, shunt fraction can be estimated by the simplified formula:

$$\frac{P(A - a)O_2}{20}$$

This formula is derived from the assumption that a 1% intrapulmonary shunt is responsible for each 20-mm Hg change in A-aDO_2. The normal shunt fraction is below 5% to 7%; clinically insignificant shunts are 10% to 19%, significant shunts are 20% to 30%, and potentially fatal shunts are greater than 30%.

Suggested References

Marini JJ. Monitoring during mechanical ventilation. Clin Chest Med 1988;9:73.

Murray J, Nadel J. Textbook of Respiratory Medicine. 2nd ed. Philadelphia, WB Saunders, 1994.

Stock MC. Respiratory function in anesthesia. In Barash PG, Cullen BF, Stoelting RK, eds. Clinical Anesthesia. 3rd ed. Philadelphia: Lippincott-Raven, 1997:747.

West JB. Respiratory Physiology: The Essentials. 6th ed. Philadelphia, Lippincott-Raven, 2000.

7
Oxygen Transport

David R. Mumme, M.D.

Oxygen transport is essentially determined by cardiac output (CO), blood oxygen content (CaO_2), and the affinity of hemoglobin (Hb) for oxygen (Fig. 7–1). Affinity determines the position of the oxyhemoglobin dissociation curve, and this is affected by pH, temperature, and 2,3-diphosphoglycerate (2,3-DPG). Five variables affect tissue oxygenation:

- Hb concentration.
- Saturation percentage (SaO_2).
- Cardiac output.
- Oxygen consumption.
- Hb affinity for oxygen (P_{50}).

CaO_2 is calculated as the sum of the oxygen bound by Hb and the oxygen dissolved in the plasma.

$$CaO_2 = (Hb \times 1.39 \times SaO_2/100) + (PaO_2 \times 0.003)$$

For example, if Hb = 15 g/dL, SaO_2 = 100%, and PaO_2 = 100 mm Hg, then

$$CaO_2 = (15 \times 1.39 \times 1) + (100 \times 0.003)$$

$$= 20.85 + 0.3 = 21.15 \text{ mL/dL}$$

Note that dissolved oxygen typically has little impact on CaO_2. Notable exceptions occur in severe anemia, carbon monoxide intoxication, and severe shock.

The oxygen content of mixed venous blood is usually 25% less than that of arterial blood. At a mixed venous O_2 saturation of 75% and O_2 tension of 40 mm Hg, mixed venous O_2 content ($C\bar{v}O_2$) is

$$C_vO_2 = (15 \times 1.39 \times 0.75) + (40 \times 0.003)$$

$$= 15.64 + .12$$

$$= 15.76 \text{ mL/dL}$$

Oxygen delivery (DO_2) to the tissues is the product of CO and CaO_2. For example, if CO = 5.0 L/min in the previous example, then the DO_2 is

$$DO_2 = 211.5 \text{ mL/L} \times 5.0 \text{ L/min}$$

$$= 1057 \text{ mL/min}$$

$$= \text{approximately 1 L/min}$$

Oxygen consumption ($\dot{V}O_2$), approximately 250 mL/min for an adult, is the difference between arterial and venous oxygen content (assuming no shunt.) The Fick principle is

$$\dot{V} = CO \times C(a - \bar{v})O_2$$

Thus, for a constant $\dot{V}O_2$, a decrease in the CO requires an increase in the $C(a - \bar{v})O_2$ by either increased CaO_2 or increased tissue oxygen extraction. Conversely, for an increased $\dot{V}O_2$, CO and/or $C(a - \bar{v})O_2$ must increase.

The Oxyhemoglobin Dissociation Curve

The oxyhemoglobin dissociation curve is the measured relationship between PO_2 and SO_2 (see Fig.

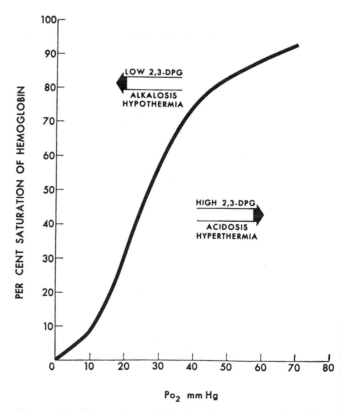

Figure 7–1. The oxyhemoglobin dissociation curve plots hemoglobin saturation (ordinate) at varying oxygen tensions (abscissa). Note that hemoglobin is approximately 80% saturated at a PaO_2 of 50 mm Hg, 75% saturated at a PaO_2 of 40 mm Hg (venous), and 30% saturated at a PaO_2 of 20 mm Hg. The normal P_{50} is 26.7 mm Hg. (From Miller RD.[1])

Table 7–1. Variables Shifting the Oxyhemoglobin
Dissociation Curve

Left	Right
Alkalosis	Acidosis
Hypothermia	Hyperthermia
Decreased 2,3-DPG	Increased 2,3-DPG
Abnormal hemoglobin (fetal)	Abnormal hemoglobin
Carboxyhemoglobin	Increased CO_2
Methemoglobin	

7–1). The position of this curve is best described by the position at which hemoglobin is 50% saturated (P_{50}), which is normally 26.7 mm Hg. Shifting this curve to the left or right has little effect on the So_2 in the normal range, where the curve is relatively horizontal; a much greater effect is seen for values in the steeper parts of the curve.

Variables shifting the oxyhemoglobin dissociation curve are listed in Table 7–1. A left-shifted oxyhemoglobin dissociation curve indicates a higher affinity of hemoglobin for oxygen and thus a higher saturation at a given PaO_2. This may require higher tissue perfusion to produce the same oxygen un-loading. A right-shifted oxyhemoglobin dissociation curve implies lower affinity, and thus lower saturation, but may permit lower tissue perfusion. Adding hydrogen ions, 2,3-DPG, and heat causes a rightward shift of the curve.

Chronic acid-base changes will cause a compensatory change in 2,3-DPG within 24 to 48 hours and return the oxyhemoglobin dissociation curve back toward normal.

Selected References

1. Miller RD. The oxygen dissociation curve and multiple transfusions of ACD blood. In Howland WS, Schweizer O, eds. Management of Patients for Radical Cancer Surgery. Clinical Anesthesia. Philadelphia: FA Davis, 1972:43.

Suggested References

Miller RD. Transfusion therapy. In Miller RD, ed. Anesthesia. 5th ed. Philadelphia: Churchill Livingstone, 2000:1613–1644.

Robertie PG, Gravlee GP. Safe limits of isovolemic hemodilution and recommendations for erythrocyte transfusion. Int Anesthesiol Clin 1990; 28:197–204.

Snyder JV. Oxygen Transport in the Critically Ill. Chicago, Year Book Medical Publishers, 1987.

8
Carbon Dioxide Dissociation Curve

Margaret R. Weglinski, M.D.

The end product of aerobic metabolism is carbon dioxide (CO_2). The amount of CO_2 in the body is a function of both CO_2 production and elimination. There is a continuous gradient of CO_2 tension as CO_2 passes from the mitochondria through the cytoplasm, extracellular fluid, venous blood, and alveolar gas, and then by way of exhalation disperses in ambient air. CO_2 elimination is dependent on pulmonary blood flow and alveolar ventilation.

CO_2 Transport in Plasma

CO_2 is transported in the blood in several forms. In plasma, CO_2 is carried in three forms (Fig. 8–1).

- A negligible amount of CO_2 combines with the amino groups of plasma proteins to form carbamino compounds according to the equation:

$$R - NH_2 + CO_2 \leftrightarrow R - NH - COOH$$

The CO_2 reaction with plasma protein is restricted to one terminal amino group in each protein and side-chain amino groups in lysine and arginine.

- A small amount of CO_2 remains in solution as CO_2 is moderately soluble in plasma (solubility coefficient is 0.03 mmol·L^{-1}·mm Hg^{-1} at 37°C). Approximately 5% of CO_2 dissolves in plasma. Of this, one molecule of CO_2 in 700 reacts with plasma water and through hydrolysis forms carbonic acid:

$$CO_2 + H_2O \leftrightarrow H_2CO_3$$

Because of the lack of carbonic anhydrase in plasma, this reaction is very slow. In fact, the concentration of CO_2 in plasma is nearly 1000 times greater than that of carbonic acid.

- The small amount of carbonic acid that is formed in plasma dissociates into hydrogen and bicarbonate ions:

$$H_2CO_3 \rightarrow H^+ + HCO_3^-$$

- It is the CO_2 in physical solution that determines blood pH. It is in this form that most of the CO_2 enters and exits the blood.

CO_2 Transport in Erythrocytes

Most of the CO_2 produced passes into the erythrocytes, where it is carried in three forms (see Fig. 8–1):

- A negligible amount of CO_2 remains in solution in erythrocyte water.
- A much larger amount of CO_2 combines with hemoglobin to form carbaminohemoglobin. This reaction is facilitated by the release of oxygen from hemoglobin, making reduced hemoglobin a 3.5-times more effective CO_2 carrier than oxyhemoglobin.
- The greatest fraction of CO_2 in the erythrocytes is hydrated to form carbonic acid, which dissociates into bicarbonate and hydrogen ions. Unlike the reaction in plasma, in the erythrocyte it is cata-

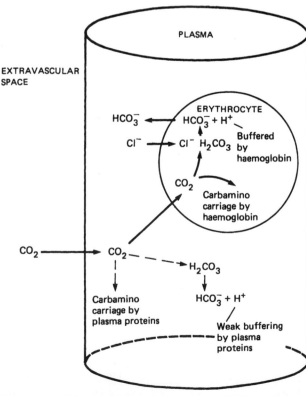

Figure 8–1. Diagrammatic representation of CO_2 transport in plasma and in the erythrocyte. (From Lumb AB.[1])

18

Table 8–1. Normal Values for Carbon Dioxide Transport in Blood

	Arterial Blood (Hb 95% Saturated)	Mixed Venous Blood (Hb 70% Saturated)	Arterial/Venous Difference
Whole blood			
PH	7.40	7.367	−0.033
P_{CO_2} (mm Hg)	40.0	46.0	+6.0
Total CO_2			
(mmol/L)	21.5	23.3	+1.8
(mL/L)	48.0	52.0	+4.0
Plasma (mmol/L)			
Dissolved CO_2	1.2	1.4	+0.2
Carbonic acid	0.0017	0.0020	+0.0003
Bicarbonate ion	24.4	26.2	+1.8
Carbamino CO_2	negligible	negligible	negligible
Total	25.6	27.6	+2.0

These values have not been drawn from a single publication but represent the mean of values reported in a large number of studies. (Modified from Lumb AB.[1])

lyzed by the enzyme carbonic anhydrase. This allows the reaction to proceed about 1000 times faster than in plasma. However, when carbonic anhydrase is inhibited, CO_2 transport remains adequate. Almost 99.9% of the carbonic acid dissociates to the bicarbonate and hydrogen ions.

□ The negatively charged bicarbonate ion produced from the dissociation of carbonic acid diffuses out of the erythrocyte into the plasma. To maintain electrical neutrality within the erythrocyte, chloride ion diffuses from plasma into the erythrocyte, in a process called the **Hamburger phenomenon** or **chloride shift**.

□ The quantity of CO_2 carried in the blood and the differences between arterial and venous blood are given in Table 8–1.

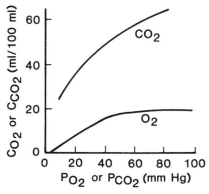

Figure 8–2. Comparison of the shape of the oxyhemoglobin and CO_2 dissociation curves. The slope of the CO_2 dissociation curve is about three times steeper than that of oxyhemoglobin dissociation curve. Cco_2 represents CO_2 content of blood, Co_2 represents oxygen content of blood, and Pco_2 and Po_2 are the partial pressures of CO_2 and O_2 in blood, respectively. (From Taylor AE, Rehder K, Hyatt RE, et al.[2])

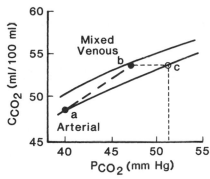

Figure 8–3. The Haldane effect, as illustrated here, is of physiologic importance in CO_2 transport. Deoxygenated blood (mixed venous) has a greater capacity to carry CO_2 than does oxygenated blood (arterial). In the absence of this shift in the CO_2 dissociation curve, tissue P_{CO_2} would need to increase considerably to load the same amount of CO_2. (From Taylor AE, Rehder K, Hyatt RE, et al.[2])

CO_2 Dissociation Curve

The CO_2 dissociation curve defines the relationship between the total CO_2 content of blood and the partial pressure of CO_2.

□ Two important differences exist between the oxyhemoglobin dissociation curve and the CO_2 dissociation curve. First, the CO_2 dissociation curve is much more linear than the O_2 dissociation curve. Second, the CO_2 dissociation curve has a steeper slope, meaning that for a given change in partial pressure, significantly more CO_2 than O_2 can be carried in blood (Fig. 8–2).

□ The degree of hemoglobin oxygenation affects the position of the CO_2 dissociation curve. The lower the saturation of hemoglobin with O_2, the higher the CO_2 content for a given P_{CO_2}. This is known as the **Haldane effect** (Fig. 8–3). This can be explained by the fact that deoxygenated hemoglobin has a higher affinity for the H^+ ions produced when carbonic acid dissociates; it has a greater ability than oxygenated hemoglobin to form carbaminohemoglobin. When hemoglobin releases O_2 in the tissues, the capacity of the blood to transport CO_2 increases (point a → point b in Fig. 8–3). When hemoglobin becomes loaded with O_2 in the lungs, the reverse process occurs (point b → point a). Without the Haldane effect, tissue P_{CO_2} would need to rise to 51 mm Hg (point a → point c) to load the same CO_2 found in mixed venous blood at a P_{CO_2} of 46 mm Hg with the Haldane effect.

Selected References

1. Lumb AB. Nunn's Applied Respiratory Physiology. 5th ed. Boston, Butterworth-Heinemann, 2000.
2. Taylor AE, Rehder K, Hyatt RE, et al. Clinical Respiratory Physiology. Philadelphia, WB Saunders, 1989.

9
Interpretation of Arterial Blood Gases

Bradly J. Narr, M.D. ▫ Steven G. Peters, M.D.

The clinical utility of arterial blood gas measurements includes assessment of oxygenation [arterial oxygen tension (PaO_2)], ventilation [arterial carbon dioxide tension ($PaCO_2$)], and acid-base status (pH). These measurements allow quantitative assessments of the life-sustaining functions of the cardiorespiratory system. Interpretation of this information permits specific diagnostic and therapeutic intervention in the operating room, intensive care, and emergency settings.

Acid-Base Disturbances

Systemic diseases are frequently associated with disturbances of acid-base status. The major extracellular buffer pair is bicarbonate/carbonic acid. A patient's pH can be determined by measuring these two variables and calculating the pH by the Henderson-Hasselbach (H-H) equation:

$$pH = 6.1 + \log \frac{HCO_3^-}{0.03 \times PaCO_2}$$

The body's physiologic response to an acid-base disturbance is threefold. Initially, the acid or base created by the systemic abnormality is **buffered** immediately by whatever buffers predominate in that body fluid compartment. Over the next several hours, **compensation** for the underlying acid-base abnormality occurs via the renal system for respiratory acid-base conditions and through the respiratory system for metabolic acid-base abnormalities. The last phase of this process is **correction** of the underlying pathophysiologic process, which in some cases eliminates the acid-base disturbance (e.g., administration of insulin for diabetic ketoacidosis) or allows the patient to return to baseline for lesions that have been exacerbated by an acute condition (e.g., pneumonia in a patient with chronic obstructive lung disease).

All simple acid-base abnormalities involve compensatory processes that minimize the effect on pH. For example, in acute metabolic acidosis, HCO_3^- decreases and respiratory compensation causes increased ventilation with a decrease in $PaCO_2$, minimizing the change in pH as dictated by the H-H equation. If this compensation does not occur, the patient has more than one acid-base abnormality, and a mixed disturbance can be diagnosed. Mixed disturbances are by far the most common clinical circumstance in critically ill or anesthetized patients.

Acid-base abnormalities are the result of different pathophysiologic processes and are not disease entities. Therefore, the differential diagnosis of any specific acid-base pattern begins with the patient's history and physical examination. Common conditions and associated disease states include:

- ▫ **Metabolic acidosis:** shock, renal failure, type I diabetes
- ▫ **Metabolic alkalosis:** diuretics, nasogastric suction, vomiting
- ▫ **Respiratory acidosis:** narcotics, neuromuscular blockade, chronic obstructive pulmonary disease
- ▫ **Respiratory alkalosis:** hyperventilation, mechanical ventilation

Ventilation

Normal $PaCO_2$ ranges between 36 and 44 torr. Production of CO_2 is relatively constant in most clinical settings, so the elimination of CO_2 is proportional to alveolar ventilation. As diagrammed in Figure 9–1, a $PaCO_2$ below 36 implies hyperventilation and a $PaCO_2$ above 44 implies hypoventilation, unless these situations occur as respiratory compensation for metabolic acid-base abnormalities.

When interpreting $PaCO_2$, the initial question is whether this $PaCO_2$ change (from 40 torr) accounts for the change in pH from 7.40. This can be estimated by the "golden rule":

For every 10 torr change in $PaCO_2$, the pH will change 0.08 unit in the opposite direction.

If the pH change can be accounted for by the $PaCO_2$ change, then the abnormality causing the $PaCO_2$ change is a respiratory disturbance. If not, then a metabolic acid-base disturbance or, more commonly, a mixed metabolic-respiratory acid-base abnormality accounts for the change.

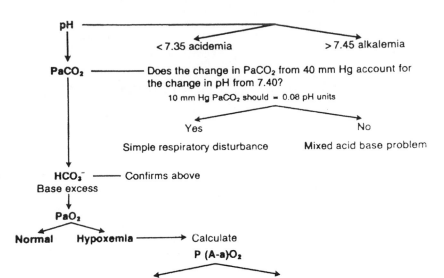

Figure 9–1. An algorithm for blood gas interpretation.

Oxygenation

Pa_{O_2} depends on inspired O_2 concentration, alveolar ventilation, mixed venous oxygen saturation (Sv_{O_2}), and ventilation/perfusion matching ($\dot{V}/\dot{Q}$). The lung is not a perfect gas-exchange unit, and to the extent that ventilation and perfusion are not matched, a gradient between the alveolar and the arterial P_{O_2} exists. Abnormalities in lung function increase this gradient and produce hypoxemia.

When interpreting the Pa_{O_2}, the first step is to determine if hypoxemia is present. In most patients this would be considered a Pa_{O_2} below 60 torr, because this is a physiologic level below which the oxyhemoglobin dissociation curve is steep and the oxygen content of the blood drops rapidly with small decreases in the Pa_{O_2}. If hypoxemia is present, then the alveolar to arterial difference for oxygen $[P(A\text{-}a)_{O_2}]$ is calculated using the simplified alveolar air equation:

$$P_{AO_2} = F_{IO_2}(P_{BP} - P_{H_2O}) - \frac{Pa_{CO_2}}{R}$$

Simplified for clinical use, this reads as follows:

$$P_{AO_2} = (F_{IO_2} \times 713) - \frac{Pa_{CO_2}}{0.8}$$

where F_{IO_2} = fractional content of inspired O_2, P_B = barometric pressure, P_{H_2O} = vapor pressure of water in alveoli at 37°C = 47 mm Hg, and R = respiratory quotient + (CO_2 production/O_2 consumption = 0.8). Pa_{O_2} and Pa_{CO_2} are determined from arterial blood gas analysis.

If the $P(A\text{-}a)_{O_2}$ gradient is normal, then the hypoxemia results from hypoventilation or decreased inspired O_2 concentration. If the $P(A\text{-}a)_{O_2}$ gradient is increased, then the hypoxemia results from a $\dot{V}/\dot{Q}$ mismatch, shunting, or, rarely, a diffusion barrier (see Fig. 9–1).

Finally, O_2 saturation should be assessed relative to the Pa_{O_2} expected for a normal oxyhemoglobin dissociation curve. If the observed saturation is less than expected for the Pa_{O_2}, then other hemoglobin abnormalities, such as carboxyhemoglobin or methemoglobin, should be considered.

10
Blood Gas Temperature Correction

John M. Van Erdewyk, M.D.

In blood gas analysis, the values of arterial carbon dioxide tension ($PaCO_2$), arterial oxygen tension (PaO_2), and pH are highly dependent on temperature. Most blood gas analysis machines are calibrated to and thus run samples at 37°C. If the patient's actual temperature is near 37°C, then the analysis machine values are approximately the same as those of the patient in vivo. The further the patient's temperature is from the machine setting of 37°C, the greater the differential in the numbers reported by the machine and the patient's actual status. **Temperature correction** refers to the process of taking the machine values and correcting them to what the patient is experiencing in vivo, either manually or automatically within the machine (given the patient's actual temperature).

As the temperature of blood decreases, the solubility of O_2 and CO_2 increases, which consequently lowers their partial pressures (i.e., decreased PO_2 and PCO_2). PCO_2 decreases by approximately 4.5% for each 1°C temperature decrease (Table 10–1). When the sample is analyzed in the machine, it is heated to 37°C, which causes a decrease in the solubility and falsely elevates partial pressure values. Temperature correction is needed to determine the patient's actual partial pressures.

Changes in temperature also affect pH. As temperature decreases, less water is dissociated into OH^- and H^+, and thus pH will rise, as will the pOH. The pH rises approximately 0.015 unit for each 1°C decrease in temperature. If the patient's temperature is less than 37°C but subsequently the blood sample is heated to 37°C in the analyzer machine, then elevated levels of H^+ (and OH) will be recorded, leading to a falsely decreased pH value compared to the patient's actual pH.

pH Stat Versus Alpha Stat

pH Stat. During cold cardiopulmonary bypass, the patient's temperature is much lower than 37°C. In a temperature-corrected system, this would produce a decreased $PaCO_2$ and an elevated pH in vivo. Two major approaches have been proposed to handle the management of blood gases during cardiopulmonary bypass–induced hypothermia. In the **pH stat** approach, CO_2 is added to the inspired gases in an attempt to keep the **corrected** $PaCO_2$ normal at 40 mm Hg and the pH normal at greater than 7.4. Proponents of this theory desire a constant pH despite varying patient temperatures. This system was used almost exclusively for the first several decades of cardiopulmonary bypass.

Alpha Stat. In the early 1980s, the **alpha stat** approach gained attention. Many physicians began using this approach because of its potential theoretical benefits, despite a lack of randomized trials or clinical outcome studies. Proponents of this approach attempt to keep a constant charge on amino acids in proteins, principally the a-imidazole ring of histidine, which functions as an important buffer on hemoglobin and other body proteins. The ratio (alpha) of dissociated to undissociated imidazole groups stays constant (alpha stat) with cooling because of changes of blood pK when CO_2 content is held constant. Constant imidazole ionization makes optimal enzyme function possible. As the patient cools, pH must rise because less H^+ is dissociated. However, equally less OH^- is available, and therefore electrochemical neutrality is maintained. Alpha stat management attempts to keep a patient's uncorrected $PaCO_2$ and pH at normal levels, believing that this represents more physiologic values by maintaining electrochemical neutrality despite varying body temperature. Temperature correction is therefore unnecessary.

Patients managed by the pH stat approach would be considered hypercarbic and have a lower pH (i.e., a respiratory acidosis) by the alpha stat approach, and alpha stat management would be considered a relative respiratory alkalosis by the pH stat system (Table 10–2). The blood of cold-blooded animals (ectotherms) undergoes pH changes during cooling parallel to that of water (alpha stat). On the other hand, homeothermic mammals in effect have "corrected" blood gases during hibernation, and their

Table 10–1. Effects of Hypothermia on PCO_2, PO_2, and pH

PCO_2	↓	4.5%/°C
PO_2	↓	
pH	↑	
		0.015 unit/°C

Table 10–2. Effects of Temperature Correction

Parameter	pH Stat as Viewed by Alpha Stat	Alpha Stat as Viewed by pH Stat
CO₂	↑	↓
pH	↓	↑
Condition	Respiratory acidosis	Respiratory alkalosis

decreased metabolic function produces anesthetic effects.

Management

Controversy exists as to which system yields a better patient outcome. Concerns include how the differing pH and P_{CO_2} levels affect cerebral and cardiac outcome. Very few studies exist in the literature. However, one recent study failed to demonstrate any important differences in outcome using these two regimens.

Suggested References

Bashein G, Townes BD, Nessly ML, et al. A randomized study of carbon dioxide management during hypothermic cardiopulmonary bypass. Anesthesiology 1990;72:7–15.

Ream AK, Reitz BA, Silverberg G. Temperature correction of P_{CO_2} and pH in estimating acid-base status: An example of the emperor's new clothes? Anesthesiology 1982;56:41–44.

Sessler DI. Temperature monitoring. In Miller RD, ed. Anesthesia. 5th ed. Philadelphia: Churchill Livingstone, 2000:1367–1389.

Shangraw RE. Acid-base balance. In Miller RD, ed. Anesthesia. 5th ed. Philadelphia: Churchill Livingstone, 2000:1390–1413.

11
Central Regulation of Ventilation

Michael P. Hosking, M.D.

Ventilation is regulated to maintain optimal and unchanging levels of pH, O_2, and CO_2 in the blood. This regulation is provided via the respiratory center, which receives input from chemical stimuli and peripheral chemoreceptors. The respiratory center is a group of nuclei within the medulla and pons that consists of three major areas:

- A **dorsal respiratory group** of neurons controlling inspiration.
- A **pneumotaxic area** in the pons assisting in regulation of inspiration.
- A **ventral respiratory group** regulating expiration.

Neural Control

Inspiratory Center. The inspiratory center located dorsally in the medulla extends its full length (Fig. 11–1). The neurons are located near the termination sites of afferent fibers from the glossopharyngeal (IX) and vagus (X) nerves. This is the site of the basic respiratory drive. It has intrinsic automaticity and normally fires for 2 seconds with a **ramp effect** of increasing intensity to the diaphragm until it abruptly ceases with a 3-second pause before initiating a new cycle.

Pneumotaxic Center. Located in the pons, the pneumotaxic center continually communicates signals to the inspiratory center to turn off inspiration (see Fig. 11–1). A strong signal results in a short (0.5- to 1-second) inspiratory cycle and consequently a more rapid respiratory rate.

- The **apneustic center** is located in the lower pons. Its role is to antagonize the effects of the pneumotaxic center, and it plays no role in normal respiration.
- In the **Hering-Breuer reflex**, bronchiolar stretch receptors feed back to the inspiratory center via the vagus nerve to limit lung overexpansion. This reflex plays a minimal role in normal ventilation but has effects when tidal volume exceeds 1.5 L.

Expiratory Center. The expiratory center extends the full length of the ventral medulla and stimulates muscles of expiration (see Fig. 11–1). It has little role in normal expiration, which is pas-

sive. With increased demand, it plays a significant role. No role in basic respiratory rhythm has been demonstrated.

Chemical Control

Central. The chemosensitive area is located bilaterally in the medulla several microns beneath the ventral surface (Fig. 11–2). This area is extremely sensitive to hydrogen ions (H^+). However, H^+ cross the blood-brain barrier poorly, and thus CO_2 indirectly controls this region through formation of carbonic acid and dissociation to H^+. When stimulated, this chemosensitive area then stimulates the inspiratory center to increase the rate of rise of the ramp effect and thus increase the rate of respiration (see Fig. 11–1):

$$CO_2 + H_2O \rightarrow H_2CO_3 \rightarrow H^+ + HCO_3^-$$

Thus Pa_{CO_2} indirectly influences the level of H^+ in the cerebrospinal fluid (CSF) and controls respiratory drive. Peak effect is reached within 1 minute. The effect begins to wane over the next several hours, and by 48 hours is only one-eighth the peak effect. Compensation is secondary to increased ac-

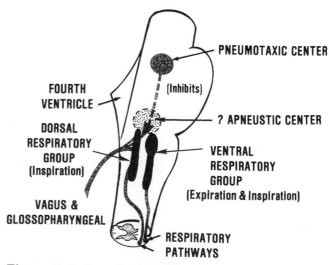

Figure 11–1. Organization of the respiratory center. (From Guyton AC, Hall JE.[1])

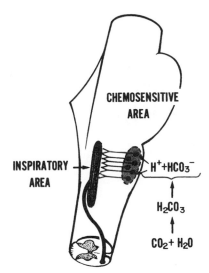

Figure 11–2. Stimulation of the inspiratory area by the chemosensitive area located bilaterally in the medulla, only a few microns beneath the ventral medullary surface. Note also that H^+ ions stimulate the chemosensitive area, whereas mainly CO_2 in the fluid gives rise to the H^+ ions. (From Guyton AC, Hall JE.[1])

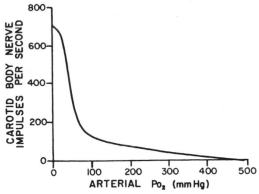

Figure 11–3. Effect of arterial Po_2 on impulse rate from the carotid body of a cat. (From Guyton AC, Hall JE.[1])

tive transport of HCO_3^- into the CSF to neutralize the H^+.

Peripheral. Peripheral chemoreceptors are located in the carotid bodies (cranial nerve IX) and aortic bodies (cranial nerve X). These areas of high blood flow are sensitive to changes in O_2, CO_2, and pH. They stimulate the inspiratory center when Pao_2 decreases; the effect is greatest between 30 and 60 mm Hg (Fig. 11–3).

Mean arterial blood pressure dropping below 70 mm Hg causes increased respiratory drive. The effect of peripheral chemoreceptors in response to hypoxia is eliminated by as little as 0.1 minimum alveolar concentration (MAC) of volatile anesthe-

tics. This may be critical in patients with chronic obstructive lung disease who are dependent on hypoxic respiratory drive. Loss of carotid body, as may occur with carotid endarterectomy, causes decreased response to hypoxia, a 30% decrease in responsiveness to changes in $Paco_2$, and no change in the resting level of respiration.

Selected References

1. Guyton AC, Hall JE. Textbook of Medical Physiology, 9th ed. Philadelphia, WB Saunders, 1996.

Suggested References

Gozal D, Shoseyov D, Keens TG. Inspiratory pressures with CO_2 stimulation and weaning from mechanical ventilation in children. Am Rev Respir Dis 1993;147:256–261.

Kelsen SG. Control of ventilation. In Baum GL, Crapo JD, Celli BR, Karlinsky JB, eds. Textbook of Pulmonary Diseases. Philadelphia: Lippincott-Raven, 1998:47–64.

12
Physiologic Effects of Hyper- and Hypocarbia

Douglas A. Dubbink, M.D.

Hypercarbia and hypocarbia have many causes. Hypercarbia exists when the Pa_{CO_2} exceeds 45 mm Hg; hypocarbia, when the Pa_{CO_2} is below 35 mm Hg.

Carbon Dioxide Transport

Bicarbonate. Between 70% and 90% of total CO_2 is in the form of bicarbonate. Bicarbonate is synthesized primarily in erythrocytes through the following reaction:

$$CO_2 + H_2O \xleftrightarrow[\text{anhydrase}]{\text{carbonic}} H_2CO_3 \leftrightarrow H^+ + HCO_3^-$$

Carbamino Compounds. Between 5% and 10% of CO_2 is found in carbamino compounds. The CO_2 is bound to the terminal amino groups of blood proteins.

Physically Dissolved. Between 5% and 10% of CO_2 is physically dissolved.

Effects of Carbon Dioxide Changes on Various Organ Systems

Central Nervous System Effects

□ For each increase of 1 mm Hg CO_2, cerebral blood flow (CBF) increases 1.8 mL·100 g^{-1}·min^{-1}, and cerebral blood volume increases 0.04 mL·100 g^{-1} within the Pa_{CO_2} range of 20 to 80 mm Hg (see Fig. 25–1).
□ The mechanism of CO_2 vasoactivity is felt to be secondary to changes in local hydrogen (H^+) in the smooth muscle cells of the arteriolar walls on the brain side of the blood-brain barrier (BBB). Initially, HCO_3^- does not cross the BBB while CO_2 does, resulting in a decreased pH of the periarteriolar cerebral spinal fluid (CSF). This leads to vasodilation within 20 to 30 seconds.[1] The pH of CSF normalizes through active changes in HCO_3^- concentration, a process with a half-life of 6 hours that is largely complete by 30 hours.

This adaptation limits the utility of prolonged hyperventilation in the treatment of increased intracranial pressure.
□ The CO_2 response in gray matter exceeds that in white matter secondary to increased vascular density. Hypercarbia has the greatest effect on vessels less than 100 microns in diameter.
□ Pathologic states may decrease the response to CO_2. For example, 12 minutes of global ischemia, BBB disruption (due to, e.g., trauma), and severe transient focal ischemia abolish CO_2 responsiveness for 24 hours.
□ Narcosis occurs when Pa_{CO_2} exceeds 90 mm Hg.
□ If Pa_{CO_2} drops below 20 to 30 mm Hg, signs of ischemia (electroencephalographic slowing and confusion) occur in nonanesthetized humans.

Respiratory System Effects

□ Maximal stimulation occurs at a Pa_{CO_2} of about 100 mm Hg. Any further increase in Pa_{CO_2} results in ventilatory depression.
□ Many anesthetic agents depress the response of the respiratory center to CO_2.
□ Hypercarbia increases pulmonary vascular resistance, and acidosis augments hypoxic pulmonary vasoconstriction.
□ Hypocarbia inhibits hypoxic pulmonary vasoconstriction and causes bronchoconstriction and decreased lung compliance.

Cardiovascular System Effects

□ The effects of hypercarbia on the cardiovascular system result from alterations in the balance between the direct depressant effects of CO_2 and increased sympathetic nervous system activity. As CO_2 rises, blood pressure and cardiac output usually increase in awake and anesthetized patients. At very high levels, hypercarbia causes a reduction in cardiac output, blood pressure, and heart rate with resultant cardiovascular collapse.

□ Arrhythmias may be associated with hypercarbia, especially during administration of halothane.

□ Hypocarbia can cause decreased cardiac output by several mechanisms. If hyperventilation occurs during positive pressure ventilation, venous return may be decreased. Depressed sympathetic activity leads to a decreased inotropic state. Increased pH causes a reduction in ionized calcium that also decreases the inotropic state.

Gastrointestinal System Effects

□ Hypercarbia (and acidosis) increases hepatic and portal venous blood flow.

□ Hypocarbia (and alkalosis) decreases hepatic and portal venous blood flow.

□ If the sympathetic adrenergic system is not completely suppressed during general anesthesia, increasing $PaCO_2$ leads to splanchnic vasoconstriction and decreased hepatic blood flow. With significant sympathetic nervous system suppression, as would occur during deep anesthesia, increased $PaCO_2$ results in increased hepatic blood flow because of vasodilation.

Renal System Effects

□ Chronic hypercarbia results in renal retention of HCO_3^- and a compensatory metabolic alkalosis.

□ Chronic hypocarbia results in HCO_3^- wasting by the kidney and a compensatory metabolic acidosis.

Metabolic Effects

□ As $PaCO_2$ rises, plasma levels of epinephrine and norepinephrine increase.

□ Hypercarbia results in increased leakage of K^+ from cells into the plasma. Reuptake of K^+ by cells is slow, and repeated episodes of hypercarbia can cause a stepwise increase in plasma K^+.

Pharmacologic Effects of Carbon Dioxide Changes

□ Hypercarbia, resulting in acidosis, can affect the pharmacokinetics of many anesthetic agents. For example, local anesthetics are weak bases, and the nonionized form is mainly responsible for transport across cell membranes. In the presence of acidemia, the relative amount of nonionized drug will decrease, resulting in less transport across cell membranes and decreased activity.

□ Increased $PaCO_2$ shifts the oxygen dissociation curve to the right (see Fig. 7–1). Decreased $PaCO_2$ has the opposite effect.

Effects of Carbon Dioxide Changes on Minimum Alveolar Concentration

There is no difference in minimum alveolar concentration (MAC) between $PaCO_2$ levels of 20 and 100 mm Hg. A $PaCO_2$ level of 245 mm Hg produces about 1.0 MAC anesthesia.

Signs and Symptoms

There are no absolute diagnostic signs of hypercarbia, but several clues may be present:

□ Flushed skin.

□ Cardiac dysrhythmias, especially ventricular extrasystoles or tachycardia.

□ Hypertension (when unexplained, always consider increased $PaCO_2$).

□ Depressed respiration.

□ Coma.

Clinical signs are not consistently present; therefore, arterial blood gas analysis or respiratory gas monitoring is often required to make the diagnosis.

Selected References

1. Snyder JV, Pinsky MR. Oxygen Transport in the Critically Ill. Chicago, Year Book Medical, 1987.
2. Michenfelder JD. Anesthesia and the Brain. New York, Churchill Livingstone, 1988.
3. Koch KA, Jackson DL, Schmiedl M, et al. Total cerebral ischemia: Effect of alterations in arterial PCO_2 on cerebral microcirculation. J Cereb Blood Flow Metab 1984;4:343.

Suggested References

Benumof JL. Respiratory physiology and respiratory function during anesthesia. In Miller RD, ed. Anesthesia. 5th ed. Philadelphia: Churchill Livingstone, 2000:578–618.
Brian, JE. Carbon dioxide and the cerebral circulation. Anesthesiology 1998;88:1365–1386.
Lumb, AB. Nunn's Applied Respiratory Physiology. 5th ed. Boston, Butterworth-Heinemann, 2000.

13
Sodium

Norman E. Torres, M.D.

Serum sodium concentration is a laboratory index representing total body water (TBW) rather than total body sodium (TBS). Therefore, disorders of TBW are reflected by an abnormal serum sodium concentration. The physical examination is the only index of TBS stores. For example, increased TBS is notable on physical examination by the presence of peripheral edema in an ambulatory patient, sacral edema in a supine patient, signs of right ventricular failure (e.g., elevated external jugular veins, hepatomegaly), and/or signs of left ventricular failure (e.g., pulmonary rales, S3, S4). The TBW equals approximately 60% of the body weight. Antidiuretic hormone (ADH), thirst, and renal medullary sodium concentration regulate the water balance.

Hypernatremia

Hypernatremia is defined as a serum sodium greater than 145 mEq/L, which usually corresponds to a deficiency in TBW. Figure 13–1 is an algorithm for the assessment and treatment of hypernatremia.

Signs and Symptoms

The manifestations of hypernatremia include mental status changes, irritability, hyperreflexia, ataxia, and seizures. Other physical findings de-

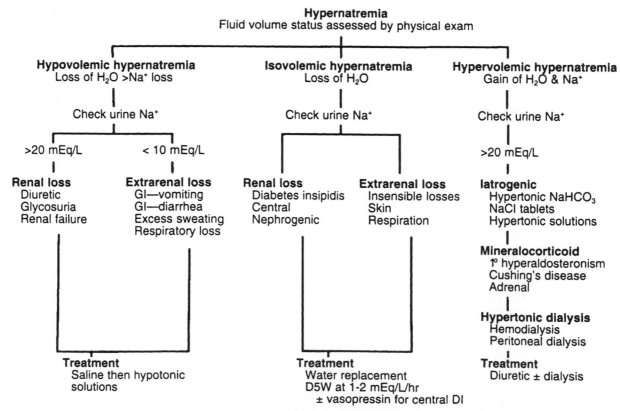

Figure 13–1. Algorithm for the causes and treatment of hypernatremia.

pend on the etiologies listed in Figure 13–1. For example, hypovolemic hypernatremia would present with hypotension, tachycardia, dry mucous membranes, loss of skin turgor, etc., whereas hypervolemic hypernatremia would present with peripheral edema, signs of right ventricular failure, and/or signs of left ventricular failure.

Treatment

Replacement of free water requires calculation of the free water deficit:

$$H_2O \text{ deficit (in liters)} = 0.6 \text{ (weight in kg)} \\ \times \text{(serum sodium/140} - 1)$$

In cases of isovolemic hypernatremia, half of the free water deficit calculated should be replaced within the first 24 hours, then the remainder replaced over the next 1 to 2 days. Treatment of severe central diabetes insipidus may involve the use of vasopressin, 5 to 10 units subcutaneously every 4 to 6 hours. In cases of hypovolemic hypernatremia, normal saline should be used first to reestablish the patient's volume status, blood pressure, and heart rate. In these situations, normal saline is relatively hypotonic to the patient's serum tonicity. Once the patient's volume is restored, recalculation of the free water deficit is used to further guide the replacement of free water. In cases with hypervolemic hy-

pernatremia, diuretics and hemodialysis may be utilized to correct the hypernatremia.

Anesthetic Management

Patients with hypernatremia should alert the anesthesiologist to the possibility of intravascular volume disorders. Management may require invasive monitoring of intravascular volume with central venous pressure, direct arterial monitoring, and/or pulmonary artery catheter monitoring.

Hyponatremia

Hyponatremia is defined as a serum sodium of less than 135 mEq/L, which usually corresponds to an excess of TBW. Determination of plasma osmolality is useful in determining the etiology of hyponatremia. The following equations are used to calculate the plasma osmolality and osmolal gap:

plasma osmolality =

$$2 \times [Na^+] + \frac{glucose}{18} + \frac{urea}{2.8}$$

$$\text{normal} \left(285\text{–}308 \, \frac{mOsm}{dL} \right)$$

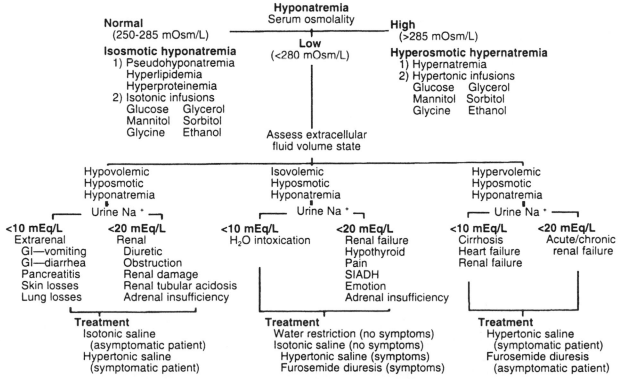

Figure 13–2. Algorithm for the causes and treatment of hyponatremia.

$$\text{osmolal gap} = \text{plasma osmolality (measured)}$$
$$- \text{plasma osmolality (calculated)}$$

$$\text{normal } (<10 \text{ mEq/L})$$

An elevated osmolal gap is indicative of the presence of toxins as ethanol, ethylene glycol, methanol, sorbitol, or isopropyl alcohol. Figure 13–2 is an algorithm for the assessment and treatment of hyponatremia.

Signs and Symptoms

Hyponatremia may present with mental status changes, lethargy, cramps, decreased deep tendon reflexes, and seizures. Other physical findings are similar to those described for hypernatremia.

Treatment

Serum sodium of less than 120 mEq/L is a severe condition and has a mortality rate of 50%. However, if the correction of the hyponatremia occurs rapidly, a demyelinating brain stem lesion may cause permanent neural damage. This illness is known as **central pontine myelinolysis**. It is believed to occur when the hyponatremia is corrected to normal or supranormal values over a short period of time. In severely symptomatic patients, correction of sodium at a rate of 1 to 2 mEq/L/hour should be done until the serum sodium reaches 125 to 130 mEq/L.

In conditions of hypovolemic or euvolemic hyponatremia, hypertonic 3% saline may be utilized for therapy in symptomatic patients. Calculation of the sodium deficit can be used to guide the volume of 3% saline used:

$$\text{sodium deficit} = 0.6 \text{ (weight in kg)}$$
$$\text{(mEq/L)} \quad \times (125 - \text{measured sodium})$$

Because 3% saline contains 513 mEq of sodium per 500 mL of water, or approximately 1 mEq of sodium per 1 mL of 3% saline, the volume of 3% NaCl (mL) needed equals the calculated sodium deficit (mEq).

For hypervolemic hyponatremia, the volume of urine required for diuresis requires estimation of the free water excess (FWE):

$$\text{FWE} = 0.6 \text{ (weight in kg)}$$
$$\times [(125/\text{measured plasma sodium}) - 1]$$

$$\text{urine volume} = \text{FWE} \times [1 - \text{urine sodium}/154]$$
$$\text{for diuresis}$$

The above formula may serve as a target goal for diuresis in the hypervolemic hypernatremic patient to obtain a serum sodium of 125 mEq/L. Further diuresis will require recalculations to guide therapy.

Selected Reference

1. Rollings ET, Rollings RC. Facts and Formulas. Nashville, TN, 1984.

Suggested References

Marino PL. Hypertonic and hypotonic syndromes. In Marino PL. The ICU Book. 2nd ed. Baltimore: Williams & Wilkins, 1998:631.

Stoelting RK, Dierdorf SF. Anesthesia and Co-Existing Disease. 3rd ed. New York, Churchill Livingstone, 1993.

14
Potassium

Norman E. Torres, M.D.

The total body potassium store in a 70-kg individual is 4200 mEq. This comprises total extracellular fluid (ECF) potassium of 60 mEq and total intracellular (ICF) potassium of 4140 mEq. The ECF potassium balance is maintained by renal function/excretion. Renal function/excretion depends on renal blood flow, renal urine output, aldosterone, antidiuretic hormone (ADH), sodium delivery to distal nephrons, and acid-base balance. The ICF potassium balance is controlled by acid-base balance, insulin, sodium-potassium ATP-dependent exchange channels, catecholamines, and aldosterone.

Hyperkalemia

The kidneys are normally able to excrete excess total body potassium and maintain plasma potassium below 5.5 mEq/L. Figure 14–1 displays causes of hyperkalemia.

Signs and Symptoms

The most significant clinical effect of hyperkalemia is on the heart's electrical conduction system. Figure 14–1 illustrates the gradual prolongation of the P-R interval (with the eventual loss of the P wave), prolongation of the QRS interval, ST segment elevation, and peaking of T-waves. The rhythm may degenerate into a sinusoidal pattern and ventricular tachycardia or fibrillation. Cardiac conduction changes usually occur with plasma potassium greater than 6.5 mEq/L but may develop at lower levels should the rise in plasma potassium occur rapidly.

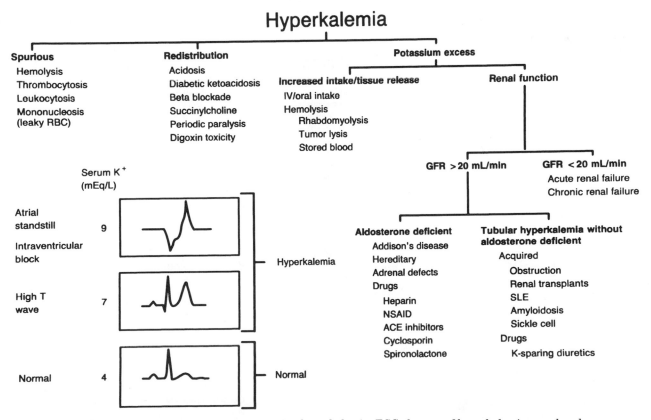

Figure 14–1. Algorithm for mechanisms causing hyperkalemia. ECG changes of hyperkalemia are also shown.

Table 14–1. Treatment Modalities for Hyperkalemia

Treatment	Dose	Mechanism	Onset	Duration
Calcium chloride	7–14 mg/kg	Direct antagonism	Instantaneous	15–30 min
Sodium bicarbonate	0.7–1.4 mEq/kg	Direct antagonism	15–30 min	3–6 hr
Glucose + insulin	25 g + 10–15 units	Redistribution	15–30 min	3–6 hr
Kayexalate	30 g po/pr	Elimination of K^+	1–3 hr	
Peritoneal dialysis		Elimination of K^+	1–3 hr	
Hemodialysis		Elimination of K^+	Rapid	

Treatment

Treatment of hyperkalemia depends on the presence of cardiac instability. Without cardiac toxicity, the therapy may be conservative with correction of the underlying cause. With cardiac instability, therapy is directed toward rapid correction of plasma potassium. Treatment modalities are listed in Table 14–1.

Anesthetic Management

Optimal plasma potassium is within the 3.5 to 5.5 mEq/L range for elective surgeries. Many factors in anesthetic management contribute to the plasma potassium. Conditions leading to acidosis will cause an increase in potassium through redistribution. Hypoventilation causes an increase in plasma carbon dioxide (CO_2), which contributes to a respiratory acidosis. Prolonged hypoxemia produces a metabolic acidosis. Administration of intubating doses of succinylcholine will increase plasma potassium by 0.5 mEq/L in normal individuals. But patients with extensive burns, trauma, upper or lower motor neuron diseases, closed-head injury, and intra-abdominal infections may have an exaggerated hyperkalemic response leading to cardiac arrest and death.

Hypokalemia

Hypokalemia is defined as plasma potassium below 3.5 mEq/L. For every 0.3 mEq/L decrease in plasma potassium, the total body potassium store decreases by 100 mEq/L. Figure 14–2 illustrates causes of hypokalemia.

Signs and Symptoms

Characteristic electrocardiographic changes, shown in Figure 14–2, include gradual P-R and

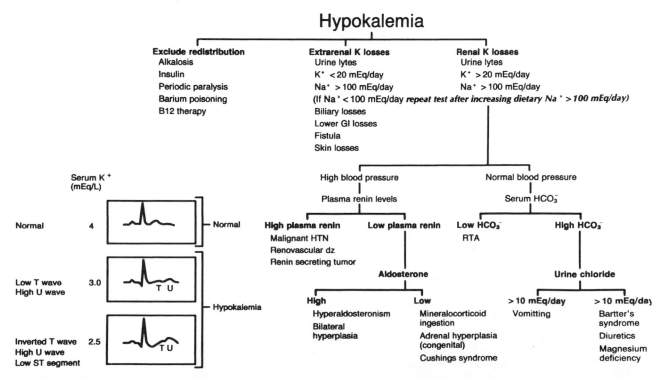

Figure 14–2. Algorithm for evaluation of mechanisms causing hypokalemia. ECG changes of hypokalemia are shown.

QRS interval prolongation with the subsequent development of prominent U waves. Hypokalemia may also induce sympathetic nervous system dysfunction in the form of orthostatic hypotension. Severe hypokalemia may also present as lower extremity weakness with more profound response to neuromuscular blocking agents. The gastrointestinal system may develop hypomotility and eventually ileus in the presence of hypokalemia.

Treatment

Therapy for hypokalemia is guided by the total body potassium and the chronicity of the hypokalemia. Chronic hypokalemia tends to be associated with a true decrease in total body potassium, whereas hypokalemia with normal body stores of potassium occurs more acutely. In the latter situation, therapy begins with correction of the underlying etiology as hyperventilation. With chronic "true" hypokalemia, treatment involves oral or intravenous replacement of potassium. Chronic hypokalemia may be associated with potassium deficits of 500 to 1000 mEq. For every 1 mEq/L decrease in plasma potassium, the total body potassium decreases by 600 to 800 mEq. Replacement of potassium in this setting would take longer than 24 hours.

Anesthetic Management

Ideally, for an elective case, plasma potassium should exceed 3.5 mEq/L. Patients with digitalis toxicity or dysrhythmia with hypokalemia may receive 0.5 to 1.0 mEq every 3 to 5 minutes until the dysrhythmia resolves. Avoidance of respiratory and metabolic alkalosis is necessary in a hypokalemic patient. Glucose loading may further exacerbate hypokalemia. Neuromuscular blocking agents may produce more relaxation than in normal individuals. An arterial line for frequent electrolyte determinations may be necessary.

Suggested References

Savarese JJ, Caldwell JE, Lien CA, et al. Pharmacology of muscle relaxants and their antagonists. In Miller RD, ed. Anesthesia. 5th ed. Philadelphia: Churchill Livingstone, 2000:412–490.

Stoelting RK, Dierdorf SF. Anesthesia and Co-Existing Disease. 3rd ed. New York, Churchill Livingstone, 1993.

Tetzlaff JE, O'Hara JF Jr, Walsh MT. Potassium and anaesthesia. Can J Anaesth 1993;40:227.

Wong KC, Schafer PG, Schultz JR. Hypokalemia and anesthetic implications. Anesth Analg 1993;77:1238–1260.

15
Calcium

Norman E. Torres, M.D.

Total serum calcium level comprises three fractions: 50% protein-bound calcium, 5% to 10% anion-bound calcium, and 40% to 45% free, or ionized, calcium. The normal range for total calcium is 8.9 to 10.1 mg/dL; the normal range for ionized calcium is 4.7 to 5.3 mg/dL. Maintenance of normal serum calcium level involves the regulatory hormones parathyroid hormone (PTH) and calcitonin (CT). These hormones regulate the release and uptake of calcium and phosphorus by the kidneys, bones, and intestines through negative feedback regulation, as illustrated in Figure 15–1.

Hypercalcemia

Large increases in extracellular calcium are buffered by the kidneys and parathyroid glands. Hypercalcemia occurs when the amount of calcium entering the extracellular fluid overwhelms the kidneys and parathyroid glands. The kidneys are able to excrete 150 to 400 mg of calcium per day. Hypercalcemia is defined as a total serum calcium greater than 10.2 mg/dL.

The measured total serum calcium is influenced by the serum albumin level. When measuring total serum calcium, a correction factor of 0.8 mg/dL increase in calcium for every 1.0 mg/dL decrease in serum albumin may be used as an approximation. Measuring ionized calcium is a direct method to obtain a true calcium level. Table 15–1 lists the symptoms of hypercalcemia.

Etiology

Common causes of moderate to severe hypercalcemia include hyperparathyroidism and malignancies. Breast cancer causes 25% to 50% of malignancy-related hypercalcemia. Other cancers associated with hypercalcemia include lung cancer; squamous cell carcinomas of the head, neck, and esophagus; gynecological tumors; renal cell carcinoma; and multiple myeloma. Solid tumors elicit a PTH-like hormone that stimulates osteoclastic activity and increases serum calcium level. In multiple myeloma, local cytokines (interleukin 1a, interleukin 1b, and tumor necrosis factor) directly stimulate bone osteoclastic activity.

Other, less common causes of hypercalcemia include vitamin D and vitamin A toxicity, thiazide diuretics (via increased calcium resorption by the kidneys), lithium therapy, sarcoidosis (via increased peripheral vitamin D conversion to 1,25 dihydroxy-vitamin D), milk-alkali syndrome (large amounts of ingested calcium), hyperthyroidism (via uncoupling of bone resorption and formation), immobilization, familial hypocalciuric hypercalcemia (a benign autosomal-dominant condition), and renal failure.

Anesthetic Management

The main emphasis in the anesthetic management of a hypercalcemic patient is on maintaining adequate hydration and urine output. Electrocardiographic monitoring may demonstrate prolonged P-R intervals, wide QRS complexes, and shortened Q-T intervals as hypercalcemia worsens. Avoidance of respiratory alkalosis may be beneficial, because alkalosis lowers plasma potassium, which would leave hypercalcemia unopposed. Although calcium enhances acetylcholine release and muscle contraction, it stabilizes the postjunctional membrane, so the response to muscle relaxants in a patient with hypercalcemia is unknown.

Hypocalcemia

Hypocalcemia is defined as total serum calcium level below 8.5 mg/dL or ionized calcium level below 4.7 mg/dL. The causes of hypocalcemia differ between the intensive care unit (ICU) patient population and the outpatient population.

Table 15–1. Symptoms of Hyper- and Hypocalcemia

Total Serum Calcium	Symptoms
<11.5	Asymptomatic
11.5–13.0	Anorexia, nausea, polyuria
>13.0	Anorexia, nausea, vomiting, lethargy, dehydration, coma, death

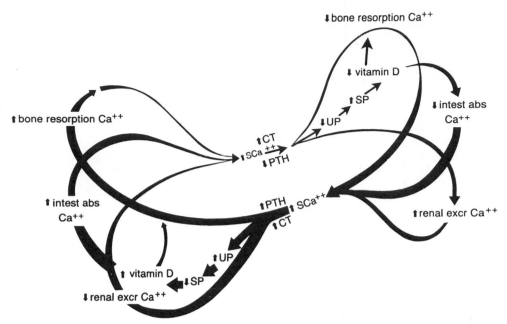

Figure 15–1. Schema of calcium homeostasis, consisting of three overlapping control loops that interlock and relate to one another through the level of blood concentrations of ionic calcium, parathyroid hormone (PTH), and calcitonin (CT). Each loop involves a calciotropic hormone target organ (bone, intestine, kidney). The limbs on the left show physiologic events that increase the blood concentration of calcium; the limbs on the right show events that decrease this concentration. UP, urine phosphate; SP, serum phosphate. (Adapted from Arnaud CD.)

Etiology

In the ICU setting, the most common causes of hypocalcemia are magnesium depletion and sepsis. Magnesium depletion diminishes the response of end organs (bones, intestines, and kidneys) to PTH hormone and inhibits PTH secretion. The inability to correct hypocalcemia through intravenous calcium administration is a hallmark of hypomagnesemia-induced hypocalcemia. This results from calcium diuresis by the kidneys from the decreased renal response to PTH. Sepsis results in hypocalcemia from calcium leakage due to microcirculatory disruption. Hypocalcemia in the setting of sepsis is considered a poor prognostic sign.

Respiratory or metabolic alkalosis induces hypocalcemia by increasing protein binding to calcium, thereby decreasing the amount of ionized calcium. Respiratory alkalosis commonly results from hyperventilation during mechanical ventilation, anxiety, and sepsis. Metabolic alkalosis may arise from nasogastric suctioning and diuretic therapy.

Renal failure decreases the conversion of vitamin D into 1,25-dihydroxy vitamin D, thereby decreasing intestinal and bone absorption while increasing serum phosphate levels. This hyperphosphatemia combines with calcium to form calcium phosphate, which precipitates within soft tissues and further decreases serum calcium.

Other causes of hypocalcemia include massive blood transfusions (through citrate binding of calcium), pancreatitis, drugs, burns, fat embolism (i.e., free fatty acids bind calcium), and cardiopulmonary bypass. In the outpatient population, hypoparathyroidism is the most common cause of hypocalcemia.

Signs and Symptoms

Hypocalcemia is often asymptomatic. However, moderate to severe hypocalcemia may produce cardiovascular and neurologic signs and symptoms. Cardiovascular signs and symptoms may include prolonged Q-T interval, bradycardia, hypotension, peripheral vasodilation, and occasionally left ventricular failure. Neurologic manifestations may include numbness around the mouth, paresthesias of all distal extremities, muscle cramps, tetany (carpopedal spasm), hyperreflexia, and seizures. On physical examination, Chvostek's sign and Trousseau's sign may be present; however, these signs lack sensitivity and specificity for hypocalcemia.

Treatment

Cardiopulmonary bypass, massive blood transfusion, tetany, pancreatitis, and post-parathyroidectomy are some of the indications for intravenous calcium replacement. Several factors guide calcium replacement therapy, including absolute serum calcium level, the rapidity of the serum calcium drop, and the underlying disease process. Intravenous calcium infusion causes vasoconstriction and in certain situations (e.g., low cardiac output or vasoconstricted state) may decrease peripheral blood flow by causing further vasoconstriction. Calcium also decreases myocardial compliance and may exacerbate underlying cardiac diastolic dysfunction. Calcium replacement in an asymptomatic hypocalcemic patient may not be indicated.

Calcium is irritating to veins and soft tissue; thus, infusion into larger central veins may be necessary. Calcium chloride (10 mL of a 10% solution) contains 272 mg (13.6 mEq) of elemental calcium; calcium gluconate (10 mL of a 10% solution) contains 90 mg (4.5 mEq) of elemental calcium. Ten mL of either solution should be diluted into 100 mL of 5% dextrose in water (D_5W) and warmed to body temperature to minimize irritation and minimize precipitation, respectively. To treat acute symptoms, a 100- to 200-mg loading dose of elemental calcium is infused over 10 minutes. Too-rapid calcium infusion may cause cardiac diastolic dysfunction. Maintenance infusion at a rate of 1 to 2 mg·kg^{-1}·hr^{-1} may then be initiated. A 15-mg/kg infusion of calcium gluconate can increase serum calcium by 2 to 3 mg/dL. The goal of acute management is to eliminate symptoms, not to return serum calcium to normal levels, however.

Suggested References

Arnaud CD. Calcium homeostasis: Regulatory elements and their integrity. Fed Proc 1978;37:2558.

Davis KD, Attie MF. Management of severe hypercalcemia. Crit Care Clin 1991;7:175.

Fauci AS, Braunwald E, Isselbacher KJ, et al. Harrison's Principles of Internal Medicine. 14th ed. New York, McGraw-Hill, 1998.

Marino PL. Calcium and phosphorus. In Marino PL. The ICU Book. 2nd ed. Baltimore: Williams & Wilkins, 1998:673.

Nussbaum SR. Pathophysiology and management of severe hypercalcemia. Endocrinol Metab Clin North Am 1993;22:343.

16
Electrolyte Abnormalities: Magnesium

Daniel R. Brown, M.D., Ph.D.

Magnesium (Mg^{2+}) is the second-most abundant cation in the body. It is intimately involved in cellular electrophysiology as well as a myriad of cellular enzymatic processes. Total body stores average 0.3 g/kg body weight, with less than 1% found in the serum and the remainder in bone and soft tissues. Primary determinants of total body magnesium are intake and renal handling. Magnesium is absorbed in the small bowel, and renal reabsorption is variable depending on magnesium stores. Under conditions of hypomagnesemia, the normal kidney will excrete less than 1 mEq/day, with more than half of the filtered load reabsorbed in the thick ascending limb of the loop of Henle.

Determination of magnesium deficiency is difficult, because magnesium is primarily an intracellular ion and serum magnesium may not reflect tissue levels. Nonetheless, therapy for magnesium disorders, almost exclusively hypomagnesemia, is often guided by serum magnesium concentration (normal 1.7 to 2.1 mg/dL).

Hypomagnesemia

Hypomagnesemia is a common electrolyte disorder, especially in the critically ill (studies have reported prevalence up to 65%). Multiple factors frequently contribute to magnesium depletion, including decreased intake, impaired intestinal absorption, and increased gastrointestinal and renal losses. Renal wasting may occur with diuresis, renal tubular disorders, and administration of certain drugs, including amphotericin B and cisplatin. Acute decreases in magnesium can occur in many clinical situations associated with catecholamine surges. It is postulated that catecholamines may cause intracellular shifting of magnesium and chelation of free magnesium by increasing serum free fatty acids. Clinically, it is important to realize that stressful clinical situations may be associated with acute hypomagnesemia.

Signs and Symptoms

Hypomagnesemia is most often asymptomatic, but life-threatening neurologic and cardiac sequelae may develop. Signs and symptoms of hypomagnesemia may often be exacerbated by other electrolyte abnormalities associated with hypomagnesemia, such as hypokalemia, hypocalcemia, and hypophosphatemia. Hypomagnesemia may cause neuromuscular excitability, mental status changes, and seizures. Considerable evidence supports an association between hypomagnesemia and cardiac arrhythmias and potentiation of digoxin toxicity. ECG changes include prolonged Q-T interval and atrial and ventricular ectopy.

Magnesium has been advocated as a treatment for torsades de pointes and digoxin toxicity arrhythmias, and also has been used to treat a wide variety of both supraventricular and ventricular arrhythmias. Indeed, evidence exists that a trial of $MgSO_4$ may be useful in the management of most arrhythmias. The exact mechanism(s) by which magnesium acts as an antiarrhythmic agent is unclear, but magnesium has class IV (calcium channel inhibition) and weak class I (sodium channel inhibition) antiarrhythmic properties. In addition, many studies suggest that magnesium has a cardioprotective effect, especially during ischemic reperfusion injury. Postulated mechanisms include a direct cellular protective effect by reducing calcium influx during ischemia and an improved myocardial oxygen supply and demand relationship by decreasing heart rate, contractility, and afterload.

Treatment

Although serum magnesium concentration may not reflect total body magnesium stores, many advocate administering $MgSO_4$ to keep serum concentration greater than 2 mg/dL. The cardiovascular effects of even rapid administration of intravenous $MgSO_4$ (4 g over 10 min) are minimal, with small decreases in blood pressure (<10%) being the most common finding. Hypotension in anesthetized patients given $MgSO_4$ may be more pronounced, because many anesthetic agents may potentiate the vasodilation and ventricular dysfunction that may be associated with rapid $MgSO_4$ administration.

Perioperative Considerations

Hypomagnesemia should be corrected before elective procedures, given the association with cardiac arrhythmias. Additionally, the possible cardioprotective actions of magnesium make normal magnesium stores desirable for elective procedures, especially for those patients at risk for myocardial ischemia.

Hypomagnesemia most frequently coexists with other electrolyte abnormalities, including hypocalcemia, hypophosphatemia, and hypokalemia. Hypomagnesemia causes suppression of parathyroid hormone release, and the resulting hypocalcemia may be severe. Magnesium is a cofactor for sodium-potassium transport, and hypomagnesemia results in cellular hypokalemia and renal potassium wasting. The mechanisms of renal potassium wasting associated with hypomagnesemia remain unclear. Replacement of potassium in the presence of hypomagnesemia is notoriously difficult, and both ions should be replaced simultaneously. In summary, clinicians should be prepared to encounter physiologic responses to multiple electrolyte disturbances in the presence of hypomagnesemia.

Hypermagnesemia

Hypermagnesemia most commonly develops in the setting of renal failure and occasionally occurs with excessive magnesium intake (such as during magnesium therapy for preeclampsia). Other causes include adrenal insufficiency and hypothyroidism.

Signs and Symptoms

Manifestations of hypermagnesemia begin to occur when serum magnesium exceeds 5 mg/dL and are primarily neurologic and cardiovascular. Hyporeflexia, sedation, and weakness are common. Hypermagnesemia has multiple actions at the neuromuscular junction, including altered presynaptic release of acetylcholine (ACh) and decreased motor end-plate sensitivity to ACh. These actions result in weakness; severe hypermagnesemia may lead to respiratory arrest. Hypotension may occur related to vasodilation, bradycardia, and myocardial depression. ECG changes are variable but often include widened QRS complex and prolonged PR interval.

Treatment

Magnesium intake should be minimized by excluding magnesium-containing antacids and magnesium in total parenteral nutrition solutions. Renal excretion can be enhanced with loop diuretics. For those patients with renal failure, dialysis may be necessary for magnesium clearance. Calcium may be administered to temporarily antagonize the effects of hypermagnesemia.

Perioperative Considerations

Close monitoring of the cardiovascular system and the neuromuscular junction is required in hypermagnesemic patients. The effects of drugs that vasodilate or depress the myocardium should be expected to be potentiated. Similarly, the actions of drugs that act on the neuromuscular junction, such as muscle relaxants and aminoglycoside antibiotics, should also be expected to be enhanced. One-half to one-third of the normal dose of nondepolarizing muscle relaxants has been recommended when magnesium is being infused.

Suggested References
Gomez MN. Magnesium and cardiovascular disease. Anesthesiology 1998;89:222–240.
Knochel JP. Disorders of magnesium metabolism. In Fauci AS, Braunwald E, Isselbacher KJ, et al, eds. Harrison's Principles of Internal Medicine. 14th ed. New York: McGraw-Hill, 1998:2263–2266.
Zaloga GP, Kirby RR, Bernards WC, Layon AJ. Fluids and electrolytes. In Civetta JM, Taylor RW, Kirby RR, eds. Critical Care. 3rd ed. Philadelphia: Lippincott-Raven, 1997:413–441.

17
Cardiac Cycle: Control and Synchronicity

William J. Davis, M.D.

The succession of atrial and ventricular events constitutes the cardiac cycle, which comprises a period of contraction (systole) followed by a period of relaxation (diastole). These two periods are further subdivided into phases. The first phase of systole is isovolemic contraction, during which the ventricle contracts with all valves closed. The second phase is the ejection phase, which brings a rapid rise in ventricular pressure and opening of the semilunar valves as ventricular pressure exceeds aortic pressure (Fig. 17–1). Diastole begins with an isovolemic relaxation phase when the aortic valve closes. Atrioventricular valves open as atrial pressure exceeds ventricular pressure during the phase of rapid inflow. This is followed by a variable phase of diastasis and the phase of atrial systole, which completes ventricular diastole.

Control

Each normal cardiac cycle is initiated by spontaneous generation of an action potential (AP) (Fig. 17–2) in the sinoatrial (SA) node (located in the posterior wall of the right atrium near the superior vena caval opening). Rhythmicity of the SA node and other parts of the conduction system is related to the less negative resting potential (-55 mV) and threshold potential of SA nodal fibers compared with ventricular muscle cells, as well as to the inactivation of fast sodium (Na) channels.

SA nodal fibers slowly leak Na into cells and potassium (K) out of cells. The resting potential gradually rises during phase 4 depolarization until it reaches a threshold voltage of -40 mV, at which point slow calcium (Ca) and Na channels open, lead-

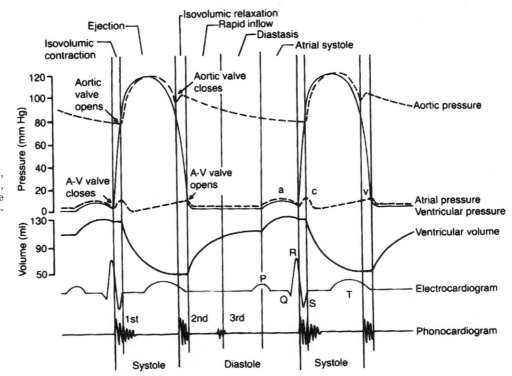

Figure 17–1. The cardiac cycle, correlating pressure changes, ventricular volume, and the electrocardiogram. (From Guyton AC, Hall JE.)

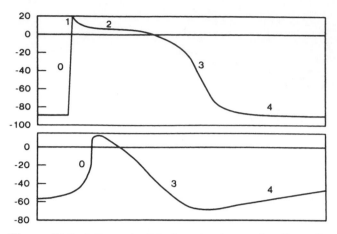

Figure 17–2. Action potentials from two types of cardiac cells. Top, AP recorded from a cell that is dependent mainly on rapid-current, fast-channel response. Bottom, AP recorded from a sinus node cell, which is dependent on slow inward current. Numbers 0–4 refer to the phases of the AP. (From Holmes DR Jr.)

ing to AP. A state of hyperpolarization then follows as K diffuses out of fibers, dropping the "resting" membrane potential down to -55 mV at the termination of AP. Finally, K channels close, with inward-leaking Na correcting outward flux of K. Thus the resting potential drifts upward to threshold level $(-40$ mV), eliciting another cycle.

The SA node controls the heart's rhythmicity, because the depolarization rate of the SA node exceeds that of other parts of the conducting system. Thus the cardiac pacemaker (SA node) loses its state of hyperpolarization more rapidly than does the rest of the conducting system (SA node rate 70 to 80/min; AV node rate, 40 to 60/min; Purkinje's fiber rate, 15 to 40/min). Sympathetic nerves are distributed to all parts of the heart, especially the ventricular muscle. These nerves (1) increase the rate of SA nodal discharge, (2) increase the rate of conduction plus excitability throughout the heart, and (3) increase the force of contraction of all cardiac musculature. (Maximal sympathetic outflow can triple the heart rate and double the strength of contraction.) The mechanism for this is norepinephrine release at sympathetic nerve endings, which is believed to increase membrane permeability to Na and Ca, increasing the tendency of the membrane potential to drift upward to the threshold for excitation. Increased calcium permeability causes increased inotropic effect.

Parasympathetic nerves are distributed via the vagus nerve mainly to the SA and AV nodes (and to a lesser extent to the atria and even less so to the ventricles). Vagal stimulation releases acetylcholine (ACh), which (1) decreases the rate of SA nodal discharge and (2) decreases the excitability of AV junctional fibers, thus slowing the impulse transmission into ventricles. Strong vagal stimulation can completely stop SA nodal discharge, leading to eventual ventricular escape beats from Purkinje fiber discharge. ACh works by increasing the permeability of muscle fibers to K, producing hyperpolarization (increased negativity inside the cells, -70 to -75 mV); thus, conduction tissue is much less excitable and takes longer to reach threshold spontaneously.

The central nervous system's vasomotor center (medullary-pontine area) contains neurons that affect chronotropic and inotropic responses from the heart. Vagal activity is reflex in origin and is aroused by impulses from carotid and aortic baroreceptors. The nucleus ambiguous contains vagal motor neurons that travel to the SA and AV nodes. Impulse activity depends mainly on baroreceptor input. Also, phasic input from the inspiratory center causes sinus arrhythmia (increased heart rate with inspiration, decreased heart rate with expiration).

Synchronicity

The action potential originating in the SA node spreads through the atrium at 0.3 m/sec; internodal pathways terminate in the AV node (1 m/sec). Delay occurs at the AV node, allowing time for the atria to empty before ventricular contraction begins. The impulse reaches the AV node 0.04 second after its origin in the SA node. The AV node's prolonged refractory period helps prevent dysrhythmias, which can occur if a second cardiac impulse is transmitted into the ventricle too soon after the first. Purkinje's fibers lead from the AV node and divide into left and right bundle branches, spreading into the apex of the respective ventricles and then back toward the base of the heart. These large fibers have a conduction velocity of 1.5 to 4 m/sec (6 times that of cardiac muscle and 150 times that of junctional fibers), which allows almost immediate transmission of cardiac impulses through the entire ventricular system. Thus, the cardiac impulse arrives at almost all portions of the ventricle simultaneously, exciting the first ventricular muscle fibers only 0.06 second ahead of the last ventricular fibers. Effective pumping by both ventricles requires this synchronous type of muscle contraction.

Suggested References

Blanck TJJ, Lee DL. Cardiac physiology. In Miller RD, ed. Anesthesia. 5th ed. Philadelphia: Churchill Livingstone, 2000:619–646.

Guyton AC, Hall JE. Textbook of Medical Physiology. 9th ed. Philadelphia, WB Saunders, 1996.

Holmes DR Jr. Cardiac arrhythmias: Anatomic and pathophysiologic concepts. In Brandenberg RO, Fuster V, Giuliani ER, McGoon DC, eds. Cardiology, Fundamentals and Practice. Chicago: Year Book Medical, 1987:739.

Opie LH. Mechanisms of cardiac contraction and relaxation. In Braunwald E, ed. Heart Disease: Textbook of Cardiovascular Medicine. 5th Ed. Philadelphia: WB Saunders, 1996:360.

18
Physiologic Determinants of Cardiac Output

William C. Oliver, Jr., M.D.

Cardiac output (CO) is the quantity of blood per minute that the heart delivers to support the metabolic demands of peripheral tissues. It indicates the condition of the entire circulatory system that is regulated by autoregulation of the tissues. CO in a normal 70-kg individual is 5 to 6 L/min with a heart rate (HR) of 80 beats/min (bpm), but it may vary from 25% below the resting supine value to an eightfold increase with exertion.[1] To compare patients of different weights, CO is also expressed as a function of body surface area (BSA). This is referred to as the cardiac index (CI):

$$CI\ (L \cdot min^{-1} \cdot m^{-2}) = CO/BSA$$

A normal CI varies between 2.5 and 3.5 $L \cdot min^{-1} \cdot m^{-2}$.

The two major determinants of CO are stroke volume (SV) and HR. These are related to CO by the following formula:

$$CO\ (L/min) = SV \times HR$$

Heart Rate

HR is determined primarily by the rate of spontaneous phase 4 depolarization of the sinoatrial (SA) node pacemaker cells. Neural and humeral mechanisms influence HR primarily. HR is important to CO in conjunction with any SV as long as preload, afterload, and contractility remain unchanged. HR may augment CO more often than SV because of recurrent sympathetic stimulation. Apart from the increase in CO secondary to HR alone, increased HR causes a positive inotropic effect. A HR exceeding 170 bpm will reduce CO because of decreased ventricular filling time.

Stroke Volume

SV is the amount of blood ejected by the ventricle with each contraction. A normal SV is 70 to 80 mL. Determinants of SV include preload, afterload, and contractility (Fig. 18–1).

Preload

The extent of myocardial fiber shortening and left ventricular size determine SV.[2] Preload is the end-diastolic myocardial fiber length, often represented as end-diastolic volume (EDV). A normal EDV is 120 mL. End-diastolic fiber length greatly affects cardiac performance, because the myocardial muscle's contractile force is related to muscle length. Cardiac muscle normally functions at the lower end of the sarcomere length. But as EDV rises, systolic pressure and the maximum rate of pressure development (dP/dt) increase, and SV increases proportionately. This provides tremendous reserve for the myocardial muscle to accommodate increased metabolic demands.

Many factors affect venous return and preload, including venous tone, total blood volume, intrathoracic pressure, body position, pulmonary vascular resistance, and atrial contraction. Venous return is primarily responsible for maintaining SV and CO. Impaired venous return (from, e.g., hemorrhage, spinal anesthesia, or positive-pressure ventilation) will depress CO. Veins have a very high capacity for volume, allowing a large amount of blood to be shifted centrally from the periphery. Although total blood volume is important to venous return and preload, the distribution of that blood volume between the extrathoracic and intrathoracic compartments is more important in terms of EDV. Atrial contraction may also augment EDV.

Ventricular volume can be determined with echocardiography, angiography, and radionuclide scan. Transesophageal echocardiography is useful perioperatively to estimate EDV, but its two-dimensional nature has limitations. Consequently, other cardiac pressure measurements are substituted for EDV and preload.[3] Left ventricular end-diastolic pressure (LVEDP) is correlated to EDV on the basis of a nonlinear, end-diastolic pressure–volume relationship. More commonly, left atrial pressure, pulmonary capillary wedge pressure (PCWP), right atrial pressure (RAP), or central venous pressure (CVP) may be used to estimate LVEDP.

The reliability of these cardiac pressures in estimating ventricular preload depends on ventricular

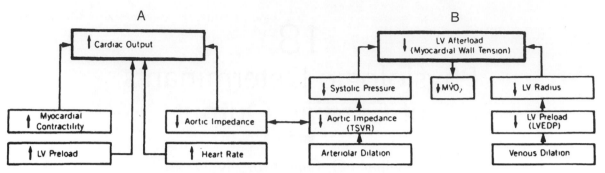

Figure 18–1. *A,* The four principal determinants of cardiac output are shown. *B,* The major factors affecting left ventricular afterload are demonstrated. (From Mason DT, Awan NA, Joyce JA, et al.[4])

compliance and heart valve integrity. Ventricular compliance (the distensibility of the chamber in response to changes in volume) is rarely normal in such disease states as coronary artery disease, cardiac tamponade, and ventricular hypertrophy. The result is a weak correlation between pressure and volume in the heart. Small increases in ventricular volume may be associated with large increases in ventricular pressure. Pulmonary artery pressure and PCWP are most commonly used to estimate preload; CVP provides the poorest estimation of left ventricular preload.

Afterload

Afterload is the force that resists muscle shortening during myocardial contraction. In the intact heart, afterload is defined as the impedance to ejection or the ventricular wall stress. Thus afterload is determined by the aortic pressure as well as the volume and thickness of the ventricle. Impedance to ejection involves aortic pressure, the aortic valve, vascular distensibility, and systemic vascular resistance (SVR).[1] SVR accounts for about 95% of the resistance to ejection and is often used clinically to estimate afterload. The formula for SVR is the following:

$$SVR = \frac{MAP - RAP}{CO} \times 80$$

where MAP is the mean arterial pressure and RAP is the right atrial pressure. Normal SVR is 900 to 1500 dynes·sec·cm^{-5}. Wood units are also used and may be expressed by dividing the SVR by 80. Blood pressure is a poor estimation of afterload.

Afterload as defined by ventricular wall stress is represented by Laplace's law:

$$T = \frac{Pr}{2h}$$

where T = tension in the left ventricular wall, P = pressure, r = radius, and h = wall thickness. Ventricular volume, left ventricular wall thickness, and systolic intraventricular pressure are primary determinants of afterload in this respect.

Intraventricular pressure has an important effect on afterload. A dilated, thin-walled ventricle generates significantly greater wall stress than does a thicker-walled, smaller ventricle. A failing ventricle will dilate and significantly increase afterload, which significantly reduces CO. Reducing afterload is an important goal in managing congestive heart failure.[1]

Contractility

Contractility refers to the myocardium's intrinsic ability to generate work from a given end-diastolic fiber length.[3] It is closely related to the availability of intracellular calcium. Contractility is defined by measurements of cardiac performance including the dP/dt, isolated papillary muscle shortening, and the work generated by isolated or whole heart preparations. Few of these definitions are clinically applicable.

No specific value represents normal contractility. Contractility may be assessed through echocardiography, angiography, and radionuclide scans. A more clinically useful index of contractility is ejection fraction (EF), the slope of the plot of SV against EDV. Although affected by changes in preload and afterload, EF is one of the most reliable and sensitive parameters of ventricular performance.

A change in contractility is considered to be a change in the heart's contractile force in the presence of unchanged diastolic dimensions and pressure. Thus it is a change in the myocardial force–velocity relation. Catecholamines, digitalis, and calcium ions increase contractility (Fig. 18–2). The adrenergic nervous system exerts the most important influence on contractility. Hypoxia, acidosis, ischemia, and certain drugs (e.g., calcium channel blockers and beta-blockers) decrease contractility.

Summary

Homeostasis of cardiac function and its instantaneous response to changing physiologic require-

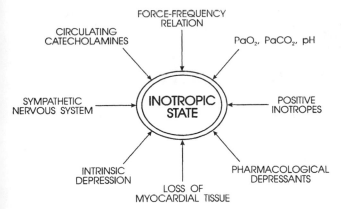

Figure 18–2. Factors affecting intrinsic inotropic state. (From Pagel PS, Warltier DC.[3])

ments are regulated by a delicate interplay among various determinants of CO. All of these factors work together to maintain sufficient CO to supply the tissue's metabolic needs. A persistent imbalance in any factor will lead to a structural adaptation of the myocardium. Although knowledge of CO is important, CO itself is not a sensitive indicator of left ventricular performance, because the circulation may adapt to maintain CO temporarily. Thus CO should be considered in concert with other phys-

iologic parameters to determine the proper course of therapy.

Selected References

1. Thys DM, Dauchot P, Hillel Z. Advances in cardiovascular physiology. In Kaplan JA, Reich DL, Konstadt SN, eds. Cardiac Anesthesia. 4th ed. Philadelphia: WB Saunders, 1999:217.
2. Braunwald E. Normal and abnormal myocardial function. In Fauce AS, Braunwald E, Isselbacher KJ, eds. Principles of Internal Medicine. 14th ed. New York: McGraw-Hill, 1998:1278.
3. Pagel PS, Warltier DC. Mechanical function of the left ventricle. In Yaksh TL, Lynch C, Zapol WM, et al, eds. Anesthesia: Biological Foundations. Philadelphia: Lippincott-Raven, 1997:1081.
4. Mason DT, Awan NA, Joyce JA, et al. Treatment of acute and chronic congestive heart failure by vasodilator-afterload reduction. Arch Intern Med 1980;140:1577.

Suggested References

Bove AA, Santamore WP. Mechanical performance of the heart. In Brandenburg RO, Fuster V, Giuliani ER, McGoon D, eds. Cardiology: Fundamentals and Practice. Chicago: Year Book Medical: 1991:150.
Little RC. Physiology of the Heart and Circulation. 4th ed. Chicago, Year Book Medical, 1989.
Stoelting RK. Pharmacology and Physiology in Anesthesia Practice. 3rd ed. Philadelphia, Lippincott-Raven, 1998.

19
Myocardial Oxygen Supply and Demand

Glenn E. Woodworth, M.D.

A concern of anesthesiologists is to prevent perioperative myocardial ischemia. Prevention is achieved by balancing myocardial oxygen supply (Table 19–1) and demand (Table 19–2).

Oxygen Supply

Coronary Blood Flow. Myocardial oxygen delivery depends on both coronary blood flow (CBF) and arterial blood oxygen content (CaO$_2$). CBF is determined by the following equation:

$$Q \propto \Delta P/R$$

where Q is CBF; ΔP is the driving pressure across the coronary vascular bed, or coronary perfusion pressure (CPP); and R is total coronary resistance. CPP is usually defined as the aortic diastolic blood pressure (AoDBP) minus the left ventricular end-diastolic pressure (LVEDP). Thus the foregoing equation may be rewritten as:

$$CBF \propto (AoDBP - LVEDP)/R$$

Coronary Perfusion Pressure. The driving pressure for CBF fluctuates with changes in aortic root blood pressure; the effect of coronary venous pressure is minimal. During the early part of systole (i.e., before ventricular ejection), the driving pressure at the coronary ostia is lower than the left ventricular systolic pressure because of a pressure gradient across the aortic valve and a Venturi effect in the aortic root. This pressure difference can be particularly pronounced in the presence of aortic stenosis.

High left ventricular pressures during systole decrease flow to the left side of the heart to less than 50% of the flow during diastole. The lower pressures in the right side of the heart yield a more uniform CBF distribution during systole and diastole; however, disease states that elevate right-sided heart pressures can produce a flow pattern similar to that of the left ventricle.

Because most CBF to the left ventricle occurs during diastole, the diastolic pressure, duration of diastole, and heart rate have been used to quantify oxygen supply using the **diastolic perfusion index.** The index is calculated from the area beneath the diastolic pressure versus time curve multiplied by the heart rate. Factors that decrease aortic diastolic pressure, decrease the time spent in diastole, or increase left ventricular diastolic pressure can produce marked reductions in CBF to the left side of the heart. Important examples include increased heart rate, which decreases the amount of time that the heart is in diastole; left ventricular failure, which increases the left ventricular diastolic pressure; and aortic stenosis, which increases left ventricular pressures and decreases aortic root pressures.

Vascular Resistance. One of the most important **extrinsic factors** affecting coronary vascular resistance is extravascular compression of the intramyocardial portion of the coronary arteries by intramyocardial pressure. Extravascular coronary artery compression is highest near the endocardium and lowest near the epicardium. Because intramyocardial pressure approaches ventricular pressure, the coronary perfusion pressure is estimated by *aortic pressure–ventricular pressure.*

Intrinsic factors contributing to coronary vascular resistance include autoregulation, degree of autonomic tone, and production of local metabolites. Coronary autoregulation maintains CBF over a wide range of perfusion pressures (i.e., between approximately 50 and 150 mm Hg). This is accomplished primarily by metabolic coupling in vessels measuring less than 150 μm. The critical metabolic mediator appears to be oxygen acting through adenosine. Specifically, decreased myocardial oxygen

Table 19–1. Determinants of Oxygen Supply

Oxygen content
Aortic root pressure
Ventricular pressure
Diastolic perfusion time (determined by heart rate)
Local vascular resistance
Autonomic innervation
Autoregulation
Coronary steal
Exogenous and endogenous substances

Table 19–2. Determinants of Myocardial Oxygen Consumption

Contractility (inotropy) = velocity of pressure development, dP/dT

Wall tension = $\dfrac{\text{pressure} \times \text{radius}}{2 \times \text{wall thickness}}$

Heart rate
Basal oxygen consumption
Work = area within systolic pressure-volume loop

tension induces adenosine-mediated coronary vasodilation by modulating calcium flux into vascular smooth muscle. Parasympathetic stimulation induces *direct* coronary vasodilation. Sympathetically mediated coronary vasodilation results from increased myocardial oxygen consumption and local metabolite production (e.g., adenosine, nitric oxide, prostaglandins, endothelin).

Arterial Blood Oxygen Content. The CaO2 is determined primarily by the hemoglobin concentration (Hb), oxygen saturation (SaO$_2$), and the amount of dissolved oxygen (PaO$_2$). Factors that affect the shape or position of the oxygen dissociation curve and availability of oxygen binding sites are also important.

$$CaO_2 = (Hb \times 1.39)(SaO_2) + (PaO_2)(0.003)$$

Other Factors. Atherosclerotic disease can increase coronary vascular resistance. In accordance with Poiseuille's law, reductions in flow are proportional to the length of the lesion and the fourth power of the radius of the lumen. This accounts for the fact that seemingly small reductions in lumen size produce critical reductions in regional blood flow. Exogenous compounds that cause coronary vasodilation include calcium channel blockers, nitrates, and dipyridamole. Catecholamines can have a dual effect. Alpha stimulation leads to vasoconstriction, whereas beta stimulation increases myocardial metabolism and causes vasodilation.

Oxygen Demand

Models used to predict myocardial oxygen consumption require estimates of basal oxygen consumption, wall tension, velocity of contraction, and mechanical work performed. Approximately 90% of myocardial oxygen consumption is for contractile activity, and less than 10% is necessary for the maintenance of cellular integrity and the electrical activity of the heart. In isolated muscle strips, oxygen consumption is proportional to the tension developed during a contraction. In the intact heart, pressure alone as a substitute for wall tension is a poor correlate of oxygen consumption. According to Laplace's law, ventricular tension is directly proportional to pressure (afterload) and chamber radius (preload), and inversely proportional to wall thickness.

One index of wall tension, calculated by determining the area under the systolic pressure versus time curve and multiplying it by the heart rate, is moderately correlated with oxygen demand. The velocity of tension development (inotropy or contractility) has also been shown to be an important determinant of oxygen consumption and can be estimated from the rate of change in pressure (dP/dT). The amount of work performed by the heart adds to its oxygen consumption and can be quantified by integrating the area under the pressure versus volume curve. In addition, the amount of work is a function of the frequency of contractions or heart rate.

To accurately assess the effects of a given intervention or change in hemodynamics, myocardial oxygen consumption must take into account all of the aforementioned factors (see Table 19–2). In the clinical setting, crude estimates are often made on the basis of systolic pressure and heart rate. These clinical estimates are often poor predictors of myocardial oxygen consumption.

Effects of Anesthetic Drugs

Given the numerous determinants of both oxygen supply and demand, evaluating a particular drug's

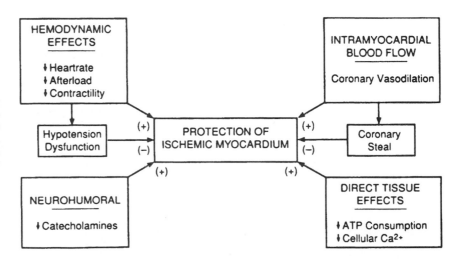

Figure 19–1. Schematic diagram showing the overall effect of anesthetics during acute myocardial infarction. Note that salvage is achieved by enhancing oxygen delivery and reducing myocardial demand by direct and indirect actions. (From Kates R, Hill R, Reves J.[1])

effects on the oxygen supply/demand ratio can be difficult. Figure 19–1 presents a schema that can be helpful when considering a drug's effects on the myocardium.

Selected Reference

1. Kates R, Hill R, Reves J. Reperfusion of the acute myocardial infarction: role of anesthesia. In Reves J, ed. Acute Revascularization of the Infarcted Heart. Orlando, FL: Grune & Stratton, 1987:35.

Suggested References

Blanck TJJ, Lee DL. Cardiac physiology. In Miller, RD, ed. Anesthesia. 5th ed. Philadelphia: Churchill Livingstone, 2000:619–646.

Ganz P, Braunwald E. Coronary blood flow and myocardial ischemia. In Braunwald E, ed. Heart Disease: A Textbook of Cardiovascular Medicine. 5th ed. Philadelphia: WB Saunders, 1997:1161–1183.

O'Brien ERM, Nathan HJ. Coronary physiology and atherosclerosis. In Kaplan JA, ed. Cardiac Anesthesia. 4th ed. Philadelphia: WB Saunders, 1999:241–270.

20
Monitoring Mixed Venous Oxygen Saturation

William G. Binegar, M.D.

Monitoring mixed venous oxygen saturation ($S\bar{v}O_2$) can provide information about the overall balance between oxygen supply and demand. $S\bar{v}O_2$ has been criticized for its lack of diagnostic specificity. However, if interpreted with other clinical information, $S\bar{v}O_2$ can provide clinically useful information.

MONITORING

The "oximetric swan" is a pulmonary artery catheter that also measures $S\bar{v}O_2$. It contains two fiberoptic channels. One channel transmits light to the pulmonary artery, where it is absorbed and reflected by red blood cells. The second channel transmits the reflected light back to a photodetector. The oxygen saturation of hemoglobin (Hb) is determined from the relative absorption of light by Hb and oxyhemoglobin (which occurs at different wavelengths). Two or three wavelength systems are used. Red light is absorbed by oxyhemoglobin at 650 nm. Infrared light at 800 nm is absorbed by both oxyhemoglobin and reduced Hb. The percent saturation is oxyhemoglobin/total Hb. A third wavelength has been added for refinement that reduces artifact.

A blood sample can be drawn from the distal lumen of the pulmonary artery catheter and analyzed in a blood gas machine. This does not give moment-to-moment values but can be used to calibrate the oximetric swan.

PHYSIOLOGY

The clinical utility of $S\bar{v}O_2$ measurement is derived from the Fick equation:

$$\dot{V}O_2 = CO\,(CaO_2 - C\bar{v}O_2)$$

where $\dot{V}O_2$ is oxygen consumption; CO is cardiac output; CaO_2 is arterial oxygen content, or $1.39 \times Hb \times SaO_2 + (0.003 \times PaO_2)$; SaO_2 is arterial oxygen saturation; PaO_2 is partial pressure of oxygen in arterial blood; and $C\bar{v}O_2$ is venous oxygen content, or $1.39 \times Hb \times S\bar{v}O_2 + (0.003 \times P\bar{v}O_2)$.

Because most of the oxygen in blood is bound to Hb, $C\bar{v}O_2$ is approximately equal to $S\bar{v}O_2$. Thus:

$$S\bar{v}O_2 = SaO_2 - \frac{\dot{V}O_2}{CO \times Hb \times 1.39}$$

Thus, the main factors that affect $S\bar{v}O_2$ are CO, Hb, $\dot{V}O_2$, and CaO_2. **The normal range is 68% to 77%.** Inherent disadvantages occur because $S\bar{v}O_2$ measures global oxygenation and does not necessarily reflect oxygenation in individual organs. Also, an increase in CO can compensate for considerable decreases in other variables.

Increased $S\bar{v}O_2$

- The most common cause is a "permanently" wedged pulmonary artery catheter.
- Hb is probably not a significant influence.
- Low $\dot{V}O_2$ can be seen with cyanide toxicity, carbon monoxide, and other types of poisoning, methemoglobinemia, sepsis, and hypothermia.
- High SaO_2 is generally not clinically significant, except during weaning or recovery from hypoxia.
- High CO may occur in patients with sepsis, burns, left-to-right shunts, AV fistulae, excessive inotropic drugs, hepatitis, or pancreatitis.

Decreased $S\bar{v}O_2$

- Decreased Hb (anemia or hemolysis).
- Low SaO_2.
- Low CO (e.g., myocardial infarction, congestive heart failure, hypovolemia, etc.).

Suggested References

Jugan E, Albaladejo P, Jayais P, et al. Continuous monitoring of mixed venous oxygen saturation during orthotopic liver transplantation. J Cardiothorac Vasc Anesth 1992;6:283.

Nelson LD. The new pulmonary artery catheters: Continuous venous oximetry, right ventricular ejection fraction, and continuous cardiac output. New Horiz 1997;5:251.

Scalea TM, Phillips TF, Goldstein AS, et al. Central venous blood oxygen saturation: An early, accurate measurement of volume during hemorrhage. J Trauma 1988;28:725.

21
Pulmonary Hypertension

William J. Davis, M.D. □ Fernando A. Zepeda, M.D.

Pulmonary hypertension (PH) describes a number of conditions that result in a chronic increase in pulmonary artery pressure (PAP). Normal PAP at sea level has a peak systolic value of 18 to 25 mm Hg, an end-diastolic value of 6 to 10 mm Hg, and a mean value of 12 to 16 mm Hg. PH is present when pulmonary artery systolic pressure exceeds 30 mm Hg and mean pressure exceeds 20 mm Hg.

Pathophysiologically, PH can be classified as primary or secondary. **Primary PH** is an uncommon disease in which no definite cause is found (a diagnosis of exclusion). It is often treated with anticoagulants (because emboli are common in these patients). Vasodilator therapy is used in an attempt to reduce pulmonary vascular resistance (PVR) with the goal of improving right ventricular function and cardiac output. About 30% of patients respond favorably to acute vasodilator therapy (e.g., nitric oxide, nitroglycerin, epoprostenol) and will improve from long-term treatment with calcium channel blockers (e.g., nifedipine, diltiazem, nicardipine, amlodipine). Continuous intravenous epoprostenol (e.g., prostacyclin, PGI_2) has been shown to improve the quality of life as well as long-term survival in patients who do not respond to conventional medical therapy (Table 21–1).[1]

Adverse effects of pulmonary vasodilator therapy include systemic hypotension and inhibition of hypoxic pulmonary vasoconstriction.

Secondary PH, by far the most common form of PH, occurs secondary to cardiac or pulmonary disease. Treatment depends on the underlying disease. An abbreviated list of causes includes the following[2]:

□ **Increased resistance to pulmonary venous drainage**—elevated left ventricular (LV) diastolic pressure (e.g., LV failure, constrictive pericarditis), left atrial hypertension (e.g., mitral stenosis or incompetence).
□ **Increased resistance to flow through the pulmonary vascular bed**—decreased pulmonary vascular bed secondary to parenchymal disease (e.g., chronic obstructive pulmonary disease, restrictive lung disease, pulmonary resection), decreased pulmonary vascular bed secondary to Eisenmenger's syndrome (i.e., patients with congenital cardiac lesions and severe PH in whom reversal of left-to-right shunt has occurred).

□ **Increased resistance to flow through large pulmonary arteries** (e.g., pulmonary thromboembolism, pulmonary stenosis).
□ **Hypoventilation** (e.g., obesity and Pickwickian syndrome, neuromuscular disorders [e.g., myasthenia gravis]) secondary to hypoxemia and acidosis-induced pulmonary vasoconstriction.
□ **Miscellaneous causes** (e.g., residence at high altitude, intravenous drug abuse).

Regardless of its cause, PH causes increased right ventricular (RV) afterload and RV enlargement (cor pulmonale). Progression of the disease may eventually result in RV failure and death. Definitive treatment of end-stage PH is lung or heart-lung transplantation.

Anesthetic Management

The anesthetic management of patients with PH can be challenging because the physiologic changes that accompany anesthesia and surgery may cause an increase in pulmonary vascular resistance, leading to acute right ventricular failure. The anesthetic goals in these patients should include[4]:

□ Defining the severity of the disase.
   Invasive monitoring of both systemic and pulmonary pressures is recommended.

Table 21–1. Dose Ranges, Routes of Administration, and Half-Lives of the Most Frequently Used Vasodilators in Patients with Primary Pulmonary Hypertension

Drug	Route	Dose Range	Half-Life
Epoprostenol*	Intravenous	2–20 ng/kg of body weight/min	3–5 min
Adenosine	Intravenous	50–200 ng/kg of body weight/min	5–10 sec
Nitric oxide	Inhaled	5–80 ppm	15–30 sec
Nifedipine†	Oral	30–240 mg/day	2–5 hr
Diltiazem†	Oral	120–900 mg/day	2–4.5 hr

*The dose range shown is for a short-term infusion; the dose range for long-term infusions often exceeds 100–150 $ng \cdot kg^{-1} \cdot min^{-1}$.
†The half-life shown refers to conventional preparations; sustained-release preparation may be administered once daily.
From Rubin LJ.[3]

A pulmonary artery catheter (PAC) allows monitoring of RV preload, RV afterload (PVR), CO, and the response to drug therapy.

This benefit must be weighed against the increased risk of PA rupture with balloon inflation.

A pulmonary artery catheter (PAC) may be difficult to insert because of low cardiac output (CO), enlarged right ventricle (RV), or the presence of tricuspid regurgitation (TR).

□ Avoiding treatable increases in PA pressure or pulmonary vascular resistance due to:

Hypoxia.	Nitrous oxide.
Hypercarbia.	α-adrenergic drugs.
Acidosis.	High airway pressures.
Hypothermia.	PEEP

□ Avoiding significant changes in right ventricular (RV) preload.

A decrease in venous return leads to a significant fall in cardiac output in the presence of a dilated and hypertrophied RV.

Volume loading is poorly tolerated and could result in RV ischemia secondary to an increase in myocardial wall tension and RV end-diastolic pressure.

□ Maintaining RV contractility.

Agents with negative inotropic properties should be used with caution.

Consider inotropic support early if the patient develops right ventricular dysfunction.

□ Maintaining LV afterload.

Avoid spinal anesthesia because of rapid onset of sympathetic blockade.

Lumbar epidural anesthesia has been successfully used for cesarean section.

Pulmonary vasodilators can be used intraoperatively to treat significant increases in pulmonary vascular resistance. Sodium nitroprusside (SNP) is an effective pulmonary vasodilator, but excessive systemic vasodilation can limit its use. Nitroglycerin has pulmonary vasodilating properties with fewer effects on the systemic vasculature than does SNP. Epoprostenol (PGI2, prostacyclin) is a short-acting agent with potent vasodilatory activity and inhibitory activity of platelet aggregation. Epoprostenol may be administered via IV or inhaled routes. Inotropic support may improve the function of a failing right ventricle in the presence of increased afterload.

Selected References

1. Gaine SP, Rubin LJ. Primary pulmonary hypertension. Lancet 1998;352:719–725.
2. Rich S, Braunwald E, Grossman W. Pulmonary hypertension. In Braunwald E, ed. Heart Disease: A Textbook of Cardiovascular Disease. Philadelphia: WB Saunders, 1997:780–806.
3. Rubin LJ. Primary pulmonary hypertension. N Engl J Med 1997;336:111–117.
4. Breen TW, Janzen JA. Pulmonary hypertension and cardiomyopathy: Anesthetic management for cesarean section. Can J Anesth 1991;38:895–899.

Suggested References

Fishman AP. Pulmonary hypertension. In Alexander RW, Schlant RC, Fuster V, eds. Hurst's The Heart, Arteries and Veins. New York: McGraw-Hill, 1998.
Gratz I. Pulmonary hypertension. Anesthesiol Clin North Am 1999;17:693–707.
Roberts NV, Keast PJ. Pulmonary hypertension and pregnancy: A lethal combination. Anaesth Intensive Care 1990;18:366–374.

22
Bradyarrhythmias

Roger D. White, M.D.

Bradyarrhythmias include sinus bradycardia, atrioventricular (AV) junctional rhythm, and heart block. Regardless of the type or etiology of the bradycardia, if the patient is symptomatic, atropine is the first drug of choice. The objective of initial therapy is to intervene quickly with a drug that is applicable to bradycardia of any type or cause. Atropine fulfills this role. The initial dose is 0.5 to 1.0 mg. If pacing is available, whether external or transvenous, it should be considered early after the initial dose of atropine, because it provides more controlled rate management without the risks of adverse drug effects.

Pharmacologic alternatives in atropine-refractory patients include dopamine, starting at 5 μg/kg/min and titrated to response or epinephrine, beginning at 2 to 10 μg/min. Isoproterenol increases myocardial oxygen demand and produces peripheral vasodilation, both of which are poorly tolerated in patients with acute myocardial ischemia. Drugs that do not decrease coronary perfusion pressure are therefore preferred (Table 22–1).

Patients with sinus bradycardia, AV junctional rhythm, or Mobitz type I second-degree block (Fig. 22–1) may respond to atropine only, based on strong vagal tone causing slow sinus node discharge or impaired AV node conduction. This may also occur

Table 22–1. Drug Therapy for Symptomatic Bradyarrhythmias

Atropine	0.5 to 1.0 mg every 3 to 5 min as needed
	Total dose 0.03 to 0.04 mg/kg (2.5 to 3.0 mg)
Dopamine	5 μg/kg/min, titrated to rate/pressure response
Epinephrine	2 to 10 μg/min, titrated as for dopamine
Isoproterenol	2 to 10 μg/min, titrated to response

in patients with complete heart block and an AV junctional escape rhythm. Patients with Mobitz type II second-degree block (Fig. 22–2) or new-onset wide–QRS complex complete heart block are much less likely to respond to atropine. In these patients the block is usually infranodal, and increased vagal tone is not a significant contributor. In patients with Mobitz II and new-onset wide–QRS complex complete heart block, pacing is the treatment of choice. Even in asymptomatic patients, pacing electrode pads or a transvenous pacing electrode should be placed prophylactically. Mobitz II block can progress without warning to complete heart block with a resultant slow and unstable idioventricular rhythm. Transvenous pacing can be accomplished by passing a pacing electrode into the right ventri-

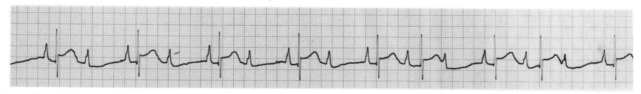

Figure 22–1. Mobitz type I (Wenckebach) second-degree AV block. The first four cycles demonstrate 2:1 block, followed by two cycles of 3:2 block, in which the increase in length of the PR interval is evident before the dropped beat. Group beating is also evident.

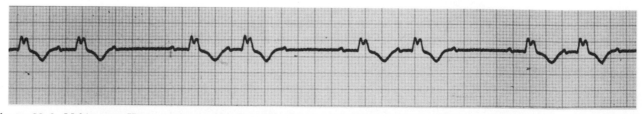

Figure 22–2. Mobitz type II second-degree AV block. The PR interval is fixed (no progressive lengthening) before the dropped beat. In addition, the QRS complex is widened, consistent with infranodal conduction system disease.

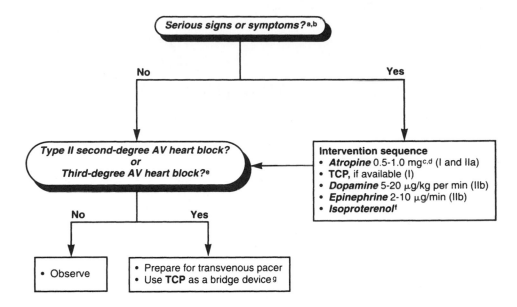

Figure 22–3. The American Heart Association's algorithm for bradycardia. (From the Textbook of Advanced Cardiac Life Support, American Heart Association, 1994, pp 1–29.)

a. Serious signs or symptoms must be related to the slow rate. Clinical manifestations include
   • Symptoms (chest pain, shortness of breath, decreased level of consciousness)
   • Signs (low BP, shock, pulmonary congestion, CHF, acute MI)
b. Do not delay TCP while awaiting IV access or for **atropine** to take effect if patient is symptomatic.
c. Denervated transplanted hearts will not respond to **atropine.** Go at once to pacing, **catecholamine** infusion, or both.
d. **Atropine** should be given in repeat doses every 3-5 min up to total of 0.03-0.04 mg/kg. Use the shorter dosing interval (3 min) in severe clinical conditions. It has been suggested that **atropine** should be used with caution in atrioventricular (AV) block at the His-Purkinje level (type II AV block and new third-degree block with wide QRS complexes) (Class IIb).
e. Never treat third-degree heart block plus ventricular escape beats with **lidocaine.**
f. **Isoproterenol** should be used, if at all, with extreme caution. At low doses it is Class IIb (possibly helpful); at higher doses it is Class III (harmful).
g. Verify patient tolerance and mechanical capture. Use analgesia and sedation as needed.

cle. If a pacing pulmonary artery catheter is in place, atrial and/or ventricular pacing probes can be inserted for rapid institution of transvenous (endocardial) pacing. External pacemakers with DDD capabilities are available to provide a spectrum of pacing choices for optimizing hemodynamics with preservation of AV synchrony. The American Heart Association's algorithm for bradycardia (Fig. 22–3) provides a convenient framework for managing patients who are bradycardic.

Suggested References

Dreifus LS, Michelson EL, Kaplinsky E. Bradyarrhythmias: Clinical significance and management. J Am Coll Cardiol 1983;1:327–338.

White RD. Acute therapy in patients with cardiac arrhythmias. In Murray MJ, Coursin DB, Pearl RG, Prough DS, eds. Critical Care Medicine: Perioperative Management. Philadelphia: Lippincott-Raven, 1997:327–340.

White RD. Pharmacologic management of arrhythmias during advanced cardiac life support. Anesthesiol Clin N Am 1995;13:849–668.

23
Supraventricular Tachyarrhythmias

Roger D. White, M.D.

Supraventricular tachyarrhythmias include arrhythmias that have a reentrant circuit (AV nodal reentrant tachycardia and atrial flutter and atrial fibrillation) and those originating from enhanced or abnormal automaticity (automatic [ectopic] atrial tachycardia and multifocal atrial tachycardia). ECG differentiation may be difficult, especially if the atrial mechanism is not evident. Tachyarrhythmias also may occur in the presence of accessory conduction pathways, most commonly in patients with Wolff-Parkinson-White syndrome.

Reentry within the AV node is the most common cause of **paroxysmal supraventricular tachycardia (PSVT).** Vagal maneuvers, such as the Valsalva maneuver, and slow AV nodal conduction can be tried first. Vagal stimulation is most effective when attempted as soon as possible after the onset of tachycardia, before reflex sympathetic tone competes with the increased vagal discharge. If vagal stimulation is ineffective, or if a vagal maneuver cannot be performed, then adenosine is the first drug of choice for pharmacologic conversion. Its safety is largely attributable to its very short half-life (6 to 10 sec).

Adenosine should be injected into a relatively proximal vein (e.g., an antecubital vein) or through a central vein. For antecubital injection, the first dose is 6 mg, followed by, if needed, 12 mg in 1 to 2 minutes. For central injection, 3 mg can be given, followed by 6 mg if needed. Adenosine is antagonized by methylxanthines such as theophylline. In patients taking theophylline-containing medications, 9 mg can be given peripherally, or 5 to 6 mg centrally. On the other hand, the action of adenosine is enhanced by dipyridamole. In patients taking dipyridamole, 2 mg can be given peripherally or 1 mg centrally. Adenosine can induce bronchospasm in patients with underlying bronchospastic disorders. Aminophylline may be the drug of choice for antagonizing adenosine-induced bronchospasm.

If adenosine is ineffective, then verapamil can be used. The dose is 2.5 to 5.0 mg IV given over 1 to 2 minutes, followed by a repeat dose of 5 to 10 mg given in 15 minutes, if needed. Verapamil should not be used if a wide–QRS complex tachycardia is present, because if the tachycardia is of ventricular origin, then verapamil is likely to cause cardiovascular collapse. Therefore, the safest course is to avoid verapamil (and diltiazem as well) in any patient with a wide–QRS complex tachycardia.

In **atrial flutter** or **atrial fibrillation,** the initial objective of therapy usually is to control a rapid ventricular rate. In hemodynamically unstable patients, cardioversion is the treatment of choice. Several drugs are available to control heart rate in atrial flutter or atrial fibrillation. These include verapamil, β-blockers such as esmolol, and the calcium-channel blocking drug diltiazem. Diltiazem is given as a bolus of 0.25 mg/kg over 2 minutes, followed as needed by a second bolus of 0.35 mg/kg in 15 minutes. An infusion of 10 to 15 mg/hr can be used for sustained control of heart rate. Adenosine can unmask the flutter or fibrillation waves, but it does not terminate atrial flutter or atrial fibrillation. Adenosine can induce enhanced AV conduction in atrial flutter, including transition from 2:1 to 1:1 conduction. Adenosine should be used only if it is considered necessary to establish the diagnosis when flutter waves are not visible or do not become evident with another maneuver, such as the Valsalva maneuver (Fig. 23–1). Ibutilide is being used to attempt pharmacologic conversion of recent-onset (<90 days) atrial fibrillation or atrial flutter. Overall success rate has been around 60% in atrial flutter and 30% in atrial fibrillation, with some reports of even higher conversion rates. Polymorphic ventricular tachycardia occurs in 3% to 5% of patients treated with ibutilide.

Automatic atrial tachycardia is a narrow-complex tachycardia with P waves different from those during sinus rhythm, though often P waves are not discernible. It is caused by either enhanced or abnormal automaticity. Adenosine can transiently suppress or slow this tachycardia.

Multifocal atrial tachycardia (MAT) is a non-reentrant tachycardia diagnosed by the presence of P waves of at least three different morphologies in the same lead with a rate greater than 100/min. Chronic obstructive pulmonary disease is the most common accompanying disease, although it can occur in various disorders, including catecholamine or theophylline excess, congestive heart failure, and hypokalemia. MAT is often mistaken for atrial fibrillation, in which case treatment is ineffective and possibly harmful. Unlike atrial fibrillation, MAT is not terminated by cardioversion, and digitalis is

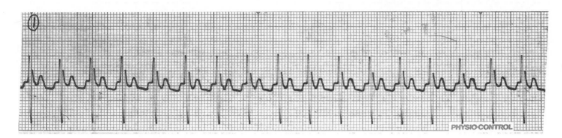

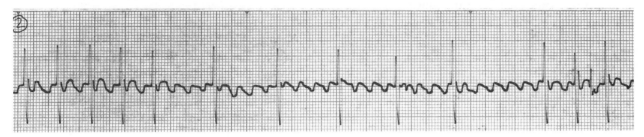

Figure 23-1. Unmasking of atrial flutter following injection of adenosine. Adenosine-induced AV block permits the flutter waves to become more evident. In fact, atrial flutter should have been considered likely by suggestive flutter waves in the baseline and the ventricular rate of 150 beats/min. Atrial flutter with 2:1 conduction is the most common presentation, with a resulting rate of 150 beats/min.

ineffective. Correction of the underlying disorder is the first step. Verapamil or diltiazem can be used to control heart rate. These drugs can convert MAT to normal sinus rhythm in some cases, but more commonly will cause slowed heart rate secondary to a decrease in atrial rate.

Patients with accessory conducting pathways can experience tachyarrhythmias. The most common form is **Wolff-Parkinson-White syndrome.** The tachycardias include orthodromic or antidromic AV reciprocating tachycardia or atrial flutter or atrial fibrillation. The most common type is orthodromic reciprocating tachycardia, in which the ventricles are depolarized via antegrade conduction through the AV node (Fig. 23–2). Retrograde conduction is via the accessory pathway. The resulting tachycardia is narrow complex. Adenosine is the drug of choice. Antidromic reciprocating tachycardia occurs much less frequently. It resembles ventricular tachycardia in that the QRS complexes are wide.

The ventricles are depolarized via the accessory connection, with retrograde return to the atria through the AV node. This tachycardia cannot be distinguished from ventricular tachycardia on ECG. Calcium-channel blockers should be avoided, because if the wide–QRS complex tachycardia is ventricular in origin, cardiovascular collapse may ensue. Again, these drugs should be avoided in the presence of any wide–QRS complex tachycardia unless one is certain that it is not ventricular in origin. Procainamide can be given at a rate of 20 to 30 mg/min to a total loading dose of up to 17 mg/kg. Amiodarone also can be used here, given in a dose of 150 mg over 10 minutes and repeated as needed.

Atrial fibrillation is the tachyarrhythmia of greatest concern in patients with Wolff-Parkinson-White syndrome; fortunately it is the least common type. The impulses from the atria are conducted into the ventricles over the accessory pathway, resulting in a wide–QRS complex tachycardia with

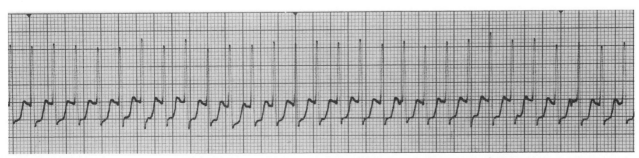

Figure 23-2. Orthodromic AV reciprocating tachycardia at a rate of 250 beats/min in a patient with Wolff-Parkinson-White syndrome. The narrow QRS complex is a result of antegrade conduction through the AV node and retrograde conduction to the atria over the accessory pathway.

very rapid ventricular rates. The tachycardia may mimic ventricular tachycardia. Cardioversion is usually the treatment of choice in patients with this tachyarrhythmia. In hemodynamically stable patients, procainamide or amiodarone can be used. Drugs that block AV nodal conduction with little or no block of conduction over the accessory pathway must be avoided; acceleration of the ventricular rate can result, increasing the risk of ventricular fibrillation. In this situation, atrial fibrillation impulses blocked in the AV node are rapidly conducted into the ventricles over the accessory pathway, resulting in very fast ventricular rates. Drugs to avoid include digoxin, β-blockers, and calcium-channel blockers. The American Heart Association's algorithms should be used to guide therapy.

Suggested References

American Heart Association in collaboration with International Liaison Committee on Resuscitation. Guidelines 2000 for Cardiopulmonary Resuscitation and Emergency Cardiovascular Care. Circulation 2000; 102 (suppl I):1.

Ganz LI, Friedman PL. Supraventricular tachycardia. N Engl J Med 1995;332:162–173.

Obel OA, Camm AJ. Accessory pathway reciprocating tachycardia. Eur Heart J 1998;19:E13–24.

Pieper SJ, Stanton MS. Narrow QRS complex tachycardias. Mayo Clin Proc 1995;70:371–375.

White RD. Pharmacologic management of arrhythmias during advanced cardiac life support. Anesthesiol Clin North Am 1995;13:849–868.

White RD. Acute therapy in patients with cardiac arrhythmias. In Murray MJ, Coursin DB, Pearl RG, Prough DS, eds. Critical Care Medicine: Perioperative Management. Philadelphia: Lippincott-Raven, 1997:327–340.

24
Ventricular Tachyarrhythmias

Roger D. White, M.D.

It is often not appreciated that ventricular tachycardia (VT) can be accompanied by hemodynamic stability. Therapeutic urgency is therefore based on the patient's hemodynamic response and not simply on the tachycardia's ventricular origin.

In monomorphic ventricular tachycardia (MVT), the QRS complexes are wide and of uniform morphology. Intermittent P waves unrelated to the QRS complexes (AV dissociation) and fusion/capture complexes are strong indicators of ventricular origin (Fig. 24–1). Other helpful evidence is a QRS width greater than 140 msec and QRS concordance across the precordium on a 12-lead ECG. Although these ECG findings should be searched for, they may not be evident. Clinical clues provide strong evidence that the tachycardia is ventricular in origin. A history of previous myocardial infarction or coronary artery disease with angina is strongly indicative of a ventricular origin of the tachycardia. Any wide–QRS complex tachycardia should be considered ventricular in origin until shown to be otherwise, and therapy should be directed with this consideration in mind.

In hemodynamically stable patients, cardioversion is the intervention of choice. Drug therapy can also be used in these patients. Lidocaine, procainamide, and amiodarone are all therapeutic options.

Polymorphic ventricular tachycardia (PVT) is characterized by irregular, wide QRS complexes that vary in amplitude and twist about the isoelectric baseline (Fig. 24–2). PVT can occur in various settings; therapy is as described for MVT.

Torsades de pointes is a form of PVT. In addition to the QRS morphologic features, there is lengthening of the QT interval (prolonged repolarization) before and after the episodes of tachycardia. Correction of the underlying cause is essential for ultimate control of the arrhythmia. Magnesium should be considered the first drug of choice in the treatment of torsades de pointes, given as magnesium sulfate 1 to 2 g over 1 to 2 minutes. If this is not effective, then overdrive pacing can be used. Traditional antiarrhythmic therapy is not likely to be successful in controlling torsades de pointes. Class IA antiarrhythmic drugs, such as procainamide, disopyramide, and quinidine, can be the cause of torsades

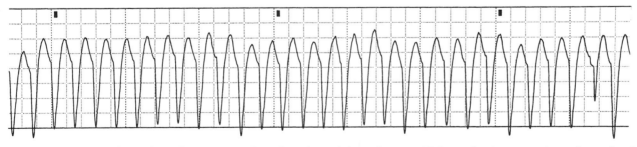

Figure 24–1. Wide-complex tachycardia at a rate of 210 beats/min. A fusion/capture QRS complex is present (second complex from the right), preceded by a P wave. Such complexes are evidence of AV dissociation and strongly support a diagnosis of VT.

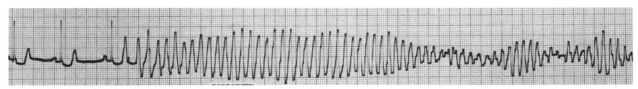

Figure 24–2. Onset of PVT in a patient with acute myocardial infarction. The characteristic twisting of the QRS complexes around the baseline is evident. PVT is identified as torsades de pointes when the QT interval is prolonged from congenital or acquired causes.

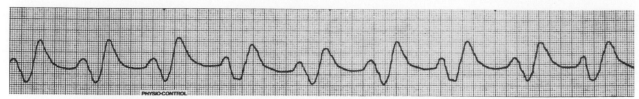

Figure 24–3. VT in the presence of hyperkalemia. The QRS complexes show a sine wave pattern.

de pointes as well as other prolonged repolarization.

VT accompanying acute hyperkalemia is often characterized by a sine wave QRS pattern (Fig. 24–3). Clinical suspicion or documentation of hyperkalemia can lead to prompt therapy with sodium bicarbonate, calcium chloride, and glucose and insulin. Such therapy can include IV sodium bicarbonate 1 to 2 mEq/kg, calcium chloride 1 g, and glucose 1 g/kg with regular insulin 0.3 U/g glucose, the latter given over 1 hour.

In the absence of evidence to support a diagnosis of VT, the assumption is that the tachycardia is ventricular in origin. Cardioversion is always a therapeutic option, especially in unstable patients.

Suggested References

Akhtar M. Clinical spectrum of ventricular tachycardia. Circulation 1990;82:1561–1573.

American Heart Association in collaboration with International Liaison Committee on Resuscitation. Guidelines 2000 for Cardiopulmonary Resuscitation and Emergency Cardiovascular Care. Circulation 2000; 102 (suppl I):1.

Miller JM. The many manifestations of ventricular tachycardia. J Cardiovasc Electrophysiol 1992;3:88–107.

Napolitano C, Priori SG, Schwartz PJ. Torsade de pointes: Mechanisms and management. Drugs 1994;47:51–65.

White RD. Acute therapy in patients with cardiac arrhythmias. In Murray MJ, Coursin DB, Pearl RG, Prough DS, eds. Critical Care Medicine: Perioperative Management. Philadelphia: Lippincott-Raven, 1997:327–340.

White RD. Pharmacologic management of arrhythmias during advanced cardiac life support. Anesthesiol Clin North Am 1995;13:849–868.

25
Factors Affecting Cerebral Blood Flow and Its Autoregulation

Scott A. Gammel, M.D.

Autoregulation, CO_2 reactivity, and O_2 reactivity are the three main factors affecting cerebral blood flow (CBF). Their relationships are depicted in Figure 25–1.

Normal CBF is 45 to 65 mL/100 g^{-1}/min^{-1}. Normal cerebral metabolic rate for oxygen ($CMRO_2$) is 3.0 to 3.8 mL/100 g^{-1}/min^{-1}. The normal $CBF:CMRO_2$ ratio is 14 to 18 at normocapnia; this relationship of CBF and $CMRO_2$ is closely maintained in physiologic conditions and is called **coupling**.

Autoregulation

Autoregulation is defined as maintenance of CBF over a range of cerebral perfusion pressures (CPP), determined as mean arterial pressure (MAP) minus intracranial pressure (ICP).

- Autoregulation in the normal brain occurs when CPP is between 50 and 100 mm Hg (see Fig. 25–1).
- Cerebral vascular resistance (CVR) varies directly with blood pressure to maintain flow, taking 1 to 2 minutes for flow to adjust after an abrupt change in pressure.
- In hypertensive patients, the autoregulatory curve is shifted to the right. The risk of ischemia could be present as the pressure falls even though the numerical value is within an acceptable range. (Several weeks of blood pressure control may be needed to return the curve to a normal range.)
- After hypotension occurs below the lower limit, autoregulation is impaired; hyperemia occurs as pressure returns to normal. But CO_2 reactivity remains intact, so inducing hypocapnia may attenuate hyperemia.
- Autoregulatory vasodilation may be limited by background sympathetic vascular tone, so inducing a chemical sympathectomy (i.e., with nitroprusside or trimethaphan) may extend the lower limit of tolerable hypotension.
- Autoregulation is also impaired in areas of relative ischemia, surrounding mass lesions, after grand mal seizures, after head injury, and during episodes of hypercarbia or hypoxemia.

CO_2 Reactivity

CO_2 levels profoundly affect CBF by changing the hydrogen ion (H^+) concentration in the extracellular fluid surrounding smooth muscle in arteriolar cell walls.

- Over the range of arterial CO_2 tension ($PaCO_2$) between 20 and 80 mm Hg, CBF quadruples. As $PaCO_2$ increases from 40 to 80 mm Hg, CBF doubles (see Fig. 25–1). As $PaCO_2$ decreases from 40 to 20 mm Hg, CBF decreases to one half of normal.
- The mechanism of CO_2 vasoactivity is felt to be secondary to changes in local H^+ in the smooth muscle cells of the arteriolar walls on the brain side of the blood-brain barrier (BBB). Initially, bicarbonate (HCO_3^-) does not cross the BBB but CO_2 does, resulting in decreased pH of the periarteriolar cerebrospinal fluid (CSF), leading to vasodilation in 20 to 30 seconds.[2] The pH of CSF normalizes with active changes in HCO_3^- concentration, a process with a half-life of 6 hours and completion by 30 hours. Chronic changes in $PaCO_2$ affect CBF for 24 to 36 hours. As the CSF pH readjusts, CBF returns toward normal. This adaptation limits the usefulness of prolonged hyperventilation in treating increased ICP.
- The CO_2 response in gray matter is greater than that in white matter secondary to increased vascular density.
- Hypercarbia has greatest effect on vessels smaller than 100 μm in diameter.
- Pathologic states decrease response to CO_2. Examples include 12 minutes of **global ischemia**, which abolishes responsiveness for 24 hours[3]; any process **disrupting the BBB** (e.g., trauma); and **transient focal ischemia**, if severe.
- A **"Robin Hood effect"** may exist in which areas of focal ischemia (where O_2 reactivity is likely lost) can receive increased flow if normal vasculature is exposed to hypocapnia; however, this effect is not predictable, and clinically normocapnia is

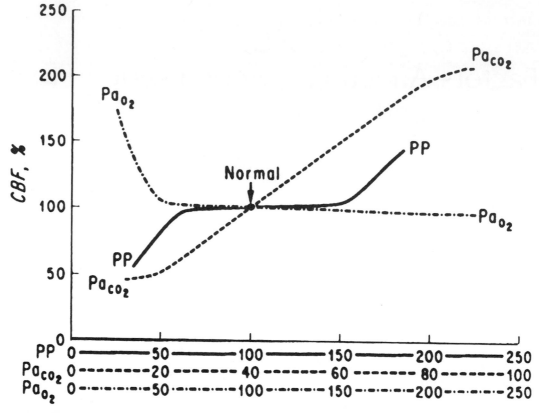

Figure 25–1. The relationship between CBF and perfusion pressure (PP), Pa_{CO_2}, and Pa_{O_2}. (From Michenfelder JD.[1])

usually maintained when regional ischemia is a risk.

▫ With Pa_{CO_2} greater than 90 mm Hg, narcosis occurs.

▫ At 20 mm Hg Pa_{CO_2}, cerebral ischemia may occur. There is a left shift in the oxyhemoglobin dissociation curve and decreased CBF. With Pa_{CO_2} below 20 mm Hg, O_2 consumption will decrease and anaerobic metabolism will increase, presumably secondary to a critical reduction in CBF.

O_2 Reactivity

Hypoxia with a Pa_{O_2} below 50 mm Hg markedly increases CBF if blood pressure is maintained (see Fig. 25–1). This effect is mediated through lactic acid and other metabolic products of acidosis. Thus, it can be said that O_2 has little direct effect on CBF. At Pa_{O_2} levels above normal, up to 1 atmosphere, only a very slight (approximately 10%) decrease in CBF has been measured.

Other Factors

Hypothermia (at levels between 28°C and 37°C) acutely reduces but does not uncouple $CMRO_2$ and CBF.[4] CO_2 reactivity is also maintained during moderate and deep levels of hypothermia. The protec-

tive effects of even mild hypothermia against ischemia are partially explained by the decrease in metabolic rate as the brain cools. However, other variables are also involved. The effects of hypothermia on $CMRO_2$ are discussed in the chapter on cerebral protection (Chapter 156).

Effects of Anesthetic Agents

▫ Autoregulation is impaired by volatile anesthetics in a dose-dependent manner.

▫ Inhalation agents reduce $CMRO_2$ and are direct cerebral vasodilators (see Chapter 41, Central Nervous System Effects of the Inhalation Agents).

▫ Clinically, most commonly used volatile agents and intravenous anesthetics preserve the CBF response to Pa_{CO_2}.[5]

▫ Opioids and other cerebral vasoconstrictors do not impair autoregulation.

▫ At 0.5 MAC of halothane or enflurane, autoregulation is partially maintained, whereas at 1.0 MAC it is abolished. Isoflurane impairs autoregulation less than halothane does.

▫ Desflurane and isoflurane are similar in terms of absolute CBF, dose-response, and preservation of CO_2 reactivity.

▫ Desflurane causes greater neurocirculatory excitation than does sevoflurane.[6]

▫ Sevoflurane's effects on CBF, $CMRO_2$, ICP, and

electroencephalogram (EEG) findings are indistinguishable from those of isoflurane in rabbits.[7, 8]

□ Halothane is the most potent cerebral vasodilator; isoflurane, the least potent.

□ Enflurane at 1.5 MAC or greater along with hypocapnia can cause seizures, thereby increasing CBF and $CMRO_2$.

□ Hyperventilation will not attenuate the increased CBF caused by halothane unless instituted before the use of halothane, whereas the effects of isoflurane and desflurane can be attenuated with simultaneous use of hyperventilation.

□ Use of isoflurane and marked hyperventilation (20 to 25 mm Hg $Paco_2$) decreases CBF, without adversely affecting cerebral metabolic balance.

□ Decreases in $CMRO_2$ caused by volatile agents are dose-dependent and nonlinear below 1 MAC; the greatest decrease occurs when the brain makes the transition from the awake state to the anesthetized state.

□ Halothane and enflurane decrease $CMRO_2$ up to 30%; isoflurane and sevoflurane decrease $CMRO_2$ by 50% (at 1 MAC end-tidal), producing an isoelectric EEG.

□ The net effect of volatile anesthetics on CBF depends on the degree of decrease in $CMRO_2$ and the degree of increase in CBF. Isoflurane produces little to no change in CBF.

□ Clinically, isoflurane must be used cautiously in patients whose cerebral metabolism is depressed by other drugs or by a pathologic process, because isoflurane may cause a greater than expected increase in CBF.

□ Nitrous oxide (N_2O) likely causes significant cerebral vasodilation, which is easily attenuated by other drugs or by hyperventilation.

Most **intravenous anesthetics** cause cerebral vasoconstriction and decrease CBF and $CMRO_2$. Ketamine is the exception; it increases CBF with a smaller change in $CMRO_2$.

□ Etomidate's effects on CBF are analogous to those of barbiturates but lead to decreased partial pressure of oxygen (Po_2) in brain tissue before occlusion of the middle cerebral artery and tissue acidosis after occlusion. In contrast, desflurane increases tissue Po_2 before occlusion and maintains tissue pH during prolonged middle cerebral artery occlusion.[9]

□ Propofol enhances neuronal damage in a rat model via N-methyl-D-aspartate (NMDA)-mediated glutamate excitotoxicity.[10]

□ Thiopental decreases, in a dose-dependent manner, CBF and $CMRO_2$ up to 50% (at induction of isoelectric EEG), and attenuates NMDA-mediated glutamate excitotoxicity.[10]

□ Benzodiazepines decrease CBF in a dose-dependent manner.

□ In animals, high-dose fentanyl and sufentanil cause seizure activity, but clinical doses are likely to cause little change in CBF.

□ Droperidol decreases CBF without a significant change in $CMRO_2$.

□ Mannitol causes an early transient increase in CBF, but CBF returns to control 10 minutes after infusion.

Selected References

1. Michenfelder JD. Anesthesia and the Brain. New York, Churchill Livingstone, 1988.
2. Snyder JV, Pinsky MR. Oxygen Transport in the Critically Ill. Chicago, Year Book Medical, 1987.
3. Koch KA, Jackson DL, Schmiedl M, et al. Total cerebral ischemia: Effect of alterations in arterial PCO_2 on cerebral microcirculation. J Cereb Blood Flow Metab 1984;4:343.
4. Black S, Michenfelder JD. Cerebral blood flow and metabolism. In Cucchiara RF, Black S, Michenfelder JD, eds. Clinical Neuroanesthesia. 2nd ed. New York: Churchill Livingstone, 2000:1–40.
5. Drummond JC, Patel PM. Cerebral physiology and the effects of anesthetics and techniques. In Miller RD, ed. Anethesia. 5th ed. Philadelphia: Churchill Livingstone, 2000:695–734.
6. Ebert TJ, Muzi M, Lopatka CW. Neurocirculatory response to sevoflurane in humans. A comparison to desflurane. Anesthesiology 1995;83:88–95.
7. Cho S, Fujgaki T, Uchiyama Y, et al. Effects of sevoflurane with and without nitrous oxide on human cerebral circulation. Transcranial doppler study. Anesthesiology 1996; 85:755–760.
8. Scheller MS, Tateishi A, Drummond JC, et al. The effects of sevoflurane on cerebral blood flow, cerebral metabolic rate for oxygen, intracranial pressure, and electroencephalogram are similar to those of isoflurane in the rabbit. Anesthesiology 1988;68:548–551.
9. Hoffman WE, Charbel FT, Edelman G, et al. Comparison of the effect of etomidate and desflurane on brain tissue gases and pH during prolonged middle cerebral artery occlusion. Anesthesiology 1998;88:1188–1194.
10. Zhu H, Cottrell JE, Kass IS. The effect of thiopental and propofol on NMDA and AMPA-mediated glutamate excitotoxicity. Anesthesiology 1997;87:944–951.

26
Anesthetic Agents and the Electroencephalogram

Donald A. Muzzi, M.D. □ Michael E. Johnson, M.D., Ph.D.

The alterations in neuroelectric activity secondary to anesthetic agents must be understood to accurately interpret the electroencephalogram (EEG) during the intraoperative period. A summary of the usual patterns of EEG changes secondary to anesthetic agents is depicted in Figure 26–1. During induction of anesthesia and at subanesthetic concentrations, an increased frequency with synchronization and some increased amplitude is commonly observed. At 1 minimum alveolar concentration (MAC) level (or the equivalent with intravenous agents), the EEG begins to slow, and, depending on the anesthetic agent, the EEG may progress to burst suppression and then to isoelectricity.[2]

Barbiturates

The barbiturates used clinically appear to yield very similar neuroelectric activity. However, differences in potency and duration of action do exist between the barbiturates.

Barbiturates initially produce fast EEG waves in the range of 20 to 30 Hz (Fig. 26–2). This pattern is known as the "initial rapid response" to barbiturates (Fig. 26–2A).[2] This fast activity begins in the frontal lobe, where it is most prominent, and spreads toward the occiput. The frequency of these fast waves decreases as the total cumulative dose of barbiturate increases. Next, spindle-shaped bursts are superimposed on the fast activity, with waves in the 5- to 12-Hz range. This pattern is commonly called "barbiturate spindles." It is at this point that the patient generally loses consciousness (see Fig. 26–2B).

A further increase in the total barbiturate dose yields a decline in the spindle bursts, at which point the EEG develops large polymorphic waves of 1 to 3 Hz (see Fig. 26–2C). If the barbiturate is injected rapidly, then the slow-wave activity will be produced with only a few traces of the fast-wave activity and barbiturate spindles. It is when this slow-wave polymorphic activity becomes dominant that the patient will tolerate skin incision. With increasing concentrations, periods of suppression begin to appear on the EEG (see Fig. 26–2D). Each of these

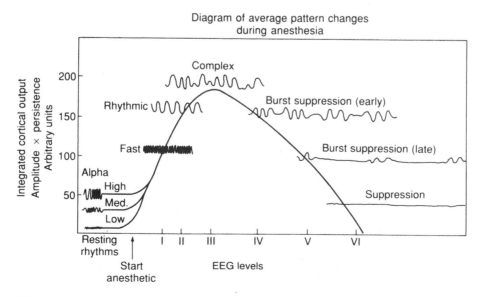

Figure 26–1. Average changes of the EEG pattern during general anesthesia. (From Martin JT, Faulconer A Jr, Bickford RG.[1])

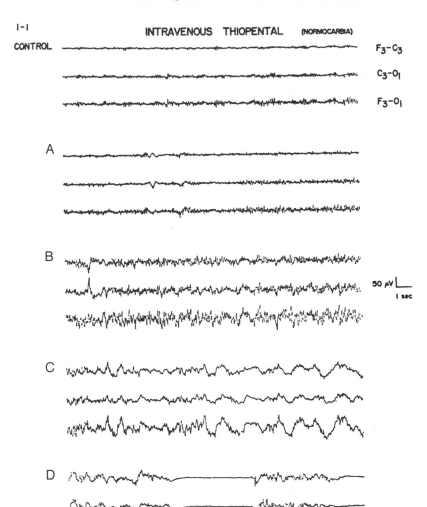

Figure 26–2. EEG effects of intravenous administration of thiopental in humans. *A,* Rapid activity. *B,* Barbiturate spindles. *C,* Slow waves. *D,* Burst suppression. (From Clark DL, Rosner BS.[2])

periods is followed by a "burst" of renewed activity that contains high-frequency components. The burst period subsides as the next period of suppression arises. Therefore, barbiturates produce this burst-suppression pattern with the burst activity starting in the 8-Hz range and decelerating to 2 to 6 Hz. The suppression period progressively lengthens with increasing dose until total electrical silence occurs.

Isoflurane

Subanesthetic concentrations of isoflurane yield 15- to 30-Hz wave activity, predominantly in the frontal areas. At the 1.0 MAC of isoflurane (1.2%), 4- to 8-Hz waves dominate the EEG. At 1.5 MAC, the waves increase in amplitude and slow to the 1- to 4-Hz range. Also at 1.5 MAC, suppressions first appear and become longer until electrical silence commences at 2 to 2.5 MAC. At times an isolated spike wave can be seen with intersuppression activity at 1.5 to 2.0 MAC isoflurane.

Enflurane

At subanesthetic concentrations, enflurane induces rapid EEG activity. The patient generally loses consciousness while this activity is prominent. At approximately 1 MAC (1.7%), large 7- to 12-Hz waves appear. When the concentration of enflurane approaches 1.5 MAC, spikes and spike waves appear followed by burst suppression. As the enflurane concentration is increased to 2 to 3 MAC, the EEG displays groups of two or three 400- to 800-V spike and wave discharges separated by 5 to 15 seconds of isoelectricity. **Electroencephalographic seizures can be seen with end-tidal concentrations of 3% enflurane with hypocapnia.[2]**

Halothane

At subanesthetic concentrations, halothane produces fast sinusoidal activity in the 10- to 20-Hz range. This pattern will persist until loss of consciousness occurs. At 1 MAC halothane (0.84%) and normocarbia, the dominant EEG frequencies are between 10 and 15 Hz. As the halothane concentration is increased, the EEG continues to slow. At 2 MAC, the predominant background rhythm is 7.5 Hz; at 2.5 MAC, it is 6 Hz. The slowing of the background rhythm continues with increasing halothane concentrations until at 4 MAC when almost all activity is in the 0.5-Hz range. One must be careful to separate the direct effects of halothane on suppression of cortical electrical activity from the attenuation in cortical activity that may be the result of decreased cerebral blood flow secondary to the cardiovascular depressant effects of halothane.

Sevoflurane

Increasing sevoflurane from 2% to 5% changes the cortical EEG pattern from high amplitude slow wave, to burst suppression, to isoelectric, to spikes interspersed with isoelectricity, reminiscent of en-

flurane.[3] Isolated cases of seizure-like movements have been reported with sevoflurane. For most, data are insufficient to determine whether the clinical picture represented akathisia or true seizure. However, in one case, incidental EEG monitoring documented a 30-second intraoperative seizure (without apparent lasting adverse effects) after sevoflurane was increased from 2% to 7%.[4]

Animal studies suggest that sevoflurane can either protect against or encourage seizures, depending on the stimulus and animal model used in the study. Sevoflurane at 1.5 MAC was similar to isoflurane in protecting against lidocaine- and penicillin-induced seizures, and protective (but less so than propofol) against bupivacaine-induced seizures.[5, 6] In a dog model where 1.5 to 2.0 MAC enflurane allowed auditory stimuli to induce seizures, 1.5 to 2.5 MAC sevoflurane did not allow such seizures. However, repetitive peripheral electrical stimulation (as would occur during somatosensory evoked potential [SSEP] monitoring) caused generalized seizures in 2 of 13 cats anesthetized with 5% sevoflurane.[3]

Nitrous Oxide

Nitrous oxide (N_2O) by itself yields characteristic dose-dependent changes in the EEG. Concentra-

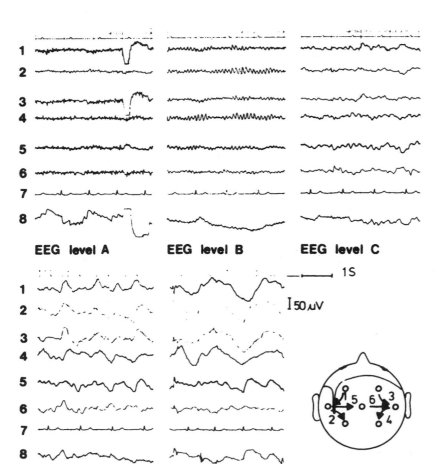

Figure 26–3. EEG after 60-ìg/kg fentanyl induction and N_2O/O_2 and lorazepam premedication. Level A, normal awake pattern, eyes open; level B, diffuse slow α-activity; level C, θ-waves with some δ-waves, some θ-activity still present; level E, some synchronized high-voltage slow δ-waves. (From Sebel PS, Bovill JG, Wauquier A, et al.[7])

tions as high as 30% rarely alter the EEG. The initial change in the EEG secondary to N_2O is the progressive loss of α-rhythm (8 to 13 Hz). As the patient loses consciousness, the α- waves disappear. As the α rhythm decreases, θ-waves (4 to 8 Hz) appear with superimposed fast activity. The fast activity is especially prominent in the frontal regions. The waves in the 4- to 8-Hz range increase in number and grow larger and come to focus in the temporal region. However, further slowing of the EEG may occur with hyperbaric administration.

Narcotics

The EEG changes produced by fentanyl are fairly consistent (Fig. 26–3). Approximately 1 minute after fentanyl induction, the α-rhythm slows and broadens. In 1 to 2 minutes, diffuse θ-waves (4 to 8 Hz) are seen with some activity (less than 3 Hz). This is followed by irregular, diffuse, slow α-waves, which can become more synchronous with a monomorphic EEG picture. At lower doses of fentanyl (30 μg/kg), the EEG exhibits significantly faster activity.

At times, patients show isolated sharp wave activity after fentanyl induction. This phenomenon is more evident with increasing doses, occurring in 20% of patients at 30 μg/kg, 60% at 50 μg/kg, and 80% at 70 μg/kg. This activity is noted mainly in the frontotemporal region.[7]

Ketamine

Ketamine produces a dissociative state of analgesia, with an altered awareness with intravenous doses of 0.25 to 0.5 mg/kg and unconsciousness at 1 to 2 mg/kg. The EEG changes appear to represent activation of thalamic and limbic structures, producing hypersynchronous δ-waves.

Benzodiazepines

Midazolam produces dose-related EEG changes, with initial increased amplitude with predominantly decreased frequency (θ, 4 to 8 Hz) activity. Increasing the dose produces high-amplitude activity below 8 Hz. Burst suppression does not appear to occur, and the EEG does not appear to become isoelectric.[8]

Selected References

1. Martin JT, Faulconer A Jr, Bickford RG. Electroencephalography. Anesthesiology 1959;20:359.
2. Clark DL, Rosner BS. Neurophysiologic effects of general anesthetics: I. The electroencephalogram and its sensory evoked responses in man. Anesthesiology 1973;38:564–582.
3. Osawa M, Shingu K, Murakawa M, et al. Effects of sevoflurane on central nervous system electrical activity in cats. Anesth Analg 1994;79:52–57.
4. Woodforth IJ, Hicks RG, Crawford MR, et al. Electroencephalographic evidence of seizure activity under deep sevoflurane anesthesia in a nonepileptic patient. Anesthesiology 1997;87:1579–1582.
5. Murao K, Shingu K, Tsushima K, et al. The anticonvulsant effects of volatile anesthetics on penicillin-induced status epilepticus in cats. Anesth Analg 2000;90:142–147.
6. Ohmura S, Ohta T, Yamamoto K, et al. A comparison of the effects of propofol and sevoflurane on the systemic toxicity of intravenous bupivacaine in rats. Anesth Analg 1999;88:155–159.
7. Sebel PS, Bovill JG, Wauquier A, et al. Effects of high dose fentanyl anesthesia on the electroencephalogram. Anesthesiology 1981;55:203–211.
8. Fleischer JE, Milde JH, Moyer TP, et al. Cerebral effects of high-dose midazolam and subsequent reversal with RO 15-1788 in dogs. Anesthesiology 1988;68:234–242.

Suggested References

Mahala M. Neurologic Monitoring. In Cucchiara RF, Michenfelder JD, Black S, eds. Clinical Neuroanesthesia. New York: Churchill Livingstone, 1998:125–176.
Scheller MS: Cerebral effects of sevoflurane in the dog: Comparison with isoflurane and enflurane. Br J Anesth 1990;65:388–392.

27
Somatosensory Evoked Potential Monitoring

Ines H. Berger, M.D.

Somatosensory evoked potentials (SSEPs) reflect the net result of neuronal activities coming from peripheral nerves through the spinal cord to the brain. They are electrical manifestations of the central nervous system response to external stimulation.

Monitoring

Repetitive electrical stimulation is applied to a major peripheral nerve via skin surface or fine-needle electrodes (square wave stimulus 0.2 to 2 msec, rate 1 to 2 Hz). The most commonly used nerves are the following:

□ Median nerve (wrist).
□ Posterior tibial nerve (ankle).
□ Peroneal nerve (popliteal fossa or below the knee).

The resulting electrical potential can be recorded at various sites along the sensory pathway to the cerebral cortex:

□ Subcortical potentials from the head, neck, spine, spinous ligaments, or epidural space.
□ Cortical potentials from the scalp or cerebral cortex (contralateral side).

Extraction of evoked potentials (EP) from background electroencephalogram (EEG) activity is done through computer signal averaging or by summation and generation of waveforms.

Transmission

The SSEP is transmitted through the following pathway:

Peripheral stimulus → peripheral nerve → dorsal root ganglia → first-order fibers in the ipsilateral posterior column to dorsal column nuclei (at the cervical medullary junction) → second-order fibers crossing to the opposite side → medial lemniscus to the thalamus → third-order fibers continuing to the frontoparietal sensimotor cortex.

The first cortical event is a negative wave over the contralateral cortex about 40 msec after posterior tibial nerve stimulation (20 msec after median nerve stimulation). By convention, this event is labeled N_{40} or N_{20}, respectively.

Evaluation

The latency and amplitude of the generated waveforms are measured (Fig. 27–1).

□ Peaks are positive or negative deflections.
□ Latency is the time from stimulation to the specific peak.
□ Amplitude is the voltage measurement from the peak apex to the succeeding trough or a designated baseline.
□ Central somatosensory conduction time (CCT) represents the difference in latency between cortical and upper cervical-spinal potential peaks ($N_{20} - N_{14}$).
□ Short-latency EPs (10 to 40 msec) arise near the side of sensory stimulation and are little influenced by physiologic or pharmacologic variables.
□ Intermediate-latency EPs (20 to 120 msec) and CCT are susceptible to anesthetic agents and physiologic variables.
□ Long-latency EPs (100 to 500 msec) arise in the cortex and are not used for monitoring.

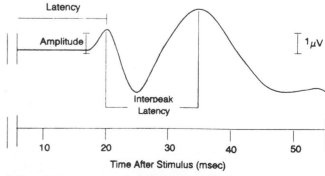

Figure 27–1. Evoked potentials are described in terms of latency (time from delivery of stimulus to onset of response) and amplitude (size in microvolts). (From Mahala ME.[1])

Intraoperative Monitoring

Intraoperative SSEP monitoring has gained popularity because it provides the ability to monitor the functional integrity of sensory pathways in anesthetized patients without relying on the "wake-up test." Baseline studies are performed preoperatively. Intraoperative SSEP monitoring is used for:

□ Procedures involving the spine (e.g., scoliosis surgery, decompressive laminectomy with fusion, fractures with instability).
□ Neurosurgical procedures (e.g., posterior fossa tumors, cervical spondylosis, vascular brainstem lesions, aneurysm clipping, carotid endarterectomy, extra- and intramedullary lesions of the spinal cord, and cauda equina lesions).

SSEP monitoring should be considered for any procedure that may involve the central sensory pathways.

Intraoperative changes in amplitude or latency or complete loss of waveforms are considered indicators of compromised sensory pathway integrity. Significant events are defined as an amplitude loss greater than 50% or a latency increase greater than 10%.

Exact tolerance limits of SSEP changes before permanent neurologic dysfunction occurs are unknown; changes lasting more than 15 minutes should be of concern. Because the spinal cord motor tracks are not monitored and have primarily a different blood supply, it is possible to have a significant postoperative motor deficit with intact SSEPs throughout the operative course.

When significant SSEP changes occur, the anesthesiologist and surgeon can try to immediately relieve or lessen the insult. Possible interventions include improving perfusion and oxygenation, decreasing the depth of anesthesia, elevating blood pressure, relieving excessive retractor pressure, and decreasing the degree of scoliosis correction.

Factors Affecting Somatosensory Evoked Potential Monitoring

Many SSEP changes are not related to surgery; some of these changes are related to anesthesia, and others are related to electrical interference in the operating room, an electrically hostile environment. Anesthesia-related factors are listed in Table 27–1. Many drugs used perioperatively can influence SSEP monitoring. Volatile agents have similar effects (in differing degrees) on SSEP which are dose-dependent and increase latency and decrease amplitude. Nitrous oxide (N_2O) causes a decreased amplitude with no change in latency when used alone or in combination with narcotics or volatile agents. Thiopental produces increased latency and decreased amplitude. Even at doses far above those required to produce an isoelectric EEG, adequate SSEP monitoring is preserved. Similar observations have been made with pentobarbital and thiamylal. In contrast, etomidate increases latency in all waves, increases CCT, and increases amplitude in all cortical waves. Thus etomidate infusions have been used to enhance SSEP recording in patients in whom pre-existing pathologies made it impossible to obtain reproducible recordings. Ketamine might also be of clinical value in SSEP signal enhancement. In contrast to diazepam, midazolam does not influence latency. Narcotics in general cause dose-dependent increases in latency and de-

Table 27–1. Effects of Anesthesia and Other Variables on SSEP Monitoring

Variable	Latency	Amplitude	Comments
Drugs			
Isoflurane	↑	↓	0.5–1.0 MAC + 60% N_2O is compatible with adequate monitoring
Enflurane	↑	↓	
Halothane	↑	↓	
Nitrous oxide	0	↓	
Thiopental	↑	↓	3–5 mg/kg has slight ↑ in LAT; SSEPs can still be monitored at 22.5 mg/kg
Etomidate	↑	↑	Bolus 0.3 mg/kg or infusion 2 mg•kg⁻•h⁻ to improve SSEPs
Ketamine	?	↑	
Droperidol	↑	↓	
Diazepam	↑	↓	0.1 mg/kg premedication allows SSEP monitoring
Midazolam	0	↓	0.3 mg/kg bolus + 0.2 mg•kg⁻¹•h⁻¹ infusion[5]
Fentanyl	↑	↓	Up to 60 μg/kg reproducible SSEPs can be recorded
Sufenta	↑	↓	Up to 5 μg/kg reproducible SSEPs can be recorded
Morphine	↑	↓	
Meperidine	↑	↑ / ↓	
Muscle relaxants	0	0	
Hypothermia	↑	↓	~25° loss of EPs; Δ of 1° → ↓ conduction time by 1 msec
Hyperthermia	0	↓	~42° loss of EPs; Δ of 1° → ↑ conduction time by 1 msec
Hypoxia	0	↓	
Hypotension	0	↓	marked loss of amplitude at MAP <40 mm Hg
Isovolemic hemodilution	↑	↓	↑ LAT significant at HCT <15% ↓ AMP significant at HCT <7%
Hypocarbia	↑	0	$ETCO_2$ <25 mm Hg

creases in amplitude. Even in relatively high doses, adequate intraoperative monitoring is possible.

A number of physiologic variables, including blood pressure, temperature, and blood gas tension, have been shown to influence SSEP recording. Decreased mean arterial pressure (MAP) to levels below cerebral autoregulation, or a rapid decline in MAP to levels within the limit of cerebral autoregulation, can produce progressive SSEP changes. Extreme isovolemic hemodilution (hematocrit levels below 15%) and hypocarbia have been shown to influence SSEP.

To distinguish possible pathologic changes from anesthetic-influenced alterations, it is necessary to follow the trend of changes in latency and amplitude. Physiologic variables should be kept as constant as possible to minimize interferences. If possible, bolus doses of drugs, as well as high doses of drugs and agents that are known to abolish the SSEP signal, should be avoided during critical phases of the operation.

Selected Reference

1. Mahala ME. Neurologic monitoring. In Cucchiara RF, Black S, Michenfelder JD, eds. Clinical Neuroanesthesia. 2nd ed. New York: Churchill Livingstone, 1998:125–176.

Suggested References

Black S, Mahala ME, Cucchiara RF. Neurologic monitoring. In Miller RD, ed. Anesthesia. 5th ed. Philadelphia: Churchill Livingstone, 2000:1324–1350.

Koht A. Anesthesia and evoked potentials: Overview. Int J Clin Mon Comp 1988;5:167.

Koht A, Schutz W, Schmidt G, et al. Effects of etomidate, midazolam, and thiopental on median nerve somatosensory evoked potentials and the additive effects of fentanyl and nitrous oxide. Anesth Analg 1988;67:435–441.

McMeniman WJ, Purcell G. Neurosurgical monitoring during anesthesia and surgery. Anaesth Intensive Care 1988;16:358.

28
Physiology of
Neuromuscular Transmission

Jerald O. Van Beck, M.D.

Motor nerve axons branch as they course distally within skeletal muscle. Ultimately, they penetrate a muscle fiber, lose their myelin sheath, and terminate at the neuromuscular junction (NMJ). In humans, each muscle fiber is focally innervated, although special muscles (e.g., extraocular muscles) have multiple NMJs per muscle fiber. Transmission from nerve to muscle is mediated by acetylcholine (ACh). ACh is synthesized in the nerve terminal and sorted in vesicles. Each nerve terminal contains approximately 500,000 vesicles arranged into transverse bands called active zones (Fig. 28–1). ACh is released into the junctional cleft after an appropriate nerve impulse reaches the nerve terminal. The transmitter then diffuses 50 to 70 nm across the cleft to bind the nicotinic cholinoceptors in the postjunctional membrane and initiate muscle contraction.

Neuromuscular Junction Function

Acetylcholine Synthesis. ACh is synthesized from acetylcoenzyme A and choline under the catalytic influence of choline-o-acetyltransferase in the axoplasm. The ACh is transported into vesicles by a specific carrier-mediated system. Approximately 80% of the ACh present in the nerve terminal is located in the vesicles, with the remainder dissolved in the axoplasm.

Nerve Terminal Depolarization. Depolarization of the nerve terminal follows the arrival of the nerve action potential and results from sodium influx through membrane sodium channels. This alters the membrane potential from -90 mV toward the membrane potential of sodium ($+50$ mV). However, at a membrane potential near 0 mV, potassium channels open and sodium channels begin to close. This results in the membrane potential going to $+10$ mV. During depolarization, calcium ions also enter the nerve terminal, where they are sequestered in the sarcoplasmic reticulum and mitochondria.

Acetylcholine Release. ACh is spontaneously released from the vesicles into the synaptic cleft. This results in small depolarizations (5 mV) at 1 to 3 Hz known as miniature endplate potentials (MEPP). Each MEPP is thought to represent the effect of the contents of a single vesicle containing 6000 to 10,000 ACh molecules, or 1 quanta. These do not result in muscle movement, and the purpose

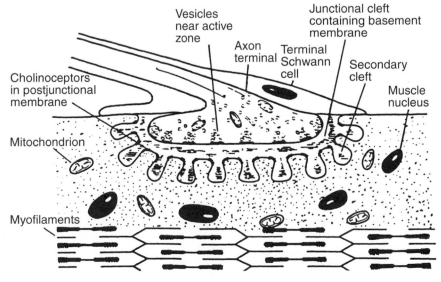

Figure 28–1. A neuromuscular junction. The axon terminal contains mitochondria, microtubules, and acetylcholine-containing vesicles. (From Bowman WC.[1])

Cholinoceptors in postjunctional membrane

Vesicles near active zone

Axon terminal

Terminal Schwann cell

Junctional cleft containing basement membrane

Secondary cleft

Muscle nucleus

Mitochondrion

Myofilaments

of a MEPP is unknown. Nonetheless, nerve terminal depolarization causes accelerated ACh release of 200 to 400 quanta by a calcium-dependent process. This results in sufficient postjunctional membrane depolarization to produce a full-sized endplate potential (EPP) and activation of the excitation-contraction sequence. Evidence exists that axoplasmic ACh is also released spontaneously and with nerve depolarization.

Transmitter Mobilization. The rate at which available ACh stores are replaced is termed **transmitter mobilization**. Evidence suggests that a positive feedback loop exists for ACh.

Postjunctional Events. Released ACh diffuses across the synaptic cleft and binds to a receptor on the postjunctional membrane. This receptor is associated with a membrane ion channel. Two molecules of ACh must bind the receptor before the receptor undergoes the conformational change necessary to open the channel to ion flow. These channels are chemically sensitive but cannot discriminate between sodium and potassium ions. Once the channels are opened, ion flow makes the immediate area more positive. Each elementary current pulse is additive and summates to produce an endplate current (EPC). The EPC depolarizes the endplate membrane to produce the EPP. Once the EPP reaches the critical threshold, a propagating action potential is triggered that is directed away from the endplate and results in the activation of muscle fiber contraction.

Junctional Cholinesterase. The neuromuscular junction contains two forms of acetylcholinesterase: a dissolved form in the nerve terminal axoplasm and a membrane-bound form anchored to the basement membrane of the junctional cleft. The enzyme acts to rapidly hydrolyze released ACh to choline and acetate. The kinetics of this enzyme in the neuromuscular junction is such that a single ACh molecule reacts with a single cholinoceptor before inactivation.

Up-and-Down Regulation

Clinical hypersensitivity and hyposensitivity (resistance) to muscle relaxants are observed in a number of pathologic states. The concept of up-and-down regulation of receptor sites has been introduced to provide a cohesive theory of receptor-drug interaction that can explain a mechanism for abnormal effects of neuromuscular blockers in the clinical setting.[2]

Up-Regulation. An increase in the number of ACh receptors develops on the postjunctional membrane in conditions involving decreased stimulation of the NMJ over time (Table 28–1). Up-regulation leads to hypersensitivity to the agonists ACh and succinylcholine (SCh), and decreased sensitivity to

Table 28–1. Conditions Associated With Acetylcholine Up-and-down Regulation

Up-regulation: ↑ agonist sensitivity, ↓ antagonist sensitivity
Upper and lower motor neuron lesions
Burns
Severe infection
Prolonged use of relaxants
Muscle trauma
Cerebral palsy
Chronic anticonvulsants

Down-regulation: ↓ agonist sensitivity, ↑ antagonist sensitivity
Myasthenia gravis
Organophosphate poisoning
Exercise-conditioning

antagonists such as nondepolarizing muscle relaxants (NDMRs). Up-regulation can lead to lethal potassium release after SCh administration in patients with motor neuron lesions, burns, prolonged use of relaxants in intensive care, and severe trauma and infections. The phenomenon can develop in 3 to 5 days when there is total loss of ACh activity at the endplate.[2] Pretreatment with NDMRs does not predictably prevent SCh hyperkalemia. In other conditions for which chronic anticonvulsant therapy is prescribed, such as cerebral palsy and epilepsy, resistance to NDMRs is seen without potassium release after SCh.

Down-Regulation. Increased sensitivity to antagonists (e.g., NDMR) and decreased sensitivity to agonists (e.g., SCh) develop in conditions of chronic agonist stimulation of receptors. These can occur with chronic reversible (e.g., neostigmine) or irreversible (e.g., organophosphorus) cholinesterase inhibitor use. Most patients with myasthenia gravis have antibodies to ACh receptors that cause the NMJ to function as if it had fewer receptors. These patients are resistant to SCh but extremely sensitive to NDMR. Down-regulation is also thought to occur in muscle groups that show a greater degree of paralysis after exercise conditioning.

Selected References

1. Bowman WC. Neuromuscular block and its antagonism: Basic concepts. In Nunn JF, Utting JE, Brown BR, eds. General Anaesthesia. 5th ed. Boston: Butterworth, 1989:151.
2. Martyn JA, White DA, Gronert GA, et al. Up-and-down regulation of skeletal muscle acetylcholine receptors: Effects on neuromuscular blockers. Anesthesiology 1992;76:822–843.

Suggested References

Azar I. Muscle Relaxants. New York, Marcel Dekker, 1985.
Bevan DR, Donati F. Muscle relaxants. In Barash PG, Cullen BF, Stoelting RK, eds. Clinical Anesthesia. 3rd ed. Philadelphia: JB Lippincott, 1997:385–412.

29
Endocrine Factors Affecting Neuromuscular Block

Wayne H. Wallender, D.O.

Endocrine disorders may affect neuromuscular blockade. Mineral, electrolyte, acid-base imbalance, and temperature alterations superimposed on these endocrinopathies can also affect the characteristics of neuromuscular-blocking agents.

Thyroid Disorders

Hyperthyroidism. Hyperthyroidism increases metabolic output and cardiac work. Anesthesia increases the risk of heart failure and arrhythmias under this circumstance. As discussed in Chapter 207, the patient should be made euthyroid, if possible, before anesthesia induction. In the selection of muscle relaxants, the impact of these drugs on the sympathetic nervous system must be considered. The secondary effects on the cardiovascular system are most important:

- Pancuronium is vagolytic and has the ability to increase heart rate.
- d-Tubocurarine, metocurine, and atracurium cause histamine release, and cardiovascular instability.
- Vecuronium, rocuronium, pipecuronium, and doxacurium appear to have little or no cardiovascular effects.

The incidence of myasthenia gravis is increased in hyperthyroid patients. A nerve stimulator should be used to guide relaxant dosing.

Hypothyroidism. In hypothyroid patients with symptoms of skeletal muscle weakness, prolonged responses to neuromuscular blockade are a consideration. These patients are at risk for postoperative respiratory failure due to respiratory muscle weakness (hypothyroid myopathy) and impaired response to hypercarbia.

The risk of postoperative respiratory failure is compounded because hypothyroid patients may be more sensitive to standard doses of nondepolarizing neuromuscular drugs because of a propensity for hypothermia, decreased hepatic metabolism, and decreased renal elimination of these drugs.

Considerations in hypothyroidism are the following:

- Increased sensitivity to depressant drugs.
- Slowed metabolism of drugs.
- Impaired ventilatory response to hypoxemia and hypercarbia.
- Presence of myopathy.
- Electrolyte abnormalities.

Lack of response to peripheral nerve stimulation before and after administration of neuromuscular-blocking agents has been reported in a normothermic, severely hypothyroid patient.[2]

Most neuromuscular-blocking agents are acceptable, but at reduced doses. A nerve stimulator should be used, keeping in mind the possibility of interference with neuromuscular excitability in the severely hypothyroid state.

Parathyroid Disorders

Hyperparathyroidism. Hypercalcemia is associated with skeletal muscle weakness, although elevated calcium level might be expected to antagonize the effects of nondepolarizing muscle relaxants. Very unpredictable responses to neuromuscular drugs are observed, and there is no evidence that one drug has any advantage over another. A conservative approach to muscle paralysis, guided by appropriate monitoring, is recommended.

Hypoparathyroidism. Concerns reflect decreased calcium level and manifestations of neuromuscular irritability (e.g., laryngospasm). Respiratory or metabolic alkalosis can rapidly decrease ionized calcium level (as can rapid blood infusion). Decreased calcium level potentiates responses to nondepolarizing neuromuscular drugs.

Adrenal Cortex Disorders

Hyperadrenocortism/Hyperaldosterism. When significant skeletal muscle weakness is present, muscle relaxants should be used with caution. Hypokalemia is also associated with skeletal muscle weakness and with increased sensitivity to the effects of pancuronium.

Adrenal Insufficiency/Mineralocorticoid Insufficiency. When skeletal muscle weakness is present, the initial dose of relaxants should be reduced.

Adrenal Medulla Disorders

Pheochromocytoma. Relaxants that are known to liberate histamine or stimulate the sympathetic nervous system should be avoided. There is no known prolongation of neuromuscular blockade.

Diabetes Mellitus

Most patients with diabetes have demonstrable neuropathic changes after several years of the disease. Autonomic nervous system dysfunction may also interfere with ventilatory control, making these patients more susceptible to the respiratory-depressant effects of drugs. Cardiovascular control may also be precarious, so muscle relaxants that liberate histamine or alter vagal tone should be avoided. End-stage renal disease can affect the elimination of relaxants. Atracurium or vecuronium clearance is unchanged in patients with renal failure; however, a report of prolonged neuromuscular blockade after long-term vecuronium use in critically ill patients with renal failure suggests that accumulation of an active metabolite, 3-desacetyl vecuronium, may be a dominant factor.[2]

Selected References

1. Miller LR, Benumof JL, Alexander LA, et al. Completely absent response to peripheral nerve stimulation in an acutely hypothyroid patient. Anesthesiology 1989;71:779–781.
2. Segredo V, Matthay M, Sharma M, et al. Prolonged neuromuscular blockade after long-term administration of vecuronium in two critically ill patients. Anesthesiology 1990;72:566–570.

Suggested References

Cook DR, Freeman AA, Lai AA, et al. Pharmacokinetics of mivacurium in normal patients and those with hepatic or renal failure. Br J Anaesth 1992;69:580.
Savarese JJ, Caldwell JE, Lien CA, et al. Pharmacology of muscle relaxants and their antagonists. In Miller RD, ed. Anesthesia. 5th ed. Philadelphia: Churchill Livingstone, 2000:412–491.
Stoelting RK, Dierdorf SF. Anesthesia and Co-Existing Disease. 3rd ed. New York, Churchill Livingstone, 1993.

30
The Sympathetic Nervous System: Anatomy and Receptor Pharmacology

James D. Hannon, M.D.

Anatomy

The sympathetic nervous system (SNS) is widely distributed throughout the body. Although afferent pathways exist and are important in relaying visceral sensory information to the central nervous system (CNS), the most clearly defined portions of the SNS are the efferent pre- and postganglionic fibers and their associated paravertebral ganglia (Fig. 30–1). The cell bodies that give rise to the preganglionic fibers of the SNS lie in the intermediolateral columns of the thoracolumbar spinal cord from T1 to L2, and the SNS is sometimes referred to as the **thoracolumbar nervous system**.

The short myelinated preganglionic fibers leave the spinal cord in the anterior nerve roots, form white rami, and synapse in sympathetic ganglia lying in three locations outside the cerebrospinal axis. The gray rami arise from the ganglia and carry postganglionic fibers back to the spinal nerves for distribution to the sweat glands, pilomotor muscles, and the blood vessels of the skin and skeletal muscle. The 22 pairs of paravertebral ganglia lie on both sides of the vertebral column. They are connected to the spinal nerves by the white and gray rami communicans and interconnected by nerve trunks to form the lateral chains. They include the upper and middle cervical ganglia, the stellate ganglia (fusion of inferior cervical and T1 ganglia), and the ganglia of the thoracic, abdominal,

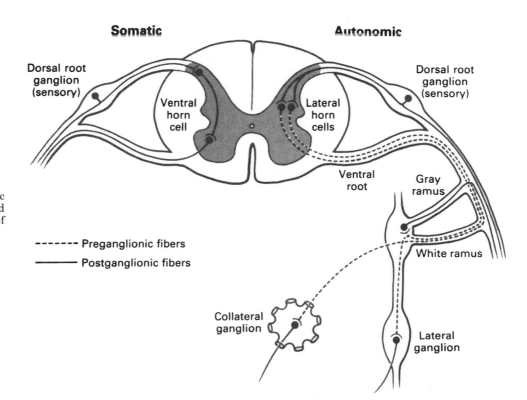

Figure 30–1. The sympathetic outflow from the spinal cord and the course and distribution of sympathetic nerves.

------ Preganglionic fibers
——— Postganglionic fibers

and pelvic sympathetic trunks. Unpaired prevertebral ganglia are found in the abdomen and pelvis near the ventral surface of the vertebral column. They are named according to the major branches of the aorta; for example, celiac, renal, superior, and inferior mesenteric ganglia. The terminal ganglia lie near the innervated organs (rectum, bladder, cervical ganglia in the neck).

The cells of the adrenal medulla are analogous to sympathetic ganglia, except that the postganglionic cells have lost their axons and secrete norepinephrine, epinephrine, and dopamine directly into the bloodstream. Preganglionic fibers may pass through several paravertebral ganglia and synapse with multiple neurons in a ganglion, a characteristic that leads to a diffused output. Postganglionic fibers arising from the sympathetic ganglia may receive input from several preganglionic fibers and innervate visceral structures in the head, neck, thorax, and abdomen. They may pass to target organs through a nerve network along blood vessels or rejoin the mixed peripheral nerve.

Receptor Pharmacology

Neurotransmitters. Acetylcholine (ACh) is the neurotransmitter of all preganglionic sympathetic fibers, including those that innervate the cells of the adrenal medulla. Norepinephrine (NE) is released by nearly all sympathetic postganglionic nerve endings; exceptions are the postganglionic cholinergic fibers that innervate sweat glands (sudomotor) and blood vessels in skeletal muscles (vasomotor). Increasing evidence indicates that neurons in the peripheral nervous system release two or more transmitters from individual nerve terminals when stimulated. Substances released with NE, such as adenosine triphosphate (ATP), may function as cotransmitters or neuromodulators.

Synthesis, Storage, Release, and Inactivation of Norepinephrine. The main site of NE synthesis is in the postganglionic nerve terminal. Tyrosine is transported actively into the axoplasm and converted to dopa (rate-limiting step) and then to dopamine by cytoplasmic enzymes. Dopamine is transported into storage vesicles, where it is converted to NE (Fig. 30–2). Exocytosis of NE is triggered by the increased intracellular calcium that accompanies an action potential. Active reuptake (uptake 1) of NE into the presynaptic terminal terminates the effect of NE at the effector site. This process accounts for nearly all of the released NE, which is then stored in vesicles for reuse. Monoamine oxidase (MAO) is responsible for metabolism of the small amount of NE that enters the cytoplasm after neuronal reuptake, and MAO and catechol-*O*-methyl-transferase (COMT) are responsible for metabolism of NE after extraneuronal uptake.

Receptor Subtypes. ACh activates nicotinic

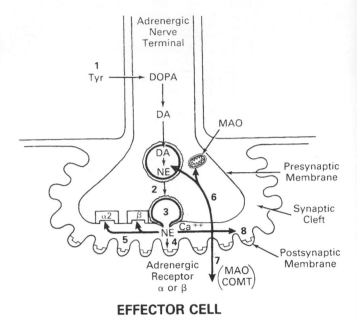

EFFECTOR CELL

Figure 30–2. Diagram of the synthesis and disposition of norepinephrine in adrenergic neurotransmission. COMT, catechol-*O*-methyltransferase; DA, dopamine; DOPA, dihydroxyphenylalanine; MAO, monoamine oxidase; NE, norepinephrine; NMN, normetanephrine; TYR, tyrosine.

cholinergic (N_N) receptors in the sympathetic ganglia and adrenal medulla. The primary sympathetic postganglionic neurotransmitter is NE. Epinephrine (E), the circulating hormone released by the adrenal medulla, and dopamine, the neurotransmitter of the less well-characterized dopaminergic system, are the other naturally occurring catecholamines that interact with peripheral adrenergic receptors. The adrenergic receptors were initially classified as α and β according to their responsiveness to NE and E. Subsequent discovery of more selective agonists and antagonists allowed the α receptors to be subdivided into α_1 and α_2, and the β receptors into β_1, β_2, and β_3. Peripheral dopaminergic (DA) receptors have also been discovered; these are classified as DA_1 or DA_2. α_1 Receptors are found in smooth muscle of vascular (contraction), genitourinary (contraction), and intestinal (relaxation) types, and in the liver (glycogenolysis, gluconeogenesis) and heart (increased contractile force, arrhythmias). α_2 Receptors are located in the pancreatic β cells (decreased insulin secretion), platelets (aggregation), nerve terminals (decreased NE release), and vascular smooth muscle (contraction). β_1 Receptors are found in the heart (increased force and rate of contraction and atrioventricular node conduction), and juxtaglomerular cells (increased renin secretion); β_2 receptors, in smooth muscle of vascular, bronchial, gastrointestinal, and genitourinary types (relaxation) and in skeletal muscle (glycogenolysis, uptake of K^+) and the liver (glycogenolysis, gluconeogenesis); and β_3 receptors, in adipose tissue (lipolysis).

Table 30–1. Adrenergic Agonists

| | Mode of Action | | | | | | |
	α1	α2	β1	β2	DA₁	DA₂	Dose
Natural							
Norepinephrine	+ + + +	+ + +	+ +	+ + +			0.05–0.3 μg/kg/min
Epinephrine	+ + +	+ +	+ + +	+ + +	+		0.05–0.2 μg/kg/min
Dopamine (low dose)					+ + + +	+ +	1–5 μg/kg/min
Dopamine (medium dose)	+	?	+ +	+	+ + + +		5–15 μg/kg/min
Dopamine (high dose)	+ + +	?	+ +	+			>15 μg/kg/min
Synthetic							
Isoproterenol	+		+ + + +	+ + + +			0.01–0.2 μg/kg/min
Dobutamine	+		+ + +	+			2.5–15 μg/kg/min
Mephentermine	+ +	?	+ + +	?			0.1–0.5 mg/kg
Ephedrine	+ +	?	+ +	+			0.2–1.0 mg/kg
Metaraminol	+ + + +	?	+ +	?			10–102 μg/kg
Phenylephrine	+ + + +		+				1–10 μg/kg/min
Methoxamine	+ + + +						0.05–0.2 mg/kg
Dopexamine			+ +	+ + +		+	1–6 μg/kg/min
Fenoldopam					+ + +		0.1–0.8 μg/kg/min

Symbols: + + + +, tremendous stimulation; + + +, marked stimulation; + +, moderate stimulation; +, slight stimulation; ?, unknown.

Receptor Stimulation. The adrenergic receptors are coupled to regulatory proteins called G proteins that stimulate (β_1, β_2, β_3, DA_1) or inhibit (α_2, DA_2) adenylyl cyclase, or stimulate (α_1) phospholipase C. Stimulation of adenylyl cyclase increases cyclic adenosine monophosphate (cAMP), which results in protein phosphorylation. Stimulation of phospholipase C causes the production of inositol trisphosphate, which increases intracellular calcium, and diacylglycerol, which activates protein kinase C. Stimulation of presynaptic α_2 and DA_2 receptors suppresses NE release from sympathetic nerve terminals, whereas stimulation of presynaptic β_2 receptors augments it.

Receptor Modulation. The responsiveness of catecholamine-sensitive cells can vary over time. Multiple mechanisms are responsible for regulating this responsiveness. *Homologous regulation* describes the case when the responsiveness is altered by the adrenergic agonists themselves (decreased receptor density or affinity). *Heterologous regulation* is when the responsiveness is altered by other factors. The density of receptors can be increased (up-regulated) by chronic administration of β-receptor antagonists, by denervation, and by hyperthyroidism. Receptors may be down-regulated by continued β-adrenergic stimulation, hypothyroidism, and possibly by corticosteroids.

Agonists

Sympathomimetic Amines. β-Phenylethylamine can be considered the parent compound. Compounds with hydroxyl groups at positions 3 and 4 of the benzene ring are called catechols; catecholamines are catechols with an ethylamine side chain. Many directly acting sympathomimetic amines stimulate both α and β receptors (Table 30-1). The ratio of activities varies among agonists along a spectrum from predominantly α (phenylephrine) to predominantly β (isoproterenol). β-receptor selectivity is enhanced by substitution of the amine group.

Antagonists

- $\alpha_1 = \alpha_2$ (nonselective): Phenoxybenzamine (irreversible), phentolamine, tolazoline
- α_1: Prazosin, terazosin, doxazosin, trimazosin
- α_2: Yohimbine
- $\beta_1 = \beta_2$ (nonselective): Propranolol, timolol, nadolol, pindolol, sotalol, labetalol (weak α_1)
- β_1: Metoprolol, atenolol, esmolol, acebutolol
- β_2: Butoxamine
- β_3: BRL 37344
- Labetalol: α_1 selective and a more potent nonselective β blocker
- Bretylium: blocks NE release
- Propofenone: β-adrenergic antagonist
- Reserpine: blocks vesicular uptake of NE
- Guanethidine: causes active release and then depletion of NE
- Cocaine and tricyclic antidepressants: block neuronal reuptake of NE
- Tyramine: causes release of vesicular and nonvesicular stores of catecholamines

Selected References

Ganong WF. Review of Medical Physiology. 19th ed. Stamford, CT, Appleton and Lange, 1999.

Landsberg L, Young JB. Physiology and pharmacology of the autonomic nervous system. In Isselbacher KJ, Braunwald E, Wilson JD, et al, eds. Harrison's Principles of Internal Medicine. 13th ed. New York: McGraw-Hill, 1994:412–425.

Lawson NW, Meyer DJ. Autonomic nervous system: Physiology and pharmacology. In Barash PG, Cullen BF, Stoelting RK, eds. Clinical Anesthesia. 3rd ed. Philadelphia: JB Lippincott, 1997:243–309.

Lefkowitz RJ, Hoffman BB, Taylor P. Neurotransmission: The autonomic and somatic nervous systems. In Hardman JG, Limbird LE, Molinoff PB, et al, eds. Goodman and Gilman's The Pharmacological Basis of Therapeutics. 9th ed. New York: McGraw-Hill, 1996:105–139.

31
The Parasympathetic Nervous System: Anatomy and Receptor Pharmacology

James D. Hannon, M.D.

Anatomy

The parasympathetic nervous system consists of preganglionic fibers that originate in the midbrain, medulla oblongata, and sacral spinal cord, and their postganglionic connections. Because of this, it is often referred to as the **craniosacral division**. Preganglionic fibers are very long; postganglionic fibers are very short. The Edinger-Westphal nucleus (in the midbrain) gives rise to the preganglionic fibers of cranial nerve III, which travel to the ciliary ganglion in the orbit. Postganglionic fibers supply the ciliary muscle and the sphincter of the iris. The parasympathetic components of cranial nerves VII, IX, and X originate in the medulla. Preganglionic fibers in cranial nerve VII form the chorda tympani, which innervates the ganglia lying on the sublingual and submandibular salivary glands, and the greater superficial petrosal nerve, which innervates the sphenopalatine ganglion. Postganglionic fibers supply the sublingual, submandibular, and lacrimal glands. The parasympathetic component of cranial nerve IX innervates the otic ganglion, and postganglionic fibers supply the parotid gland. Cranial nerve X contains preganglionic fibers that do not synapse until they reach many small ganglia directly on or in the viscera of the thorax and abdomen. It accounts for about 75% of parasympathetic activity and innervates the heart, tracheobronchial tree, liver, spleen, kidney, and the entire gut except the distal colon. Preganglionic vagal fibers synapse in the plexuses of Auerbach and Meissner in the intestinal wall. The preganglionic parasympathetic sacral outflow (S2, S3, S4) forms the pelvic nerves (nervi erigentes) that supply the distal colon, urinary bladder, and genitalia.

Receptor Pharmacology

Neurotransmitters. Acetylcholine (ACh) is the preganglionic and postganglionic neurotransmitter in the parasympathetic nervous system. Nerves that release ACh are said to be cholinergic. Increasing evidence indicates that neurons in the peripheral nervous system release two or more transmitters from individual nerve terminals when stimulated. Substances such as vasoactive intestinal peptide (VIP) released with ACh may function as cotransmitters or neuromodulators.

Synthesis, Storage, Release, and Inactivation of Acetylcholine. Two enzymes, choline acetyl transferase and acetylcholinesterase (AChE) are involved in the synthesis and degradation of ACh. Two precursors are needed, acetyl coenzyme A, formed in mitochondria from pyruvate, and choline, taken up from the extracellular space by active transport. ACh is formed by choline acetyl transferase in the cytoplasm and sequestered in synaptic vesicles. ACh synthesis is capable of supporting a very high rate of synaptic release; uptake of choline is the rate-limiting step. Continuous small amounts of ACh (quanta) are released from the cholinergic nerve ending even without depolarization, resulting in miniature end-plate potentials (mepps) in the postsynaptic membrane. These potentials are below the threshold required to cause firing. Depolarization of the nerve terminal by an action potential permits the influx of calcium ions, which facilitates the release of 100 or more quanta of ACh by exocytosis. ACh is not taken up by the cholinergic nerve endings. Instead, it is rapidly (almost immediately) hydrolyzed to choline by AChE, which is present in high concentrations at all cholinergic junctions (Fig 31–1).

Receptor Subtypes. Cholinergic receptors are classified as nicotinic (N) or muscarinic (M) according to their response to nicotine and muscarine. N receptors can be subclassified as N_N and N_M types. N_M receptors are found at the neuromuscular junction in skeletal muscle; N_N receptors, in autonomic ganglia (sympathetic and parasympathetic), the adrenal medulla, and the central nervous system (CNS). There are at least five different subtypes of M receptors, all found in the CNS. In the periphery, M_1 receptors are located in autonomic ganglia and various secretory glands. M_2 receptors are found mainly in the heart, and also in smooth muscle. They slow spontaneous depolarization in the sinoatrial node, shorten the duration of the action potential in the atrium, and decrease conduc-

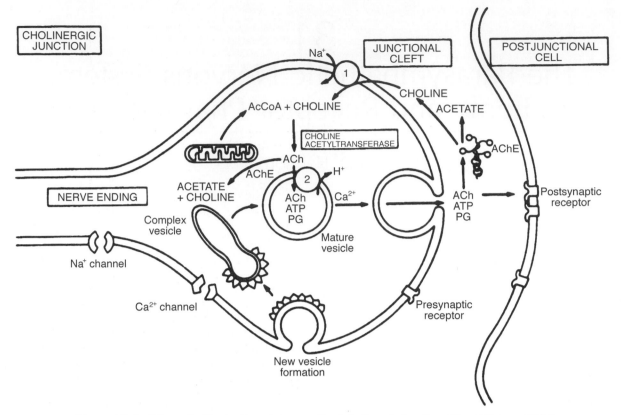

Figure 31–1. Schematic illustration of a generalized cholinergic junction. (From Katzung BG.[1])

tion velocity in the atrioventricular node. They also may provide presynaptic regulation of ACh release from nerve endings in smooth muscle tissue and the CNS. M_3 receptors are located in smooth muscle, where they cause contraction, and in secretory glands, where they cause increased secretion. No agonists with a high degree of selectivity among receptor subtypes are currently available for clinical use.

Receptor Stimulation. N receptors are ligand-gated ion channels that respond rapidly and cause increased permeability to Na^+ and Ca^{2+}, depolarization, and excitability. In contrast, M receptors belong to the class of G protein-coupled receptors, are slower to respond, and can cause either excitation or inhibition. Stimulation of M_1 and M_3 receptors activates phospholipase C and causes hydrolysis of phosphoinositides and mobilization of intracellular Ca^{2+}. M_3 receptors located on endothe-

lial cells in vascular beds are responsible for relaxation. Stimulation causes the release of nitric oxide (NO), which diffuses to adjacent smooth muscle cells and causes them to relax. Activation of M_2 and M_4 receptors inhibits adenylyl cyclase and regulates ion channels through G proteins.

Receptor Modulation. If nicotinic receptor activation is prolonged, the effector response is abolished. ACh released from parasympathetic nerves inhibits release of norepinephrine from sympathetic nerve endings.

Cholinergic Agonists. ACh has a limited therapeutic value because of its widely distributed response, its lack of penetration into the CNS, and its rapid hydrolysis by AChE and plasma butyrylcholinesterase (plasma or pseudocholinesterase). Nicotine is the prototypical ganglionic stimulant, but it is of limited clinical use because of its many side effects. Muscarinic agonists include synthetic ana-

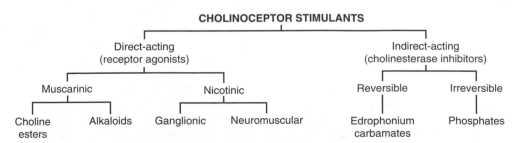

Figure 31–2. The major classes of cholinoceptor-activating drugs. (From Watanabe A.[2])

logs of ACh such as methacholine, bethanechol, and carbachol, and natural alkaloids such as pilocarpine, muscarine, and arecoline. Often, sustained cholinergic agonism is achieved with drugs that increase ACh by inhibiting AChE (Fig 31–2). Most act on true cholinesterase and butyrylcholinesterase. Neostigmine is used for antagonism of neuromuscular blockade and to treat myasthenia gravis. Physostigmine, a tertiary amine that crosses the blood-brain barrier, is used to overcome atropine toxicity in the CNS through an indirect muscarinic effect. Organophosphate insecticides block cholinesterase permanently.

Muscarinic Antagonists. All of the actions of ACh and cholinergic agonists at M receptors can be blocked by atropine and related drugs (scopolamine, belladonna alkaloids). In general, these antagonists cause little effect at the N receptors. Tertiary amines such as atropine and scopolamine cross the blood-brain barrier (atropine less than scopolamine), whereas the quaternary amine glycopyrrolate does not. Ipratropium is a quaternary ammonium compound that when inhaled produces bronchodilation similar to atropine but without inhibiting mucociliary clearance.

Nicotinic Antagonists. These include neuromuscular relaxants (e.g., curare, succinylcholine, pancuronium) that antagonize ACh at the neuromuscular junction but have variable potencies at the autonomic ganglia, and ganglionic-blocking drugs (mecamylamine and trimethaphan), which are still used to control blood pressure in patients with dissecting aortic aneurysm because they also inhibit sympathetic reflexes.

Selected References

1. Katzung BG. Introduction to anatomic pharmacology. In Katzung B, ed. Basic and Clinical Pharmacology. 4th ed. Norwalk, CT: Appleton and Lange, 1989:61.
2. Watanabe A. Cholinoceptor-activating drugs. In Katzung B, ed. Basic and Clinical Pharmacology. 4th ed. Norwalk, CT: Appleton and Lange, 1989:70.

Suggested References

Lawson NW, Meyer DJ. Autonomic nervous system: Physiology. Philadelphia: JB Lippincott, 1997:243–309.

Lefkowitz RJ, Hoffman BB, Taylor P. Neurotransmission: The autonomic and somatic nervous systems. In Hardman JG, Limbird LE, Molinoff PB, et al, eds. Goodman and Gilman's The Pharmacological Basis of Therapeutics. 9th ed. New York: McGraw-Hill, 1996:105–139.

Moss J, Renz CL. The autonomic nervous system. In Miller RD, ed. Anesthesia. 5th ed. Philadelphia: Churchill Livingstone, 2000:523–577.

32
Mechanisms of Hepatic Drug Metabolism and Excretion

Joseph J. Sandor, M.D.

Drug clearance is defined as the theoretical volume of blood from which a drug is completely removed in a given time interval. Total drug clearance is the sum of multiple elimination pathways and is dependent on liver blood flow, extraction ratios, and protein binding. Intrinsic extraction ratios in turn are affected by **genetic factors**, **enzyme induction**, **hepatocellular dysfunction**, and **hepatic congestion.**

Enzyme Systems

Enzyme systems are genetically determined and are affected by age and hepatocellular disease. Hepatic microsomal enzymes, including cytochrome P-450, are a complex set of enzymes and pigmented hemoproteins located in the smooth endoplasmic reticulum which are capable of metabolizing hundreds of compounds. Nonmicrosomal enzymes have the capacity for **conjugation**, **hydrolysis**, and to a lesser extent, **oxidation** and **reduction**. Nonmicrosomal enzyme systems are located in the liver, plasma, and gut. Unlike the microsomal enzymes, they do not undergo induction. Nonspecific esterases are nonmicrosomal enzymes.

Microsomal enzymes may be induced by hundreds of agents, including:

- Phenobarbital.
- Polycyclic hydrocarbons (tobacco).
- Rifampin.
- Phenytoin.
- Chronic ETOH.

Enzyme systems may be inhibited by:

- Competitive inhibition.
- Blockade of drug-cytochrome binding sites (e.g., the effect of cimetidine on the metabolism of meperidine, diazepam, propranolol, and lidocaine).
- Hepatocellular injury (toxins, infections, tumor, congestion).

Pathways of Metabolism

Most pharmacologically active compounds are **lipid soluble** and must cross cell membranes to reach their sites of action. Lipid solubility allows rapid absorption from the foregut and distal renal tubules. Thus, excretion of lipid-soluble drugs is difficult unless they are biotransformed to more polar water-soluble compounds, which facilitates excretion in bile and urine.

Biotransformation Reactions

Phase I reactions involve alterations of, addition to, or splitting off an existing functional group and include **oxidation**, **reduction**, and **hydrolysis**. Phase II reactions include **conjugation reactions** in which a drug is coupled to a polar chemical group, enhancing water solubility (Fig. 32–1).

Phase I reactions include the following:

- **Oxidation** (90% of all hepatic reactions) results in removal of electrons from a molecule through NADPH as an intermediary, ultimately adding them to an oxygen molecule. This results in the

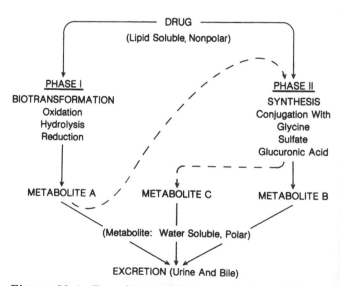

Figure 32–1. Two phases of drug metabolism—biotransformation and synthesis—generally result in the formation of more water-soluble metabolites that are readily excreted in the urine and bile. (From Baden JM, Rice SA.[1])

formation of H_2O and an oxygen atom (usually as OH^-), which is inserted into a drug molecule. **Hydroxylation** creates an unstable compound that splits spontaneously (e.g., dealkylation, deamination, oxidation, dehalogenation, dehydrogenation, desulfuration).

□ **Reduction** reactions result in the direct addition of electrons to a molecule, resulting in instability or polarity. This occurs in the absence of oxygen.

□ **Hydrolysis** is the addition of H_2O into a drug molecule creating an unstable compound that ultimately splits (e.g., amidases, esterases).

Conjugative or synthetic reactions that form a water-soluble compound (phenol, alcohol, carboxylic acids) are termed phase II reactions. They result from an enzymatically mediated combination of various endogenous compounds (e.g., amino acids, acetate, glucoronic acid, methyl groups, sulfates) with parent drugs or metabolites. The polar groups are often the result of phase I reactions.

Hepatic Drug Elimination

Hepatic drug elimination is dependent on **hepatic blood flow** and **extraction ratio** for the unbound fraction of the particular drug. Elimination of drugs with high extraction ratios (e.g., bupivacaine, fentanyl, ketamine, lidocaine, meperidine, metoprolol, naloxone, propranolol, sufentanil) is more dependent on hepatic blood flow than drug metabolism. Elimination of drugs with low extraction ratios is more sensitive to changes in the liver's ability to metabolize the drug. This includes drugs such as diazepam, lorazepam, phenytoin, theophylline, thiopental, and Coumadin (warfarin). Drugs with an intermediate extraction ratio include alfentanil, vecuronium, methohexital, and midazolam.

Selected Reference

1. Baden JM, Rice SA. Metabolism and toxicity of inhaled anesthetics. In Miller RD, ed. Anesthesia. 5th ed. Philadelphia: Churchill Livingstone, 2000:147–173.

Suggested References

Hudson RJ. Basic principles of clinical pharmacology. In Barash PG, Cullen BF, Stoelting RK (eds). Clinical Anesthesia. 3rd ed. Philadelphia: Lippincott-Raven, 1997:221–242.

Parks DA, Skinner KA, Gelman S, Maze M. Hepatic Physiology. In Miller RD, ed. Anesthesia. 5th ed. Philadelphia: Churchill Livingstone, 2000:647–661.

Stoelting RK. Pharmacology and Physiology in Anesthetic Practice. 3rd ed. Philadelphia, JB Lippincott, 1999.

33
Hepatic Physiology and Preoperative Evaluation

Frank D. Crowl, M.D.

Patients with severe hepatic dysfunction are known to be at risk for significant perioperative mortality. Some patients also develop unexpected hepatic dysfunction in the perioperative period. Schemel[1] found that 1 in 700 healthy asymptomatic ASA I and II patients admitted for elective surgery had unexplained abnormalities in preoperative liver function tests. After cancellation of their surgery, one-third of these patients developed clinical jaundice. The reported incidence of postoperative hepatic dysfunction as demonstrated by abnormalities in liver function tests is between 1 in 239 and 1 in 1091 anesthetics. Frequently, elevated bilirubin can be attributed to transfusion or hematoma resorption.

Metabolic Function

- **Glucose homeostasis** is maintained in the liver by a combination of glycogenesis (glucose → glycogen, 75 g stored in liver ~ 24-hr supply), the conversion of fats and proteins to glucose by gluconeogenesis, and the release of glucose from glycogen by glycogenolysis. Insulin stimulates glycogenesis and inhibits gluconeogenesis and the oxidation of fatty acids. Glucagon and epinephrine have the opposite effect by inhibiting glycogenesis and stimulating gluconeogenesis.
- **Fat metabolism** (beta oxidation of fatty acids) provides a large proportion of body energy requirements and reduces the need for gluconeogenesis.
- **Protein synthesis.** All plasma proteins are produced in the liver except gammaglobulins, which are synthesized in the reticuloendothelial system, and antihemophiliac factor VIII.
- **Drug biotransformation.**
- **Bilirubin formation and excretion.**

Hepatic Blood Flow

Total hepatic blood flow (HBF) is approximately $100 \text{ mL} \times 100 \text{ g}^{-1} \times \text{min}^{-1}$. Of this, 75% is delivered by the portal vein, which is rich in nutrients from the gut, is partially deoxygenated, and supplies 50% to 55% of hepatic oxygen requirements (see Fig. 43–1). The remaining 25% of HBF is delivered by the hepatic artery, which supplies 45% to 50% of hepatic oxygen requirements.

Splanchnic vessels supplying the portal vein receive sympathetic innervation from T3-11. Stimuli such as arterial hypoxia, hypercarbia, and catecholamines produce hepatic artery and portal vein vasoconstriction and decreased HBF. β-adrenergic blockade, positive end-expiratory pressure, positive-pressure ventilation (increased hepatic vein pressure decreases HBF), inhalation anesthetics, regional anesthesia with a sensory level above T5, and surgical stimulation (proximity of surgery to the liver determines the degree of HBF reduction) can all cause a reduction in HBF.

Liver Function Tests

Albumin

- The normal level is 3.5 to 5.5 g/dL.
- It is an indirect measure of the synthetic capacity of the liver and may have a predictive value for survival in hepatic disease.
- T½ ~ 14 to 21 days.
- Functions include drug, hormone, and bilirubin transport and binding; maintenance of plasma oncotic pressure; and nutrition.
- A level below 2.5 g/dL may signify severe hepatic disease.
- Other causes of decreased albumin include decreased synthesis (malnutrition), and increased losses (e.g., nephrotic syndrome, burns, ascites, and protein-losing enteropathies).
- Decreased serum albumin may increase the free fraction of protein-bound drugs and increase drug sensitivity.
- Total body albumin can be elevated in patients with cirrhosis who have a low serum albumin level but a large amount of albumin in ascitic fluid.

Table 33–1. Liver Function Tests and Differential Diagnosis

Hepatic Dysfunction	Bilirubin	Transaminase Enzymes	Alkaline Phosphatase	Causes
Prehepatic	Increased unconjugated fraction	Normal	Normal	Hemolysis Hematoma resorption Bilirubin overload from whole blood
Intrahepatic (hepatocellular)	Increased conjugated fraction	Markedly increased	Normal to slightly increased	Viral Drugs Sepsis Hypoxemia Cirrhosis
Posthepatic (cholestatic)	Increased conjugated fraction	Normal to slightly increased	Markedly increased	Stones Sepsis

From Stoelting RK, Dierdorf SF.[2]

Prothrombin Time

□ Normal prothrombin time (PT) is 8.4 to 12.0 seconds.

□ PT is the most important qualitative measure of the liver's function and ability to synthesize proteins. All coagulation factors except factor VIII are synthesized in the liver. Prothrombin's half-life is 6 hours; therefore, it can reflect acute hepatic injury. The PT measures not only prothrombin but the entire extrinsic coagulation pathway. A PT prolonged by more than 4 seconds is associated with a poor 6-month survival in patients with hepatic disease.

□ Other causes of an increased PT include vitamin K deficiencies (e.g., malnutrition, cystic fibrosis), drug effects, decreased plasminogen levels, and fibrinolysis and disseminated intravascular coagulation.

Bilirubin

□ Normal unconjugated (indirect) bilirubin level is 0.2 to 0.8 mg/dL. Unconjugated bilirubin is water insoluble, has minimal urinary excretion, and is neurotoxic.

□ Normal conjugated (direct) bilirubin level is 0.0 to 0.3 mg/dL. Conjugated bilirubin is water soluble and is excreted in the urine.

□ Normal total bilirubin level is less than or equal to 1.1 mg/dL.

□ Bilirubin is produced by the breakdown of heme (hemoglobin, myoglobin, and cytochrome enzymes) and is then bound to albumin for transport to the liver, where it is conjugated via glucuronyl transferase and subsequently excreted into biliary canaliculi. Overt jaundice occurs with total bilirubin levels above 3 mg/dL. This may be accompanied by itching, encephalopathy, and renal insufficiency. Hemolysis causes an increase in unconjugated bilirubin with a decrease in hemoglobin and an increase in reticulocyte count. Gilbert's syndrome is a genetic defect in the conjugation pathway of bilirubin, resulting in an increase in indirect bilirubin without a decrease in hemoglobin or an increase in reticulocyte count. Intrinsic hepatic disease is reflected by an increase in direct bilirubin.

Transaminases

□ Normal level of aspartate aminotransferase (AST, formerly SGOT) is 12 to 31 U/L.

□ Normal level of alanine amino transferase (ALT, formerly SGPT) is 10 to 32 U/L.

□ Transaminases are released in response to acute hepatic injury. The magnitude of rise in serum concentration does not always correlate with the severity of the disease.

□ Transaminase levels may be normal or decreased in patients who underwent gastrointestinal bypass surgery and in patients with hemochromatosis, fatty liver of obesity, or end-stage hepatic disease.

□ Skeletal muscle injury can produce marked increases in transaminase levels.

Alkaline Phosphatase

□ Normal alkaline phosphatase level is 90 to 240 U/dL.

□ Alkaline phosphatase is released from bile ducts in response to acute injury.

□ Alkaline phosphatase level is markedly elevated in obstructive jaundice. This helps differentiate obstructive jaundice from jaundice due to parenchymal hepatic disease.

□ Alkaline phosphatase is also present in the skeleton, gastrointestinal tract, pancreas, and placenta.

□ Elevated alkaline phosphatase level can occur in the absence of hepatic disease (e.g., metastatic bone disease, hyperparathyroidism, rickets and osteomalacia, pregnancy, and pancreatic carcinoma).

□ Hepatic cause can be confirmed by measuring serum levels of 5-nucleotidase.

Liver function tests may be useful for the differential diagnosis of liver disease, as depicted in Table 33–1.

Selected References

1. Schemel WH. Unexpected hepatic dysfunction found by multiple laboratory screening. Anesth Analg 1976;55:810–812.
2. Stoelting RK, Dierdorf SF. Diseases of the liver and biliary tract. In [AU1]Anesthesia and Co-Existing Disease. 3rd ed. New York: Churchill Livingstone, 1993:251–275.

Suggested References

Hudson RJ. Basic principles of clinical pharmacology. In Barash PG, Cullen BF, Stoelting RK, eds. Clinical Anesthesia. 3rd ed. Philadelphia: Lippincott-Raven 1997:221–242.

34
Renal Physiology

William J. Davis, M.D.

Blood Flow, Glomerular Filtration, Tubular Reabsorption, and Secretion

Renal Blood Flow. At rest, the kidneys receive 20% to 25% of cardiac output (1.5 L/min) (the renal cortex receives 75% of renal blood flow [RBF]). The efferent arteriole has considerable resistance to blood flow, resulting in a high-pressure glomerular capillary system for filtration into Bowman's capsule. **Autoregulation** maintains near-constant RBF and glomerular filtration rate (GFR) through a wide range of mean arterial blood pressures (i.e., between approximately 70 and 170 mm Hg) (Fig. 34–1). Although the exact mechanism has yet to be elucidated, autoregulation is thought to be mediated by a myogenic response in preglomerular afferent arterioles; that is, renal vascular resistance of the afferent arteriole increases and decreases in response to increased and decreased mean arterial blood pressure.

Glomerular Filtration. The GFR is the amount of glomerular filtrate formed per minute by nephrons (average, 125 mL/min, or 180 L/day). Filtration pressure in the glomerular capillaries (± 60 mm Hg) is opposed by colloid osmotic pressure in capillary blood and pressure in Bowman's capsule (normal filtration pressure is ± 10 mm Hg).

Factors Affecting GFR

- **Renin** is a proteolytic enzyme synthesized by juxtaglomerular cells of afferent arterioles. It is secreted in response to decreased renal artery perfusion pressure (i.e., hypotension stimulates baroreceptors located in afferent arterioles), increased sympathetic nervous system stimulation, and increased chloride flow past macula densa cells in the distal tubules. Renin is responsible for converting angiotensinogen to angiotensin I (ATI). Angiotensin I is then converted to angiotensin II (ATII) by pulmonary enzymes. Angiotensin II is a potent direct arterial vasoconstrictor that also stimulates adrenal cortical release of aldosterone.
- **Cardiac output** affects RBF, which in turn in-

fluences GFR. For example, increased cardiac output increases RBF and GFR.
- **Sympathetic** stimulation causes preferential afferent arteriolar constriction, thereby lowering pressure in glomerular capillaries and decreasing GFR. Decreased sympathetic stimulation in turn increases urine output via an opposite mechanism.
- **Permeability** of glomerular capillaries is 50 times that of skeletal muscle capillaries. Neutral substances with molecular diameters smaller than 4 nm are freely filtered (inulin), whereas substances greater than 8 nm in diameter are not filtered. Albumin is negatively charged; therefore, although it is 7 nm in diameter, negative charges in the glomerular capillaries repel anionic albumin, limiting the glomerular concentration to only 0.2% of plasma albumin concentration.

Tubular Reabsorption and Secretion

Approximately 80% of water, sodium, and chloride passing in glomerular filtrate is reabsorbed from proximal renal tubules into peritubular capillaries. Sodium transfer is against a gradient and

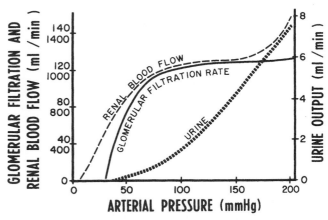

Figure 34–1. Autoregulation keeps glomerular filtration rate and renal blood flow relatively unchanged when arterial pressure is increased. Urine output varies directly with arterial pressure. (From Guyton A, Hall J.[1])

requires an energy-dependent sodium pump to overcome this concentration gradient (this is the greatest energy expenditure by the kidneys). Water and chloride transfer is passive and follows the sodium to maintain isotonicity of ultrafiltrate—more than 99% of water is normally reabsorbed. Glucose and amino acids are almost completely reabsorbed. Potassium, calcium, and phosphate ions are also actively absorbed. Most drugs are either weak acids or bases and exist in the filtrate as water-soluble ions and undissociated lipid-soluble acids or bases. As water is reabsorbed, drug concentration increases, building up a gradient encouraging diffusion. Lipid-soluble drugs are easily absorbed, ions less so.

In **tubular secretion**, H^+ and K^+ are actively secreted into the renal tubules as are some drugs (e.g., salicylate, atropine, morphine, neostigmine, and meperidine). Water reabsorption out of renal tubules is mainly by osmotic diffusion because of diffusion or reabsorption into peritubular capillaries. Two-thirds of the water is reabsorbed in the proximal renal tubules. Further reabsorption occurs in the loop of Henle via the countercurrent mechanism, and antidiuretic hormone-mediated reabsorption in the collecting ducts conserves further water.

Most cations are transported actively through the renal tubule lining. Anions usually are passively transported as a result of electrical potential differences developed by cation transport; for example, sodium ions are actively transported, with chloride following passively. HCO_3^- is thought to be reabsorbed as CO_2 (HCO_3^- combines with H^+ secreted into tubular fluid, forming carbonic acid, which dissociates into water and CO_2). The highly lipid-soluble CO_2 diffuses into peritubular capillaries.

Selected Reference

1. Guyton A, Hall J. Textbook of Medical Physiology. 9th ed. Philadelphia, WB Saunders, 1996.

Suggested References

Bevan D. Renal function. In Nimmo W, Smith G, eds. Anaesthesia. London: Blackwell Scientific 1994:272–287.
Massry SG, Glassock RJ. Normal anatomy, physiology and metabolism of the kidney. In Textbook of Nephrology. 3rd ed. Baltimore: Williams & Wilkins, 1995:3–160.
Sladen RN. Renal physiology. In Miller RD, ed. Anesthesia. 5th ed. Philadelphia: Churchill Livingstone, 2000:663–693.
Stoelting RK. Kidneys. In Stoelting RK, ed. Pharmacology and Physiology in Anesthetic Practice. 3rd ed. Philadelphia: JB Lippincott, 1999:722–735.

35
Renal Function Tests

C. Thomas Wass, M.D.

Evaluation of Renal Function

Urinalysis. Urinalysis is a useful noninvasive diagnostic tool available to assess renal function. Testing includes visual inspection (Table 35–1); dipstick determination of pH, blood, glucose, and protein; specific gravity; and examination of urinary sediment. The pH is rarely diagnostic, but in conjunction with serum pH and bicarbonate it is useful in evaluating renal tubule acidification function.

Dipstick determinations register glucose but not other reducing sugars; elevations suggest diabetes mellitus (when filtered glucose load exceeds tubular reabsorption capacity) or a tubule defect (e.g., Fanconi's syndrome or isolated glycosuria). Blood is detected with great sensitivity but not specificity because myoglobin is detected along with hemoglobin. Protein testing is not sensitive for albumin on dipstick analysis.

Urine should be carefully examined microscopically, especially if dipstick testing indicates an abnormality. Hematuria may be confirmed or white blood cells found, signifying inflammation within the kidney or urinary tract. Casts can be more significant in localizing the level of renal injury.

Creatinine. An end-product of skeletal muscle catabolism, creatinine is excreted solely by the kidneys. Normal serum creatinine value ranges from 0.7 to 1.2 mg/dL. Because creatinine production is proportional to skeletal muscle mass, elderly patients may have normal serum creatinine concen-

trations despite substantial reductions in renal function.

Blood urea nitrogen. Blood urea nitrogen (BUN) is a byproduct of protein metabolism. Normal value ranges from 8 to 20 mg/dL. BUN values may increase independent of renal function as a result of dehydration, a high-protein diet, degradation of blood from a large hematoma or the gastrointestinal tract, or accelerated catabolism (e.g., a metabolic state observed in patients sustaining trauma, sepsis, or burns).

Both creatinine and BUN tend to be insensitive measures of changing renal function. That is, increases in their concentration typically do not occur until the glomerular filtration rate (GFR) is reduced by as much as 75%. Accordingly, both are late indicators of impaired renal function. Dehydration is suspected in patients with a BUN-to–serum creatinine ratio exceeding 20:1.

Creatinine Clearance. This measures glomerular ability to filter creatinine and is the most reliable clinical measure of GFR. Normal value ranges from 110 to 150 mL/min. Mild, moderate, and severe impairment have corresponding values of approximately 40 to 60 mL/min, 20 to 40 mL/min, and less than 20 mL/min. Serial measurement of GFR is important in determining the severity of renal dysfunction and monitoring disease progression. It is estimated using the following formula:

$$GFR = \frac{(140 - age)\,(body\ weight\ in\ kg)}{(serum\ creatinine)\,(72)}$$

More precise measurement requires collection of timed urine samples and use of the following formula:

$$GFR = UV/P$$

where U is the urinary creatinine concentration in mg/dL, V is the volume of urine in mL/min, and P is the plasma creatinine concentration.

Renal Blood Flow. Renal blood flow (RBF) can be experimentally calculated by measuring para-aminohippurate (PAH) clearance. PAH is an organic acid and is filtered by the glomerulus and secreted by the proximal tubule with a first-pass clearance close to 100%.

Table 35–1. Urine Colors and Their Causes

Color	Common Cause(s)
Yellow	Normal
Red	Hemoglobinuria, myoglobinuria, hematuria, beets, rifampin
Orange	Bilirubin, pyridium (phenazopyridine)
Brown	Bilirubin, methemoglobin (Hb in acid urine)
Black	Melanin, hemoglobinuria, homogentisic acid (alkaptonuria)
Blue, blue-green, green	Amitriptyline, methylene blue
White	Chyluria

From Gonin J, Molitoris B.[1]

Tubular Function Tests. These tests reflect the kidney's ability to perform its homeostatic functions. They include urinary sodium and fractional excretion of sodium. Urinary sodium (UNa) is useful in assessing volume status. UNa below 20 mEq/L suggests intravascular volume depletion, whereas UNa above 40 mEq/L suggests decreased ability of renal tubules to reabsorb sodium (e.g., acute tubular necrosis).

Fractional excretion of sodium (FE_{Na}) reflects renal tubular sodium reabsorption. FE_{Na} describes sodium clearance as a percentage of creatinine clearance:

$$FE_{Na} = \text{sodium clearance/creatinine clearance} \times 100\%$$

FE_{Na} below 1% is seen in normal or hypovolemic patients; FE_{Na} above 1% indicates tubular damage (e.g., acute tubular necrosis).

Urine-Concentrating and Diluting Ability. This is assessed by measuring urine osmolality (normal 300 mOsm/kg, but it can range from 50 to 1200 mOsm/kg) and can be evaluated as "appropriate or inappropriate" with respect to serum osmolality (or tonicity; normal range is approximately 278 to 298 mOsm/kg). Normally, as serum tonicity increases, antidiuretic hormone release from the posterior pituitary causes water conservation, and urine osmolality increases. The opposite occurs with dilution of the vascular space, with water diuresis causing urine osmolality to decrease.

Urinary Acidification Capacity. The kidneys excrete nonvolatile acids produced by protein catabolism, thereby preventing systemic acidosis. On a usual American diet, random urine pH is typically below 6.5. An acidification defect can be tested by giving ammonium chloride orally. If the urine pH is not below 5.5 when serum pH is below 7.35 and HCO_3^- is below 20 mEq/L, then a renal tubule acidification defect is present.

Radiologic Tests to Evaluate the Renal System

Table 35–2 describes radiologic tests used to evaluate the renal system.

Table 35–2. Tests for Evaluation of Renal System and Their Uses

Test	Primary Uses
Abdominal flatplate	Determine kidney size
Excretory urogram (IVP)	Best scan of entire renal and excretory system; evaluate hematuria, screen for stones and renal masses
Antegrade pyelogram	View upper tract in cases of obstruction
Retrograde pyelogram	Evaluate obstruction; obtain image of ureters
Computed tomography	Evaluate masses and renal morphology; examine retroperitoneum
Ultrasound	Visualize renal size and location, screen for obstruction, evaluate renal masses
Magnetic resonance imaging	Renal vein thrombosis, masses
Arteriogram	Detect renal artery stenosis (RAS), renal vein thrombosis, evaluation of renal masses
Venogram	Detect renal vein thrombosis
^{131}I-OIH	Evaluate RBF, obstruction, split renal function
^{99m}Tc-DTPA	Evaluate GFR, obstruction, split renal function, RAS
^{99m}Tc-DMSA	Morphology
^{67}Gallium citrate	Assess for infection, ?interstitial nephritis

RBF, renal blood flow; IVP, intravenous pyelogram; DTPA, diethylene triaminopentacetic acid; DMSA, dimercaptosuccinate; ^{131}I-OIH, ^{131}I-orthoiodohippurate.
Modified from Gonin J, Molitoris B.[1]

Selected References

1. Gonin J, Molitoris B. Laboratory evaluation of renal disorders. In Kelly W, ed. Textbook of Internal Medicine. 3rd ed. Philadelphia: Lippincott-Raven, 1997:1042–1048.

Suggested References

Payne RB. Creatinine clearance: A reluctant clinical investigation. Ann Clin Biochem 1986;23:243–250.
Reiser I, Porush J. Evaluation of renal function. In Massry SG, Glassock RJ, eds. Textbook of Nephrology. 3rd ed. Baltimore: Williams & Wilkins, 1995:1780–1788.

36
Chronic Obstructive Pulmonary Disease and Restrictive Lung Disease

David O. Warner, M.D.

The separation of lung disease into obstructive and restrictive patterns is based on the results of pulmonary function tests (see Chapter 1). To summarize, **obstructive disease** is characterized by an increase in expiratory airflow resistance, which causes an increase in total lung capacity (TLC), residual volume (RV), and functional residual capacity (FRC) and a decrease in the forced expiratory volume in 1 second normalized to forced vital capacity ratio ($FEV_1\%$). **Restrictive disease** is associated with decreased lung volumes and is characterized by a decrease in TLC, RV, and FRC and a normal $FEV_1\%$.

Clinical Features of Chronic Obstructive Pulmonary Disease

Approximately 5% of Americans suffer from chronic obstructive pulmonary disease (COPD). The most important cause is cigarette smoking, which accelerates normal age-related declines in pulmonary function to where it produces symptoms (Fig. 36–1). Classically, COPD is subdivided into emphysema and chronic bronchitis, although many patients experience features of both types.

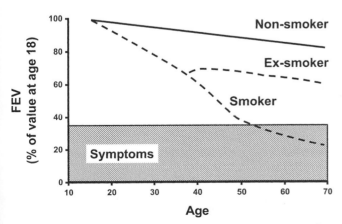

Figure 36–1. Declines in $FEV_1\%$ in a nonsmoker, an ex-smoker who quit at age 35, and a smoker. When $FEV_1\%$ drops below threshold, symptoms develop. (Modified from Celli BR.)

Emphysema implies the destruction of lung parenchyma with normal airways. The loss of tissue produces hyperinflation of the lungs, which distorts the chest wall and contributes to dyspnea, loss of diffusing capacity, and increased expiratory airflow resistance, as the forces which normally exert radial traction on the airways are lost.

Chronic bronchitis is caused by inflammation of the airways, which produces increased mucus secretions and thickening of the airway mucosa. The resulting airway obstruction leads to ventilation-perfusion mismatch and, in severe cases, to hypoxia and CO_2 retention.

Chronic Management

Optimal management of COPD includes smoking cessation (which usually halts the accelerated decline of pulmonary function; see Fig. 36–1), inhaled bronchodilators in patients with a reversible component of airway obstruction (anticholinergic drugs, such as ipratropium, may be particularly useful), and theophylline for severe cases. In general, corticosteroids, mucokinetic agents, and respiratory stimulants are not helpful. Chronic oxygen therapy may be necessary for advanced disease. Contrary to legend, oxygen will not increase $PaCO_2$ in most patients; any increases are most likely caused by changes in ventilation-perfusion distribution rather than reductions in hypoxic ventilatory drive. Acute exacerbations may require mechanical ventilatory support, which with recent advances in "noninvasive ventilation" technology can often be effectively provided without endotracheal intubation. Lung volume reduction surgery is currently being investigated to improve chest wall mechanics in patients with severe hyperinflation.

Perioperative Considerations

Pulmonary function should be optimized in these patients with appropriate use of bronchodilators and treatment of any active infections. Preoperative pulmonary function tests do not predict postoperative pulmonary outcomes and should be obtained only as necessary to optimize preoperative function. The only intervention demonstrated to improve respiratory outcomes in these patients is incentive spirometry, which should be instituted preoperatively and maintained for at least the first week postoperatively. Smoking cessation is desirable, although several weeks of abstinence may be required to demonstrate a benefit. Although tradition holds that regional anesthesia is preferable in these patients, there are no data supporting this assertion, and even patients with severe COPD can safely undergo general anesthesia with endotracheal intubation. Postoperative regional analgesia can provide excellent pain control, but there is no evidence that it reduces the frequency of postoperative respiratory complications.

Clinical Features of Restrictive Lung Disease

Many processes produce restrictive disease, including those that affect the lung parenchyma itself (such as pulmonary fibrosis) and those that affect the chest wall surrounding the lung (such as obesity, pleural effusion, and respiratory muscle weakness from whatever cause). These two types of restriction can be distinguished by testing lung compliance and diffusing capacity, which are both decreased with parenchymal disease and are normal with chest wall disease (because the underlying lung is normal). Chronic management of restrictive lung disease depends on the cause but often involves supportive care only, because many of the underlying processes are themselves not amenable to cure.

Perioperative Considerations

As with chronic therapy, perioperative management varies with the etiology of restriction. As with obstructive disease, optimization of preoperative function and cessation of smoking is desirable. Regional techniques may be appropriate, although their benefits are unproven. In addition, patients with severe dyspnea may not be able to tolerate prolonged surgical positioning. In general, patients needing mechanical ventilation may only tolerate relatively low tidal volumes because of decreased respiratory system compliance, and high breathing frequencies may be required to maintain adequate minute ventilation. Patients with respiratory muscle weakness may require prolonged postoperative ventilatory support to overcome the normal decrease in pulmonary function produced by surgery and anesthesia.

Suggested References

American Thoracic Society. Standards for the diagnosis and care of patients with chronic obstructive pulmonary disease. Am J Respir Crit Care Med 1995;152:S77–120.

Celli BR. Clinical aspects of chronic pulmonary disease. In Baum GL, Crapo JD, Celli BR, Karlinsky JB. Textbook of Pulmonary Diseases. 6th ed. Philadelphia: Lippincott-Raven, 1998;843–863.

Taylor AE, Rehder K, Hyatt RE, Parker JC. Clinical Respiratory Physiology. Philadelphia, WB Saunders, 1989.

Warner DO, Warner MA, Offord KP, et al. Airway obstruction and perioperative complications in smokers undergoing abdominal surgery. Anesthesiology 1999;90:372–379.

37

Preparation for Anesthesia: Tobacco and Caffeine Withdrawal

Brad J. Narr, M.D. □ Steve G. Peters, M.D.

Caffeine

Physiologic Effects

Caffeine is one of the most commonly ingested substances in the world. It is present in coffee, tea, many soft drinks, chocolate, and hundreds of nonprescription medications. Perioperative fasting can lead to unpleasant physical symptoms related to caffeine withdrawal, such as moderate to severe headache, lack of energy, and fatigue that may prolong postoperative hospitalization.[1]

Caffeine is a methylxanthine with stimulatory effects due to blockade of adenosine receptors that stimulate GABA-nergic neurons.[2] Initially, caffeine increases blood pressure and plasma catecholamine levels, increases urine production, and augments gastric acid secretion. Epidemiologic studies seeking a link to cardiac arrhythmia or an increased risk for solid tumors have yielded no convincing evidence.

Conditions for Caffeine Withdrawal

A recent set of double-blind experiments attempted to characterize caffeine withdrawal symptoms.[3] There was no difference in symptoms with 300 mg of caffeine (the equivalent of approximately 3 cups of coffee) consumed in one morning dose or in three 100-mg increments over the course of a day. The range of symptoms as a function of maintenance dose (100, 300, and 600 mg/day) increased proportionately with caffeine intake; however, even abstaining from the lowest dose caused significant caffeine withdrawal symptoms. A duration of exposure as short as three days can still produce withdrawal symptoms. The severity of these symptoms increases with longer exposures.

Treatment Options

The most common caffeine withdrawal symptom is headache. This symptom is likely to occur in relatively healthy patients scheduled for elective outpatient surgery; however, narcotics are often administered in the perioperative period, and thus patients typically do not complain of headache. The American Society of Anesthesiologists Task Force on Preoperative Fasting allows clear liquids until 2 hours before surgery.[4] Drinking coffee or another caffeine-containing beverage early in the morning of surgery has been reported to mitigate symptoms. Intravenous caffeine is available for piggyback infusion. A dose of 100 mg can alleviate symptoms without adversely affecting heart rate or blood pressure in most patients.

Tobacco

Epidemiology and Physiologic Effects of Tobacco Smoke

At least one-third of surgical patients smoke tobacco.[5] Tobacco use has acute and chronic systemic effects. Acute effects include increased carbon monoxide blood levels (i.e., carboxyhemoglobin; elimination half-life of 4 to 6 hours) and nicotine-induced increased sympathetic tone. Chronic effects include cardiovascular disease, respiratory dysfunction, immune system abnormalities, and possibly hemostatic changes.

Anesthetic Complications

The cardiopulmonary effects of recent tobacco use are most likely related to increased carboxyhemoglobin levels and nicotine-related changes in oxygen delivery and myocardial oxygen balance.[6] Such problems can be ameliorated by relatively short-term smoking cessation. For example, smoking cessation 12 to 18 hours before surgery results in a dramatic drop in carboxyhemoglobin levels and sympathetic tone and normalization of the oxyhemoglobin dissociation curve. Long-term (e.g., 6 to 8 weeks) benefits of smoking cessation include return of normal mucociliary function, airway reactivity, airway secretion, and immune function. A blinded study of preoperative smoking cessation in patients scheduled for elective cardiac surgery revealed that patients who stopped smoking for 2 months or less had four times the rate of pulmonary complications than those who had stopped for longer than 2 months before the surgery.[7] In fact, patients who had stopped smoking for longer than 6 months had the same rates of pulmonary complications as patients who had never smoked.

Patients with severe smoking-related lung disease are thought to be at increased risk for pulmonary complications. Advances in anesthetic care (e.g., pulse oximetry and end-tidal CO_2 monitoring) may modify the applicability of findings from earlier studies. A recent study of smokers undergoing abdominal surgery reported that preoperative airway obstruction predicted the occurrence of bronchospasm, but not prolonged endotracheal intubation, prolonged ICU admission, or the need for readmission to the ICU.[8]

Treatment Options

Abstinence from smoking during the perioperative period may provide an excellent opportunity for long-term smoking cessation. Recent advances in the pharmacotherapy of smoking cessation (e.g., nicotine nasal spray, nicotine inhalers, bupropion hydrochloride, nicotine gum, and nicotine dermal patches) are available. However, care must be exercised when using these adjuncts. Controlled animal studies have demonstrated failure of tissue grafting in subjects exposed to systemic nicotine.

Selected References

1. Silversman K, Evans SM, Strain EC, Griffiths RR. Withdrawal syndrome after the double-blind cessation of caffeine consumption. N Engl J Med 1992;327:1109–1114.
2. Daly JW, Fredholm BB. Caffeine: An atypical drug of dependence. Drug Alcohol Depend 1998;51:199–206.
3. Evans SM, Griffiths RR. Caffeine withdrawal: A parametric analysis of caffeine dosing conditions. J Pharmacol Exp Ther 1999;289:285–294.
4. American Society of Anesthesiologists Task Force on Preoperative Fasting. Practice guidelines for preoperative fasting and the use of pharmacologic agents to reduce the risk of pulmonary aspiration: Application to healthy patients undergoing elective procedures. Anesthesiology 1999;90:896–905.
5. Moller AM, Pedersen T. The effect of tobacco smoking on risks in connection with anesthesia and surgery. Development of complications and the preventive effect of smoking cessation. Ugeskrift for Laeger 1999;161:4273–4276.
6. Warner MA, Offord KP, Warner ME, et al. Role of preoperative cessation of smoking and other factors in postoperative pulmonary complications: A blinded prospective study of coronary artery bypass patients. Mayo Clin Proc 1989;64:609–616.
7. Warner DO, Warner MA, Offord KP, et al. Airway obstruction and perioperative complications in smokers undergoing abdominal surgery. Anesthesiology 1999;90:372–379.
8. Hughes JR, Goldstein MG, Hurt RD, et al. Recent advances in the pharmacotherapy of smoking. JAMA 1999;281:72–76.

38
Thermoregulation and Perioperative Hypothermia

C. Thomas Wass, M.D.

Thermoregulation

As with any other neurally mediated physiologic process, thermoregulation involves afferent thermal sensing, central processing, and efferent responses.[1, 2] Thermal receptors are distributed throughout the body (e.g., skin, abdominal and thoracic tissues, spinal cord, hypothalamus), with cold and warm impulses transmitted to the central nervous system via $A\delta$ and C fibers, respectively. Central processing (primarily in the hypothalamus) results in voluntary (e.g., wearing appropriate attire, adjusting ambient temperature) and involuntary (autonomic) efferent responses.

In unanesthetized patients, *cold*-induced autonomic defenses follow a hierarchical pattern that progresses from vasoconstriction to nonshivering thermogenesis and finally shivering thermogenesis (Fig. 38–1).[1, 2] Vasoconstriction decreases cutaneous blood flow and heat loss primarily in the fingers and toes. Although its effects are minimal in adults, nonshivering thermogenesis can double metabolic heat production in the mitochondria-rich brown fat of neonates and infants. Shivering thermogenesis results from involuntary skeletal muscle activity that increases metabolic rate and heat production.

Warmth-induced autonomic responses also occur in an orderly manner.[1, 2] For example, sweating occurs before vasodilation. Each gram of evaporated sweat dissipates approximately 580 calories of heat to the environment.[1]

Core temperatures between the first cold-induced (i.e., vasoconstriction) and warmth-induced (i.e., sweating) responses define the *interthreshold range*.[1–3] Temperatures within this 0.2°C range do not trigger thermoregulatory defense mechanisms.

Effects of Anesthesia on Thermoregulation

General Anesthesia

Intravenous and inhalation anesthetics inhibit thermoregulation in a dose-dependent manner.[1–3] That is, general anesthetics increase the thresholds for warmth-induced thermoregulatory responses and decrease the thresholds for cold-induced defenses. Accordingly, there is a 20-fold increase (i.e., from 0.2°C to 4.0°C) in the interthreshold range. These changes result in a broader poikilothermic range, greater heat loss, and an increased frequency and magnitude of perioperative hypothermia.

Regional Anesthetics

As discussed earlier, thermoregulatory defenses are neurally mediated. Nerve blocks disrupt these neural pathways and interfere with thermoregulation. During spinal or epidural anesthesia, thermoregulation is lost to the lower half of the body. Thermoregulation remains intact above the level of the block, and thus the interthreshold range increases only from 0.2°C to 0.8°C (i.e., a fourfold increase).[1, 3]

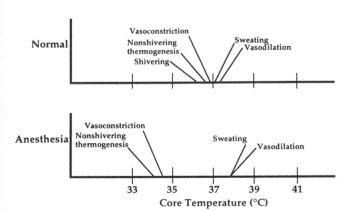

Figure 38–1. Thermoregulatory thresholds in unanesthetized (upper panel) and anesthetized (lower panel) individuals. Core temperatures between the first cold-induced (i.e., vasoconstriction) and warmth-induced (i.e., sweating) responses define the *interthreshold* (IT) *range*. General anesthesia increases the IT range 20-fold (i.e., from 0.2°C to 4.0°C) when compared with that of unanesthetized patients. (From Sessler DI.[2])

Systemic Side Effects of Perioperative Hypothermia

Central Nervous System

A large amount of experimental evidence indicates that hypothermia protects the brain from ischemic and traumatic injury.[2, 4] In contrast, fever has been reported to worsen outcomes following cerebral ischemia or head trauma.[2, 4] Hypothermia produces a slowed electroencephalogram and increased somatosensory evoked potential (SSEP) latency.[4] Changes in SSEP amplitude are less clearly defined.

Cardiovascular

Decreased core temperature can slow intracardiac conduction, predispose patients to lethal cardiac arrhythmias, increase pulmonary and systemic vascular resistance, decrease myocardial contractility, decrease cardiac output, induce myocardial ischemia, and interfere with normal functioning of platelets and the coagulation cascade.[4–8] Interestingly, myocardial ischemia does not appear to be related to increases in whole-body metabolism that result from shivering.[5] Rather, it is likely due to other mechanisms (e.g., increased norepinephrine concentrations).[5, 6]

Wound Infections

Decreased cutaneous blood flow and impaired leukocyte mitogenesis, motility, and phagocytosis result in impaired oxidative killing of bacteria by neutrophils.[1, 4, 8] This has been shown to increase the risk of wound infections threefold in patients undergoing colon resection, increasing the duration of hospitalization by approximately 20% in patients who become hypothermic.[9]

Miscellaneous

Systemic hypothermia also causes a leftward shift of the oxyhemoglobin dissociation curve, decreased O_2 consumption and CO_2 production, slowed metabolism of anesthetic drugs, and a predisposition to citrate toxicity.

Mechanisms and Prevention of Perioperative Hypothermia

Perioperative hypothermia develops via several mechanisms: redistribution, convection, radiation, conduction, and evaporation. Although all of these mechanisms are important to some extent, the ini-

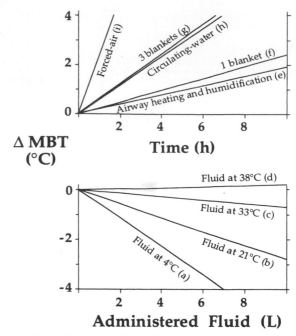

Figure 38–2. Relative effects of warming methods on body temperature. The y-axis depicts changes in mean body temperature (ΔMBT) as a function of time (upper panel) or fluid administered (lower panel). (From Sessler DI.[3])

tial drop in core temperature is predominantly due to redistribution of heat from the core to peripheral tissues.[1, 3]

Prevention and treatment of hypothermia may be achieved using *passive* techniques (e.g., applying cotton blankets, sterile drapes, reflective "space" blankets) or *active* techniques (e.g., using forced-air convective warmers, conductive circulating water mattress, IV fluid warmers, radiant infrared lamps, airway heating and humidification).[1, 3] Of these techniques, heat conservation is most effectively achieved using forced-air convective surface warming (Fig. 38–2).

Selected References

1. Sessler DI. Mild perioperative hypothermia. N Engl J Med 1997;336:1730–1737.
2. Sessler DI. Deliberate mild hypothermia. J Neurosurg Anesthesiol 1995;7:38–46.
3. Sessler DI. Perioperative thermoregulation and heat balance. Ann N Y Acad Sci 1997;813:757–777.
4. Wass CT, Lanier WL. Hypothermia-associated protection from ischemic brain injury: Implications for patient management. Int Anesthesiol Clin 1996;34:95–111.
5. Frank SM, Fleisher LA, Olson KF, et al. Multivariate determinants of early postoperative oxygen consumption in elderly patients. Anesthesiology 1995;83:241–249.
6. Frank SM, Higgins MS, Breslow MJ, et al. The catecholamine, cortisol, and hemodynamic responses to mild perioperative hypothermia. Anesthesiology 1995;82:83–93.
7. Frank SM, Fleisher LA, Breslow MJ, et al. Perioperative maintenance of normothermia reduces the incidence of morbid cardiac events. JAMA 1997;277:1127–1134.
8. Schubert A. Side effects of mild hypothermia. J Neurosurg Anesthesiol 1995;7:139–147.
9. Kurtz A, Sessler DI, Lenhardt R. Perioperative normothermia to reduce the incidence of surgical-wound infection and shorten hospitalization. N Engl J Med 1996;334:1209–1215.

39
Molecular and Cellular Mechanisms of Anesthesia

Carlos B. Mantilla, M.D. □ Gilbert Y. Wong, M.D.

Despite considerable advances in the field of anesthesia, our understanding of the underlying mechanism(s) of general anesthesia is still incomplete. A general anesthetic state is obtained with a combination of **amnesia, analgesia,** and **lack of response to noxious stimuli.**

Potent anesthetic agents include small molecules (e.g., nitrous oxide), alcohols, halogenated ethers, and complex compounds (e.g., barbiturates and propofol). The diversity in chemical structure suggests **multiple modes of action.** Anesthetic agents share certain characteristics, including *hydrophobicity* (i.e., low water solubility, expressed as a lipid-to-water partition coefficient) and *lack of specific antagonists* capable of reversing anesthetic effects. Anesthetics have generally been considered to act nonspecifically on lipid membranes in the central nervous system (CNS). However, recent findings suggest that most anesthetics have *specific* effects on membrane proteins, contributing to their complex mechanisms of action.

Central Nervous System Effects

Anesthetic drugs have been shown to exert inhibitory and excitatory effects on various CNS structures. In general, anesthetics **inhibit brainstem reticular formation, resulting in loss of consciousness.** The interaction between inhibitory and excitatory effects on various CNS structures probably determines the behavioral and physiologic changes observed during anesthesia.

Cellular Effects

Since the discovery of a direct relationship between lipid solubility and anesthetic potency, it has been maintained that anesthetics act nonselectively on neuronal membranes (the **Meyer-Overton rule;** Fig. 39–1). According to this theory, hydrophobic anesthetics are concentrated in the lipid membranes, which contain proteins required for electrical conduction. Once in the lipid membrane, anes-

thetics could potentially change the order and fluidity of the neuronal lipid bilayer, interact with membrane proteins directly, or alter the protein-lipid interface. **Synaptic transmission is sensitive to anesthetics** and may be affected at both presynaptic and postsynaptic sites (Fig. 39–2). However, **axonal conduction is not altered** by clinically relevant concentrations of anesthetics.

The **unitary hypothesis** of anesthesia proposes the existence of **a common mechanism for the action of all anesthetics.** Although this hypothesis is attractive, our current understanding of the molecular and cellular basis of consciousness, memory, and perception suggests diverse anesthetic effects, which does not support this hypothesis.

Lipid-Based Hypotheses

Based on the Meyer-Overton rule, the **lipid solubility hypothesis** suggests that anesthesia is produced when sufficient numbers of molecules disrupt neuronal lipid membranes. Several findings are inconsistent with the lipid solubility hypothesis. First, some hydrophobic molecules, chemically similar to

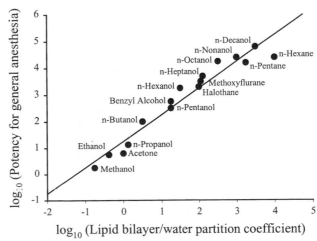

Figure 39–1. Relationship between anesthetic potency and hydrophobicity of alcohols and other anesthetics. (From Franks NP, Lieb WR.[1])

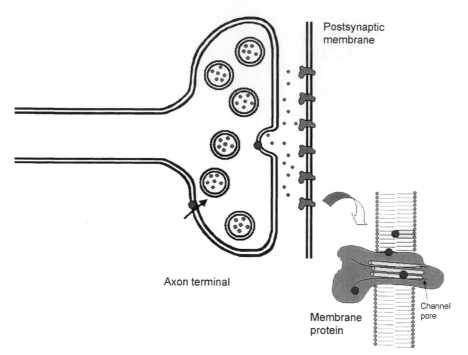

Figure 39–2. Potential sites of anesthetic action include presynaptic and postsynaptic targets (shown in large filled circles). *Presynaptic* inhibition of Ca^{2+} entry in the axon terminal following the action potential and direct inhibition of neurotransmitter vesicle release leads to decreased availability of neurotransmitter in the synaptic cleft and reduced impulse transmission. *Postsynaptic* effects (see inset) may result from direct effects on the lipid membrane, lipid-protein interface, or hydrophobic pockets within transmembrane proteins, leading to altered protein function.

anesthetics, are either much less potent than predicted or altogether nonanesthetic. Second, application of increased pressure to membranes does not alter the lipid solubility of anesthetic agents, whereas this increased pressure antagonizes the anesthetic state (a phenomenon termed the **pressure-reversal effect**). Third, *n*-alcohols exhibit increasing anesthetic potency and hydrophobicity as the carbon chain is elongated, but an additional carbon molecule past 12 or 13 is associated with loss of anesthetic action (the **cutoff effect**).

Modifications of the lipid solubility hypothesis attempt to account for these phenomena by including lipid perturbation effects. The **critical volume hypothesis** suggests that anesthesia occurs when anesthetics cause lipid membrane expansion, thereby disrupting membrane protein function. At clinically relevant anesthetic concentrations, the membrane expands approximately 0.4%. This has similar effects to a 1°C increase in temperature, which is not associated with anesthesia. In addition, although this hypothesis would explain the pressure-reversal effect, it still fails to explain the anesthetic cutoff effect.

The **lipid fluidity hypothesis** arises from the disordering effect that anesthetics exert on membranes, which can interfere with the function of membrane proteins. Anesthetic potency correlates with the disordering effect on cholesterol membranes. The cutoff parallels the altered membrane-disordering ability of alcohols, and pressure increases reverse the anesthetic-induced changes in membrane fluidity. Nevertheless, the assumption that changes in the lipid membrane result in altered protein function has yet to be proven.

Protein-Based Hypotheses

Recent evidence suggests protein-based effects of anesthetics. First, stereoselective effects for barbiturates, ketamine, and isoflurane have been shown. (The S isomer is more potent than the R isomer.) Second, the steep dose-response curve for volatile anesthetics suggests receptor occupancy, given that 1 MAC (minimum alveolar concentration) is effective in 50% of subjects, whereas 1.3 MAC is effective in 95% of subjects. Third, general anesthetic potency correlates well with protein inhibition (Fig. 39–3). Finally, the existence of hydrophobic pockets in pro-

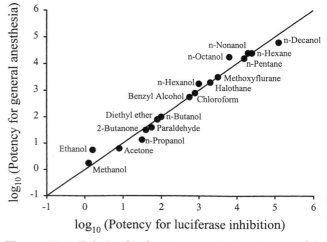

Figure 39–3. Relationship between anesthetic potency and inhibition of the firefly enzyme luciferase for alcohols and other anesthetics. (From Franks NP, Lieb WR.[1])

teins could explain the correlation of potency with hydrophobicity and the anesthetic cutoff.

Studies on ligand- and voltage-gated ion channels show selective anesthetic effects. For example, ketamine-induced anesthesia is mediated by antagonism of N-methyl-D-aspartate (NMDA) receptors. Nitrous oxide also inhibits NMDA receptors. Moreover, most anesthetics augment GABA activity. Furthermore, anesthetics decrease presynaptic neurotransmitter release to a small degree, probably by decreasing Ca^{2+} entry. Despite the effects of general anesthetics on Ca^{2+}, Na^+, and K^+ channels at high concentrations, voltage-gated channels are largely insensitive to anesthetics.

Increasing evidence from studies using clinically relevant concentrations of anesthetics suggests a more selective mechanism of action possibly on a more limited number of CNS targets. **Direct postsynaptic effects on ligand-gated ion channels are likely the primary effect**, altering protein conformation by binding to discrete hydrophobic regions. Clearly, further research in this field is needed.

Selected Reference

1. Franks NP, Lieb WR. Molecular and cellular mechanisms of general anesthesia. Nature 1994;367:607–614.

Suggested References

Forman SA, Raines DE, Miller KW. The interactions of general anesthetics with membranes. In Yaksh TL, ed. Anesthesia: Biologic Foundations. Philadelphia: Lippincott-Raven, 1998:5–18.

Jenkins A, Franks NP, Lieb WR. Effects of temperature and volatile anesthetics on $GABA_A$ receptors. Anesthesiology 1999;90:484–491.

Mihic SJ, Ye Q, Wick MJ, et al. Sites of alcohol and volatile anaesthetic action on $GABA_A$ and glycine receptors. Nature 1997;389:385–388.

Pocock G, Richards CD. Excitatory and inhibitory synaptic mechanisms in anaesthesia. Br J Anaesth 1993;71:134–147.

40
Cardiovascular Effects of the Inhalation Agents

Timothy S.J. Shine, M.D.

There is no one perfect anesthetic agent. The inhalation agents come closest to providing the components of a complete anesthetic (i.e., analgesia, amnesia, hypnosis, and muscle relaxation) as a single agent. All of the inhalation agents depress the cardiovascular system. However, differences exist in their hemodynamic effects. The overall effect of inhaled anesthetics is a reduction in mean arterial pressure. The blood pressure drop with halothane is primarily due to a reduction in myocardial contractility and heart rate and a slight reduction in systemic vascular resistance. Enflurane not only decreases myocardial contractility, it also reduces systemic vascular resistance. Isoflurane, sevoflurane, and desflurane cause a blood pressure drop primarily through a decrease in systemic vascular resistance. Figure 40–1 shows that blood pressure

is decreased by halothane, enflurane, and isoflurane in direct proportion to the dose. At 2 MAC (minimal alveolar concentration) isoflurane, arterial blood pressure is approximately 50% of control.

Systemic Vascular Resistance. Isoflurane and desflurane are potent vasodilators, as shown in Figure 40–2. Halothane and enflurane cause a modest reduction in systemic vascular resistance. Isoflurane causes up to a 50% reduction in systemic vascular resistance at 1.9 MAC.

Heart Rate. Heart rate may be increased by isoflurane, desflurane, and enflurane. The heart rate increase with desflurane is more pronounced at deeper levels of anesthetic, whereas halothane may cause no change or cause a decrease in heart rate. The explanation for this is that baroreceptor function is impaired under halothane anesthesia, whereas isoflurane is less depressant to the baroreflex. Also, there is some evidence that isoflurane causes depression of vagal and preganglionic sympathetic activity in cats. However, vagal activity was more depressed than sympathetic activity. During isoflurane anesthesia, heart rate increased from

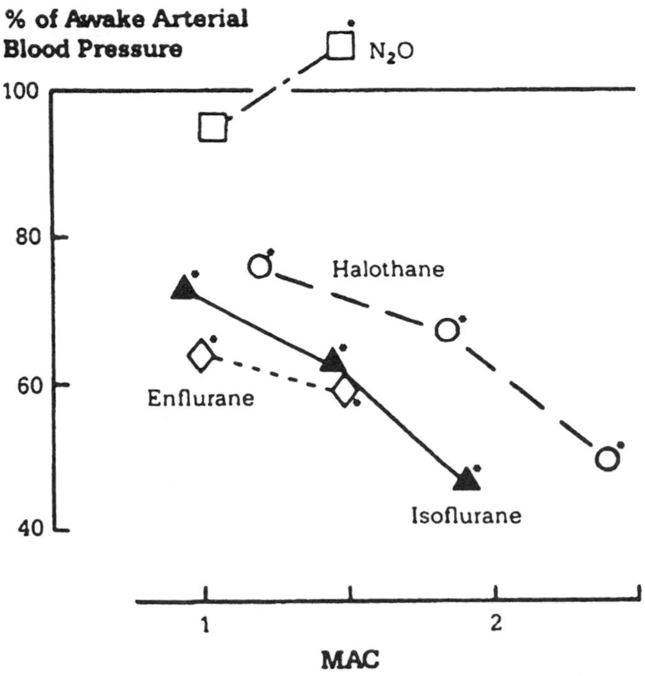

Figure 40–1. Isoflurane, halothane, and enflurane (but not nitrous oxide) significantly (*) decrease arterial blood pressure from the preanesthesia value in a dose-related fashion. (From Eger EI II.[1])

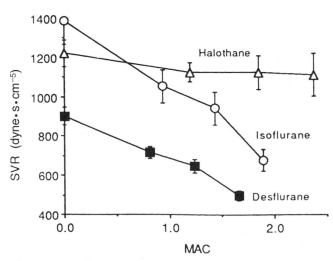

Figure 40–2. Comparison of the effects of desflurane (■) with those of isoflurane (O) and halothane (Δ) on systemic vascular resistance (SVR) in healthy young men. (From Weiskopf RB et al.[2])

the preoperative value in patients under age 40, but did not change in older patients.

Myocardial Contractility. Cardiac output is depressed by enflurane and halothane in a dose-related fashion. Isoflurane and desflurane have little or no effect on cardiac output (Fig. 40–3). A decrease in stroke volume produces lower cardiac output with enflurane and halothane. The decreased stroke volume with isoflurane is compensated for by an increased heart rate. The inhalation anesthetics depress myocardial contraction in the following order:

$$halothane = enflurane > isoflurane$$
$$isoflurane = desflurane = sevoflurane$$

The mechanism of this cardiac depression involves alterations of intracellular calcium (Ca^{2+}) homeostasis at several subcellular targets in the normal cardiac muscle cell.

Thus it can be said that whereas halothane depresses the cardiovascular system by decreasing contractility and isoflurane decreases peripheral vascular resistance, enflurane causes more hypotension by decreasing both contractility and peripheral vascular resistance (Table 40–1). Because cardiac output is preserved with isoflurane, desflurane, and sevoflurane, perfusion of the myocardium and brain is relatively preserved during anesthesia with these agents.

Sensitivity to Epinephrine. All of the volatile agents sensitize the myocardium to epinephrine. The effect is greatest for halothane, followed by enflurane, isoflurane, and desflurane. Children are

Table 40–1. Cardiovascular Effects of the Inhalation Agents

	Contractility	Peripheral Resistance	Systolic Blood Pressure
Halothane	↓	—	↓
Enflurane	↓	↓	↓↓
Isoflurane, desflurane, and sevoflurane	—	↓	↓

less likely to exhibit this effect than adults. Drugs that block the reuptake of norepinephrine such as cocaine and ketamine also increase the arrhythmogenicity of the volatile agents. Johnston et al[3] assumed that one-half the dose of epinephrine required to produce three or more premature ventricular contractions (PVCs) is unlikely to produce PVCs, so that 1 μg/kg of epinephrine during halothane anesthesia and 3 μg/kg during isoflurane anesthesia are unlikely to cause dysrhythmias (Fig. 40–4).

Coronary Vasodilation. Enflurane, halothane, and isoflurane have all been shown to have some coronary vasodilating properties. In isolated vessels, halothane relaxed coronary arteries more than isoflurane. The mechanism of coronary artery relaxation is through an effect on intracellular Ca^{2+} regulation at several locations in vascular smooth muscle cells. At one time there was controversy as to whether isoflurane might "steal" coronary blood flow away from areas of myocardial ischemia; multiple animal studies have refuted this. Studies have shown that isoflurane and halothane do not change collateral-dependent or ischemic zone myocardial

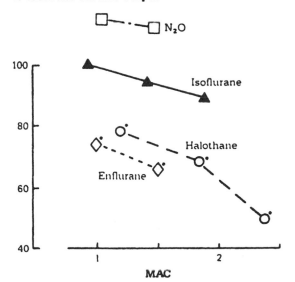

Figure 40–3. In volunteers, neither isoflurane nor nitrous oxide anesthesia depressed cardiac output below levels found during the awake state. In contrast, both halothane and enflurane decreased output significantly (*) and did so to a greater extent at deeper levels of anesthesia. (From Eger EI II.[1])

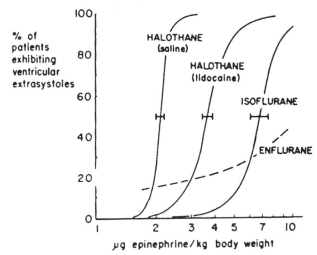

Figure 40–4. Results of a subcutaneous dose of epinephrine showing the percentage of patients with at least three ventricular extrasystoles. (From Johnston RR, Eger EI II, Wilson C.[3])

blood flow when diastolic arterial pressure is kept constant.

Selected References

1. Eger EI II. Isoflurane (Forane). A Compendium and Reference. 2nd ed. Madison, WI, Anaquest, 1988.
2. Weiskopf RB, Cahalan MK, Eger EI II, et al. Cardiovascular actions of desflurane in normocarbic volunteers. Anesth Analg 1991;73:143.
3. Johnston RR, Eger EI II, Wilson C. A comparative interaction of epinephrine with enflurane, isoflurane, and halothane in man. Anesth Analg 1976;55:709.

Suggested References

Bollen BA, Tinker JH, Hermsmeyer K. Halothane relaxes previously constricted isolated porcine coronary artery segments more than isoflurane. Anesthesiology 1987;66:748.

Forrest JB, Buffington C, Cahalan MK, et al. A multi-centre clinical evaluation of isoflurane. Can J Anaesth 1982;29:S15.

Pagel PS, Farber NE, Warltier DC. Cardiovascular pharmacology. In Miller RD, ed. Anesthesia. 5th ed. Philadelphia: Churchill Livingstone, 2000:96–124.

Sill JC, Bove AA, Nugent M, et al. Effects of isoflurane on coronary arteries and coronary arterioles in the intact dog. Anesthesiology 1987;66:273.

41

Central Nervous System Effects of the Inhalation Agents

Margaret R. Weglinski, M.D.

The inhalation anesthetics produce dose-related reversible depression and/or excitation of brain function, resulting in unconsciousness and analgesia. This change in central nervous system (CNS) function is associated with alterations in cerebral metabolic rate (CMR), cerebral blood flow (CBF), electroencephalogram (EEG), and evoked potentials. Alterations in CMR and CBF can have clinical significance, especially in patients with neurologic disorders. Although the CMR and CBF effects of inhalation agents can be manipulated in some instances to improve the clinical outcome of patients with CNS diseases, they also have the potential to adversely affect the diseased brain and the performance of neurosurgery.

Here the effects of the inhalation agents on CMR, CBF, intracranial pressure (ICP), EEG, and evoked potentials are discussed in a general sense, and then specific properties of each agent are considered.

Flow-metabolism coupling is defined as a constant matching of oxygen and glucose delivery to metabolic demand. This is demonstrated by parallel changes in CBF as CMR changes. A misconception about the volatile agents is that, because they increase CBF and decrease CMR, they "uncouple" flow and metabolism. In fact, although increasing concentrations of volatile agents result in a higher CBF for a given CMR, a coupled relationship between these variables persists (Fig. 41-1).

This relationship between CMR and CBF is apparent only if adequate blood pressure is maintained; if blood pressure is allowed to decrease, the increase in CBF will be attenuated or abolished. This is because volatile anesthetics tend to inhibit autoregulation and to actually abolish it at high doses (Fig. 41-2). The inhalation anesthetics do not inhibit CO_2 reactivity and actually appear to exaggerate it. Thus in the normal brain, the cerebral

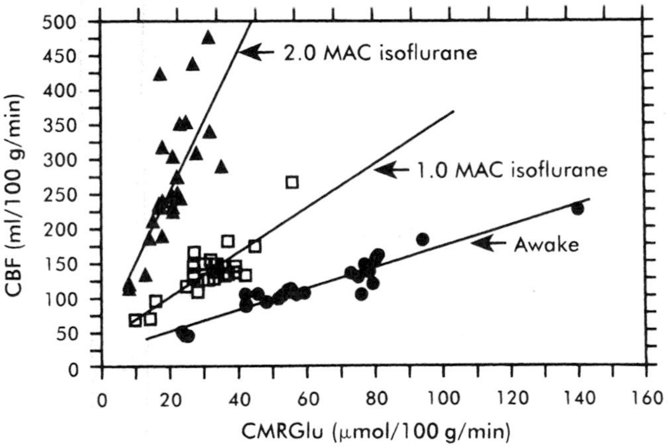

Figure 41-1. Regression plots of regional cerebral metabolic rate for glucose (CMRGlu) versus regional cerebral blood flow (rCBF) in the rat. As the concentration of isoflurane is increased, the slope of the regression line increases (i.e., a higher CBF for a given CMRGlu value). This indicates that isoflurane is a cerebrovasodilator in the rat brain but that it does not uncouple flow and metabolism, even at 2 MAC. (From Todd MM, Warner DS, and Maktabi MA[1]; data from Maekawa T, Tommasino C, Shapiro HM, et al.[2])

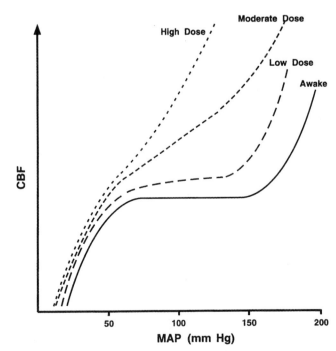

Figure 41-2. Schematic representation of the effect of a progressively increased dose of a typical volatile anesthetic agent on CBF autoregulation. Both upper and lower thresholds are shifted to the left. (From Drummond JC, Patel PM.[3])

vasodilation that occurs in response to a volatile anesthetic can be blunted, abolished, or reversed by increasing hypocapnia. These responses may not apply in the presence of intracranial pathology.

Because the inhalation agents cause an increase in CBF (and in cerebral blood volume [CBV]), the use of these anesthetics in patients at risk for increased ICP was initially a concern. However, numerous studies have confirmed that hypocapnia attenuates or blocks the increase in ICP that otherwise would occur in patients at risk.

Anesthetic-induced EEG changes follow a common pattern (as discussed in Chapter 26). Anesthesia induction causes increased frequency with synchronization and increased amplitude. At about 1 minimum alveolar concentration (MAC), the EEG slows progressively; depending on the anesthetic, burst suppression, an isoelectric pattern, or seizures may evolve as the anesthetic concentration is increased.

Critical regional cerebral blood flow is defined by Michenfelder as "that flow below which the majority of subjects develop ipsilateral EEG changes indicative of ischemia within 3 minutes following carotid occlusion."[4] Table 41–1 lists the critical blood flow of various agents reported in multiple studies.[5]

The inhalation agents also affect evoked potentials, but only minimally at concentrations below 1 MAC. All anesthetics tend to increase evoked potential latencies and decrease amplitudes. Evoked potentials of cortical origin are particularly sensitive to anesthetics; brain stem auditory evoked potentials are the most resistant. Although more sensitive to anesthetics, somatosensory evoked potentials (SSEPs) can be adequately monitored at less than 1 MAC of the volatile anesthetics.

Nitrous Oxide

Cerebral Metabolic Rate and Cerebral Blood Flow. Although nitrous oxide (N_2O) is still mistakenly perceived as being inert physiologically and pharmacologically, it is a cerebral vasodilator that can cause increased ICP. This effect can be clinically significant in neurosurgical patients with increased intracranial elastance. The effect of N_2O on ICP is blocked or blunted by narcotics, barbiturates, and hypocapnia. Its effect on CMR in humans is less clear, although most data suggest that it causes an increase. Cerebrovascular autoregulation

Table 41–1. Critical Regional Cerebral Blood Flow for Anesthetic Agents in Patients Receiving Volatile Agent with Nitrous Oxide

Halothane	20 mL · 100 g^{-1} · min^{-1}
Enflurane	15 mL · 100 g^{-1} · min^{-1}
Isoflurane	10 mL · 100 g^{-1} · min^{-1}
Desflurane	≤10 mL · 100 g^{-1} · min^{-1}
Sevoflurane	11.5 mL · 100 g^{-1} · min^{-1}

and CO_2 reactivity are maintained during N_2O anesthesia.

Electroencephalogram. N_2O concentrations above 50% cause most subjects to lose consciousness, and α-activity is replaced by fast-wave activity. Concentrations near 75% elicit slow-wave activity (4 to 8 Hz) with background fast-wave activity superimposed on it. In hyperbaric conditions, fast-wave activity is abolished, and progressive slowing is evident.

Evoked Potentials. A N_2O concentration below 1 atmosphere has a minimal effect on evoked potentials. Its primary effect is to decrease the amplitude of the evoked response; it has little or no effect on latency.

Pneumocephalus. Pneumocephalus can occur during posterior fossa or cervical spine surgery done under N_2O anesthesia with the patient in the sitting position. When the dura is open, cerebrospinal fluid (CSF) can drain continuously due to gravity and will be replaced by air (an effect known as the inverted pop-bottle phenomenon). This results in a progressive accumulation of air in the ventricles and/or over the cortical surfaces. Because N_2O will equilibrate with any air-filled space in the body, and because its blood solubility is 30 times greater than that of nitrogen, this, will lead to a transient, but significant net increase of gas molecules in the space and hence an increase in its volume or pressure once the dura is closed. Thus N_2O may cause tension pneumocephalus of sufficient significance to produce major cerebral compromise, manifested by seizures, altered consciousness, or specific neurologic deficits.

If a tension pneumocephalus is suspected, N_2O should be discontinued. Patients receiving a second anesthetic within the first three weeks after undergoing supratentorial craniotomy are at risk for complications if N_2O is used. A significant number of these patients will still have significant intracranial air collection.[6]

Halothane

Cerebral Metabolic Rate and Cerebral Blood Flow. Among the volatile anesthetics in use today, halothane is the most potent cerebral vasodilator. It produces a dose-related decrease in CMR. Michenfelder et al. found that in dogs on cardiopulmonary bypass at a concentration of about 4.5% halothane, the EEG became isoelectric.[7] However, in contrast to the effects of high-dose barbiturates or high-dose isoflurane, the CMR did not plateau with the onset of EEG isoelectricity but instead continued to decrease despite the absence of any brain functional work. These findings are thought to reflect a toxic effect of high halothane concentrations on oxidative phosphorylation. No study has shown any evidence of a cerebral toxic effect from halothane concentrations below 2.3%.

Intracranial Pressure. Halothane can increase ICP in patients at risk by causing increases in CBF and cerebral blood volume (CBV). But the establishment of hypocapnia (PaCO$_2$ below 30 mm Hg at normothermia) before the introduction of halothane consistently blocks halothane's effect on ICP. The simultaneous initiation of hyperventilation and halothane administration does not reliably prevent ICP increases. Halothane decreases CSF production but increases the resistance to CSF reabsorption.

Electroencephalogram. At clinically relevant concentrations, halothane cannot produce an isoelectric EEG.

Evoked Potentials. In normal subjects, effective recording of SSEPs can be accomplished with 0.5 to 0.75 MAC halothane (with 60% N$_2$O). A higher halothane concentration can be used if N$_2$O is omitted.

Enflurane

Cerebral Metabolic Rate and Cerebral Blood Flow. Enflurane has cerebral vasodilating effects, but less so than halothane. Enflurane causes decreased CMR. However, seizures can be produced with enflurane at high concentrations (1.5 to 2 MAC), especially when combined with hypocapnia. With the onset of seizure activity, CMR increases approximately 50%. Because enflurane is used clinically at much lower doses and without extreme hypocapnia, its use is not contraindicated in patients with a history of seizure activity.[4]

Intracranial Pressure. Enflurane's potential to increase ICP can be blocked by inducing hypocapnia before administering enflurane, keeping in mind the increased risk of seizures from the combination of extreme hypocapnia and high enflurane concentrations. Enflurane increases CSF production as well as the resistance to CSF reabsorption.

Evoked Potentials. As discussed for halothane, effective recording of SSEPs can be accomplished in normal subjects at 0.5 to 0.75 MAC enflurane (with 60% N$_2$O).

Isoflurane

Cerebral Metabolic Rate and Cerebral Blood Flow. Isoflurane is the least potent cerebral vasodilator of the volatile agents. CO$_2$ reactivity may be greater with isoflurane than with halothane, and isoflurane appears to maintain cerebral autoregulation better than halothane (up to 1 MAC). Isoflurane depresses CMR more than halothane and enflurane do. At 2.0 MAC, isoflurane causes an isoelectric EEG and up to 50% decrease in CMR. Doubling the isoflurane concentration to 4.0 MAC has been shown to cause no further decrease in CMR (in contrast to what occurs with

halothane); there is no evidence of toxicity from deep levels of isoflurane anesthesia.

Intracranial Pressure. Isoflurane's potential to increase ICP can be blocked by simultaneous induction of hypocapnia. It is not necessary to induce hypocapnia before administering isoflurane (as it is for halothane). Isoflurane has no effect on CSF production, and it decreases the resistance to CSF reabsorption.

Electroencephalogram. See the previous section, "Cerebral Metabolic Rate and Cerebral Blood Flow" above.

Evoked Potentials. Isoflurane's effects on evoked potentials are similar to those discussed earlier for halothane and enflurane.

Desflurane

Cerebral Metabolic Rate and Cerebral Blood Flow. The cerebral metabolic and vascular effects of desflurane are similar to those of isoflurane. Desflurane is a cerebral arteriolar dilator and produces a dose-dependent decrease in cerebrovascular resistance and CMR. Like isoflurane, it may be used to induce controlled hypotension. But desflurane may be associated with a greater elevation in heart rate and arterial blood pressure during anesthetic induction than is isoflurane.

Intracranial Pressure. As is true for all volatile anesthetic agents, desflurane may increase ICP in certain patients. This potential is commonly blocked by induction of hypocapnia. However, one study in humans showed a sustained elevation in lumbar CSF pressure after administration of 1 MAC desflurane despite previous establishment of hypocapnia. Desflurane has been shown to produce an increase in CSF formation and no significant effect on CSF reabsorption in dogs.

Electroencephalogram. Desflurane produces a dose-related depression of EEG activity. In swine, prominent burst suppression was observed at MAC levels above 1.24. Although EEG tolerance to the cerebral effects of desflurane has been observed in dogs, it has not been seen in either humans or swine.

Sevoflurane

Cerebral Metabolic Rate and Cerebral Blood Flow. The effects of sevoflurane on CMR and CBF resemble those of isoflurane. Both at normocarbia and at hypocarbia, in most animal models sevoflurane produces little change in global CBF. Cerebral autoregulation and cerebral vascular responsiveness to changes in CO$_2$ are preserved in patients with cerebrovascular disease up to a concentration slightly below 1 MAC.

Intracranial Pressure. Earlier institution of hypocapnia blocks sevoflurane's potential to increase ICP at concentrations up to 1.5 MAC in dogs. The effect of simultaneous institution of hyperventilation and administration of sevoflurane has not been studied.

Electroencephalogram. At a concentration of approximately 2 MAC, sevoflurane can cause burst suppression. EEG monitoring for cerebral ischemia is feasible with 0.6% to 1.2% sevoflurane.[8]

Selected References

1. Todd MM, Warner DS, Maktabi MA. Neuroanesthesia: A critical review. In Longnecker DE, Tinker JH, Morgan GE Jr, eds. Principles and Practice of Anesthesiology. Vol. 2. 2nd ed. St. Louis: Mosby, 1998:1607–1658.
2. Maekawa T, Tommasino C, Shapiro HM, et al. Local cerebral blood flow and glucose utilization during isoflurane anesthesia in the rat. Anesthesiology 1986;65:144–151.
3. Drummond JC, Patel PM. Cerebral physiology and the effects of anesthetic techniques. In Miller RD, ed. Anesthesia. 5th ed. New York: Churchill Livingstone, 2000:695–734.
4. Michenfelder JD. Anesthesia and the Brain. New York, Churchill Livingstone, 1988.
5. Weglinski MR, Losasso TJ, Sharbrough FW, Perkins WJ. Regional cerebral blood flow (rCBF) and EEG with carotid cross clamping in desflurane-N_2O anesthetized patients. Anesthesiology 1996;85:201.
6. Reasoner DK, Todd MM, Scamman FL, Warner DS. The incidence of pneumocephalus after supratentorial craniotomy: Observations on the disappearance of intracranial air. Anesthesiology 1994;80:1008–1012.
7. Michenfelder JD, Theye RA. In vivo toxic effects of halothane on canine cerebral metabolic pathways. Am J Physiol 1975;229:1050–1055.
8. Grady RE, Weglinski MR, Sharbrough FW, Perkins WJ. Correlation of regional cerebral blood flow with electroencephalographic changes during sevoflurane-nitrous oxide anesthesia for carotid endarterectomy. Anesthesiology 1998;88:892–897.

42
Renal Effects of the Inhalation Agents

Jerry A. Hall, M.D.

Inhalation anesthetics can adversely affect renal function during their administration. This is usually secondary to their physiologic effects on the cardiovascular, endocrine, and sympathetic nervous systems. These effects are almost always transient, and •renal function parameters return to normal soon after the cessation of anesthesia.

Because the volatile anesthetics used today are all fluorinated, their metabolism theoretically can also cause renal damage from the release of inorganic fluoride (F⁻). This fluoride-induced nephrotoxicity (high-output renal failure) was most noticeable with methoxyflurane, which was 50% to 75% metabolized by the liver—the primary reason why it is no longer used clinically.

Physiologic Effects

- The volatile anesthetics produce dose-dependent reductions in renal blood flow, glomerular filtration rate (GFR), and urine output.
- These changes are secondary to the volatile anesthetics' effects on blood pressure and cardiac output.
- Halothane has no effect on the autoregulation of renal blood flow.
- Renal function post-transplant is not affected by the choice of volatile agent.
- The aforementioned adverse effects can be abolished or decreased by **preoperative hydration**.

Fluoride-Induced Nephrotoxicity

Inorganic fluoride is produced by oxidative dehalogenation of volatile anesthetics. In addition to fluoride, trifluoroacetic acid (TFA) is a byproduct of the metabolism of the volatile anesthetics. Serum TFA and urine TFA excretion increase after desflurane administration, but some 1000 times less than they do after halothane administration. Isoflurane metabolism produces intermediate levels of TFA in humans.

The toxic fluoride level is 50 to 60 μM/L; toxicity depends on the volatile anesthetic used and on the duration of exposure. Fluoride toxicity impairs the ability to concentrate urine, resulting in polyuria, hypernatremia, and elevated serum osmolality. Possible causative mechanisms include the following:

- Fluoride-induced inhibition of adenylate cyclase activity prevents normal action of antidiuretic hormone on distal convoluted tubules.
- Fluoride ions cause intrarenal vasodilation, leading to shunting of renal blood flow from cortical to medullary nephrons, interfering with the countercurrent multiplier mechanism.

Fluoride-induced nephrotoxicity is most likely with the use of methoxyflurane, sevoflurane, and enflurane; halothane, isoflurane, and desflurane do not release sufficient fluoride on metabolism to present any theoretical risk.

Enflurane

Short-term administration (less than 4.9 minimum alveolar concentration [MAC]-hours) of either enflurane or halothane does not alter renal concentrating ability. Prolonged administration (9.6 MAC-hours or longer) of enflurane causes small but detectable decreases in renal concentrating ability despite average serum fluoride levels of 15 μM/L.

Should enflurane be avoided in patients with pre-existing renal disease?

- Because fluoride excretion depends on GFR, patients with decreased GFR have the potential to develop increased fluoride levels for longer durations.
- Mazze et al.[1] could not demonstrate decreased renal function in patients with chronic renal disease receiving either enflurane or halothane. In fact, they noted decreased serum creatinine and increased creatinine clearance with both agents.

Desflurane

Metabolism of desflurane is one-tenth that of isoflurane, so postoperative serum fluoride levels are not elevated in most studies, despite the fact that the desflurane molecule contains six fluoride atoms (Fig. 42–1).[2] A study comparing desflurane

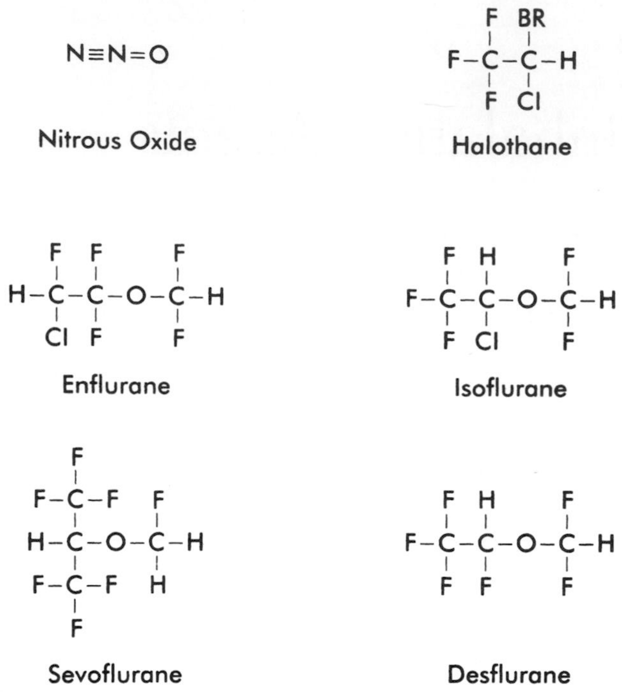

N≡N=O

Nitrous Oxide

F BR
| |
F–C–C–H
| |
F Cl

Halothane

F   F   F
| | |
H–C–C–O–C–H
| | |
Cl F   F

Enflurane

F   H   F
| | |
F–C–C–O–C–H
| | |
F   Cl   F

Isoflurane

F
|
F–C–F   F
| |
H–C–O–C–H
| |
F–C–F   H
|
F

Sevoflurane

F   H   F
| | |
F–C–C–O–C–H
| | |
F   F   F

Desflurane

Figure 42–1. Chemical structures of the volatile anesthetics.

and isoflurane showed no changes in hepatic or renal function in patients with chronic hepatic and renal disease.[3]

Sevoflurane

The sevoflurane molecule contains seven fluoride atoms. Human studies have shown that biotransformation of sevoflurane can produce elevated peak inorganic fluoride levels, especially after prolonged exposure.[4, 5] However, no increases in postoperative creatinine or blood urea nitrogen have been demonstrated.[4, 5]

Summary

□ All volatile anesthetics cause decreased renal function that can be attenuated or abolished by preoperative hydration.
□ Fluoride-induced nephrotoxicity, a problem with methoxyflurane, is rare at usual anesthetic concentrations and duration of enflurane use.
□ After isoflurane and desflurane administration, fluoride release does not affect the kidneys.
□ The use of enflurane and sevoflurane in patients with renal disease is controversial.

Selected References

1. Mazze RI, Sievenpiper TS, Stevenson J. Renal effects of isoflurane in patients with abnormal renal function. Anesthesiology 1984;60:161–163.
2. Koblin DD. Characteristics and implications of desflurane metabolism and toxicity. Anesth Analg 1992;75:S10.
3. Zaleski L, Abello D, Gold MI. Desflurane versus isoflurane in patients with chronic hepatic and renal disease. Anesth Analg 1993;76:353–356.
4. Frink EJ Jr, Ghantous H, Malan TP, et al. Plasma inorganic fluoride with sevoflurane anesthesia: Correlation with indices of hepatic and renal function. Anesth Analg 1992;74:231–235.
5. Kobayashi Y, Ochiai R, Takeda J, et al. Serum and urinary inorganic fluoride concentrations after prolonged inhalation of sevoflurane in humans. Anesth Analg 1992;74:753–757.

Suggested References

Malhotra V, Diwan S. Anesthesia and the renal and genitourinary systems. In Miller RD, ed. Anesthesia. 5th ed. New York: Churchill Livingstone, 2000:1934–1959.
Stoelting RK. Pharmacology and Physiology in Anesthetic Practice. 3rd ed. Philadelphia, Lippincott-Raven, 1999.

43
Hepatic Effects of the Inhalation Agents

Gregory A. Nuttall, M.D.

Anatomy

The liver is the only major organ in the body that receives a dual afferent blood supply (Fig. 43–1). It receives both high-pressure saturated blood (via the hepatic artery) and low-pressure desaturated blood (via the portal vein). Because of this anatomy, the cells adjacent to the hepatic venules are very susceptible to hypoxia, which results in centrilobular necrosis. The liver receives a total hepatic blood

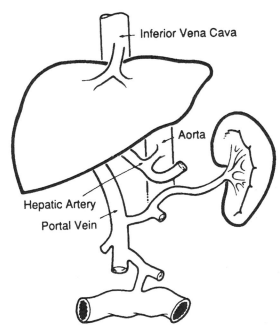

Figure 43–1. The liver receives a dual afferent blood supply, with about 75% of hepatic blood flow provided by the low-pressure portal vein. The remainder of hepatic blood flow is derived from the hepatic artery. Autoregulation of hepatic blood flow is controversial. If autoregulation does occur, it seems to influence only that blood flow delivered by the hepatic artery. The two afferent blood supplies to the liver join at the hepatic sinusoids, and venous effluent enters the hepatic veins and subsequently the inferior vena cava. Total hepatic blood flow is determined by the perfusion pressure across the liver (mean portal vein or arterial pressure minus hepatic vein pressure) and splanchnic vascular resistance. Cirrhosis of the liver increases resistance to flow through the portal vein and decreases hepatic blood flow. (From Stoelting RK, Dierdorf SF.[3])

flow (THBF) of about 1450 mL/min, which represents about 25% of the cardiac output (Table 43–1). THBF is determined by hepatic perfusion pressure (HPP). HPP depends on mean hepatic artery or portal vein pressure minus hepatic vein pressure (5 mm Hg) and splanchnic vascular resistance. Causes of decreased THBF include:

- Decreased mean hepatic artery pressure secondary to decreased systemic mean arterial pressure or increased splanchnic vascular resistance.
- Decreased portal perfusion pressure secondary to decreased systemic pressure or increased hepatic vein pressure.

The occurrence of autoregulation of hepatic blood flow is controversial. In dogs, autoregulation of hepatic blood flow occurs during the fed, metabolically active state but not during fasting. Splanchnic vessels are innervated by sympathetic vasoconstrictor fibers (T3-11). Multiple hormones affect hepatic blood flow.

Anesthetic Effects on Total Hepatic Blood Flow

Halothane and Isoflurane. Gelman et al[1] demonstrated that changes in hepatic arterial blood flow in pigs were more closely associated with changes in mean arterial pressure (MAP) and cardiac output during halothane anesthesia than during isoflurane or fentanyl anesthesia. Hepatic oxygen uptake was maintained at baseline levels during both halothane and isoflurane anesthesia. Oxygen content of the hepatic venous blood was maintained at baseline levels during isoflurane anesthesia and was decreased by halothane anesthe-

Table 43–1. Hepatic Blood Flow

	% THBF	% O$_2$ Supply	Mean Pressure (mm Hg)
Hepatic arterial	30	50	80
Portal venous (PV)	70	50	10

sia. Thus, the hepatic oxygen supply/demand ratio was maintained at baseline levels during isoflurane anesthesia (which induced a 30% decrease in MAP), but decreased during halothane anesthesia.

The foregoing results correlate well with a previous study by Gelman et al[2] in dogs in which THBF was decreased less by isoflurane than by halothane. Halothane unmasks the direct relaxant effect of carbon dioxide on vascular smooth muscle so that hypercarbia leads to decreased splanchnic vascular resistance.

Enflurane. Enflurane has effects similar to those of halothane at equipotent doses, but it has not been thoroughly studied.

Other Anesthetic Techniques. In **spinal** anesthesia, a drop in THBF parallels a decreased MAP. Anesthesia to T7-10 leads to a 20% decrease in THBF; anesthesia to T2-3 leads to a greater than 25% decrease in THBF. **Epidural** anesthesia is similar to spinal anesthesia in causing a decrease in MAP. **Controlled ventilation** with high peak pressures and positive end-expiratory pressure decreases THBF by increasing hepatic venous pressure.

Effect of Operative Site. Surgery near the liver (cholecystectomy) induces a greater decrease in THBF than surgery far from the liver. The decrease in THBF induced by a cholecystectomy was greater than the effect of halothane anesthesia inducing a 50% decrease in MAP.

Effect of Total Hepatic Blood Flow on Drug Metabolism. The elimination of a drug that has a high extraction ratio will be influenced more directly by changes in THBF than by changes in intrinsic clearance or protein binding.

Anesthetic Effects on Hepatic Function

Many studies have reported changes in liver function tests after anesthesia and surgery. It is important to understand that liver function tests are rarely specific, and because of the liver's enormous reserve, considerable damage must occur before the tests are altered. Halothane, but not isoflurane or enflurane, is associated with transient elevations of bromosulfophthalein retention following 8.8 MAC-hours without surgical stimulation. Enflurane is associated with transient elevations of plasma serum glutamic oxaloacetic transaminase (SGOT) after 8.8 MAC-hours without surgical stimulation. The site of the operation has a greater effect on liver function than does the type of anesthetic, as reflected in perioperative measurements of the liver-specific lactate dehydrogenase isozyme 5.

Anesthetic Biotransformation by the Liver

Biotransformation of inhalation anesthetics by the liver occurs through the cytochrome P_{450} oxidase system. About 10% to 20% of halothane is metabolized. Enflurane is metabolized about one-tenth, isoflurane about one-hundredth, and desflurane one-thousandth as much as halothane.[4] Products of metabolism include trifluoroacetic acid, organic fluorides, and other ions, which in the case of halothane have been implicated in rare but severe hepatic dysfunction and necrosis (halothane hepatitis). The mechanism is probably multifactorial and may be related to an immune response to the metabolites aggravated by cellular hypoxia and decreased hepatic perfusion.[5]

Selected References

1. Gelman S, Dillard E, Bradley EL Jr. Hepatic circulation during surgical stress and anesthesia with halothane, isoflurane, or fentanyl. Anesth Analg 1987;66:936.
2. Gelman S, Fowler KC, Smith LR. Liver circulation and function during isoflurane and halothane anesthesia. Anesthesiology 1984;61:726.
3. Stoelting RK, Dierdorf SF. Anesthesia and Co-Existing Disease. 3rd Ed. New York, Churchill Livingstone, 1993.
4. Sutton TS, Koblin DD, Gruenke LD, et al. Fluoride metabolites after prolonged exposure of volunteers and patients to desflurane. Anesth Analg 1991;73:180.
5. Stock JGL, Strunin L. Unexplained hepatitis following halothane. Anesthesiology 1985;63:424.

Suggested References

Parks DA, Skinner KA, Gelman S, et al. Hepatic physiology. In Miller RD, ed. Anesthesia. 5th ed. Philadelphia: Churchill Livingstone, 2000:647–661.

44
Nitrous Oxide

Renee E. Caswell, M.D.

Nitrous oxide (N_2O) is a colorless, odorless gas with a molecular weight of 44. It is the only inorganic gas used for anesthesia. It is manufactured by heating ammonium nitrate in a controlled process. The maximum standards for contaminants permitted in N_2O are nitrogen dioxide, 1.0 parts per million (ppm); halogens, 1.0 ppm; and ammonia, 25 ppm.

N_2O is not flammable but will support combustion as actively as oxygen. The blood/gas partition coefficient is low (0.47). Surgical anesthesia is not possible with N_2O alone, because the drug has low potency as an anesthetic agent; the minimum alveolar concentration (MAC) value in humans is 104%. N_2O is most often used in concentrations of 50% to 70% as an adjuvant to more potent inhaled anesthetics or in addition to intravenous anesthetics.

Respiratory Effects

N_2O decreases tidal volume and increases respiratory rate in a spontaneously breathing patient. N_2O reduces the ventilatory response to both carbon dioxide (CO_2) and hypoxia.

Central Nervous System Effects

Although not a potent anesthetic, N_2O has good analgesic properties. Maximum analgesic effects are noted at a concentration of 35%. At a concentration of 75% N_2O, 50% of patients are unaware of their surroundings. N_2O concentrations exceeding 60% can increase cerebral blood flow and potentially increase intracranial pressure.

Cardiovascular Effects

Compared with other inhalation agents, N_2O has only minimal cardiovascular effects. The slight direct myocardial depression is usually offset by sympathetic stimulation, so that little effect is observed. Adjuvant opioids can block the sympathomimetic effects of N_2O, and some circulatory depression can be seen when narcotics are used with N_2O.

Metabolism and Toxicity

N_2O was previously thought to not be metabolized or undergo any degree of biotransformation, being excreted entirely unchanged through the lungs with a small amount diffusing through the skin. Anaerobic bacteria in the bowel metabolize it through a reductive pathway with the production of free radicals. There is no convincing evidence that these free radicals cause any specific organ injury.

N_2O inactivates methionine synthetase by oxidizing the cobalt in vitamin B_{12}. This can affect deoxyribonucleic acid (DNA) synthesis. A picture similar to pernicious anemia can be seen in laboratory animals after prolonged exposure to N_2O. Megaloblastic hematopoiesis and degenerative neurologic changes are noted. N_2O has also been implicated in the impairment of immune function by decreasing neutrophilic chemotaxis and mucociliary transport. Retrospective epidemiologic studies have consistently shown an increased incidence of spontaneous abortion in women working in operating rooms. No cause-and-effect relationship has been proved, and it is unclear whether trace levels of anesthetic agents, infectious factors, or even stress levels might be implicated. Multiple studies have failed to show mutagenic or carcinogenic effects of N_2O or other anesthetics in humans.

Nitrous Oxide and Closed Air Spaces

N_2O can diffuse into closed air spaces with significant clinical consequences. N_2O moves quickly, whereas nitrogen (N_2) moves slowly. Although relatively insoluble compared to other anesthetics, N_2O is 30 times more soluble than N_2. The blood/gas coefficient of N_2O is 0.47, whereas that of N_2 is 0.015. As a result, at any given partial pressure, far more N_2O can be carried to or removed from a closed gas space. The air space will expand, increasing volume, increasing pressure, or both.

Compliant Spaces Increase Volume

The maximum change in volume that can result is **geometrically** related to the concentration of N_2O in the alveoli (Fig. 44-1).

$$\frac{\text{Change in}}{\text{volume (\%)}} = \frac{\text{nitrous oxide in alveoli (\%)}}{1 - \text{fractional \% of nitrous oxide}}$$

$$100\% = \frac{50\%}{1 - 0.50}$$

50% N_2O: 100% increase in volume

80% N_2O: 400% increase in volume

Noncompliant Spaces Increase Pressure

The maximum change in pressure is arithmetically related to the partial pressure of N_2O in the alveoli.

50% nitrous oxide increases pressure 0.5 atm
75% nitrous oxide increases pressure 0.75 atm

These principles hold true for any anesthetic used, but they are clinically relevant for N_2O because of its low solubility and the high concentrations used (i.e., isoflurane would not show an effect on closed air spaces, because it is used at only 1% to 2% concentration).

Examples

Bowel Gas/Bowel Obstruction. Usually the bowel contains small volumes of gas, so that the increase in volume is of no consequence. For example, 100 mL of bowel gas resulting from swallowing and bacteria could increase two to three times without any problems. On the other hand, the stomach and intestine can contain 5 to 10 L of air; 1 to 2 L is not uncommon. Doubling or tripling this volume

can crowd the operative area, limit diaphragm movement and compromise respiration, make abdominal closure difficult, and increase abdominal pressure during laparoscopy with CO_2 inflation. Even with obstruction, changes in volume occur slowly. Surgery lasting less than 1 hour will cause insignificant changes in volume.

Pneumothorax and Communicating Blebs. Because of the high blood flow in the lungs, the effect of N_2O on a pneumothorax occurs rapidly. N_2O (75%) can double the size of a pneumothorax in 10 minutes, and triple it in 30 minutes.

Venous Air Emboli. An animal study by Munson and Merrick[1] showed that the 50% lethal dose for volume of air embolism was decreased 3.4 times by N_2O anesthesia. If N_2O is being used intraoperatively, it should be discontinued immediately when a venous air embolism is suspected.

Balloon-Tipped Catheters. It was observed that when trying to float a pulmonary artery catheter in a patient anesthetized with N_2O, a greater volume could be withdrawn from the balloon than was injected. Kaplan et al[2] determined that the volume change in the catheter tip was maximal at 5 to 10 minutes depending on the N_2O mixture. This increased volume can cause a problem if a wedged balloon expands. It is advisable to deflate the balloon and reinflate it every few minutes if N_2O is being used and to always deflate the balloon after the wedge pressure is determined.

Endotracheal Tube Cuffs. N_2O can also diffuse into endotracheal tube cuffs, causing increases in volume and pressure. Overexpansion of the endotracheal tube cuffs secondary to N_2O diffusion may cause airway obstruction and glottic and subglottic trauma. Volume increase depends on concentration and length of time exposed. Four hours of N_2O at 100% will increase cuff volume by 300% to 350%.

Middle Ear. N_2O enters the middle ear cavity, elevating middle ear pressure. Normally, any increase in middle ear pressure is vented via the eustachian tube into the nasopharynx. Narrowing of the eustachian tube by acute inflammation, scar tissue, or surgery in the vicinity of the eustachian tube impairs this venting. Increases in pressure can cause:

□ Disruption of previous middle ear surgery.
□ Displacement of the tympanic membrane graft during tympanoplasty surgery.

Intraocular Pressure. Sulfur hexafluoride (SF_6) and perfluoropropane (C_3F_8) are sometimes used in the surgical management of retinal disease, including retinal detachments and macular holes. The gases are injected into the vitreous cavity at varying concentrations. N_2O is 117 times more soluble than SF_6. Pressure has been shown to increase by 14 to 30 mm Hg if N_2O is used. This increased pressure can compromise retinal blood flow and cause retinal ischemia or infarction. Reabsorption of N_2O from the ocular cavity may cause underfilling of the therapeutic gas mixtures, and thus potentially compromise the success of surgery.

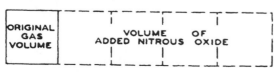

Figure 44–1. Volume changes in a closed space when alveolar N_2O is 50% *(A)* or 80% *(B)*. (From Eger EI, Saidman LJ.[3])

Dural Closure. It is not necessary to discontinue N$_2$O before closing the dura during craniotomy to avoid expanding intracranial air and increasing intracranial pressure.[4]

Selected References

1. Munson ES, Merrick HC. Effect of nitrous oxide on venous air embolism. Anesthesiology 1966;27:783–787.
2. Kaplan R, Abramowitz MD, Epstein BS. Nitrous oxide and air-filled balloon-tipped catheters. Anesthesiology 1981;55:71–76.
3. Eger EI II, Saidman LJ. Hazards of nitrous oxide anesthesia in bowel obstruction and pneumothorax. Anesthesiology 1965;26:61–66.
4. Domino KB, Hemstad JR, Lam AM, et al. Effect of nitrous oxide on intracranial pressure after cranial-dural closure in patients undergoing craniotomy. Anesthesiology 1992;77:421–425.

Suggested References

Eger EI. Nitrous Oxide. New York, Elsevier Science, 1985.
Gillman MA. Haematological changes caused by nitrous oxide. Cause for concern? Br J Anaesth 1987;59:143.
Nunn JF. Clinical aspects of the interaction between nitrous oxide and vitamin B$_{12}$. Br J Anaesth 1987;59:3.
Roizen MF, Plummer GO, Lichtor J. Nitrous oxide and dysrhythmias. Anesthesiology 1988;66:427–431.

45
Factors Affecting Anesthetic Gas Uptake

Mary B. Jedd, M.D.

Blood/Gas Partition Coefficients

The blood/gas partition coefficient can be thought of as the "blood solubility" of an anesthetic. It describes the relative affinity of an anesthetic for the gas and for the blood. For example, isoflurane has a blood/gas partition coefficient of 1.4. This means that at equilibrium, the isoflurane concentration in the blood would be 1.4 times the concentration in the gas (alveolar) phase. By definition, the partial pressures of the agent in blood and gas are equal at equilibrium, but the blood contains more isoflurane. The coefficient describes how the anesthetic agent partitions itself between blood and alveolar gas at equilibrium. The blood/gas partition coefficients of commonly used inhalation anesthetics are listed in Table 45–1.

Uptake

Anesthetic solubility, cardiac output, and the alveolar to venous partial pressure difference are the three major factors affecting uptake and distribution. Their relationship is expressed by the formula:

$$\text{Uptake} = \lambda \cdot Q \cdot \frac{P_A - P_V}{P_B}$$

where λ = solubility, Q = cardiac output, $(P_A - P_V)$ = alveolar to venous partial pressure difference, and P_B = barometric pressure.

Table 45–1. Partition Coefficients at 37°C

Anesthetic	Blood/Gas Partition Coefficient
Desflurane	0.45
Nitrous oxide	0.47
Sevoflurane	0.65
Isoflurane	1.4
Enflurane	1.8
Halothane	2.5
Diethyl ether	12.0
Methoxyflurane	15.0

Modified from Eger EI.[1]

A higher blood/gas partition coefficient will cause increased uptake of anesthetic gas by the blood. Increased uptake will keep the alveolar to inspired gas ratio (F_A/F_I) low (Fig. 45–1). Because the anesthetic partial pressures in all body tissues approach that in alveoli, the higher the solubility, the more delayed the onset of anesthetic effect in the brain when the blood/gas partition coefficient is high. Although more anesthetic agent is taken up by the blood, the partial pressure of the agent rises slowly because of the blood's greater capacity for the agent. Uptake of the more soluble volatile agents can be increased by anesthetic overpressuring, delivering a higher concentration of inspired gas than is aimed for in the alveoli.

Ventilation

The alveolar partial pressure (P_A) of an anesthetic influences the partial pressure in the brain. The

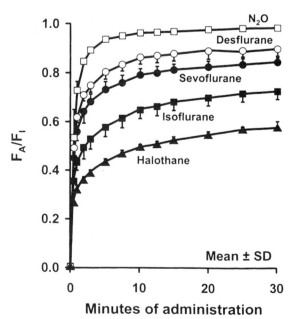

Figure 45–1. The pharmacokinetics of modern inhalation anesthetics defined as the ratio of end-tidal anesthetic concentration (F_A) to inspired anesthetic concentration (F_I) (mean ± SD). The rate of rise of F_A/F_I over time for most agents correlates inversely with the relative solubility of the anesthetics. (From Yasuda Lockhart SH, Eger EI, et al.[2])

inspired concentration of the anesthetic gases and alveolar ventilation are the two factors influencing the rate at which the alveolar concentration of the anesthetic increases. Increasing the inspired concentration (FI) or alveolar ventilation increases the rate of alveolar concentration (FA) increase. The rate of FA increase is also influenced by the concentration effect and the second gas effect (see Chapter 48).

During **hyperventilation**, more anesthetic is delivered to the lungs, increasing the rate of FA/FI increase. This change is more pronounced with more soluble anesthetics, because a large portion of highly soluble anesthetic delivered to the lungs is taken up by the blood. During **hypoventilation**, the rate of alveolar concentration increase is slowed because of decreased delivery of anesthetic gas to the lungs.

An increased **functional residual capacity** (FRC) results in slower dilution of anesthetic gas with the residual air and subsequent slower rate of alveolar concentration increase because of this dilution. Decreased FRC has the opposite effect. Thus, uptake is more rapid for patients with disease conditions that reduce FRC.

Cardiac Output

Increased Cardiac Output. As cardiac output increases, more blood travels through the lungs, thereby removing more anesthetic from the gas phase and resulting in a lower alveolar concentration and a **slower** rate of FA increase. Changes in cardiac output have the most pronounced effect on the uptake of more soluble anesthetic gases. The alveolar to venous anesthetic gradient results from tissue uptake. As this gradient approaches 0 and tissues are fully saturated, uptake of anesthetic by the blood ceases, and the FA/FI ratio more rapidly approaches unity.

Decreased Cardiac Output. With decreasing blood flow through the lungs, less anesthetic is taken up by the blood, and alveolar concentration **increases** more rapidly. Again, highly soluble agents are most affected. With a poorly soluble agent, the rate of FA/FI increase is rapid regardless of the cardiac output and thus is little affected by a decrease in cardiac output. With highly soluble agents, a potentially dangerous positive feedback exists in that anesthetic-induced cardiac depression decreases uptake, increases alveolar concentration, and further depresses cardiac output.

Distribution of Cardiac Output. Anesthetic in the blood distributed to the vessel-rich group

Table 45–2. Tissue Group Characteristics

	Group			
	Vessel-Rich	Muscle	Fat	Vessel-Poor
Percentage of body mass	10	50	20	20
Perfusion as percentage of cardiac output	75	19	6	0

From Eger EI.[1]

(Table 45-2) equilibrates rapidly with that in the vessel-rich tissues. After blood returns to the lungs, it soon has the same partial pressure that it had on leaving the lungs. As the gradient for the uptake of anesthetic approaches 0, alveolar concentration rises rapidly. Because children have greater perfusion of the vessel-rich group than adults, FA/FI rises more rapidly, so anesthesia is achieved more rapidly in these patients.

Ventilation/Perfusion Mismatch. $\dot{V}/\dot{Q}$ mismatch tends to increase the alveolar-anesthetic partial pressure and decrease the arterial anesthetic partial pressure. With the less soluble anesthetics, the arterial partial pressure of the anesthetic decreases markedly because of mixing with blood from areas with inadequate ventilation. With more highly soluble anesthetics, blood from the relatively hyperventilated alveoli contains more anesthetic, which compensates for blood emerging from underventilated alveoli, resulting in less effect on arterial partial pressure.

Cardiac Shunts. A left-to-right shunt in the presence of normal tissue perfusion does not affect anesthetic uptake. With a right-to-left shunt, a fraction of blood does not pass through the lungs and cannot take up anesthetic. This results in a slower rate of increase in arterial concentration of anesthetic and slower induction, with the least soluble agents affected most (see Chapter 47).

Selected References

1. Eger EI II. Uptake and distribution. In Miller RD, ed. Anesthesia. 5th ed. Philadelphia: Churchill Livingstone, 2000:74–95.
2. Yasuda N, Lockhart SH, Eger EI, et al. Comparison of kinetics of sevoflurane and isoflurane in humans. Anesth Analg 1991;72:316–324.

Suggested References

Eger EI. Anesthetic Uptake and Action. Baltimore, Williams & Wilkins, 1974.

46
Minimum Alveolar Concentration

Richard Belmont, D.O. □ Brian A. Hall, M.D.

Dosing for most routes of administration of pharmacologic agents can be measured by the mass of the drug per kilogram of the patient's weight. However, for inhalation agents, the weight of the drug and the weight of the patient have little to do with the intensity of a drug's effect. Therefore, a system for quantifying the amount of volatile agent necessary for anesthesia was devised.

Minimum alveolar concentration (MAC) is the alveolar concentration of volatile anesthetic in volumes percent necessary to prevent purposeful movement in 50% of patients during skin incision. It should be noted that different noxious stimuli require variable volatile partial pressures to prevent purposeful movement. For example, Zbinden and colleagues found that 1.03% isoflurane was required to prevent purposeful movement in response to 50-Hz electrical tetanus, whereas 1.76% isoflurane was required for laryngoscopy with intubation. The term **MAC-awake** is the MAC of a given volatile anesthetic at which a patient will open his or her eyes to command. This concentration is generally 0.3 to 0.4 the usual MAC value (0.3 MAC for isoflurane, 0.5 MAC for halothane). **MAC-intuba-** **tion** is the MAC of anesthetic that will inhibit movement and coughing during endotracheal intubation. **MAC block adrenergic response** (MAC-BAR) is the MAC necessary to blunt the sympathetic response to noxious stimuli. This is generally 1.5 times the standard MAC value.

Alveolar partial pressure is used as the measure of anesthetic concentration because the partial pressure in the alveolus quickly equilibrates with that in the blood and brain because of the brain's high blood flow. At equilibrium, partial pressures of anesthetics are equal in all body tissues. End-tidal anesthetic concentrations can be measured, and they correlate directly with those in the brain. Defined in terms of percentage of 1 atmosphere, MAC is unaffected by altitude and remains the same at high elevations and in a hyperbaric chamber.

Determination of MAC

MAC is determined in humans by anesthetizing them with the anesthetic alone in oxygen and

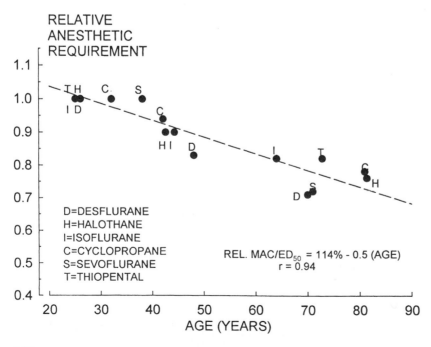

D=DESFLURANE
H=HALOTHANE
I=ISOFLURANE
C=CYCLOPROPANE
S=SEVOFLURANE
T=THIOPENTAL

REL. MAC/ED$_{50}$ = 114% - 0.5 (AGE)
r = 0.94

Figure 46–1. Anesthetic requirement decreases with advancing age, whether the requirements are expressed as MAC for inhalation agents or as ED$_{50}$, the relative median effective dose, for intravenous agents. (From Muravchic S.[2])

Table 46–1. MAC Values for Commonly Used Inhalation Agents

Agent	MAC (Volumes %, 30–55 Years Old)
Isoflurane	1.15
Enflurane	1.68
Halothane	0.75
Desflurane	7.25
Sevoflurane	2.05
Nitrous oxide	105–110

Adapted from Stoelting RK, Miller RD.[1]

Table 46–3. Impact of Physiologic and Pharmacologic Factors on MAC

No change in MAC
 Duration of anesthesia
 Gender
 Anesthetic metabolism
 Thyroid gland dysfunction
 Hyperkalemia or hypokalemia
 $PaCO_2$ 15–95 mm Hg
 PaO_2 above 38 mm Hg
 Blood pressure above 40 mm Hg

Increase MAC
 Hyperthermia
 Drugs that increase CNS catecholamine levels (monoamine oxidase inhibitors, tricyclic antidepressants, acute cocaine ingestion, acute amphetamine ingestion)
 Infants
 Hypernatremia
 Chronic ethanol abuse (?)

Decrease MAC
 Hypothermia
 Preoperative medication
 Intravenous anesthetics
 Neonates
 Elderly
 Pregnancy
 α_2 agonists
 Acute ethanol ingestion
 Lithium
 Cardiopulmonary bypass
 Neuraxial opioids (?)
 PaO_2 below 38 mm Hg

From Stoelting RK, Miller RD.[1]

allowing 15 minutes for equilibration at a single preselected concentration. A single skin incision is made, and the patient is observed for the presence or absence of purposeful movement. A group of patients must be tested in this fashion over a range of anesthetic concentrations that allow and prevent patient movement. The percent of patients in groups of four or more that show a positive response to surgical stimulation is plotted against the average alveolar concentration for that group. A best-fit line is drawn through these points and the concentration at which half of the subjects move with skin incision, and MAC is determined (Table 46–1).

Of the characteristics of inhalation anesthetics, the oil:gas partition coefficients correlate most closely with MAC. The product of the oil:gas partition coefficient and MAC ranges from 100 to 150, as shown in Table 46–2.

The dose-response curve for volatile anesthetics is steep; 1 MAC prevents skeletal muscle movement on incision in 50% of patients, whereas 1.3 MAC prevents movement in 95% of patients. The influence of two inhalation agents administered concomitantly can be determined by understanding that MAC values are additive. If 0.75 MAC N_2O is coadministered with 0.75 MAC isoflurane, then the resulting effect is 1.5 MAC.

Clinical Correlation to MAC

Using MAC as an index of anesthetic potency is reproducible and provides a measure of the partial pressure of drug necessary to produce anesthesia. It is important to remember that MAC is an average value for a population rather than an absolute for each individual. Caution should be used when comparing MAC values obtained from the response of a single preparation to the clinical response when other drugs are being used concurrently.

Factors Affecting MAC

MAC is age-dependent. The MAC value for full-term neonates is less than that for infants; otherwise, MAC steadily decreases with increasing age (Fig. 46–1).

Numerous physiologic and pharmacologic factors, disease states, and conditions can raise or lower MAC (Table 46–3). Some drugs may have opposite effects, depending on chronicity of administration. For example, acute cocaine ingestion raises MAC,

Table 46–2. Correlaton of Minimum Alveolar Concentration (MAC) with Oil/Gas Partition Coefficients

Agent	N₂O	Isoflurane	Enflurane	Desflurane	Halothane	Sevoflurane
MAC (age 30–55) (%)	104	1.15	1.68	6.0	0.75	2.05
Oil:gas partition coefficients	1.4	98	98	18.7	224	47.2
Product	146	113	165	112	168	97

whereas chronic cocaine ingestion lowers MAC. Alcohol lowers MAC acutely but raises it chronically.

Selected References

1. Stoelting RK, Miller RD. Basics of Anesthesia. 3rd ed. New York, Churchill Livingstone, 1994.
2. Muravchick S. Anesthesia for the elderly. In Miller RD, ed. Anesthesia. Vol. 2. 5th ed. Philadelphia: Churchill Livingstone, 2000:2140–2156.

Suggested References

Barash PG, Cullen BF, Stoelting RK. Clinical Anesthesia. 3rd ed. Philadelphia, Lippincott-Raven, 1997.

Quasha AL, Eger EI, Tinker JH. Determination and applications of MAC. Anesthesiology 1980;53:315.

Stanski DR. Monitoring Depth of Anesthesia. In Miller RD, ed. Anesthesia. Vol. 1. 5th ed. Philadelphia: Churchill Livingstone, 2000:1087–1116.

Zbinden AM, Maggiorini M, Peterson-Felix S, et al. Anesthesia depth defined using multiple noxious stimuli during isoflurane/oxygen anesthesia. Anesthesiology 1994;80:253.

47
Effect of Intracardiac Shunts on Inhalation Induction

David J. Cook, M.D.

Intracardiac shunts may alter the rate of induction of inhaled anesthetic agents. This alteration depends on the direction and size of the shunt and on the solubility of the anesthetic used.

Induction of anesthesia is a function of the equilibration of three factors: the rate of anesthetic inflow into the lungs (as determined by minute ventilation and inspired fraction of anesthetic), the rate of transfer of anesthetic from lungs to arterial blood, and the rate of transfer of anesthetic from blood to brain:

$$P_A \leftrightarrow P_a \leftrightarrow P_b$$

where P_A = alveolar partial pressure of the inhaled anesthetic, P_a = arterial partial pressure of the inhaled anesthetic, and P_b = brain partial pressure of the inhaled anesthetic. P_v = mixed venous partial pressure of the inhaled anesthetic

- Shunts primarily alter the $P_A \leftrightarrow P_a$ relationship. The determinants of anesthetic uptake from alveoli are the blood/gas partition coefficient of the anesthetic agent (P_c), cardiac output (CO), and the alveolar to mixed venous partial pressure difference of the anesthetic agent ($P_A - P_v$).
- The **blood/gas partition coefficient** is a distri-

bution ratio between two phases at equilibrium (relative solubility). High solubility slows the rate of P_A and P_a increase and subsequently slows induction.

- During the period of induction, P_A is **much** greater than P_v, and P_A-P_v does not limit the rate of induction.
- Assuming no change in ventilation or inspired fraction of anesthetic (F_I) and normal tissue perfusion, the rate of induction is determined primarily by anesthetic solubility and the effective pulmonary blood flow.

Right-to-Left Shunt

With a right-to-left shunt, a portion of the CO bypasses the lung. This slows induction, because less anesthetic can be transferred from the alveoli to blood per unit time.

- This slowed induction is proportional to the degree of shunting.
- The impact of the shunt is greater with the less soluble anesthetic agents (Figs. 47–1 and 47–2).

For a soluble anesthetic (e.g., ether):

- If ventilation is 5 L/min with 10% ether, then 500 mL/min of ether is delivered to the alveoli.

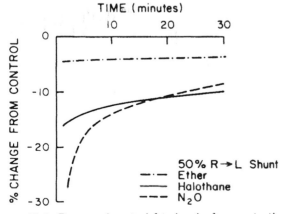

Figure 47–1. Decrease in arterial-to-inspired concentration ratio caused by a 50% right-to-left shunt from control for three anesthetics of different solubility (ether, halothane, and N_2O). (From Tanner G.[1])

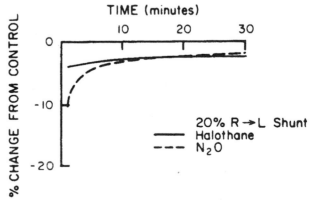

Figure 47–2. Decrease in arterial-to-inspired concentration ratio from control for two anesthetics (halothane and N_2O) caused by a 20% right-to-left shunt. (From Tanner G.[1])

□ If CO is 5 L/min, then the blood can absorb 5000 mL/min of ether before equilibrium is reached.
□ If pulmonary blood flow is 2.5 L (50% right-to-left shunt), then the pulmonary blood flow can still take up 2500 mL/min of ether.

For a **poorly soluble** anesthetic (e.g., N_2O):

□ If ventilation is 5 L/min with 50% N_2O, then 2500 mL/min of N_2O is delivered to the alveoli.
□ If CO = 5 L/min, then the blood can absorb 1250 mL/min until equilibrium is reached.
□ In the presence of a 50% shunt, the pulmonary blood flow can take up only 625 mL/min of N_2O.

With highly soluble agents, uptake is limited primarily by ventilation. With poorly soluble agents, uptake is limited primarily by blood flow. Subsequently, the impact of shunting is greater with agents of lower solubility (see Figs. 47–1 and 47–2).

Left-to-Right Shunt

With a left-to-right shunt, there is no significant change in the speed of induction, assuming that systemic blood flow is normal. If tissue perfusion is decreased because of the left-to-right shunt, then induction will initially be slowed, because less anesthetic will be delivered to the brain per unit time. Usually CO increases to compensate for the shunting, and local control of vasculature maintains cerebral perfusion and minimizes the effect of the shunt (Fig. 47–3).

Mixed Shunt (Right-to-Left and Left-to-Right)

A left-to-right shunt attenuates the slowed anesthetic induction that may occur with right-to-left shunting because of an increase in effective pulmonary blood flow.

Summary

□ With right-to-left intracardiac shunts, anesthetic induction may be slowed in proportion to the size of the shunt.

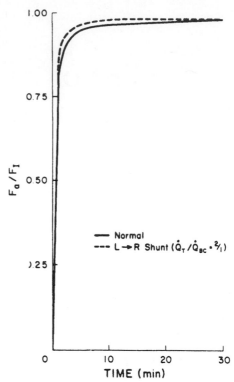

Figure 47–3. Arterial-to-inspired concentration ratio for N_2O modeled with and without a 50% left-to-right shunt and normal tissue perfusion. $\dot{Q}_T$ = total cardiac output; $\dot{Q}_{BC}$ = systemic cardiac output perfusing body compartments; Fa = arterial anesthetic fraction; FI = inspired anesthetic fraction (From Tanner G.[1])

□ With left-to-right shunts with normal cerebral perfusion, there is little effect on induction.
□ In mixed shunts, the shunting effect is attenuated.
□ These effects are most marked for insoluble gases, with only small or moderate effects seen with gases of intermediate solubility.

Selected References

1. Tanner G. Effect of left to right, mixed left to right and right to left shunts on inhalation induction in children: A computer model. Anesth Analg 1985;64:101–107.

Suggested References

Eger EI II. Anesthetic Uptake and Action. Baltimore, Williams & Wilkins, 1974.

48
Concentration Effect and Second Gas Effect

William J. Davis, M.D.

Concentration Effect

Increasing the inspired concentration of a gas produces a more rapid rise in alveolar concentration of that gas. This phenomenon is termed the **concentration effect,** which results from two factors. The first factor is confusingly referred to as the **concentrating effect;** the second factor is an **effective increase in alveolar ventilation**.

Concentrating Effect. The total lung volume is decreased by the amount of gas taken up by the blood (i.e., uptake). This reduction in volume concentrates the gas remaining within the lung. The magnitude of this effect is influenced by the concentration of gas within the lung. For example, when the lung is filled with 1% nitrous oxide (N_2O), if one-half is taken up, then the remaining concentration is 0.5% (0.5 parts in 99.5 parts) (Fig. 48–1, A and B). If the same lung is filled with 80% N_2O and one-half is taken up, then the remaining concentration is 67% (40 parts in a total of 60) (see Fig. 48–1, C and D).

Effective Increase in Alveolar Ventilation. The negative pressure created by the uptake of N_2O into the blood causes inflow of additional gas (i.e., draws gas down the trachea), which replaces N_2O lost by uptake. Increasing alveolar ventilation makes alveolar gas more like inspired gas, thereby decreasing the inspired (F_i) to alveolar (F_A) concentration difference. Because inspired gas contains 80% N_2O (see the example cited earlier), this further raises the alveolar concentration of N_2O from 67% to 72% (see Fig. 48-1, D and E).

Second Gas Effect

Uptake of large volumes of a first or primary gas (usually N_2O) from alveoli increases the rate of increase in alveolar concentration of a second gas given concomitantly. This phenomenon is known as the **second gas effect**. Factors responsible for the concentration effect also govern the second gas effect. Because uptake of the first gas (N_2O) increases the inspiratory volume, this effective increase in alveolar ventilation should increase the alveolar concentration of all concomitantly inspired gases regardless of their inspired concentration. Moreover, uptake of the first gas reduces the total gas volume, thereby increasing the concentration of the second gas (Fig. 48–2) .

The fractional uptake of the second gas determines the relative importance of increased ventilation versus the concentrating effect. Increased ventilation plays the greater role in raising the second gas concentration when the fraction of the second gas removed by uptake into the blood is large (i.e., with more soluble second gases). The concentrating effect plays the greater role when uptake into the blood is small (i.e., with less soluble agents).

The concentration and second gas effects both hasten inhalation induction (i.e., increase the rate of F_A/F_i increase). Uptake of large volumes of anesthetic, usually N_2O, concentrates the remaining gases regardless of whether they are N_2O (**concentration effect**) or a second gas concomitantly administered (**second gas effect**). Uptake of large volumes also increases the effective alveolar ventilation. The concentrating action plus an increase in alveolar ventilation tend to increase the concentration of both N_2O and a second gas. Because uptake

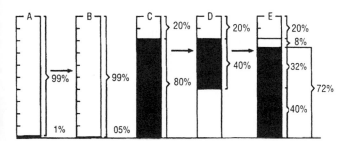

Figure 48–1. Each rectangle *(A to E)* illustrates the lung gas concentrations. The **filled areas** represent N_2O, and the **open areas** represent O_2. At a low concentration, uptake of one-half of the N_2O halves the alveolar anesthetic concentration *(A & B)*. At a high concentration, uptake of one-half of the anesthetic reduces the concentration by a smaller amount *(C & D)*, and even this amount is further decreased by the drawing in of sufficient gas to replace that taken up *(D & E)*. Thus, uptake of one-half of the anesthetic reduces an 80% starting concentration by one-tenth instead of one-half. (From Eger EI II.[1])

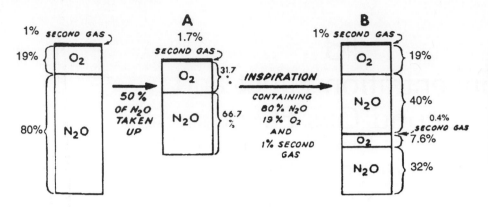

Figure 48–2. A lung is filled with 80% N_2O and 1% of a second gas. Uptake of 50% of the N_2O increases the concentration of the second gas to 1.7% (*A*). Restoration of the lung gas volume by addition of more of the original 80% to 1% mixture changes the second gas concentration to 1.4%. (From Eger EI II.[1])

of large volumes of N_2O is limited to the first 5 to 10 minutes of induction, these effects are of importance only during this period.

While acknowledging the usefulness of the original descriptions[1] of the concentration and second gas effects for teaching purposes, Korman and Mapleson[2] suggested that these explanations are too simplistic and do not consider alternative volume effects of gas uptake. It should also be pointed out that a 1999 study[3] reported that N_2O did not affect the alveolar or blood concentrations of a second gas (enflurane) under controlled constant volume ventilation, leading the authors to conclude that the second gas effect is not a valid concept.

Diffusion Hypoxia

Diffusion hypoxia can cause patients to desaturate on termination of an anesthetic that includes N_2O. The scientific basis for this phenomenon can be found in the discussion of the second gas effect and concentration effect of N_2O, both of which result from the low blood/gas solubility of N_2O.

Because N_2O has such a low blood/gas partition coefficient (0.47), large volumes of N_2O diffuse from the blood to the alveoli upon termination of N_2O administration. During 5 to 10 minutes after the N_2O has been turned off, a sufficient volume of N_2O can diffuse into the alveoli to actually displace oxygen. If room air were the only gas being adminis-

tered during this time frame, then the fraction of alveolar oxygen can fall below 0.21 and put the patient at risk for hypoxia. An additional means of producing hypoxia is the displacement of CO_2 by N_2O. If dilution by N_2O causes the fraction of alveolar CO_2 to fall below the level needed to maintain $PaCO_2$ sufficient to drive ventilation, then hypoventilation could cause further hypoxia. These factors become more important when residual narcotics depress ventilation, or in patients with chronic lung disease.

Diffusion hypoxia is prevented by administering 100% oxygen for 5 to 10 minutes on termination of N_2O. Patients should be observed for adequate ventilation during this period.

Selected References

1. Eger EI II. Effect of inspired anesthetic concentration on the rate of rise of alveolar concentration. Anesthesiology 1963;24:153–157.
2. Korman B, Mapleson WW. Concentration and second gas effects: Can the accepted explanation be improved? Br J Anaesth 1997;78:618–625.
3. Sun X, et al. The "second gas effect" is not a valid concept. Anesth Analg 1999;88:188–192.

Suggested References

Eger EI II. Anesthetic Uptake and Action. Baltimore, Williams & Wilkins, 1974.
Eger EI II. Uptake and distribution. In Miller RD, ed. Anesthesia. 5th ed. Philadelphia: Churchill Livingstone, 2000:74–95.

49
Thiopental

C. Thomas Wass, M.D.

Barbituric acid (2,4,6,-trioxohexahydropyrimidine) (Fig. 49–1) was first synthesized by von Baeyer in 1864. Although this molecule is the structural framework from which barbiturates are derived, it is devoid of anesthetic properties. Structural modification at the number 2 and 5 carbon atoms results in barbiturate drugs that have sedative-hypnotic properties. For example, replacement of the oxygen atom with a sulfur atom at the C2 position and adding a large aliphatic carbon group to the C5 atom transforms barbituric acid into thiopental. Clinically, sodium thiopental was first administered in 1934 by John Lundy at the Mayo Clinic in Rochester, Minnesota and by Ralph Waters at the University of Wisconsin, Madison.

Thiopental [5-ethyl-5-(1-methyl-butyl)-2-thiobarbituric acid] is commercially prepared as water-soluble, highly alkaline sodium salts with a pKa of 7.6 and pH of 10.5. Decreased pH may result in precipitation. Reconstitution with Ringer's lactate solution is not recommended. Refrigerated thiopental is stable for approximately 1 week following reconstitution with sterile water.

As with many intravenous anesthetics, stereoisomerism plays a significant role in thiopental's biologic activity. For example, thiopental is commercially prepared as a racemic mixture; however, its *l* isomer is nearly twice a potent as its *d* isomer. Both isomers exert their biologic activity by enhancing and mimicking the action of γ-aminobutyric acid (GABA) at GABA_A receptors.

Pharmacokinetics

Distribution of intravenous drugs throughout body tissues is determined by tissue blood flow, blood-tissue concentration gradient, lipid solubility, extent of protein binding, and degree of ionization. Thiopental is very lipid soluble, and thus readily crosses the blood-brain barrier. Other pharmacokinetic properties of thiopental are listed in Table 49–1.

Because the brain is a highly perfused (i.e., belongs to the vessel-rich organ group), relatively low-volume organ, cerebral thiopental concentrations equilibrate rapidly with the central blood pool (Fig. 49–2), resulting in depressed electroencephalographic (EEG) activity—and induction of anesthesia—within 20 to 40 seconds.

After achieving maximal concentration within the central nervous system, thiopental follows its concentration gradient back into the central blood pool and is subsequently *redistributed* to a relatively large skeletal muscle reservoir. As a result, EEG activity returns toward baseline—and patients emerge from anesthesia—within 5 to 8 minutes. That is, *redistribution* is the primary mechanism responsible for prompt awakening following an induction dose of thiopental. But when thiopental is administered in multiple doses or as an infusion, skeletal muscle becomes progressively saturated and eventually equilibrates with the central blood pool, thereby preventing further uptake by this large tissue reservoir. At that point, further decreases in blood thiopental concentrations occur more slowly and become dependent on uptake by less well-perfused organs (e.g., adipose) and metabolism.

Thiobarbiturate *metabolism* occurs primarily in hepatic endoplasmic reticulum; however, a small fraction of drug may undergo extrahepatic (e.g., kidney) biotransformation. Biologic reactions responsible for the production of inactive water-soluble me-

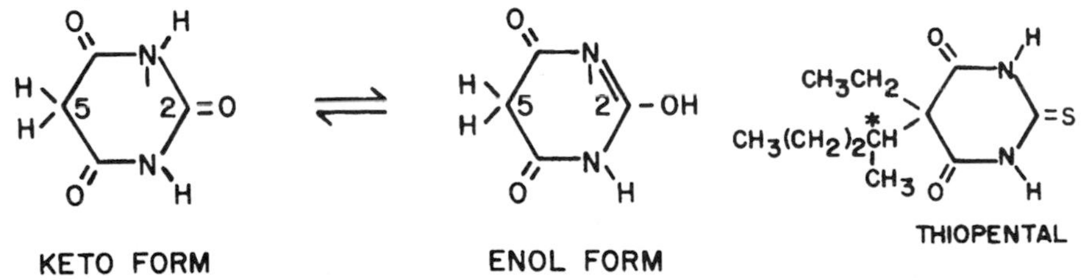

Figure 49–1. Keto and enol forms of barbituric acid, and thiopental. (Modified from Fragen RJ, Avram MJ.)

Table 49–1. Pharmacokinetic Properties of Thiopental

V_{dss} (L/kg)	Cl_E (mL/min/kg)	$t_{1/2\alpha}$ (min)	$t_{1/2\beta}$ (h)	Protein Binding (%)	Estimated Hepatic Extraction Ratio
2.5 ± 1.0	3.4 ± 0.5	3–5	11.6 ± 6.0	72–86	0.15

V_{dss} = volume of distribution at steady-state; Cl_E = elimination clearance; $t_{1/2\alpha}$ = redistribution half-life; $t_{1/2\beta}$ = elimination half-life. (Modified from Fragen RJ, Avram MJ.[2])

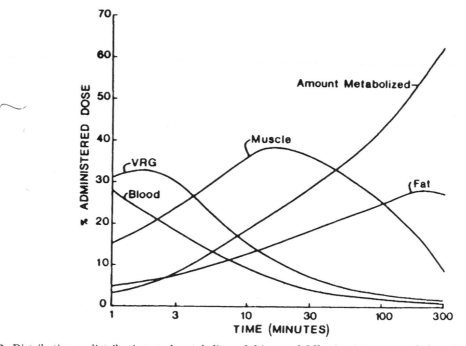

Figure 49–2. Distribution, redistribution, and metabolism of thiopental following intravenous bolus. (Modified from Stoelting RK.)

tabolites include oxidation of substituents on the C5 atom, desulfurization on the C2 atom, and hydrolytic opening of the barbituric acid ring. Of additional interest, hepatic clearance is characterized as a *low hepatic extraction ratio* (see Table 49–1), and thus thiopental metabolism is more dependent on hepatic enzyme (e.g., P450 oxidase) activity than on hepatic blood flow.

Finally, thiopental metabolites are eliminated from the body by renal *excretion*. Less than 1% of thiopental is recovered unchanged in the urine. The degree of protein binding substantially affects renal glomerular filtration and tubular reabsorption. For example, competitive displacement of thiopental from plasma proteins (primarily albumin) by aspirin, phenylbutazone, or uremic toxins results in enhanced drug effect because of increased free drug fraction and greater renal tubular reabsorption

Suggested References

Fragen RJ, Avram MJ. Barbiturates. In Miller RD, ed. Anesthesia. 5th ed. New York: Churchill Livingstone, 2000:209–227.

Morgan GE, Mikhail MS. Nonvolatile anesthetics. In Morgan GE, Mikhail MS, eds. Clinical Anesthesiology. Stamford, CT: Appleton and Lange, 1996:128–148.

Russo H, Bressolle F. Pharmacodynamics and pharmacokinetics of thiopental. Clin Pharmacokinet 1998;35:95–134.

Stoelting RK. Barbiturates. In Stoelting RK, ed. Pharmacology and Physiology in Anesthetic Practice. Philadelphia: JB Lippincott, 1991:102–117.

Wood M. Intravenous anesthetic agents. In Wood M, Wood AJJ, eds. Drugs and Anesthesia. Baltimore: Williams & Wilkins, 1990:179–223.

50
Propofol

Joseph G. Weber, M.D.

Propofol (2,6,-diisopropylphenol) is an intravenous anesthetic that belongs to the family of sterically hindered phenols (Fig. 50–1). It is water insoluble and has been made available in two formulations to allow intravenous use. The first formulation was a 1% solution solubilized in Cremophor EL, a castor oil derivative. This formulation was withdrawn because of anaphylactoid reactions associated with the solubilizing agent. The current formulation is a 1% emulsion containing 10% soybean oil, 2.25% glycerol, and purified 1.2% egg phosphatide, similar to parenteral lipid formulations. This emulsion has not been reported to cause histamine release, but persons **allergic to egg whites** may have an allergic reaction to the emulsion.

Purported advantages of propofol include rapid induction of anesthesia, rapid metabolism that allows continuous infusion with little drug accumulation, rapid emergence from anesthesia, and a low incidence rate of postoperative nausea and vomiting. The antiemetic effects and clear emergence are most pronounced when anesthesia is maintained with propofol, not merely induced with propofol. Antiemetic effects are strong enough so that propofol is occasionally used postoperatively in nauseated patients.

Disadvantages of propofol include hypotension, respiratory depression, pain on injection, and expense. The prevalence rate of pain on injection ranges from 10% to 50%, although the incidence rate of thrombophlebitis is low. Pain on injection can be attenuated by intravenous use of local anesthetics or narcotics and slow administration of propofol into a large vein with rapidly running intravenous fluids.

Effects on Major Organ Systems

Central Nervous System. The exact mechanism of action has yet to be fully elucidated; however, stimulation of γ-aminobutyric acid (**GABA**) **receptors** is likely responsible for propofol's anesthetic properties. Propofol 2 mg/kg induces unconsciousness in less than 1 minute. This is comparable to thiopental, etomidate, or methohexital. Induction is smooth, with excitatory effects seen less often than with methohexital, although more often than with thiopental. An induction bolus of propofol will produce anesthesia lasting approximately 4 minutes, a duration comparable to that of thiopental. Propofol produces electroencephalographic changes characteristic of general anesthesia. This decrease in cerebral function is accompanied by **decreased cerebral metabolism, cerebral blood flow, and intracranial pressure**.

Cardiovascular. Propofol causes a **dose-dependent decrease in blood pressure** comparable to that caused by thiopental. This hypotension is caused by reductions in systemic vascular resistance and myocardial contractility. Cardiac output is decreased.

Respiratory. Propofol produces **dose-dependent respiratory depression** that ultimately results in apnea. This respiratory depression is thought to be from a decrease in central inspiratory drive. The ventilatory response to carbon dioxide is decreased.

Other Organ Systems. Propofol has not been reported to have adverse effects on liver function, renal function, coagulation, or steroidogenesis. Administration of propofol increases the depth, but not the duration, of neuromuscular blockade produced with atracurium or vecuronium. There are anecdotal reports of profound metabolic acidosis associated with bradyarrhythmia, progressive myocardial failure, and death in children sedated with propofol infusions for prolonged periods. It is not known how

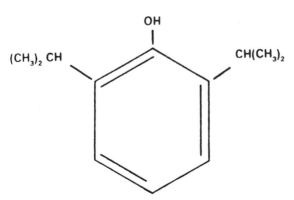

Figure 50–1. Propofol, 2,6,-diisopropylphenol.

propofol infusion played a role in the development of the acidosis, although mechanisms have been proposed.

Pharmacokinetics and Pharmacodynamics

The concentration of propofol decreases rapidly following an intravenous bolus due to redistribution of drug (i.e., $t_{1/2\alpha}$ = 2 to 8 min). The elimination half-life ($t_{1/2\beta}$ = approximately 1 hr) is markedly shorter than that of thiopental ($t_{1/2\beta}$ = approximately 11 hr). Both two-compartment and three-compartment models have been proposed. The volume of distribution is large, but becomes significantly smaller with increasing age. Thus, dosages should be reduced in elderly patients.

Propofol is excreted from the body as glucuronide and sulfate conjugates primarily in the urine. Because clearance of propofol exceeds hepatic blood flow, extrahepatic mechanisms have been proposed.

Blood concentrations of 2.5 to 6 μg/mL are required for major surgery; concentrations of 1.5 to 4.5 μg/mL are adequate for minor surgery. Movement on skin incision is prevented in 50% of premedicated patients (on 66% N_2O) by blood levels of 2.5 μg/mL.

Dosages

The dosage for induction of anesthesia is 1.5 to 2.5 mg/kg. This should be reduced in patients who are elderly, who are hypovolemic, or who have poor cardiac reserve. Anesthesia can also be induced with 20 to 40 mg given every 10 seconds until onset of unconsciousness. Anesthesia can be maintained with frequent intermittent boluses of propofol 0.5 mg/kg, titrated to clinical effect, or with a propofol infusion, 100 to 300 μg/kg/min. A good starting dose for conscious sedation is 50 μg/kg/min.

Suggested References

Reves JG, Glass PSA, Lubarsky DA. Nonbarbiturate intravenous anesthetics. In Miller RD, ed. Anesthesia. 5th ed. Philadelphia: Churchill Livingstone, 2000:228–272.

Schuttler J, Ihmsen H. Population pharmacokinetics of propofol: A multicenter study. Anesthesiology 2000;92:727–738.

Sebel PS, Lowdon JD. Propofol: A new intravenous anesthetic. Anesthesiology 1990;72:393–396.

Smith I, White PF, Nathanson M, Gouldson R. Propofol: An update on its clinical use. Anesthesiology 1994;81:1005–1043.

Stoelting RK. Nonbarbiturate induction drugs. In Stoelting RK, ed. Pharmacology and Physiology in Anesthetic Practice. 3rd ed. Philadelphia: Lippincott-Raven, 1999:140–157.

Wood M. Intravenous anesthetic agents. In Wood M, Wood AJJ, eds. Drugs and Anesthesia. 2nd ed. Baltimore: Williams & Wilkins, 1990:179–223.

51
Ketamine

Scott A. Lockwood, M.D.

When introduced in the 1960s, ketamine was thought to be the "complete" anesthetic drug that would provide all of the components of anesthesia necessary for surgery: pain relief, immobility, amnesia, and loss of consciousness. Side effects soon proved that ketamine was not the ultimate anesthetic drug, however.

Ketamine is a central nervous system depressant that produces dissociative anesthesia thought to be due to electrophysiologic inhibition of thalamocortical pathways and stimulation of the limbic systems. Clinically, patients remain in a cataleptic state in which the eyes are open with a slow gaze. Intense analgesia (somatic greater than visceral) is present, as well as amnesia (anterograde), but not necessarily loss of consciousness.

Structure

Ketamine is available as a slightly acidic (pH 3.5 to 5.5) racemic mixture containing equal amounts of the two optical isomers. When studied separately, the plus isomer is more potent and less likely to cause emergence reactions than the minus isomer. Ketamine is metabolized by the hepatic cytochrome P-450 system.

Mechanism of Action

Ketamine interacts with N-methyl-D-aspartate (NMDA), opioid, nicotinic and muscarinic receptors, and with voltage-sensitive calcium channels.[1] Antagonism of NMDA receptors is thought to account for most of ketamine's analgesic, psychomimetic, and amnestic effects (Fig. 51–1).[2] Intense analgesia is thought to occur through the selective depression of the medial thalamic nuclei, as well as suppression of spinal cord activity necessary for transmission of pain to higher centers. Physostigmine may reverse some actions of ketamine.

Pharmacokinetics

Onset of Action. Ketamine has a rapid onset of action. Peak plasma concentrations are reached in less than 1 minute after intravenous (IV) administration, in less than 5 minutes after intramuscular (IM) administration, and in 7 to 30 minutes after rectal administration.

Dosages. Ketamine is given in the following dosages: IV, 1 to 2 mg/kg; IM, 5 to 10 mg/kg; rectally, 8 mg/kg.

Solubility. Ketamine is 5 to 10 times more lipid soluble than thiopental. This results in rapid transfer across the blood-brain barrier.

Duration of Action. Ketamine has a relatively short duration of action. Consciousness returns 10 to 15 minutes after IV induction doses, but analgesia requires far lower levels and persists into the postoperative period. Rapid redistribution from the brain to inactive sites is primarily responsible for the termination of unconsciousness. Half-life is $T_{1/2\alpha} = 10$ minutes and $T_{1/2\beta} = 1$ to 2 hours. A cumulative effect may be seen with repeated or continuous administration.

Metabolism. Ketamine is metabolized extensively by hepatic microsomal enzymes. More than 90% is demethylated to form the active metabolite norketamine (which is one-third as potent as ketamine). More than 4% is excreted unchanged in urine, and fecal excretion accounts for less than 5% of the dose. Chronic administration results in enzyme induction with subsequent tolerance to the analgesic effects. This is commonly seen in burn

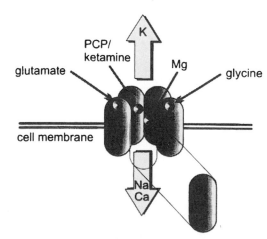

Figure 51–1. Schematic diagram of the molecular structure of the NMDA glutamate receptor/channel complex. The receptor consists of five subunits surrounding a central ion channel permeable to Ca, K, and Na. Binding sites for the agonist glutamate and the obligatory coagonist glycine are indicated. Competitive glutamate and glycine antagonists act on these sites. One of the subunits has been removed to allow a view inside the ion channel, in which binding sites for ketamine and Mg are located. These compounds block NMDA receptor functioning noncompetitively. PCP = phencyclidine. (From Kohrs R, Durieux ME.)

Table 51–1. Circulatory Effects of Ketamine

	Control	Ketamine (2 mg/kg IV)	% Change
Heart rate (beats/min)	74	98	+33
Mean arterial pressure (mm Hg)	93	119	+28
Cardiac index (L/min/m²)	3.0	3.8	+29
Systemic vascular resistance (pru)	16.2	15.9	
Right atrial pressure (mm Hg)	7	8.9	
Pulmonary artery pressure (mm Hg)	17	24.5	+44
Tension-time index (mm Hg sec)	2700	4640	+68

Modified from Stoelting RK.

patients who receive repeated dosages. Dependence also may occur.

Systemic Effects

Cardiovascular. Ketamine produces cardiovascular (CV) effects that resemble sympathetic nervous system (SNS) stimulation with increases in blood pressure, heart rate, cardiac output, and myocardial oxygen demand. Blood pressure increases 20 to 40 mm Hg during the first 3 to 5 minutes of IV administration and then declines to normal over the next 10 to 20 minutes. Ketamine should be used with caution in hypertensive patients (Table 51–1).

In vitro, ketamine produces direct myocardial depression, emphasizing the importance of an intact SNS for cardiac stimulation. Ketamine causes direct central sympathetic stimulation, inhibits norepinephrine reuptake into postganglionic sympathetic nerve endings, and depresses the baroreceptor reflex, causing increases in SNS activity. Critically ill patients may experience decreased blood pressure and cardiac output with ketamine, reflecting depletion of catecholamine stores and exhaustion of SNS compensating mechanisms. CV stimulation may be absent if ketamine is used with volatile anesthetics, β-blockers, or benzodiazepines.

Central Nervous System. Ketamine is a potent **cerebral vasodilator,** causing a 60% increase in cerebral blood flow and leading to increased intracranial pressure. This effect may be blunted by pretreatment with thiopental or diazepam. However, ketamine is contraindicated in patients with space-occupying intracranial lesions.

Ketamine by itself does not alter the seizure threshold. However, ketamine in combination with aminophylline does decrease the seizure threshold.

Emergence delirium occurs 5% to 30% of the time. Incidence rate is increased when (1) the patient is over age 16; (2) dosages are greater than 2 mg/kg; (3) the drug is rapidly administered, and (4) the patient has preexisting personality problems. Emergence reactions usually occur early during emergence from anesthesia, persist for a few hours, and are characterized by visual, auditory, proprio-

ceptive, and confusional illusions often with associated feelings of excitement, fear, or euphoria.

The incidence rate of delirium can be decreased by pretreatment with diazepam (0.15 to 0.3 mg/kg) before ketamine induction (although this will not reliably prevent dreaming). Atropine and droperidol may increase the incidence rate of delirium; thus, if an anticholinergic is indicated, glycopyrrolate should be chosen.

Ketamine causes a dose-dependent decrease in the MAC of halothane. Conversely, the administration of a drug that reduces hepatic blood flow such as halothane will decrease the clearance of ketamine.

Respiratory. Ketamine does not produce significant ventilatory depression, and the response to CO_2 is preserved. Respiratory rate decreases for 2 to 3 minutes after administration; apnea can occur from a large dose of ketamine given rapidly or from using ketamine with opioids. Upper airway skeletal muscle tone is well maintained, as are upper airway reflexes, yet airway protection is still required in patients at risk for vomiting and aspiration.

Salivary and tracheobronchial mucous gland secretions are increased. Glycopyrrolate is preferable to atropine to decrease secretions.

Bronchodilation equivalent to that seen with potent inhalation agents occurs in patients with reactive airway disease. The mechanism for this effect is probably sympathomimetic stimulation, although there may be a direct effect on bronchial smooth muscle as well.

Miscellaneous. An analgesic dose of ketamine (0.2 to 0.5 mg/kg) administered during labor does not depress the newborn. Ketamine has been used safely in patients with myopathies and susceptibility to malignant hyperthermia.

Low-dose Ketamine for Postoperative Pain Relief. In the late 1990s multiple prospective, randomized, controlled studies showed the efficacy of low-dose (0.1 to 0.2 mg/kg IV given intraoperatively or at the time of anesthetic induction) ketamine for postoperative pain relief.[3] The drug is most effective when used as an adjunct to narcotics and local anesthetics. Studies showing the effectiveness of preemptive ketamine are promising as well. Synergistic and additive effects have been described. These effects are believed to be the result of ketamine's NMDA blockade, which acts to reduce windup and other pain mechanisms.[3]

Selected References

1. Reich DL, Silvay G. Ketamine: An update on the first twenty-five years of clinical experience. Can J Anaesth 1989;36:186.
2. Tweed WA, Minuck M, Mymin D. Circulatory responses to ketamine anesthesia. Anesthesiology 1972;37:613–619.
3. Schmid RL, Sandler AN, Katz J. Use and efficacy of low-dose ketamine in the management of acute postoperative pain: a review of current techniques and outcomes. Pain 1999;82:111–125.

Suggested References

Kohrs R, Durieux ME. Ketamine: Teaching an old drug new tricks. Anesth Analg 1998;87:1186–1193.
Stoelting RK. Pharmacology and Physiology of Anesthetic Practice. 3rd ed. Philadelphia, Lippincott-Raven, 1999.

52
Opioid Pharmacology

Richard H. Rho, M.D. □ Gilbert Y. Wong, M.D.

Opioids are a structurally related class of natural or synthetic agents ranging from endogenous peptides to alkaloid derivatives that have morphine-like properties. They may be classified into three major groups based on pharmacodynamic activity: pure agonists, pure antagonists (e.g., naloxone), and mixed agonists/antagonists (e.g., butorphanol, nalbuphine).

The clinical effects of a particular opioid depend on which specific receptor type(s) that it binds. Several opioid receptor subtypes have been characterized according to their differences in affinity, anatomic location, and functional responses:

μ_1: Supraspinal analgesia, bradycardia, sedation, pruritus.

μ_2: Respiratory depression, euphoria, physical dependence, pruritus.

κ: Spinal analgesia, respiratory depression, sedation, miosis.

σ: Hypertension, tachycardia, dysphoria, delirium, mydriasis.

δ: Spinal analgesia, respiratory depression.

The analgesic effects from systemic administration of opioids may result from receptor activity at several different nervous system sites, including:

□ The sensory neuron of the peripheral nervous system.

□ The dorsal horn of the spinal cord, which inhibits the transmission of nociceptive information involving substance P.

□ The brainstem medulla, which potentiates descending inhibitory pathways that modulate ascending pain signals.

□ The cortex of the brain, which decreases the perception and emotional response to pain.

Central Nervous System Effects

High doses of opioids may cause deep sedation or hypnosis; however, opioids do not reliably produce amnesia. Opioids reduce the minimum alveolar concentration of volatile anesthetics required during balanced general anesthesia.

Seizures can result from the neuroexcitatory effects of normeperidine, a metabolite of meperidine. Normeperidine-induced seizures are more likely in patients who have received chronic meperidine therapy, have received large doses of meperidine over a short period, and/or have impaired renal function with decreased ability to eliminate this metabolite.

Opioids can reduce cerebral metabolic oxygen requirements, cerebral blood flow, and intracranial pressure if ventilation is unchanged.

Opioids cause miosis by stimulating the Edinger-Westphal nucleus of the oculomotor nerve. In patients in whom ventilation is not controlled, opioid-induced respiratory depression can produce hypoxemia, resulting in pupillary dilation.

Nausea and vomiting can occur with opioid administration. Opioids stimulate the chemoreceptor trigger zone located in the area postrema of the brain stem, which can result in vomiting.

Respiratory Effects

Opioid administration decreases minute ventilation by decreasing the respiratory rate (as opposed to tidal volume).

Opioids have a direct effect on the respiratory centers in the medulla, producing a dose-dependent depression of the ventilatory response to carbon dioxide. A decreased slope and rightward shift is noted on the carbon dioxide response curve (Fig. 52–1). The apneic threshold, defined as the highest Pa_{CO_2} without ventilatory effort, is increased with opioids. Opioids also blunt the increase in ventilation in response to hypoxemia.

Musculoskeletal Effects

Opioids can produce generalized skeletal muscle rigidity (see Chapter 54). Loss of chest wall compliance and contraction of laryngeal and pharyngeal muscles can be severe, resulting in ventilatory difficulty even with positive-pressure ventilation. The mechanism of opioid-induced muscle rigidity is believed to be mediated by the $\mu-$ receptors at the supraspinal level by increasing dopamine synthesis and by inhibiting γ-aminobutyric acid activity. This muscle rigidity can be prevented by decreasing the

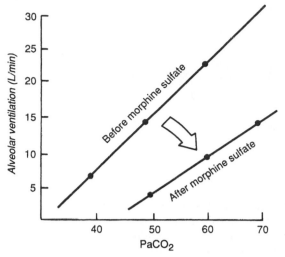

Figure 52–1. Opioid depression of ventilation is depicted by a shift of the CO_2 response curve downward and to the right. (From Morgan GE Jr, Mikhail MS.)

rate of opioid administration or by administering a muscle relaxant.

Postoperative shivering can be improved with meperidine, which may act through a κ-receptor mechanism. Only 12.5 to 25 mg IV is usually needed to produce this effect in an adult.

Cardiovascular Effects

At clinically relevant doses, opioids do not cause significant myocardial depression; however, opioids can cause a dose-dependent bradycardia that results in decreased cardiac output. One exception is meperidine, which may cause tachycardia because of its structural similarities to atropine. Meperidine may also cause a decrease in myocardial contractility. Most opioids exert their cardiovascular effects both by sympatholysis via vasomotor centers in the medulla and by increased parasympathetic tone via vagal pathways.

Gastrointestinal Effects

Opioids can cause an ileus by both vagal and peripheral mechanisms. There is an increase in nonperistaltic smooth muscle tone in the small and large bowel, but this ineffective nonpropulsive activity leads to an overall increase in bowel transit time. Opioids generally increase common bile duct pressure and delay gall bladder emptying; however, these effects are less pronounced with meperidine.

Hormonal Effects

Opioids may decrease the stress response to pain and surgery by acting on the hypothalamus. The inhibition of gonadotropin-releasing hormone and corticotropin-releasing factor results in decreased release of endogenous cortisol.

Histamine Release

Although true allergic responses to opioids are rare, opioids may cause a non–IgE-mediated release of histamine from mast cells. This decreases systemic vascular resistance, with resultant decreases in blood pressure and tachycardia.

Suggested References

Coda BA. Opioids. In Barash PG, et al, eds. Clinical Anesthesia. Philadelphia: Lippincott-Raven, 1997:329–358.

McQuay H. Opioids in pain management. Lancet 1999;353:2229–2232.

Morgan GE Jr, Mikhail MS. Nonvolatile anesthetic agents. In Morgan GE Jr, Mikhail MS, eds. Clinical Anesthesiology. 2nd ed. Stamford, CT: Appleton and Lange, 1996:128–148.

53
Cardiovascular Effects of Narcotics

Kent H. Rehfeldt, M.D.

Anesthesiologists frequently administer narcotics preoperatively, intraoperatively, and postoperatively. Intraoperatively, an opioid-based anesthetic is often selected for hemodynamically unstable patients because, compared with other classes of anesthetic drugs, opioids usually cause few serious perturbations in the cardiovascular system. Nonetheless, narcotics, especially in large doses, can alter hemodynamics. Changes in heart rate, cardiac conduction, blood pressure, and myocardial contractility are possible. Whether these effects are beneficial or detrimental depends on the specific narcotic, the dose, and the clinical setting.

Administration of narcotics (with the exception of meperidine) usually results in decreased heart rate. This negative chronotropic effect represents narcotic stimulation of μ_2-receptors in medullary vagal nuclei and can be eliminated by bilateral vagotomy. Sinoatrial (SA) node depression and prolonged atrioventricular (AV) node conduction can occur, as can sinus arrest and even asystole. Fortunately, these serious, life-threatening reactions are rare and may be more likely when narcotics are given in conjunction with other potentially vagotonic medications (e.g., succinylcholine) or vagotonic stimuli (e.g., peritoneal traction). Earlier administration of drugs such as pancuronium or atropine diminishes the likelihood of narcotic-induced decreases in heart rate.

Besides bradycardia, narcotic administration can lower blood pressure. Decreased sympathetic tone probably accounts for most of the blood pressure reduction. A direct narcotic effect on vascular smooth muscle has also been postulated. In addition, morphine and meperidine trigger histamine release, which can contribute to hypotension. The tone of both venous capacitance vessels and arteriolar resistance vessels may decrease. Hypotensive effects are most prominent in patients with increased sympathetic tone, such as those with congestive heart failure or hypovolemia. Blood pressure changes are less common in isovolemic, supine patients. However, orthostatic hypotension may be seen in patients with an autonomic nervous system impairment (e.g., autonomic neuropathy in diabetics). Decreased blood pressure is not due to myocardial depression; narcotics, with the exception of meperidine, have no significant negative inotropic properties at clinical doses.

Hypertension is occasionally observed in patients receiving opioid medications intraoperatively. Most frequently seen in patients with preserved left ventricular function, hypertensive responses probably result from either too low of a narcotic dose or inadequate administration of other types of anesthetics.

Morphine

Similar to most narcotics, morphine tends to decrease heart rate through central vagal stimulation. A negative chronotropic influence on both the SA and AV node is noted, although the former is probably more important at clinical concentrations. This vagotonic property results in an antiarrhythmic effect as the threshold for ventricular fibrillation is raised. Morphine does not potentiate the effects of catecholamines on the myocardium.[1] Both venous and arterial dilation occur, though venodilation generally lasts longer and can be sufficient to decrease cardiac output, especially at larger doses. Morphine's ability to decrease preload, lower heart rate, and diminish myocardial oxygen demands make it a useful drug in the setting of myocardial ischemia.

Morphine administration results in elevation of plasma histamine levels in proportion to the rate of injection. The hypotensive effects of histamine are partially offset by histamine-stimulated release of epinephrine from the adrenal medulla. Increased epinephrine levels may explain the increased myocardial contractility associated with morphine doses of 1 to 2 mg/kg. Earlier treatment with a combination of H_1 and H_2 receptor antagonists limits the hemodynamic effects of histamine.

Meperidine

Like morphine, meperidine causes histamine release. In fact, compared with morphine, equipotent doses of meperidine result in a greater elevation of plasma histamine levels. Orthostatic hypotension associated with meperidine may also be more severe than that seen with morphine. Intrathecal meperidine decreases blood pressure in women in labor.[2]

Meperidine has a number of cardiovascular effects that are unique among the opioids. First, because of its structural similarity to atropine, meperidine may elevate heart rate after intravenous administration. This vagolytic property can lead to increased ventricular rate in patients with atrial fibrillation and accelerated conduction of atrial flutter waves.[3] Second, unlike other narcotics, meperidine in large doses has negative inotropic effects. Third, like class III antiarrhythmics, meperidine can prolong the duration of action potential,[4] thereby potentiating class I antiarrhythmics such as quinidine and procainamide.

Fentanyl

Fentanyl tends to decrease heart rate to a greater degree than morphine. Indeed, the vagally mediated heart rate decline may be sufficient to contribute to hypotension. Blood pressure may also drop in response to diminished sympathetic tone. Fentanyl depresses neonatal baroreceptor reflexes, potentially contributing to hypotension.[2] Intrathecal fentanyl given to women in labor lowers blood pressure slightly from prelabor values.[5] Unlike meperidine, fentanyl does not have any direct negative inotropic properties and does not trigger histamine release.

Sufentanil

Like fentanyl, sufentanil does not release histamine and has no negative inotropic effects. Bradycardia is often noted in association with sufentanil administration. Decreased cardiac output may accompany the bradycardia. Compared with equipotent doses of fentanyl, sufentanil appears more likely to produce hypotension. Nonetheless, hemodynamic disturbances are generally minimal in patients with preserved left ventricular function. Like fentanyl and meperidine, intrathecal sufentanil decreases blood pressure in women in active labor.[1]

Alfentanil

Like fentanyl and sufentanil, alfentanil does not cause histamine release or direct myocardial depression. Administration results in a decreased heart rate and a dose-dependent decline in blood pressure. However, alfentanil may be less efficacious than fentanyl and sufentanil in preventing unwanted hemodynamic responses to surgical stimulation.

Remifentanil

Remifentanil administration is usually associated with a 15% to 20% decline in mean arterial pressure and bradycardia.[6] However, severe bradycardia following remifentanil boluses of 1 μg/kg has been reported.[7] Dose-dependent decreases in blood pressure occur in response to remifentanil boluses and infusions. Remifentanil appears to be about 31 times more potent than alfentanil with respect to its ability to lower blood pressure.[8] Plasma histamine level does not increase in response to a remifentanil bolus. When used as a sedative during regional anesthesia, remifentanil provides more stable hemodynamics than propofol.[9]

Selected References

1. Stoelting RK. Opioid agonist and antagonist. In Stoelting RK, ed. Pharmacology and Physiology in Anesthetic Practice. 3rd ed. Philadelphia: Lippincott-Raven, 1999:77–112.
2. Honet JE, Arkoosh VA, Norris MC, et al. Comparison among intrathecal fentanyl, meperidine, and sufentanil for labor analgesia. Anesth Analg 1992;75:734–739.
3. Collins VJ. Opiate and narcotic drugs. In Collins VJ, ed. Physiologic and Pharmacologic Bases of Anesthesia. Baltimore: Williams & Wilkins, 1996:544–562.
4. Brown DV, Tuman KJ. Morphine compounds. In White PF, ed. Textbook of Intravenous Anesthesia. Baltimore: Williams & Wilkins, 1997:191–202.
5. Mandell GL, Jamnback L, Ramanathan S. Hemodynamic effects of subarachnoid fentanyl in laboring parturients. Reg Anesth 1996;21:103–111.
6. Bürkle H, Dunbar S, Van Aken H. Remifentanil: A novel, short-acting, μ-opioid. Anesth Analg 1996;83:646–651.
7. DeSouza G, Lewis MC, TerRiet MF. Severe bradycardia after remifentanil. Anesthesiology 1997;87:1019–1020.
8. Warner DS, Hindman BJ, Todd MM, et al. Intracranial pressure and hemodynamic effects of remifentanil versus alfentanil in patients undergoing supratentorial craniotomy. Anesth Analg 1996;83:348–353.
9. Desmonts JM, Aitkenhead AR, Camu F, et al. Comparison of remifentanil and propofol as adjunct therapy during regional anesthesia. Anesthesiology 1995;83:A857.

54
Perioperative Narcotic Problems: Muscle Rigidity and Biliary Colic

Pamela A. Mergens, M.D.

Muscle Rigidity

It is well established that all clinically useful opioids have the potential to cause extreme rigidity. Higher narcotic doses provoke rigidity more frequently, as do high rates of infusion. N_2O, alfentanil, and older patients are also more often associated with rigidity after narcotic administration. The following doses and incidences have been reported:

□ Alfentanil: 175 μg/kg produced rigidity in 10 of 10 patients.
□ Fentanyl: 12 μg/kg produced rigidity in 9 of 10 patients.
□ Sufentanil: 2.6 μg/kg and 3.5 μg/kg produced muscle rigidity in individual patients.

Clinical Features

Musculature. Onset of rigidity can be abrupt, involving upper extremity flexion, lower extremity extension, immobility of the head, abdominal rigidity, and severe chest wall rigidity that can lead to ineffective ventilation. Myoclonic or athetoid movements have also been noted, as has vertical nystagmus. Rigidity has been reported to be provoked or increased with adjustments of the mask, loud noise, or passive movement of a limb.

Electromyogram. Onset of rigidity produces increased electromyographic activity, which correlates with loss of consciousness and unresponsiveness.

Electroencephalogram. Recent studies have determined that rigidity after opioid administration is not related to seizure activity. During craniotomy and electrocorticography procedures for epilepsy, however, alfentanil (50 μg/kg) is used to amplify pathological seizure spikes on the electroencephalogram.

Treatment

Muscular rigidity leading to respiratory compromise has been documented on narcotic induction, in an awake and extubated patient during transport to the recovery room, and as delayed as 24 hours postoperatively. Thus the interventional approach taken will depend on when rigidity occurs.

Induction. If muscular rigidity develops during induction and leads to an inability to ventilate, a muscle relaxant should be used to maintain the positive aspects of the narcotic induction and abolish the rigidity. Rigidity will cease shortly after administration of muscle relaxants.

Postoperatively. In an awake and extubated patient, naloxone, a pure narcotic antagonist, will reverse all receptor-mediated effects of opioids, including rigidity and pain relief. The usual starting dose of naloxone is 40 μg intravenously, with incremental dosing thereafter until the desired endpoint is reached. In a mechanically ventilated patient, use of either a muscle relaxant or naloxone has been reported to be efficacious.

Neonatal Procedures. Muscle rigidity and jerking severe enough to impair ventilation were described in neonates given 9 to 15 μg/kg alfentanil before treatment procedures.[1] It was concluded that alfentanil should not be used without muscle relaxants in this setting.

Prevention

Pharmacologic agents reported to decrease the incidence and/or severity of rigidity include midazolam, methocarbamol, etomidate, thiopental, benztropine, succinylcholine, and pancuronium. Concomitant use of nitrous oxide with a narcotic has been cited as a contributing factor in narcotic-induced rigidity. Giving primary doses of nondepolarizing relaxants and avoiding rapid injection of large doses of opioids are effective prevention strategies.

Neuropharmacology of Opioid Muscle Rigidity

Narcotics are thought to produce muscle rigidity through some mechanism not involving a direct effect on the muscle fiber or on the neuromuscular junction. The physiology of opioid-induced muscle rigidity is still poorly understood, but a mechanism involving the central nervous system is most likely responsible. Neurochemical research in animals provides evidence that dopaminergic neurons within the basal ganglia may be involved. The nucleus pontis raphae and striatonigral GABA pathways have also been implicated.

Biliary Colic

Narcotics are known to cause spasm of the choledochoduodenal sphincter of Oddi and increased common bile duct pressure in a dose-dependent fashion. When administered as premedicants, narcotics may precipitate pain that mimics acute cholecystitis or myocardial infarction.

Intra- or perioperative administration of narcotics has also been reported to significantly retard the passage of contrast medium into the duodenum during operative cholangiography. Failure to appreciate this phenomenon may lead to an unnecessary surgical exploration of the common bile duct with an attendant increased operative time and postoperative morbidity. Narcotic-induced smooth muscle sphincter spasm is a μ-opioid receptor–mediated phenomenon. It peaks within 6 minutes of administration of intravenous fentanyl and dissipates within 30 minutes.[2] Bile duct narrowing has been shown to be more significant after morphine than fentanyl and other narcotics.[3]

Treatment

Naloxone has been given to reverse "narcotic-induced" biliary colic. This clearly is not a first-line choice for the patient under general anesthesia, because significant cardiovascular alterations may occur secondary to reversal of narcotic-induced anesthesia and/or analgesia.

Glucagon (2 mg IV) is also effective in relieving sphincter spasm. Glucagon administration is associated with occasional hypersensitivity reactions. Glucagon is believed to increase smooth muscle cell cyclic adenosine monophosphate levels. Narcotic-induced biliary spasm may be reduced by nitroglycerin.

Summary

Opioids can produce muscle rigidity in a dose-dependent fashion. Although easily blocked by muscle relaxants, this effect can be a serious problem in unanesthetized patients.

The evidence that narcotic administration before intraoperative cholangiography increases the incidence of biliary tract pseudo-obstruction is controversial. Some studies have shown very temporary increases in CBDP after narcotic bolus injection, especially when morphine is used.

Selected References

1. Pokela ML, Ryhanen PT, Loivisto ME, et al. Alfentanil-induced rigidity in newborn infants. Anesth Analg 1992;75:252.
2. Hynynen MJ, Turunen MT, Kortilla KT. Effects of alfentanil and fentanyl on common bile duct pressure. Anesth Analg 1986;65:370.
3. Vierra ZG, Duarte B, Renigers SA, et al. Double-blind ultrasonographic study of the effect of five analgesics on the common bile duct. Anesthesiology 1989;71:A232.

Suggested References

Benthuysen J, Smith N, Sanford T, et al. Physiology of alfentanil-induced rigidity. Anesthesiology 1986;64:440.
Mirenda J, Tabatabai M, Wong K. Delayed and prolonged rigidity greater than 24 h following high-dose fentanyl anesthesia. Anesthesiology 1988;69:624.

55
Nonsteroidal Anti-Inflammatory Drugs

Jack L. Wilson, M.D.

Nonsteroidal anti-inflammatory drugs (NSAIDs) are used frequently during the perioperative period as well as in the treatment of acute and chronic pain conditions. Although these medications have potent anti-inflammatory and analgesic properties, their use is not without risk.

Mechanism of Action

The anti-inflammatory effects of NSAIDs are largely due to the inhibition of cyclooxygenase, which prevents formation of inflammatory mediators such as prostaglandins and thromboxanes. Some NSAIDs also inhibit lipoxygenase, preventing production of leukotrienes (Fig. 55–1). Two forms of the cyclooxygenase enzyme (COX) have been identified. The first, COX-1, is present in all tissues, including gastric mucosa, where it is thought to play a protective role. The second, COX-2, is produced primarily at the site of inflammation.

Older NSAIDs, such as ibuprofen, block both forms of the COX enzyme. COX-2 inhibitor–specific drugs introduced in the late 1990s have a reduced likelihood of gastrointestinal toxicity. Initial studies indicated analgesic efficacy similar to that of older, nonspecific NSAIDs.

Traditionally, it was believed that NSAIDs exerted an anti-inflammatory effect peripherally, preventing production of localized inflammatory mediators. There may be a central analgesic mechanism as well. Following spinal NMDA receptor activation, accumulation of arachidonic acid metabolites occurs. NSAIDs injected intrathecally in rats have resulted in decreased pain behaviors following intraperitoneal injection of an irritant. There may be a role for intrathecal use in humans, particularly for conditions related to central sensitization. This remains in the investigational stage.

Indications

Acute and chronic pain conditions may both respond to NSAIDs, and these medications have a strong role in the outpatient pain clinic. Chronic use of NSAIDs necessitates repeated patient follow-up and observation for toxicity.

Nonopioid analgesics have a role as perioperative adjuncts. Ketorolac is the sole NSAID with United States Food and Drug Administration approval for parenteral use. When given intravenously in the perioperative period and used along with reduced opioid doses, or in place of opioids, ketorolac may decrease the risk of sedation, respiratory depression, nausea, vomiting, and pruritus. This may be especially beneficial in an outpatient surgical setting.

Toxicity

NSAIDs are some of the most widely prescribed medications. Each year, more than 70 million prescriptions, and 30 billion nonprescription tablets, are sold in the United States. The toxicities of NSAIDs are potentially life-threatening. The most clinically relevant toxicities relate to the gastrointestinal, renal, hematologic, and hepatic systems.

Gastrointestinal System. Dyspepsia is commonly related to NSAID use. Gastrointestinal bleeding, perforation, and silent ulceration are also associated with NSAID use and must be carefully monitored. The risk of GI toxicity increases linearly with patient age. Other risk factors include previous peptic ulcer disease, corticosteroid use, excessive alcohol use, and concurrent multiple NSAID use. Dyspepsia resulting from NSAIDs can generally be treated empirically with an H_2 receptor antagonist or a proton-pump inhibitor. If NSAIDs are strongly indicated but the patient has risk factors for gastrointestinal toxicity, misoprostol or a proton-pump inhibitor can be used concurrently. Alternatively, the patient can be treated with a COX-2 selective antagonist.

Renal System. Reduced renal blood flow resulting in medullary ischemia may result when patients with prostaglandin-regulated renal blood flow receive NSAIDs. This may include patients with heart failure, renal insufficiency, or hepatic disease. Allergic nephritis and tubulointerstitial nephritis may also result from NSAID use.

Hepatic System. Hepatic toxicity related to NSAID use is uncommon, and the mechanism of

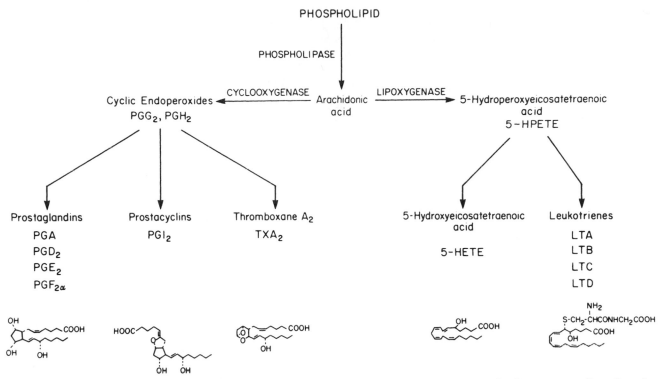

Figure 55–1. Arachidonic acid metabolism. Five major groups of metabolites are formed: prostaglandins, prostacyclins, thromboxanes, 5-HETE, and leukotrienes. (From Katz N, Ferrante FM.)

toxicity is not well defined. Reportedly, 3% of patients receiving these medications may experience hepatic toxicity, making clinical observation with occasional liver function tests appropriate.

Hematologic System. Nonacetylated salicylates, salsalate, and choline magnesium trisalicylate do not affect platelet function, but aspirin (through COX inhibition) impairs platelet function for the life of the platelet (7 to 10 days). Other NSAIDs reversibly inhibit platelets for their duration of action (a matter of hours). The mechanism of this decreased platelet function relates to inhibition of thromboxane synthesis, a prostaglandin involved in platelet aggregation and adhesion. NSAID use appears to present no significant risk to the patient undergoing epidural or spinal anesthesia. When NSAIDs are used concurrently with other antiplatelet medications, bleeding complications may be more likely, although data on this combination are lacking.

Respiratory System. NSAIDs can precipitate a potentially life-threatening exacerbation of reactive airway disease with severe respiratory compromise in patients with aspirin-induced asthma. These patients typically have a history of perennial vasomotor rhinitis, with development of nasal polyps.

Suggested References

Abramowicz D, ed. Rofecoxib for osteoarthritis and pain. Med Lett Drugs Ther 1999;41:59–61.

Cousins MJ, Bridenbaugh PO. Neural Blockade in Clinical Anesthesia and Management of Pain. 3rd ed. Philadelphia, Lippincott-Raven, 1998.

Katz JA. Opioids and nonsteroidal antiinflammatory analgesics. In Raj PP, ed. Pain Medicine: A Comprehensive Review. St. Louis: Mosby, 1996:126–141.

Katz N, Ferrante FM. Nociception. In Ferrante FM, VadeBoncouer TR, eds. Postoperative Pain Management. New York: Churchill Livingstone, 1993;17–67.

Urmey WF, Rowlingson J. Do antiplatelet agents contribute to the development of perioperative spinal hematoma? Reg Anesth and Pain Med 1998;23 Suppl 2:146–151.

Wolfe MM, Lichtenstein DR, Singh G. Gastrointestinal toxicity of nonsteroidal antiinflammatory drugs. N Engl J Med 1999;340:1888–1898.

Yaksh TL. Spinal Drug Delivery. Amsterdam, Elsevier, 1999.

56
Succinylcholine Side Effects

Thomas J. Christopherson, M.D.

Succinylcholine (SCh) is a depolarizing neuromuscular-blocking drug that acts at the postjunctional neuromuscular membrane to produce rapid skeletal muscle relaxation. Several side effects have been associated with SCh administration, including massive hyperkalemia, malignant hyperthermia, anaphylaxis, cardiac dysrhythmias, prolonged apnea, phase II blockade, and postoperative myalgias, as well as increases in intraocular, intragastric, and intracranial pressures.

Massive Hyperkalemia

Depolarizing neuromuscular-blocking drugs produce sustained opening of the nicotinic cholinergic receptor channel. Under normal conditions, postjunctional membrane depolarization results in leakage of potassium ions from the interior of cells sufficient to produce an average increase of 0.5 to 1.0 mEq/L in serum potassium concentration.[1] However, when SCh depolarizes muscle that has been traumatized (e.g., crush injury) or denervated (e.g., upper motor neuron lesion), enough potassium may extrude from cells to produce systemic hyperkalemia and cardiac arrest. This susceptibility to hyperkalemia is thought to be caused by **proliferation of junctional and extrajunctional cholinergic receptors**. Receptor upregulation provides more postjunctional sites for succinylcholine to interact with, causing increased release of potassium. Patient populations at risk for SCh-induced hyperkalemia include patients with **upper motor neuron lesions** resulting from stroke, brain or spinal cord tumors, other intracerebral or spinal cord mass lesions, closed head injury, or encephalitis. Other disease processes implicated in predisposing patients to succinylcholine-induced hyperkalemia include unhealed third-degree burns, severe intra-abdominal infections, severe metabolic acidosis with hypovolemia, crush injuries, and prolonged nondepolarizing muscle blockade or immobility. Because the precise point at which SCh induces hyperkalemia after burns and other trauma cannot be known with certainty, it is advisable to not administer SCh to such patients beyond the first 24 hours postinjury.[2] Pretreatment with a defasciculating dose of neuromuscular-blocking drug does *not* seem to influence the magnitude of potassium release evoked by SCh.

Rhabdomyolysis

Patients with Duchenne's muscular dystrophy (DMD) may develop rhabdomyolysis, hyperkalemia, and intractable cardiac arrest after receiving SCh. This scenario has led to death in a number of children with undiagnosed DMD. In males under age 5 years, the use of SCh should be reserved for situations where it is clearly indicated, such as emergency pediatric intubations and laryngospasm.

Malignant Hyperthermia

SCh is a known triggering agent for malignant hyperthermia and should be avoided in the anesthetic management of all patients known to be susceptible to or who have a strong family history of malignant hyperthermia.

Anaphylactic Reactions

Numerous case reports describe severe, and sometimes fatal, reactions to SCh. Several studies have demonstrated the reliability of skin testing, leukocyte histamine-release assay, and detection of IgE antibodies to succinylcholine in aiding diagnosis of allergic reactions to SCh even when these tests are performed several years after the initial anaphylactic reaction.[3]

Cardiac Arrhythmias

SCh is capable of producing diverse cardiac dysrhythmias. Not only does it directly stimulate muscarinic receptors of the sinus node, but it also stimulates autonomic and nicotinic receptors in both sympathetic and parasympathetic ganglia. Therefore, sympathotonic children will be prone to bradycardia after a single dose, whereas adults, who are relatively vagotonic, will likely experience increased heart rate.

In addition, it has been demonstrated that successive boluses of SCh, given 2 to 10 minutes apart, can result in sinus bradycardia, junctional rhythms, and even sinus arrest. This relationship of the second dose suggests a possible role of the SCh metabolites succinylmonocholine and choline in enhancing the slowing of heart rate.[4] Administration of a nondepolarizing drug approximately 3 minutes before the first dose of SCh greatly reduces the incidence of bradycardia.

Succinylcholine Apnea

Some patients who receive a conventional dose of SCh may experience a prolonged neuromuscular block due to the presence of **atypical plasma cholinesterase**. Homozygotes of this atypical enzyme (approximately 1 in every 3,200 patients) can anticipate a greatly prolonged duration of SCh-induced neuromuscular blockade, whereas heterozygotes (approximately 1 in every 480 patients) will experience only a modest prolongation. **Dibucaine**, an amide-linked local anesthetic, inhibits 80% of the activity of normal plasma cholinesterase, compared with only a 20% inhibition of the homozygote atypical enzyme. A dibucaine number of 80 (i.e., percent inhibition) thus confirms the presence of normal plasma cholinesterase. However, the dibucaine number does not reflect the *quantity* of pseudocholinesterase present, but rather the *quality* of the enzyme and its ability to hydrolyze SCh.

Phase II Blockade

Infusion of large doses of SCh over a prolonged period of time may result in a phase II blockade ("desensitizing SCh neuromuscular blockade"). Clinically, similar to the neuromuscular block produced by nondepolarizing muscle relaxants, phase II blockade may produce unexpected weakness on emergence from anesthesia. On a cellular level, the muscle cell membrane repolarizes gradually, but neuromuscular transmission remains blocked. The response of a phase II blockade to reversal is unpredictable.

Postoperative Myalgias

Skeletal muscle myalgias of the neck, back, and abdomen can occur after SCh administration. These myalgias may be secondary to fasciculation-induced muscle spindle stretching, or they may result from prejunctional repetitive motor nerve firing.[5] Myoglobinuria may also occur. Small doses of a nondepolarizer, which acts presynaptically to suppress these repetitive discharges, will attenuate muscle fasciculations. Debate still persists, however, as to whether preventing fasciculations necessarily correlates with a reduction in SCh-induced muscle aches.[6]

Intraocular Pressure Increase

SCh causes a modest transient increase in intraocular pressure that persists for 5 to 10 minutes after administration. Although patients with treated glaucoma are at minimal risk, administration of SCh to patients with recent ocular incisions or with penetrating eye injuries may result in vitreous expulsion and visual loss. Whether pretreatment with a nondepolarizer attenuates dangerous rises in intraocular pressure remains controversial.[7, 8]

Intragastric Pressure Increase

SCh can cause on average a 40 cm H_2O increase in intragastric pressures, presumably due to abdominal muscle contraction. Studies have shown that pretreatment with a nondepolarizer decreases this rise in pressure. It has been shown that lower esophageal sphincter pressure also increases following SCh, resulting in maintained gastroesophageal barrier pressures.[9] Whether SCh during induction causes increased susceptibility to esophageal reflux and possible pulmonary aspiration (secondary to increased intragastric pressures) remains debatable.

Intracranial Pressure Increases

Several studies suggest that succinylcholine may increase intracranial pressure (ICP), whereas others have been unable to demonstrate this phenomenon. This ambiguity has spawned a variety of clinical recommendations and considerable debate.[10] The mechanism responsible for this phenomenon has yet to be fully elucidated, but proposed mechanisms include decreased venous effluent from the brain due to fasciculation-induced increases in intrathoracic pressure, neck muscle contraction with resultant jugular venous compression, and SCh-induced increases in afferent muscle spindle activity that cause increased cerebral blood flow, cerebral blood volume, and intracranial pressure. It has been suggested that succinylcholine should not be deleted from the therapeutic armamentarium for emergency airway management based solely on ICP concerns.[10, 11]

Selected References

1. Gronert GA, Theye RA. Pathophysiology of hyperkalemia induced by succinylcholine. Anesthesiology 1975;43:89–99.

2. Tolmie JD, Joyce TH, Mitchell GD. Succinylcholine danger in the burned patient. Anesthesiology 1967;28:467–470.

3. Didier A, Benzanti M, Senft M, et al. Allergy to suxamethonium: Persisting abnormalities in skin tests, specific IgE antibodies, and leukocyte histamine release. Clin Allergy 1987;17:385–392.

4. Schoenstadt DA, Whitcher CE. Observations on the mechanism of succinylcholine-induced cardiac arrhythmias. Anesthesiology 1963;24:358–362.

5. Hartman GS, Giamengo SA, Riker WF. Succinylcholine: Mechanism of fasciculations and their prevention by d-tubocurarine or diphenylhydantoin. Anesthesiology 1986;65:405–413.

6. Manchikant L, Grow JB, Colliver JA, et al. Atracurium pretreatment for succinylcholine-induced fasciculations and postoperative myalgia. Anesth Analg 1985;64:1010–1014.

7. Miller RD, Way WL, Hickey RF. Inhibition of succinylcholine-induced increased intraocular pressure by nondepolarizing muscle relaxants. Anesthesiology 1968;29:123–126.

8. Meyers EF, Kaupin T, Johnson M, et al. Failure of nondepolarizing neuromuscular blockers to inhibit succinylcholine-induced increased intraocular pressure. A controlled study. Anesthesiology 1978;48:149–151.

9. Smith G, Dalling R, Williams TIR. Gastro-esophageal pressure gradient changes produced by induction of anesthesia and suxamethonium. Br J Anaesth 1978;50:1137–1143.

10. Kovarik WD, Mayberg TS, Lam AM, et al. Succinylcholine does not change intracranial pressure, cerebral blood flow velocity, or the electroencephalogram in patients with neurologic injury. Anesth Analg 1994;78:469–473.

11. Silber SH. Rapid sequence intubation in adults with elevated intracranial pressure: A survey of emergency medicine residency programs. Am J Emerg Med 1997;15:263–267.

57
Prolongation of Succinylcholine Effect

Ronald J. Faust, M.D.

Pharmacology

At the motor nerve ending, the nerve action potential normally causes calcium channels to open, leading to the release of acetylcholine from storage vesicles. Acetylcholine diffuses across the junctional cleft to react with receptor proteins in the end plate to initiate muscle contraction. Molecules released from the end plate are quickly (in less than 1 msec) metabolized by **acetylcholinesterase** molecules attached to the end plate outside the cell via stalks of collagen.

Succinylcholine consists of two molecules of acetylcholine linked by methyl groups (see Fig. 59–1). Succinylcholine attaches to the nicotinic cholinergic receptor and mimics the action of acetylcholine, thus producing depolarization of the postjunctional membrane. Compared with acetylcholine, the hydrolysis of succinylcholine is slow, resulting in a sustained depolarization. Yet compared to other relaxants, the duration of action of succinylcholine is brief (3 to 5 minutes), due to hydrolysis by **pseudocholinesterase** (PChE), also known as plasma cholinesterase. This rapid breakdown of succinylcholine permits only a fraction of administered dose to reach the neuromuscular junction. Action of succinylcholine is terminated by diffusion from the end plate to extracellular fluid. The initial metabolite, succinylmonocholine, is only 1/20th to 1/90th as potent as the parent compound. Succinylmonocholine is subsequently hydrolyzed to succinate and choline.

Phase 1 Versus Phase 2 Block

A phase 2 neuromuscular blockade can cause prolongation of the action of succinylcholine; it is a risk of using repeated doses or an infusion of succinylcholine. Responses to neuromuscular stimulation that characterize a phase 1 block (normal after succinylcholine administration) include:

- Decreased contraction in response to a single twitch stimulus.
- Decreased amplitude but sustained response to a continuous stimulus.
- Train-of-four (TOF) ratio greater than 70%.

- Absence of posttetanic facilitation.
- Augmentation of neuromuscular blockade by anticholinesterase.

Phase 2 blockade may occur when the dose (usually >6 mg/kg) or duration of succinylcholine use is excessive. The exact mechanism for the transition from phase 1 to phase 2 blockade is not known but is thought to occur when the postjunctional membrane has become repolarized but still does not respond normally to acetylcholine. The pattern of neuromuscular stimulation is similar to that of a nondepolarizing drug, characterized by:

- Decreased contraction in response to a single twitch.
- Tetanic fade.
- TOF ratio less than 30%.
- Posttetanic facilitation.
- Reversal of neuromuscular blockade with anticholinesterases.

Phase 2 blockade can be avoided if succinylcholine administration is stopped when TOF fade becomes evident. Reversal of a phase 2 blockade is controversial; it should not be attempted until spontaneous recovery of the twitch has occurred.

Pseudocholinesterase

PChE is a serine hydrolyase capable of hydrolyzing esters including acetylcholine, succinylcholine, mivacurium, trimethaphan, and ester-type local anesthetics. PChE is found in plasma, liver, pancreas, heart, and brain. It is distinct from acetylcholinesterase, which is found in nerve endings and in red blood cells. The physiologic role of PChE is obscure, but it may be involved in lipid metabolism, choline homeostasis, or slow nerve conduction. Low plasma or tissue levels or even complete absence of PChE is compatible with normal health and development. PChE is synthesized by the liver, has a serum half-life of 8 to 12 days, and is an α_2-receptor globulin that exists in aggregate form, usually as a tetramer. The four subunits are identical, with each one having an active catalytic site. The tetramer weighs 320,000 d. The concentration of PChE in plasma is about 5 mg/L.[1]

Table 57–1. Dibucaine Number and Duration of Block

Pseudocholinesterase Type	Incidence	Dibucaine Number	Response to Succinylcholine
Homozygous typical	Normal	70–80	Normal
Heterozygous atypical	1/480	50–60	Lengthened by 50%–100%
Homozygous atypical	1/3,200	23–30	Prolonged to 4–8 hours

Adapted from Savarese JJ, Caldwell JE, Lien CA, et al.[2]

Clinical interest in PChE abnormalities and pharmacology stemmed from observations that certain patients given succinylcholine developed prolonged apnea. The first assays to determine PChE activity and biochemical characteristics were developed by Kalow in 1957. PChE activity is determined by colorimetric assay using benzylcholine as a substrate. Quantitative PChE activity from a patient's serum is compared to that in pooled control serum to determine units of activity. The qualitative tests, **dibucaine number** (DN) and **fluoride number**, reflect reduced PChE activity resulting from the addition of dibucaine or sodium fluoride to the assay.

Pseudocholinesterase Abnormalities

Inherited PChE Abnormalities. Deoxyribonucleic acid techniques have been used to elucidate the genetic causes of PChE variants. It was determined that there is only one PChE gene and that its location is on chromosome 3, and all variants are determined by mutations of one gene.

Atypical variants were originally described by Kalow who identified individuals whose PChE could not metabolize succinylcholine and were only partially inhibited by dibucaine. Whereas a normal individual's hydrolysis of benzylcholine was inhibited 70% by dibucaine, affected individuals showed only 30% inhibition of hydrolysis (Table 57–1). When prolonged paralysis occurs after succinylcholine administration, a PChE quantitative assay and DN should be obtained. The patient's ventilation should be supported mechanically and sedative/amnesic drugs administered until neuromuscular function returns. Although some texts still recommend blood transfusion to replace PChE, the risks of transfusion are far higher than those associated with a few hours of mechanical ventilation.

Fluoride-resistant variants have been found whose enzyme was inhibited by sodium fluoride but not by dibucaine. Several extremely rare **silent variants** have little or no PChE. More common **K variants** inherit genes producing low levels of normal PChE; similar **J and H variants** also have been discovered. **High-activity variant** families have been identified with cholinesterase activity three times normal.

Physiologic Variances in PChE Activity. The amount of PChE is age dependent under normal circumstances. From birth to age 6 months, the activity is 50% of that in nonpregnant adults. Activity reaches 70% of adult activity by age 6 and normal adult levels at puberty. Pregnancy is associated with 25% to 30% decreased PChE activity from week 10 to postpartum week 6. This reduction has no clinical significance.

Acquired PChE Defects. Decreased PChE activity can be seen in a number of disease states and with administration of various drugs. Hepatitis, cirrhosis, malnutrition, cancer, myxedema, acute infection, and myocardial infarction are associated with decreased PChE activity in plasma. Certain drugs, including acetylcholinesterase inhibitors, pancuronium, procaine, hexafluorenium, and organophosphate insecticides, inhibit PChE, whereas other drugs, including steroids and chemotherapeutic agents, can cause decreased PChE synthesis. Decreasing PChE activity to 25% control, as seen in severe liver disease, prolongs succinylcholine duration from 3.0 ± 0.15 minutes to only 8.6 ± 0.7 minutes, an increase that is usually undetectable in the clinical setting. Other diseases, such as thyrotoxicosis and nephrotic syndrome, are associated with increased PChE activity of probably no clinical significance.

Clinically significant PChE abnormalities are uncommon, with succinylcholine-induced prolonged apnea occurring in 1 in 2,500 patients. Viby-Mogensen studied 225 patients with prolonged apnea after succinylcholine administration and found that 66% had an inherited PChE abnormality.[3] Succinylcholine apnea from the various abnormal PChE phenotypes is usually of shorter duration than the surgical procedure.

Selected References

1. Pantuck EJ. Plasma cholinesterase: Gene and variations. Anesth Analg 1993;77:380.
2. Savarese JJ, Caldwell JE, Lien CA, et al. Pharmacology of muscle relaxants and their antagonists. In Miller RD, ed. Anesthesia. 5th ed. Philadelphia: Churchill Livingstone, 2000:412–490.
3. Viby-Mogensen J. Correlation of succinylcholine duration of action with plasma cholinesterase activity in subjects with the genotypically normal enzyme. Anesthesiology 1980; 53:517.

Suggested Reference

Nelson T, Burritt M. Pesticide poisoning, succinylcholine-induced apnea and pseudocholinesterase. Mayo Clin Proc 1986;61:705.

58
Nondepolarizing Muscle Relaxants

Mark T. Keegan, M.D.

The introduction of nondepolarizing muscle relaxants (NDMRs) into clinical practice marked a significant advance in anesthesia and surgery. The 1990s saw the appearance of new drugs, free from many of the undesirable side effects of the older relaxants. In recent years, some of these new agents have threatened succinylcholine's position as the drug of choice for rapid-onset, short-acting muscle relaxation.

Mechanism of Action

By competing with acetylcholine for binding to nicotinic receptor alpha subunits, NDMRs cause skeletal muscle relaxation. The relaxants may also be capable of blocking the ion channel directly, thus stopping the flux of Na^+ through the ion pore.

Characteristics of Nondepolarizing Neuromuscular Blockade

Muscle relaxation caused by NDMRs is characterized clinically by a train of four T1:T4 ratio <1 (with <0.7 representing adequate surgical relaxation), tetanic "fade," posttetanic potentiation, absence of fasciculations, potentiation by other NDMRs, and antagonism of the block by acetylcholinesterase inhibitors. Blockade by NDMRs affects rapidly moving small muscles (e.g., laryngeal muscles) initially, then muscles of the limbs and trunk (e.g., adductor pollicis) and, finally, diaphragmatic muscles.

Alterations in Sensitivity

Enhanced NDMR effects occur with administration of volatile anesthetics, local anesthetics, diuretics, antiarrhythmics, aminoglycosides, magnesium, and lithium. Hypothermia, acidosis, and hypokalemia also increase the potency of NDMRs. Patients with myasthenia gravis are very sensitive to the effects of NDMRs. In contrast, due to proliferation of nicotinic receptors (upregulation), patients with burn injuries are resistant. Administration of 10% of the intubating dose of NDMR 2 to 4 minutes before a second large dose is known as priming. Priming may accelerate the onset of muscle relaxation.

Chemical Structure

Currently used NDMRs include benzylisoquinolinium and aminosteroid compounds (Tables 58–1, 58–2). All have one or more positively charged quaternary ammonium groups. (Acetylcholine has a single quaternary ammonium.) NDMRs may also be classified on the basis of duration of action into short-, intermediate-, and long-acting medications. The aminosteroids have no hormonal properties.

Histamine Release

Some muscle relaxants, especially benzylisoquinolines, may cause histamine release when injected rapidly intravenously. For example, d-tubocurarine, mivacurium, atracurium, and metocurine cause significant histamine release. The mechanism is not well defined, but the effect is more pronounced with larger doses. Erythema, tachycardia, and hypotension may occur. Bronchospasm is rare.

Cardiovascular and Autonomic Effects

Because of their structural similarity to acetylcholine, certain muscle relaxants act at muscarinic and nicotinic receptors in the autonomic nervous system. Pancuronium, for example, causes mild increases in mean arterial pressure, heart rate, and cardiac output from its vagolytic effects on the cardiac muscarinic receptors and its ability to act as an indirect sympathomimetic. The newer steroidal muscle relaxants (e.g., rocuronium, rapacuronium) do not have these properties. Vagolysis is prominent with the trisquaternary relaxant gallamine.

Table 58–1. Commonly Used Nondepolarizing Muscle Relaxants Arranged According to Structural Class and Duration of Action

	Short Action	Intermediate Action	Long Action
Benzylisoquinolinium	Mivacurium	Atracurium Cisatracurium	d-Tubocurarine Metocurine Doxacurium
Aminosteroid	Rapacuronium	Vecuronium Rocuronium	Pancuronium Pipecuronium

Metabolism

Mivacurium is hydrolyzed by plasma cholinesterase at 80% of the rate of succinylcholine metabolism. Its action is prolonged in patients with pseudocholinesterase deficiency (e.g., patients with hepatic cirrhosis or atypical pseudocholinesterase). Atracurium is metabolized chemically by the Hofmann elimination (to laudanosine and monoacrylate) and enzymatically by nonspecific plasma esterases. Laudanosine causes central nervous system excitement in experimental animals, but this is unlikely to be clinically significant in humans. Pancuronium is excreted largely unchanged in the urine, and its action may be prolonged in patients with renal failure. Vecuronium undergoes predominantly biliary excretion. Atracurium, cisatracurium, and mivacurium are good choices in patients with renal impairment.

New Nondepolarizing Muscle Relaxants

Cisatracurium

One of the 10 stereoisomers of atracurium, the 1R-cis, 1R'-cis form comprises approximately 15% of the atracurium mixture. The purified preparation, known as cisatracurium, is a muscle relaxant that is four times more potent than the parent compound. Cisatracurium does not cause histamine release; hence it has minimal cardiovascular effects. Metabolism is by the Hofmann degradation, but nonspecific esterases have no role in its elimination.

Rocuronium

Rocuronium is a monoquaternary aminosteroid with a structure similar to that of vecuronium. When administered at three times ED_{95}, rocuronium has an onset of action similar to that of succinylcholine, although the laryngeal muscles are relatively more resistant to rocuronium's effects. Doses used for rapid tracheal intubation (0.9 to 1.2 mg/kg) typically cause neuromuscular blockage that may last for an hour or more. The liver is the primary route of elimination, and rocuronium's action may be prolonged in patients with hepatic disease.

Rapacuronium (ORG 9487)

This new monoquaternary synthetic steroid was released in the United States in late 1999. Because of its low potency, it has a rapid onset of action, similar to that of succinylcholine. A dose of 1.5 mg/kg will produce good intubating conditions in 60 seconds, and the neuromuscular block lasts for about 20 minutes. Early administration of neostigmine significantly reduces the duration of paralysis. Rapacuronium is devoid of the side-effect profile of succinylcholine (see Chapter 56), but does cause some histamine release. Metabolism of rapacuronium yields 3-desacetylrapacuronium, a muscle relaxant that is twice as potent as the parent molecule. Rapacuronium has the potential to replace succinylcholine as a means of achieving brief-onset muscle relaxation.

Table 58–2. Characteristics of the Commonly Used Muscle Relaxants

Agent	Intubating Dose (mg/kg)	Infusion Rate (μg/kg/min)	Onset (sec to intubation)	Duration	Vagolysis	Histamine Release	Elimination
Succinylcholine	1.5	NA	30–90	Very short	Variable	Slight	Pseudocholinesterase
Mivacurium	0.15	3–12	90–150	Short	No	Yes	Pseudocholinesterase
Rapacuronium	1.5	NA	45–90	Short	Yes	Yes	Kidney, ester hydrolysis
Rocuronium	0.9–1.2	9–12	60–90	Intermediate	Yes	No	Liver, kidney
Cisatracurium	0.15–0.2	1–3	90–120	Intermediate	No	No	Hofmann degradation
Atracurium	0.5	3–12	90–150	Intermediate	No	Yes	Hofmann, ester hydrolysis
Vecuronium	0.08–0.12	1–2	90–150	Intermediate	No	No	Liver, kidney
Pancuronium	0.08–0.12	NA	Slow	Long	Yes	No	Kidney, liver

Suggested References

Fleming NW, Chung F, Glass PSA, et al. Comparison of the intubation conditions provided by rapacuronium (ORG 9487) or succinylcholine in humans during anesthesia with fentanyl and propofol. Anesthesiology 1999;91:1311.

Haspel KL, Ali HH. Physiology of neuromuscular transmission and mechanism of action of neuromuscular blocking agents. In: Longnecker DE, Tinker JH, Morgan GE, eds. Principles and Practice of Anesthesiology. 2nd ed. St. Louis: Mosby, 1998: 755.

Saverese JJ, Caldwell JE, Lien CA, Miller RD. Pharmacology of muscle relaxants and their antagonists. In: Miller RD, ed. Anesthesia. 5th ed. Philadelphia: Churchill Livingstone, 2000:412.

Stoelting RK. Neuromuscular blocking drugs. In: Stoelting RK, ed. Pharmacology and Physiology in Anesthetic Practice. 3rd ed. Philadelphia: Lippincott-Raven, 1999:182–223.

59
Nonrelaxant Side Effects of Nondepolarizing Muscle Relaxants

Jerald O. Van Beck, M.D.

Nondepolarizing muscle relaxants include a variety of agents that can be classified according to chemical class (the steroidal compounds and the benzylisoquinolinium substances). Steroidal compounds include pancuronium, pipecuronium, vecuronium, rocuronium, and rapacuronium. Benzylisoquinolinium compounds include d-tubocurarine, metocurine, doxacurium, atracurium, cisatracurium, and mivacurium (Fig. 59–1). All block acetylcholine competitively at the neuromuscular junction. Additional cholinoceptive sites include nicotinic receptors of autonomic ganglia; muscarinic receptors in the sinus node of the heart, bowel, bladder, and other sites; and esteratic receptors, such as the active site of acetylcholinesterase.

Nonrelaxant Side Effects

Interference with Autonomic Function. Autonomic ganglia are blocked by d-tubocurarine at

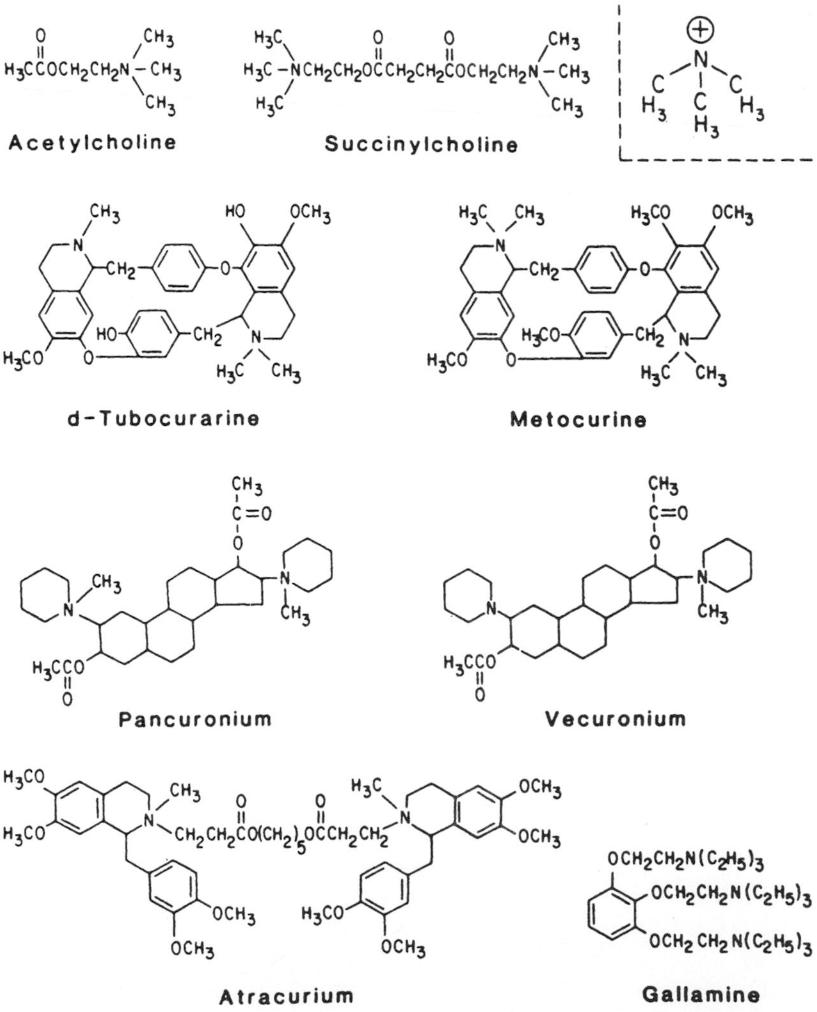

Figure 59–1. Chemical structures of acetylcholine, succinylcholine, and six nondepolarizing neuromuscular blocking agents. (From Lebowitz PW, Ramsey FM.)

doses slightly higher than that required for blockade of the neuromuscular junction. Metocurine has one-third the potency of d-tubocurarine as a ganglionic blocker, whereas the other agents have no effect. d-Tubocurarine and metocurine may impair autonomic reflexes and contribute to hypotension in high doses.

Muscarinic receptors are also affected by some agents. Pancuronium and gallamine have a vagolytic effect on the nodal cells of the heart. Parasympathetic muscarinic receptor blockade in other organs does not appear to be clinically significant.

The sympathetic nervous system contains at least three sets of muscarinic receptors. Blockade of these receptors on dopaminergic interneurons decreases modulation of ganglionic traffic (disinhibition), and blockade of adrenergic neurons results in removal of a negative feedback system for catecholamine release (Fig. 59–2). Pancuronium and gallamine inhibit norepinephrine reuptake by adrenergic nerves and may cause norepinephrine release independent of muscarinic blockade.

These mechanisms contribute to an increase in heart rate after pancuronium administration. Muscarinic blockade at sympathetic adrenergic neurons represents the mechanism behind the exaggerated response sometimes seen with pancuronium during light anesthesia. Although these agents do not directly induce cardiac arrhythmias, pancuronium or gallamine administration may predispose a patient to arrhythmias because of (1) vagal block with shift toward adrenergic tone, (2) indirect sympathomimetic activation, and (3) atrioventricular nodal blockade greater than sinoatrial nodal blockade. d-Tubocurarine, on the other hand, may increase the threshold for epinephrine-induced arrhythmias, as shown in a dog model with nitrous oxide and halothane anesthesia.

Histamine Release. The benzylisoquinolinium compounds cause nonimmunologic release of histamine and possibly other mediators from mast cells (d-tubocurarine > metocurine > atracurium and mivacurium). Histamine release is a function of dose and rate of administration. The physiologic effects of histamine include positive chronotropy (H_2 receptors), inotropy (H_1 receptors, negative; H_2 receptors, vasodilation), coronary artery effects (H_1 receptors, vasoconstriction; H_2 receptors, vasodilation), and peripheral vasodilation. Plasma histamine concentrations equal to or greater than 1,500 pg/mL are associated with hypotension and tachycardia. Duration is generally 1 to 5 minutes. Atracurium has no significant hemodynamic effect at doses equal to or less than 0.4 mg/kg but may have such an effect at doses greater than 0.6 mg/kg. Slow administration over 75 seconds will prevent hemodynamic response, as will earlier administration of antihistamines (Table 59–1).

Other. Laudanosine, a metabolite of atracurium, causes CNS stimulation and possibly seizures in high concentrations.

Allergic reactions are rare. Potential for allergy

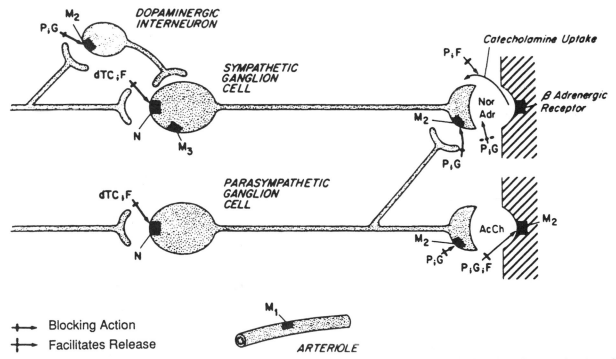

Figure 59–2. Diagrammatic representation of the autonomic nervous system with respect to the heart, and sites of action of some neuromuscular blocking drugs on this system. The muscarinic receptors have been divided into three subclasses (M1, M2, and M3). Abbreviations: N = nicotinic receptor; P = pancuronium; G = gallamine; F = fazadinium; Dtc = d-tubocurarine. (From Scott R, Savarese J.)

Table 59–1. Effects of a 100% Blocking Dose of Nondepolarizing Muscle Relaxants in Humans Under Halothane Anesthesia

Drug	Ganglion Block	(Muscarinic) Vagal Block	Histamine Release	SVR	CO	Under Anesthesia BP	HR
Tubocurarine	**	—	***	↓	↓	↓	—
Metocurine	*	—	**	↓	—	↓	—
Pancuronium	—	**	—	—	↑	↑	↑
Gallamine	—	***	—	—	↑	↑	↑
Alcuronium	*	*	—	↓	↑	↓	↑
Fazadinium	**	**	—	↓	↑	↓	↑
Vecuronium	—	—	—	—	—	—	—
Atracurium	—	—	—	—	—	—	—

Abbreviations: SVR = systemic vascular resistance; CO = cardiac output; BP = blood pressure (mean arterial pressure); HR = heart rate. * = mild; ** = moderate; *** = major.
From Scott R, Savarese J.

exists in patients with history of seafood or iodine allergy if they receive Metubine Iodide, or gallamine trethiodide. Sulfites are present in commercial preparations of d-tubocurarine and gallamine.

The potential for **carcinogenicity, mutogenicity,** or **teratogenicity** in humans is unknown. Of these agents, gallamine crosses the placenta to the greatest extent, but no adverse effects have been noted in neonates from administration during cesarean section.

Suggested References

Lebowitz PW, Ramsey FM. Muscle relaxants. In Barash PG, Cullen BF, Stoelting RK, eds. Clinical Anesthesia. Philadelphia: JB Lippincott, 1989:339.

Schnider SM, Levinson G. Anesthesia for Obstetrics. 3rd ed. Baltimore, Williams & Wilkins, 1993.

Scott R, Savarese J. The cardiovascular and autonomic effects of neuromuscular blocking agents. In Katz RL, ed. Muscle Relaxants: Basic and Clinical Aspects. 2nd ed. New York: Grune & Stratton, 1985:117.

60
Neostigmine, Pyridostigmine, and Edrophonium

Lawrence J. Winikur, M.D.

Classification

Acetylcholinesterase inhibitors are commonly administered to accelerate the reversal of nondepolarizing muscle relaxant blockade of the neuromuscular junction. Acetylcholinesterase breaks down acetylcholine into choline and acetic acid. Acetylcholinesterase is one of the most efficient enzymes known; a single molecule has the capacity to hydrolyze an estimated 300,000 molecules of acetylcholine per minute. Neostigmine, pyridostigmine, and edrophonium are reversible inhibitors of acetylcholinesterase. When the enzyme is inhibited, the concentration of acetylcholine in the junctional cleft is increased. This allows acetylcholine to compete for acetylcholine receptor sites, as nondepolarizing muscle relaxants diffuse into the cleft, and bind to the sites as an agonist.

Structure

The active center of the acetylcholinesterase molecule consists of a negative subsite, which attracts the quaternary group of choline through both coulombic and hydrophobic forces, and an esteratic subsite where nucleophilic attack occurs.

Neostigmine, pyridostigmine, and edrophonium are quaternary ammonium ions that do not cross the blood-brain barrier. Neostigmine and pyridostigmine bind to the acetylcholinesterase molecule through formation of a carbamyl-ester complex at the esteratic site of the enzyme that acts as a competitive substrate for acetylcholine. This chemical reaction is similar to the hydrolysis of acetylcholine that forms an acetylated, rather than a carbamylated, enzyme. In both cases, water will cleave the covalent bond, but this occurs much more slowly (minutes rather than nanoseconds) for the carbamylated enzyme.

Edrophonium has neither a carbamate nor an ester group and is not hydrolyzed. It binds to the acetylcholinesterase molecule by virtue of its electrostatic attachment to the anionic site of the molecule and is further strengthened by hydrogen bonding at the esteratic site. This blockade is of brief duration; it is the duration of the drug in the body, rather than the duration of molecular action, that is important. Individual edrophonium molecules leave the enzyme rapidly, but are immediately replaced by another molecule as long as the drug is present in the body.

Pharmacokinetics and Pharmacodynamics

Edrophonium, neostigmine, and pyridostigmine do not differ in terms of pharmacokinetics. This similarity means that the difference in their potencies is most likely explained on a pharmacodynamic basis.

Because all three drugs are quaternary ammonium ions, they are poorly lipid soluble and do not effectively penetrate lipid cell membrane barriers, such as the gastrointestinal tract or blood-brain barrier. In contrast, lipid-soluble drugs with anticholinesterase activity, such as physostigmine (a tertiary amine) and organophosphates, are readily absorbed from the gastrointestinal tract and other mucous membranes and have predictable central nervous system effects.

Neostigmine, pyridostigmine, and edrophonium have very large volumes of distribution because of extensive tissue storage in organs such as the liver and kidneys.

The reported shorter onset of action of edrophonium may reflect a presynaptic (i.e., acetylcholine release) rather than a postsynaptic (i.e., acetylcholinesterase inhibition) action. Neostigmine has been shown to be more rapid and effective than edrophonium in reversing profound neuromuscular block, especially when the relaxant being reversed is pancuronium or vecuronium. These differences are decreased if a larger (1.0 mg/kg) dose of edrophonium is administered.[1]

Renal excretion accounts for about 50% of the elimination of neostigmine and about 75% of the elimination of pyridostigmine and edrophonium. All three agents have similar elimination half-lives.

The prolongation of their elimination half-lives by renal failure is similar to that affecting clearance of the muscle relaxants; thus "recurarization" is rarely a problem in patients suffering from renal disease.

Pharmacologic Effects

Although the nicotinic effects of these agents are desirable for reversing neuromuscular blockade, muscarinic effects on the gastrointestinal, pulmonary, and cardiovascular systems can be problematic. These effects are blocked by administration of atropine or glycopyrrolate.

The predominant effect on the heart is bradycardia from slowed conduction velocity of the cardiac impulse through the atrioventricular node. Hypotension may result, reflecting decreases in peripheral vascular resistance.

Anticholinesterase drugs enhance gastric fluid secretion and motility of the entire gastrointestinal tract. This is probably from the effect of accumulated acetylcholine at the ganglion cells of Auerbach's plexus and on smooth muscle cells.

Bronchial, lacrimal, salivary, gastric, and sweat gland secretion is increased.

Clinical Uses

Routine use of acetylcholinesterase antagonists is somewhat controversial. Although the side effects must be considered, reversal may offer a margin of safety. The degree of blockade is not always accurately assessed. Even when the "train-of-four" response on a peripheral nerve stimulator appears normal, up to 70% of the postjunctional receptors may be occupied by nondepolarizing muscle relaxant.

Recommendations for Use of Acetylcholinesterase Antagonists

□ Maintain neuromuscular blockade at 70% to 90% twitch depression. Profound blockade is rarely necessary for surgical procedures and will render antagonists ineffective.
□ Use anticholinesterase reversal agents after the return of 10% of control twitch.
□ Muscles of the face are more resistant to neuromuscular blockers than those of the upper extremity.

□ Clinical assessment should be done along with peripheral nerve stimulators. The maximum inspiratory pressure (MIP) and sustained head lift are recommended clinical guides. An MIP of -25 cm H_2O or greater is sufficient for adequate ventilation. An MIP less than or equal to -45 cm H_2O correlates with a normal CO_2 response curve and sustained head lift.
□ After endotracheal extubation, patients require careful monitoring for residual blockade and assessment of airway adequacy.
□ If the neuromuscular block is not antagonized by a reasonable dose of antagonist (edrophonium 35 to 70 mg/70 kg, neostigmine 2.5 to 5.0 mg/70 kg, or pyridostigmine 10 to 20 mg/70 kg), assess for factors that affect neuromuscular blockade and reversal. Factors that may delay or inhibit antagonism of blockade include hypothermia, profound blockade, respiratory acidosis, presence of certain antibiotics (e.g., aminoglycosides), hypokalemia, and hypermagnesemia.

The time required to antagonize neuromuscular blockade depends on at least four factors[1]:

□ The degree of paralysis.
□ The pharmacokinetics and pharmacodynamics of the muscle relaxant.
□ The specific antagonist.
□ The dose of antagonist.

Neostigmine and pyridostigmine are the standard anticholinesterase drugs used in the treatment of myasthenia gravis. These drugs increase the response of skeletal muscles to repetitive impulses by increasing the availability of endogenous acetylcholine.

Selected Reference

1. Rupp SM, McChristian JW, Miller RD, et al. Neostigmine and edrophonium antagonism of varying intensity neuromuscular blockade induced by atracurium, pancuronium or vecuronium. Anesthesiology 1986;64:711–717.

Suggested References

Cronnelly R, Morris RB: Antagonism of neuromuscular blockade. Br J Anaesth 1982;45:183.
Savarese JJ, Caldwell JE, Lien CA, Miller RD. Pharmacology of muscle relaxants and their antagonists. In Miller RD, ed. Anesthesia. 5th ed. Philadelphia: Churchill Livingstone, 2000:415–490.
Stoelting RK. Anticholinesterase drugs and cholinergic agonists. In Stoelting RK, ed. Pharmacology and Physiology in Anesthetic Practice. 3rd ed. Philadelphia: Lippincott-Raven, 1998;224–236.

61
Atropine, Scopolamine, and Glycopyrrolate Pharmacology

Niki M. Dietz, M.D.

Atropine

Atropine is a naturally occurring tertiary amine antimuscarinic.[1] It competitively inhibits the action of acetylcholine or other cholinergic stimuli at autonomic effectors innervated by postganglionic cholinergic nerves.[2] At usual doses, the principal effect is antagonism of cholinergic stimuli at muscarinic receptors, with little or no effect at nicotinic receptors.

Atropine is an alkaloid of belladonna plants (deadly nightshade and jimson weed). It was used as eye drops by Venetian women to produce mydriasis, which was thought to enhance beauty (belladonna, translated, is "beautiful woman"). In the Roman Empire, atropine was used to produce obscure and prolonged poisoning; hence the name atropine, after Atropos, the oldest of the three fates, who cuts the thread of life.

Pharmacokinetics

Absorption. Atropine is well absorbed from the gastrointestinal tract from the upper small intestine. It is also well absorbed following intramuscular administration or inhalation.

Distribution. Atropine undergoes rapid distribution throughout the body, and 50% is plasma protein bound. Atropine crosses the blood-brain barrier and the placenta.

Elimination. Atropine's plasma half-life is 2 to 3 hours. Metabolism is hepatic. It is excreted in the urine 30% to 50% unchanged.

Pharmacologic Properties

Gastrointestinal. Atropine reduces the volume of saliva. It reduces the volume of gastric secretions and inhibits motility of the gastrointestinal tract from esophagus to colon, prolonging transit time. It relaxes the lower esophageal sphincter.

Cardiovascular. The effect is dose dependent. A dose of 0.4 to 0.6 mg initially causes a slight decrease in heart rate because of central vagal stimulation before peripheral cholinergic blockade. A dose of 1 to 3 mg causes progressively increased tachycardia by blocking normal vagal inhibition of the sinoatrial node; by the same mechanism, atropine can reverse sinus bradycardia secondary to extracardiac causes but has little or no effect on sinus bradycardia caused by intrinsic disease of the sinoatrial node. Atropine may cause cutaneous vasodilation, especially at toxic doses. This is referred to as atropine flush.

Respiratory. Atropine reduces the volume of secretions from the nose, mouth, pharynx, and bronchi. It relaxes smooth muscles of bronchi and bronchioles with resultant decreases in airway resistance.

Central Nervous System. Atropine stimulates the medulla and higher cerebral centers. Toxic doses can cause restlessness, irritability, disorientation, hallucination, and coma. This constellation of symptoms is called central anticholinergic syndrome. Physostigmine can be used to treat this problem.

Genitourinary. Atropine decreases the tone and amplitude of ureter and bladder contractions; this effect is more pronounced in neurogenic bladders. Bladder capacity is increased and incontinence is relieved as uninhibited contractions are reduced. Pelves, calyces, and ureters are dilated.

Ophthalmic. Atropine blocks responses of the sphincter muscle of the iris and the ciliary muscle of the lens to cholinergic stimulation, resulting in mydriasis (pupil dilation) and cycloplegia (paralysis of lens accommodation). It usually has little effect on intraocular pressure except in patients with angle-closure glaucoma, in whom intraocular pressure may increase.

Scopolamine

Scopolamine, another belladonna alkaloid, has stronger antisalivary actions and more potent central nervous system effects (Table 61–1). It is a strong amnesic that usually also produces sedation

Table 61–1. Comparison of Antimuscarinic Drugs

	Duration		CNS	Gastrointestinal Tone	Gastric Acid	Airway Secretions	Heart Rate
	IV	IM					
Atropine	15–30 min	2–4 hr	+ +	– –	–	–	+ + +*
Scopolamine	30–60 min	4–6 hr	+ + +†	–	–	– – – –	–0*
Glycopyrrolate	2–4 hr	6–8 hr	0	– – –	– – –	– – –	+0

*May decelerate initially.
†CNS effect often manifests as sedation before stimulation.
Adapted from Lawson NW, Meyer J.

and euphoria. Restlessness and delirium are not unusual and can make patients difficult to manage. Elderly patients can be injured from falls when unsupervised. Scopolamine produces less cardiac acceleration than atropine, and both drugs can produce paradoxical bradycardia when used in low doses, possibly through a weak peripheral cholinergic agonist effect.

Glycopyrrolate

Glycopyrrolate is a synthetic antimuscarinic with a quaternary ammonium structure.[3] Its structure prevents it from crossing lipid barriers; thus it does not cross the blood-brain barrier, and central nervous system toxicity is unlikely. The anticholinergic properties of glycopyrrolate are similar to those of atropine (see Table 61–1). Glycopyrrolate is a more potent antisialogogue and has a longer duration of action than atropine. It has minimal effects on heart rate.

Selected References

1. Moss J, Renz CL. The autonomic nervous system. In Miller RD, ed. Anesthesia. 5th ed. New York: Churchill Livingstone, 1999:523–577.
2. Lawson NW, Meyer J. Autonomic nervous system physiology and pharmacology. In Barash PG, Cullen BF, Stoelting RK, eds. Clinical Anesthesia. 3rd ed. Philadelphia: Lippincott Williams & Wilkins, 1997:243–327.
3. Stoelting RK. Pharmacology and Physiology in Anesthetic Practice. 3rd ed. Philadelphia, Lippincott-Raven, 1998.

62
Sodium Bicarbonate

Stephen T. Gott, M.D.

The acid-base system is one of the most precisely regulated constituents of body fluid. The body is divided into a two-compartment system, an intracellular compartment and an extracellular compartment, where fluids within each are supplied with buffers to stabilize [H^+] with the addition of acid or base. The bicarbonate buffer is the most important extracellular buffer, representing 40% to 50% of the body's total buffering capacity. Other intracellular and extracellular buffers include hemoglobin, proteins, and phosphates. All of the buffer pairs are in equilibrium with one another, reflecting the isohydric principle as defined by the following relationship:

$$[H+] = K_{a1}\frac{0.03\ PCO_2}{[HCO_3^-]} = K_{a2}\frac{[H_2PO_4^-]}{[HPO_4^{-2}]} = K_{a3}\frac{[IIA]}{[A^-]}$$

where [H^+] = hydrogen ion concentration, K_{a1} = dissociation constant, PCO_2 = arterial CO_2, [HCO_3^-] = bicarbonate concentration, [$H_2PO_4^-$] = phosphoric acid concentration, K_{a2} = dissociation constant, [HPO_4^{-2}] = hydrogen phosphate concentration, K_{a3} = dissociation constant, [HA] = acid, and [A^-] = conjugate base.

The Bicarbonate System

$$CO_2 + H_2O \rightleftharpoons H_2CO_3 \rightleftharpoons HCO_3^- + H^+$$

This buffer system depends on hydration of CO_2 to H_2CO_3 (carbonic acid). Carbonic anhydrase is the enzyme responsible for this conversion in erythrocytes and certain tissues. This conversion also occurs slowly in plasma. Carbonic acid is in equilibrium with bicarbonate and hydrogen ions. The hydrogen ion formed is buffered by reduced hemoglobin, which can also transport CO_2 as carbaminohemoglobin. The bicarbonate formed then diffuses into plasma in exchange for chloride ion (chloride shift):

$$H^+ + Hb^- \rightleftharpoons HHb$$

At a given pH, the ratio of bicarbonate to carbonic acid is constant. At pH = 7.4, this ratio is 20:1. The bicarbonate:carbonic acid buffer can be expressed through the **Henderson-Hasselbalch equation:**

$$pH = 6.1 + \log \frac{[HCO_3^-]}{[H_2CO_3] + [\text{dissolved } CO_2]}$$

Because the concentration of dissolved CO_2 in plasma is in equilibrium with alveolar CO_2, the concentration of CO_2 in plasma can be calculated from the partial pressure of CO_2 using the following equation:

$$CO_2\,(\text{mmole/L}) = 0.03 \times P_ACO_2\,(\text{mmHg})$$

The Henderson-Hasselbalch equation can be expressed as follows:

$$pH = 6.1 + \log \frac{[HCO_3^-]}{0.03 \times PaCO_2}$$

([H_2CO_3] can be ignored, because [dissolved CO_2] is much greater than [H_2CO_3].)

In the presence of an acid load, such as in metabolic acidosis, three processes are involved in an attempt to maintain normal arterial pH:

- Intracellular and extracellular buffers.
- Regulation of renal H+ excretion, which keeps plasma [HCO_3^-] within narrow limits.
- Variations in alveolar ventilation, which controls $PaCO_2$.

Extracellular buffering of excess H^+ by HCO_3^- occurs almost immediately. Within several minutes, the respiratory compensation occurs through hyperventilation. Within 2 to 4 hours, the intracellular buffers provide further buffering as H^+ ions enter the cells in exchange for intracellular potassium and sodium ions (K^+ and Na^+). These processes initially help prevent a significant reduction in arterial pH until acid-base homeostasis can be restored by the renal excretion of the H^+ load as ammonium ion (NH_4^+) and titratable acid (which may take days to achieve).

The response to changes in pH induced by increased $PaCO_2$ (respiratory acidosis) is somewhat different. There is virtually no extracellular buffering, because HCO_3^- cannot effectively buffer H_2CO_3. Similarly, there is no compensatory change in alveolar ventilation, because the primary disturbance is one of abnormal respiration. Thus the intracellular buffers and changes in renal H+ excretion constitute the only protective mechanisms against respiratory acidosis. These buffers increase plasma [HCO_3^-] by only 1 mEq/L for each 10 mm Hg increase in PCO_2 and are usually ineffective in maintaining normal pH. If hypercapnia persists, within hours there will be an increase in renal excretion of H^+, producing further elevation of plasma [HCO_3^-]. But although this renal compensation will increase the pH toward normal, acid-base homeostasis will not be restored until ventilation is normalized.

Uses

Compensatory physiologic mechanisms and correction of the underlying cause of the metabolic disturbance are usually sufficient to restore acid-base balance. Generally, administration of sodium bicarbonate is not necessary, unless the acidosis is severe enough to overcome the compensatory mechanisms (pH less than 7.1 to 7.2 or plasma bicarbonate concentration of 8 mEq/L or less).

Sodium bicarbonate is primarily used as an alkalizing agent in the treatment of severe metabolic acidosis that occurs in a number of conditions, such as lactic acidosis, ketoacidosis, cardiopulmonary resuscitation (CPR), and severe respiratory acidosis. It is not recommended for routine use during CPR because of the problems mentioned later.

If treatment is indicated, the bicarbonate dose is based on the calculated deficit determined from arterial blood gas measurements, as well as on the patient's age, weight, and clinical condition.

$$NaHCO_3 \text{ (mEq)} = 0.3 \times \text{body weight (kg)} \times \text{base deficit (mEq/L)}$$

$NaHCO_3$ is available for injection in an 8.4% solution (1 mEq/mL). Only one-half of the calculated deficit should be replaced at one time. Fractional doses may be repeated as necessary. The [HCO_3^-] obtained is dictated by the amount remaining after **all** extracellular buffers are titrated, its apparent volume of distribution (approximately 40% to 60% of body weight), the compensatory ventilatory response, and eventually the compensatory renal response. Frequent laboratory determinations and clinical evaluations are necessary to monitor fluid and electrolyte and acid-base status.

Potential Problems

▫ Inadvertent extravasation of $NaHCO_3$ into the tissues may cause a chemical cellulitis.
▫ Excessive $NaHCO_3$ administration may result in metabolic alkalosis with a leftward shift of the oxyhemoglobin dissociation curve and subsequent impairment of oxygen release to the tissues. Metabolic alkalosis may be accompanied by hyperirritability or tetany, because a bicarbonate-induced increase in pH increases the binding of free calcium to albumin, resulting in decreased free calcium ion concentration. Hypokalemia may result because of an exchange of K^+ for H^+ in the tissues in an attempt to offset the metabolic alkalosis. Severe bicarbonate-induced alkalosis should be treated with intravenous calcium gluconate and/or an acidifying agent such as ammonium chloride.
▫ During cardiac arrest, the PCO_2 of cardiac venous blood is higher than mixed venous PCO_2. Use of sodium bicarbonate may exacerbate this acidosis. In addition, the use of hypertonic solution may cause a decrease in coronary perfusion pressure and have adverse effects on the resuscitation effort.
▫ HCO_3^- and H^+ do not readily cross the blood-brain barrier. The [HCO_3^-] is similar in blood and cerebrospinal fluid (CSF). However, arterial pH (~7.40) normally is higher than CSF pH (~7.32) and PCO_2 is higher in the CSF than in arterial blood (48 mm Hg versus 40 mm Hg). Because CO_2 crosses the blood-brain barrier, an increase in $PaCO_2$ may result in a paradoxical CSF and tissue acidosis.
▫ Because each gram of sodium bicarbonate contains about 12 mEq of sodium, sodium and water retention and edema may occur with sodium bicarbonate treatment, especially when large doses are given or when $NaHCO_3$ is given to patients with renal insufficiency or congestive heart failure or to those receiving corticosteroids.
▫ Sodium bicarbonate is generally contraindicated in patients with metabolic or respiratory alkalosis, hypocalcemic patients, patients with excessive chloride loss (vomiting, gastrointestinal suctioning), and patients at risk for developing diuretic-induced hypochloremic alkalosis.

Pediatric Precautions

Rapid injection (10 mL/min) of hypertonic sodium bicarbonate solutions in children less than 2 years of age may predispose to hypernatremia, decreased CSF pressure, and potential intraventricular hemorrhage. It is recommended for children that the intravenous rate of infusion of $NaHCO_3$ should not exceed 8 $mEq \cdot kg^{-1} \cdot day^{-1}$ and that slow intravenous administration of a 4.2% solution be used.

Suggested References

Feldman GM, Ripley EBD. Acid-base homeostasis. In Carlson RW, Geheb MA, eds. Principles and Practice of Medical Intensive Care. Philadelphia: WB Saunders, 1993:1219.

Sendak MJ. Monitoring and management of perioperative electrolyte abnormalities, acid-base disorders, and fluid replacement. In Longnecker DE, Tinker JH, Morgan GE Jr.,eds. Principles and Practice of Anesthesiology. 2nd ed. St. Louis: Mosby, 1998:942.

Shangraw RE. Acid-base balance. In Miller R, ed. Anesthesia. 5th ed. Philadelphia: Churchill Livingstone, 2000:1390–1413.

Stoelting RK. Acid-base balance. In Stoelting RK, ed. Pharmacology and Physiology in Anesthetic Practice. 3rd ed. Philadelphia: Lippincott-Raven, 1998:703–707.

63
Vasopressors and Inotropes

Pamela Jensen-Bundy, M.D.

A **vasopressor** is a drug used to elevate arterial blood pressure above the existing level. Once synonymous with only arterial vasoconstriction, the principle hemodynamic effects of vasopressors are now known to include changes in heart rate (**chronotropism**), contractility (**inotropism**), myocardial conduction (**dromotropism**), rhythm, and peripheral vascular dilation or constriction, influencing preload and afterload. An **inotrope** is a drug that influences the contractility of the myocardium. The uses of vasopressors in anesthesia include (1) maintenance of organ perfusion until definitive therapy can be initiated, (2) treatment of anaphylaxis, (3) prolongation of local anesthetic action, and (4) cardiopulmonary resuscitation.

Characteristics of the ideal positive inotrope are listed in Table 63–1. Elevation of the blood pressure alone has repeatedly been demonstrated to be an insufficient goal in the treatment of low cardiac output syndromes. The goal is to reestablish blood flow to vital organs. Understanding the importance of the patient's intravascular volume is also crucial to resuscitation efforts and has ushered in a rational approach using volume therapy in conjunction with vasoactive drugs. Because 80% of the circulating volume is contained in the veins, venoconstriction has also become an important consideration. Venoconstriction adds little to total vascular resistance, but it produces small changes in capacitance vessels that can produce large shifts in intravascular volume.

Table 63–1. Characteristics of the Ideal Positive Inotropic Agent

Enhances contractile state by increasing velocity and force of myocardial fiber shortening
Lacks tolerance
Does not produce vasoconstriction
Does not cause cardiac dysrhythmias
Does not affect heart rate
Controllability—immediate onset and termination of action
Elevates perfusion pressure by raising cardiac output rather than systemic vascular resistance
Redistributes blood flow to vital organs
Direct acting—not dependent on release of endogenous amines
Compatible with other vasoactive drugs
Effective orally or parenterally

From Lawson NW, Meyer DJ Jr.

Adrenergic vasopressors exert their influence through adrenergic-autonomic receptors. Adrenergic agents are also classified as catecholamines and noncatecholamines.

☐ **α-receptors** respond preferentially to norepinephrine (NE) more than or equal to epinephrine. α-receptors are classified as α_1 or α_2. α_1-receptors mediate smooth muscle contraction and vasoconstriction, as well as the nonhemodynamically significant functions of salivation, gastrointestinal relaxation, sweating, gluconeogenesis, and glycogenolysis. Stimulation of α_2-receptors inhibits NE release presynaptically in the central nervous system (CNS). Additional α_2 actions include platelet aggregation and inhibition of insulin and renin release. **β-receptors** respond preferentially to isoproterenol more than epinephrine and more than or equal to NE. β_1-receptor actions mediate increased heart rate, contractility, and conduction as well as lipolysis. β_2-receptor stimulation causes glycogenolysis, gluconeogenesis, smooth muscle relaxation, and insulin and amylase secretion. **Dopaminergic** (DA) receptors respond to dopamine and are found in the CNS and in renal, coronary, and mesenteric vessels. DA_1-receptor stimulation produces renal and mesenteric vascular relaxation, whereas DA_2-agonists inhibit presynaptic release of NE.
☐ The net effects of the sympathomimetics are equal to the sum of their α, β, and dopaminergic effects. The adverse effects are related to excessive α (decreased peripheral perfusion, tachyphylaxis) and β (arrhythmias, increased myocardial oxygen consumption) effects.
☐ Tachyphylaxis occurs with increasing plasma volume loss and downregulation of adrenergic receptors. Precapillary sphincters relax in hypoxic and acidotic conditions, whereas postcapillary sphincters remain contracted. Hydrostatic pressure then extravasates fluid into the interstitial space, producing edema.

Specific Agents

Doses of the specific agents described in the following list are given in Table 63–2:

Table 63–2. Dosage Schedules for the Sympathomimetic Amines

Drug (listed from α to β)	Dosages	
	IV Push Adults	*IV Infusion*
Methoxamine	5–10 mg	Not recommended
Phenylephrine	50–100 μg	a. 10 mg/250 mL
		b. 40 μg/mL
		c. $0.15–0.75\ \mu g \cdot kg^{-1} \cdot min^{-1}$
		d. $0.15\ \mu g \cdot kg^{-1} \cdot min^{-1}$
Norepinephrine	Not recommended	a. 4 mg/250 mL
		b. 16 μg/mL
		c. $0.01–0.1\ \mu g \cdot kg^{-1} \cdot min^{-1}$
		d. $0.1\ \mu g \cdot kg^{-1} \cdot min^{-1}$
Metaraminol	Not recommended	a. 100 mg/250 mL
		b. 400 μg/mL
		c. $0.5–7\ \mu g \cdot kg^{-1} \cdot min^{-1}$
		d. $0.5\ \mu g \cdot kg^{-1} \cdot min^{-1}$
Epinephrine	0.3–0.5 mg SubQ for asthma or IV for anaphylaxis 0.5–1.0 mg for cardiac arrest q 5 min	a. 1 mg/250 mL
		b. 4 μg/mL
		c. $0.01–0.30\ \mu g \cdot kg^{-1} \cdot min^{-1}$
		d. $0.015\ \mu g \cdot kg^{-1} \cdot min^{-1}$
Ephedrine	5–10 mg	Not recommended
Mephentermine	15–30 mg	a. 500 mg/250 mL
		b. 2000 μg/mL
		c. $4–8\ \mu g \cdot kg^{-1} \cdot min^{-1}$
		d. $4\ \mu g \cdot kg^{-1} \cdot min^{-1}$
Dopamine	Not recommended	a. 200 mg/250 mL
		b. 800 μg/mL
		c. $2–20\ \mu g \cdot kg^{-1} \cdot min^{-1}$
		d. $2\ \mu g \cdot kg^{-1} \cdot min^{-1}$
Dobutamine	Not recommended	a. 250 mg/250 mL
		b. 1000 μg/mL
		c. $2–30\ \mu g \cdot kg^{-1} \cdot min^{-1}$
		d. $5\ \mu g \cdot kg^{-1} \cdot min^{-1}$
Isoproterenol	Not recommended	a. 1 mg/250 mL
		b. 4 μg/mL
		c. $2–10\ \mu g \cdot min^{-1}$ to desired effect
		d. $0.015\ \mu g \cdot kg^{-1} \cdot min^{-1}$

a, mixture; b, concentration $(\mu g/mL)$; c, dose range $(\mu g \cdot kg^{-1} \cdot min^{-1})$; d, standard rate of infusion $(\mu g \cdot kg^{-1} \cdot min^{-1})$.
Modified from Lawson NW, Meyer DJ Jr.

□ **Methoxamine**: Pure α_1-receptor agonist; used to treat paroxysmal atrial tachycardia. Reduces cardiac output (CO).

□ **Phenylephrine**: Pure α_1-receptor agonist; venoconstrictor. Causes decreased CO in patients with ischemic heart disease. Good for weaning patients from cardiopulmonary bypass and for treating symptoms in patients with tetralogy of Fallot.

□ **Norepinephrine** (NE): Direct-acting α- and β-receptor agonist. It is the natural mediator of the sympathetic nervous system.

□ **Metaraminol**: Direct α- and β-receptor agonist with indirect action by causing NE release.

□ **Epinephrine**: An endogenous catecholamine with α- (skin, muscle, kidney) and β-receptor (muscle) effects. Inhalation anesthesia sensitizes myocardium to catecholamines, causing arrhythmias. The maximum dose of epinephrine is 6.7 μg/kg when using 1.2 minimal alveolar concentration (MAC) isoflurane, less with halothane and enflurane.

□ **Ephedrine**: Acts directly but primarily indirectly to cause release of NE. It is used primarily to increase blood pressure following spinal or epidural anesthesia. It has little adverse effect on uterine blood flow and so can be used in obstetrics. Tachyphylaxis may occur.

□ **Mephentermine**: Has direct β-receptor effects to increase inotropy and indirect α-receptor effects.

□ **Dopamine**: A precursor of NE that has α, β, and dopaminergic effects. A dose of 0.5 to 3 $\mu g \cdot kg^{-1} \cdot min^{-1}$ produces renal effects, primarily dopaminergic, increasing renal blood flow; 2 to 10 $\mu g \cdot kg^{-1} \cdot min^{-1}$ produces primarily β effects; 10 to 20 $\mu g \cdot kg^{-1} \cdot min^{-1}$ produces primarily α effects.

□ **Dobutamine**: This exerts primarily β effects, with β_1 greater than β_2. It produces minimal changes in heart rate and systemic vascular resistance. It inhibits hypoxic pulmonary vasoconstriction. It is used for inotropic effect in congestive heart failure from coronary artery disease. Because it has β_1 effects, it can produce tachyarrhythmias.

□ **Isoproterenol**: This pure β-receptor agonist is used to decrease pulmonary hypertension, as a temporary pacemaker, as a bronchodilator, and to reverse β blockade.

□ **Amrinone**: Phosphodiesterase inhibitor that increases cyclic AMP, calcium influx, and vasodilation. Side effects include thrombocytopenia, ventricular arrhythmias, and centrilobular necrosis. Dose: bolus, 0.75 mg/kg over 2 to 3 min; infusion, 3 to 10 μg·kg^{-1}·min^{-1}.

□ **Milrinone**: Phosphodiesterase inhibitor. Side effects include ventricular arrhythmias. Like amrinone, hypotension may occur if the loading dose is given too quickly. Dose: bolus, 50 μg/kg over 10 min; infusion, 0.4 to 0.8 μg·kg^{-1}·min^{-1}.

□ **Aminophylline**: Has both β_1 and β_2 effects. Inhibition of phosphodiesterase raises cyclic AMP levels, yielding a β response. It is used as a bronchodilator for its smooth muscle relaxation. It also has positive inotropic and chronotropic effects and reduces afterload. Dose: bolus, 6 mg/kg over 20 to 30 min; maintenance, 0.5 to 0.7 mg·kg^{-1}·h^{-1}.

□ **Glucagon**: Exerts β_1 effects. It is used for enhancing atrioventricular nodal conduction, particularly in digitalis toxicity. Side effects include nausea, vomiting, glucose disturbances, and hypokalemia. Dose: bolus, 50 μg/kg; infusion, 5 to 10 μg·kg^{-1}·min^{-1}.

□ **Digoxin**: Positive inotrope, but slows impulse propagation. It blocks the Na-K-ATPase pump and calcium influx. Dose: 0.25 to 1 mg.

□ **Calcium** (CaCl$_2$): Positive inotrope and vasopressor whose effects last 10 to 20 minutes. It is useful as a mild inotrope, after cardiopulmonary bypass or when massive transfusion of blood depresses myocardial contractility from citrate toxicity, and when calcium channel blocker overdose is suspected. Dose: 2 to 10 mg/kg.

Selected Reference

1. Lawson NW, Meyer DJ Jr. Autonomic nervous system: Physiology and pharmacology. In Barash P, Cullen B, Stoelting R, eds. Clinical Anesthesia. 3rd ed. Philadelphia: Lippincott-Raven, 1997:243–309.

Suggested References

Fontes ML, Hines RL. Pharmacologic management of perioperative left and right ventricular dysfunction. In Kaplan JA, ed. Cardiac Anesthesia. 4th ed. Philadelphia: WB Saunders, 1999:1155–1191.

Moss J, Renz CL. The autonomic nervous system. In Miller RD, ed. Anesthesia. 5th ed. Philadelphia: Churchill Livingstone, 2000:523–577.

64
Nitroglycerin

William G. Binegar, M.D.

Mechanism of Action for Vasodilation

Nitroglycerin (NTG) is metabolized to nitric oxide (NO) in the vascular smooth muscle wall and acts to stimulate cyclic GMP (cGMP) production. This leads to dephosphorylation of the myosin light chain and relaxation of smooth muscle, which is associated with decreased intracellular calcium. Sulfhydryl (SH) groups are required to produce the NO. Vascular tolerance can occur when excessive SH groups are metabolized by prolonged exposure to NTG. NTG may have greater effects as a venodilator because of greater uptake in veins compared to arteries.

Metabolism

Metabolism occurs in the liver by glutathione organic nitrate reductase; inactivated metabolites are excreted by the kidney. NTG also appears to be taken up by the endothelium of vessel walls and metabolized there. NTG has a half-life of 1.9 to 2.6 minutes.

Cardiovascular Effects

Higher blood levels and greater tissue uptake have been shown on the venous side. NTG acts primarily on venous capacitance vessels, causing peripheral pooling of blood, reduced heart size, and decreased cardiac ventricular wall tension. With increased concentrations, relaxation of arterial vessels occurs, first affecting conductance vessels and then the smaller resistance vessels.

Cardiac performance depends on the underlying status. With a **normal** or **low** ventricular filling pressure, cardiac output (CO) may decrease because of inadequate preload. In congestive heart failure (CHF), CO increases as a result of reduced systolic wall tension or afterload. NTG also improves CO in CHF in patients with mitral regurgitation. In patients with **coronary artery disease**, NTG causes decreased wall tension and decreased myocardial oxygen demand, which in turn results in increased myocardial contractility and CO.

Myocardial blood flow is affected indirectly via hemodynamic changes and directly by coronary arterial dilation. Coronary perfusion increases from lowering left ventricular end diastolic pressure (LVEDP) more than aortic diastolic pressure. A decrease in LVEDP also reduces extrinsic tissue compression of coronary vessels in the subendocardium. Therapeutic doses of NTG dilate large coronary arteries but not coronary arterioles, benefiting collateral and subendocardial blood flow to ischemic areas. NTG produces less coronary steal than agents that produce intense vasodilation of the small coronary resistance vessels. High NTG doses (9 to 32 $\mu g \cdot kg^{-1} \cdot min^{-1}$) cause direct coronary arteriolar vasodilation, overriding any coronary autoregulation. Part of NTG's action on coronary vasodilation may involve its effects on stimulating prostacyclin.

Therapeutic Uses

Antianginal effects are multifactorial. Decreased myocardial oxygen demand is the primary factor achieved by reductions in preload and systolic wall tension. Also, increased oxygen delivery will occur with coronary arterial dilation.

- With **partial** occlusion, the patient will probably benefit from decreased myocardial oxygen consumption.
- With **total** occlusion, the patient will probably benefit from redistribution.
- With **spastic** vessels, the patient will benefit from coronary vascular relaxation.

In the **acute myocardial infarction** setting, NTG was once considered contraindicated because of hypotension and tachycardia. Studies now show an increase in collateral blood flow to ischemic regions and decreased infarction size. Maximum benefit is probably attained when CHF coexists. As long as hypotension is avoided, patients with acute myocardial infarction without heart failure also benefit. Beneficial effects appear greater with inferior infarctions than with anterior infarctions (possibly because the right coronary artery is more prone to spasm). NTG works better if started within 10 hours. The starting dose is 0.5 $\mu g \cdot kg^{-1} \cdot min^{-1}$.

Perioperative indications are myocardial ischemia, CHF, systemic and pulmonary hypertension, and coronary artery spasm. Preoperative oral or transcutaneous nitrates are to be continued until time of surgery. Transcutaneous administration is probably not effective intraoperatively, because absorption is not reliable. Intranasal NTG has been used to treat the pressor response to tracheal intubation. Intraoperative indications for intravenous NTG include hypertension greater than 20% of preoperative levels in patients with coronary artery disease, LVEDP greater than 18 to 20 mm Hg, ST changes greater than 1 mm, acute right or left ventricular dysfunction, or coronary artery spasm. Intraoperative doses below 1.0 $\mu g \cdot kg^{-1} \cdot min^{-1}$ are not considered effective.

Prophylactic NTG has been evaluated in patients with coronary disease undergoing a variety of surgical procedures. Although it reduced the incidence rate of wall motion abnormalities as detected by transesophageal echocardiography, several studies showed that prophylactic NTG was ineffective in reducing the incidence rate of ischemia as evidenced by electrocardiography.

Adverse Effects

Adverse effects of NTG include the following:

□ Nitrate **tolerance** may occur with repeat oxidation of SH groups; cross-tolerance with possible decreased effect in patients previously given isosorbide dinitrate.

□ Drug **dependence** is evident at industrial doses, with ammunition workers developing chest pain 2 to 3 days after being off work. Although clinical evidence does not yet exist, abrupt cessation of nitrate therapy should be avoided.

□ **Nitrate**, a metabolite, converts oxyhemoglobin to methemoglobin.

□ Polyethylene tubing is recommended, because polyvinylchloride tubing absorbs NTG.

□ **Relative** contraindications include increased intracranial pressure, hypovolemia, and angina associated with aortic stenosis, idiopathic hypertrophic subaortic stenosis, and tachyarrhythmias.

Suggested References

Dodds TM, Stone JG, Coromilas J, et al. Prophylactic nitroglycerin infusion during noncardiac surgery does not reduce perioperative ischemia. Anesth Analg 1993;76:705–713.

Harrison DG, Bates JN. The nitrovasodilators. New ideas about old drugs. Circulation 1993;87:1461.

Lell W, Johnson P, Plagenhoef J, et al. The effect of prophylactic nitroglycerin infusion on the incidence of regional wall-motion abnormalities and ST segment changes in patients undergoing coronary artery bypass surgery. J Card Surg 1993;9:228.

Royster RL, Zvata DA. Anti-ischemic drug therapy. In Kaplan JA, ed. Cardiac Anesthesia. 4th ed. Philadelphia: WB Saunders, 1999:95.

Stoelting RK. Peripheral vasodilators. In Stoelting RK, ed. Pharmacology and Physiology in Anesthetic Practice. 3rd ed. Philadelphia: Lippincott-Raven, 1998:313–330.

65
Sodium Nitroprusside

Scott A. Gammel, M.D.

Pharmacology

The mechanism of action of sodium nitroprusside (SNP) is relaxation of vessel wall smooth muscle. Specific mechanisms include the following:

☐ SNP is metabolized to nitric oxide, activating guanylate cyclase and increasing levels of cyclic GMP and causing relaxation of arteriolar and venule smooth muscle.
☐ SNP is also reported to interfere with sulfhydryl receptors and/or intracellular calcium activation, leading to smooth muscle relaxation.
☐ At the tissue level, it has been found that during SNP administration tissue PO_2 is markedly reduced (in skeletal and cardiac muscle and in liver), whereas arterial PO_2 is normal. This results from dilation of precapillary sphincters on the arterial side of the capillary bed but not on (or not as great on) the venule side, resulting in decreased blood flow. Also, a significant volume of blood is diverted through functional arterial-venous shunts during SNP administration. SNP's molecular structure is shown in Figure 65–1. Its metabolism is summarized in Figure 65–2.
☐ The conversion of SNP to the SNP radical is not limited by enzyme activity, and the conversion to free cyanide ions occurs very rapidly and is not inhibited by hypothermia.
☐ The conversion of cyanide ion to thiocyanate is inhibited by hypothermia and requires adequate vitamin B_{12} (thought to be deficient in Leber's optic atrophy and tobacco amblyopia). Cysteine is needed to produce thiosulfate.

SNP toxicity results from cytochrome oxidase poisoning and cessation of oxidative metabolism.

☐ The maximum recommended dose is 8.0 $\mu g \cdot kg^{-1} \cdot min^{-1}$ over 1 to 3 hours or 500 $\mu g \cdot kg^{-1} \cdot hr^{-1}$ chronically; the usual perioperative rate of 0.5 to 2.0 $\mu g \cdot kg^{-1} \cdot min^{-1}$ is about 1/16th to 1/4th the maximum dose (administered chronically).
☐ Children or young adults have greater risk of toxicity because they have pronounced baroreceptor reflexes, necessitating larger doses of SNP.
☐ Propranolol, captopril, and volatile anesthetics blunt receptor reflexes and reduce the amount of SNP needed.
☐ Infusion should be discontinued if tachyphylaxis,

metabolic acidosis, or increased mixed venous oxygen saturation develops.

Cardiovascular Effects

☐ SNP decreases blood pressure, systemic vascular resistance, and right atrial pressure.
☐ SNP causes reflex increases in heart rate and contractility.
☐ SNP causes an increase in cardiac output secondary to decreased left ventricular impedance and reflex increased sympathetic activity.
☐ SNP can lead to myocardial ischemia and associated infarction via coronary steal and decreased diastolic blood pressure.

Pulmonary Effects

SNP is known to attenuate hypoxic pulmonary vasoconstriction. The resulting increase in shunt fraction is likely to be greater in those with normal lungs versus those with chronic obstructive pulmonary disease, in whom the shunt fraction is already increased.

Central Nervous System Effects

☐ SNP has no known direct effects on the central or autonomic nervous system.

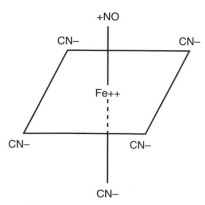

Figure 65–1. Sodium nitroprusside. (From Tinker JH, Michenfelder JD.)

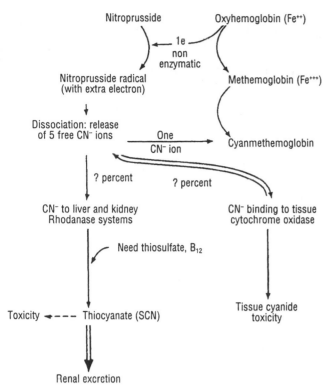

Figure 65–2. Schematic representation of nitroprusside breakdown releasing cyanide, with cyanide taking three paths: (1) reacting with methemoglobin; (2) reacting with tissue cytochrome oxidase (cyanide toxicity); (3) converted by rhodanase into thiocyanate for excretion. (From Tinker JH, Michenfelder JD.)

- □ SNP is generally thought to increase cerebral blood flow (CBF) and, more importantly, cerebral blood volume (CBV).
- □ SNP dilates capacitance vessels regardless of anesthetic background and dilates resistance vessels when autoregulation has been blunted (e.g., by volatile anesthetics), so that CBV increases and thereby increases intracranial pressure (ICP), particularly if there is a preexisting decreased intracranial compliance.
- □ When correlated with percent reduction in mean arterial pressure (MAP), ICP increases maximally with moderate reduction (<30%) in MAP.

- □ In normal animals, CBF autoregulation is impaired by SNP, so blood flow is directly related to cerebral perfusion pressure.
- □ Cyanide ions in cerebrospinal fluid may cross the blood-brain barrier, causing cyanide encephalopathy and toxic edema or even brain damage, particularly in patients with impaired autoregulation and reduced CBF and poor collateral circulation.

Coagulation Effects

- □ SNP decreases the number and aggregation of platelets 1 to 6 hours postinfusion in patients with congestive heart failure. Platelet count and function return to preinfusion values in 24 hours. Controlled hypotension using SNP reduces epinephrine-induced (and spontaneous) aggregation of platelets.[1]
- □ During general anesthesia, systemic SNP significantly reduces blood flow to free musculocutaneous flaps, but local infusion into the flap significantly increases flow.[2]

Selected References

1. Dietrich GV, Heesen M, Boldt J, et al. Platelet function and adrenoreceptors during and after induced hypotension using nipride. Anesthesiology 1996;85:1334–1340.
2. Banic A, Krejci V, Erni D, et al. Effects of sodium nitroprusside and phenylephrine on blood flow in free musculocutaneous flaps during general anesthesia. Anesthesiology 1999;90:147–155.

Suggested References

Stoelting RK. Pharmacology and Physiology in Anesthetic Practice. 3rd ed. Philadelphia, Lippincott-Raven, 1998.
Tinker JH, Michenfelder JD. Sodium nitroprusside: Pharmacology, toxicology and therapeutics. Anesthesiology 1976;45:340.
Van Aken H, Miller ED. Deliberate hypotension. In Miller RD, ed. Anesthesia. 5th ed. Philadelphia: Churchill Livingstone, 2000:1470–1490.
Woodside J Jr, Garner L, Bedford RF, et al. Captopril reduces the dose requirement for sodium nitroprusside induced hypotension. Anesthesiology 1984;60:413.

66
Deliberate Hypotension

Beth A. Elliott, M.D.

Deliberate hypotension is an adjunctive technique used during surgery to decrease blood loss and facilitate the surgical procedure. As early as 1917, Harvey Cushing first noted the "bloodless field" and improved neurosurgical operating conditions in patients with low blood pressure. Over the ensuing decades, many different techniques have been used to produce deliberate intraoperative hypotension: in the 1940s, phlebotomy and high spinal anesthesia; in the early 1950s, ganglionic blocking agents and epidural anesthesia; in the mid-1970s, intravenous vasodilators; and in the 1980s, adrenergic blocking agents. Today, the diversity of agents used to create deliberate hypotension is impressive, but a single "ideal" hypotensive agent remains elusive.

The "ideal" hypotensive agent should be easily administered and controlled. It should have a rapid, predictable onset with a dose-dependent effect. It should have a short biologic half-life or be easily reversible, should be nontoxic and produce no toxic metabolites, should not alter blood flow to vital organs, and should produce no untoward physiologic response.

Purported advantages of deliberate hypotension include:

□ Decreased surgical blood loss.
□ Improved visibility in the surgical field.
□ Decreased operating time.
□ Decreased number of blood products transfused.

Indications for deliberate hypotension include:

□ Neurosurgery: aneurysm clipping, arteriovenous malformation resection, tumor resection.
□ Orthopedics: total hip arthroplasty, spinal fusion/instrumentation.
□ Ear, nose, and throat/oral surgery: head and neck tumor resection, major facial reconstruction, orthognathic procedures, middle ear procedures.
□ Gynecologic/urologic: radical pelvic surgery, prostatectomy.
□ Miscellaneous: religious blood refusal, rare blood type, difficult cross-match.

Risks Associated with Deliberate Hypotension

Regardless of method, deliberate hypotension is ultimately achieved by reduction in systemic vascular resistance and/or cardiac output. The morbidity associated with deliberate hypotension is related to inadequate perfusion of vital end organs, such as the central nervous system and myocardium. The widely accepted "safe" lower limit for mean arterial blood pressure (MAP) during deliberate hypotension is between 50 and 55 mm Hg for healthy patients. This value represents the lower limit of cerebral autoregulation. Chronically hypertensive patients may experience loss of autoregulation at higher MAP values, but this can normalize with effective antihypertensive therapy. Patients with increased intracranial pressure (ICP) and/or intracranial pathology will also be susceptible to insult at higher MAP values. MAP reduction to 20% to 30% below baseline (with an absolute lower limit of 50 mm Hg in healthy patients) is considered usual clinical practice.

Retinal artery thrombosis, persistent hypotension, oliguria, anuria, and hemorrhage have also been reported as complications of this technique. Mortality directly attributable to deliberate hypotension is very low.

Relative Contraindications for Deliberate Hypotension

□ Cerebrovascular disease: stroke or a history of transient ischemic attack.
□ Spinal cord compression.
□ Cardiovascular disease: angina, history of myocardial infarction, untreated hypertension, peripheral vascular disease.
□ Aortic stenosis.
□ Renal or hepatic dysfunction.
□ Increased ICP.
□ Pregnancy.
□ Severe pulmonary disease.
□ Hypovolemia and severe anemia.

Monitoring During Deliberate Hypotension

Vigilant monitoring of vital organ function is necessary for the successful outcome of the hypotensive technique. Standard intraoperative monitors (electrocardiogram, blood pressure cuff, stethoscope, temperature, pulse oximetry, end-tidal CO_2) are required for all patients. Direct arterial blood pressure monitoring should be mandatory for all patients undergoing deliberate hypotension. Arterial blood gases, serum electrolytes, and hematocrit should be measured periodically during the case. An indwelling urinary catheter should be considered for most patients, and a central venous line is helpful in those cases involving large fluid shifts and/or blood loss, or if preexisting disease warrants. Evoked potential monitoring (somatosensory or motor evoked potentials) may be helpful during spinal fusion/instrumentation to assess spinal cord integrity.

Pharmacologic Agents Used to Achieve Deliberate Hypotension

Vasodilators

Sodium nitroprusside (SNP) is one of the more widely used agents for inducing hypotension because of its rapid onset and short biologic half-life. Vasodilation occurs primarily in the arteriolar resistance vessels. Onset of effect is measured in seconds, and duration of effect is 1 to 3 minutes, making SNP responsive to rapid titration. Mechanism of action involves interaction with sulfhydryl groups to block intracellular calcium activation and nitric oxide stimulation of cyclic GMP, which produces smooth muscle relaxation in vessel walls. Dosage titration should begin at 0.05 to 0.10 µg/kg/min and adjusted as needed to achieve the desired blood pressure (see Chapter 65).

The SNP molecule contains five cyanide ions that are released on breakdown of the drug. Cyanide binds to intracellular cytochrome oxidase and results in tissue hypoxia. Cyanide toxicity is related to total dose per unit of time. The risk of toxicity is reduced if the dose is kept below 8 µg/kg/min. Signs of toxicity include tachycardia, metabolic acidosis, and tachyphylaxis. If toxicity is suspected, the drug should be discontinued immediately.

Other problems associated with the use of SNP include activation of the renin-angiotensin system and the release of vasopressin. This activation contributes to resistance to the hypotensive effect of SNP, tachyphylaxis, and rebound hypertension occurring after SNP is discontinued. Alteration of cerebral autoregulation and abolition of hypoxic pulmonary vasoconstriction may cause significant problems in susceptible patients. Reflex tachycardia and impaired platelet function can also occur with SNP use.

Nitroglycerin (NTG) can be used to produce deliberate hypotension, primarily through vasodilation of venous capacitance vessels. Resistance vessels are also affected, but to a much lesser degree. Onset of action occurs within minutes, and duration of effect is limited by the short biologic half-life ($t_{1/2}$ = 2.6 minutes). NTG is less reliable than SNP in producing hypotension; however, it does have some advantages. NTG is not associated with tachyphylaxis or rebound hypertension, and it has no toxic effects. Dosing is typically started at 0.2 µg/kg/min, with titration as needed to achieve the desired effect. Like SNP, NTG is a potent cerebral vasodilator that has the potential to produce deleterious effects in patients with increased ICP.

Ganglionic Blocking Agents

The only ganglionic blocker available in the United States, **trimethaphan** has long been used to produce deliberate hypotension. Because it nonselectively occupies receptors in the autonomic ganglia, it produces both sympathetic and parasympathetic blockade. Onset of effect occurs within seconds, and rapid metabolism by plasma cholinesterase limits its duration to 1 to 2 minutes. Titration is begun at 0.03 to 6 mg/min, with adjustments made as needed to achieve the desired effect. Potential problems with trimethaphan include tachyphylaxis, histamine release (related to rate of administration), bronchospasm, and potentiation of succinylcholine myoneural blockade. Side effects related to unwanted parasympathetic blockade include mydriasis, cycloplegia, tachycardia, reduced gastrointestinal activity, and urinary retention. In addition, there is evidence of cerebral toxicity (electroencephalogram burst suppression, slowing, high voltage, and increased brain lactate) in animal models at a MAP of 55 mm Hg. The pupillary effects alone (fixed, dilated pupils) keep many practitioners from using this drug in neurosurgical patients. Moreover, large doses may result in prolonged hypotension.

Adrenergic Blocking Agents

Esmolol is a short-acting cardioselective β-adrenergic blocking agent. It has a rapid onset of action and short duration ($t_{1/2}$ = 9 minutes) because of rapid metabolism by cholinesterase. As with other β-blocking agents, esmolol's hypotensive effect is achieved primarily through reduced chronotropy and inotropy. Plasma renin activity is reduced, there is no rebound hypertension after discontinuation of the drug, and there are no toxic effects. Dosage should begin with an initial bolus of 0.5 to 1.0 mg/kg to establish appropriate blood levels, followed by an infusion of 50 to 300 µg/kg/min to achieve the desired effect. Young, healthy patients may be resistant to the hypotensive effects of esmolol alone. Addition of a vasodilating agent may produce synergy and establish adequate levels of hypotension at reduced dosages for both drugs, obviating many of the negative effects of each.

Labetolol has both α-blocking and nonspecific β-blocking activity. Blood pressure reduction results from decreased cardiac output and peripheral vascular resistance. Onset of effect is seen within 5 minutes, but a long half-life (4 to 5 hours) may limit labetolol application in certain clinical scenarios where rapid titration is important. Dosing can occur with intermittent 5- to 10-mg boluses IV every 10 minutes until the desired effect is achieved. Advantages include reduction in plasma renin activity, no rebound hypertension, and no increased ICP (even in the setting of reduced intracranial compliance).

Inhalation Anesthetics

Isoflurane decreases blood pressure primarily by reducing peripheral vascular resistance. Its rapid onset, ease of use, absence of toxic side effects, and ability to maintain cardiac output make it a popular adjunct for producing deliberate hypotension. Doses associated with usual anesthetic concentrations (~1 MAC) have been shown to decrease the cerebral metabolic rate for oxygen and preserve cerebral autoregulation. Newer inhalation anesthetics have not been as well investigated. Agents that produce vasodilation without significantly reducing cardiac output are theoretically safer, because they preserve flow to the CNS and myocardium.

Other Pharmacologic Agents

Purine derivatives (adenosine and adenosine triphosphate) have been advocated for deliberate hypotension because of their extremely short half-life (10 to 20 seconds). Potent vasodilators, these agents provide rapid reductions in blood pressure at doses of 0.06 to 0.35 mg/kg/min. Purine derivatives can maintain cardiac filling pressures and heart rate with little change in plasma renin activity or catecholamines. Purines are also potent cerebral and coronary vasodilators; this effect may produce unwanted increases in CBF or intracoronary steal with resultant myocardial ischemia.

Urapidil (not available in the United States) is an antihypertensive agent that interacts with peripheral α-adrenergic receptors and 5-hydroxytryptamine receptors in the CNS. It produces peripheral vasodilation without stimulating the sympathetic nervous system. It shows promise as an adjunctive agent for deliberate hypotension, because intracranial pressure and compliance are not affected and rebound hypertension does not occur.

Summary

A growing body of evidence indicates that deliberate hypotensive techniques can be used to decrease surgical blood loss and transfusion requirements. However, widespread application of these techniques to all clinical scenarios is unjustified. Despite the degree of interest in and investigation into deliberate hypotensive techniques, to what degree blood pressure can be safely lowered yet still produce a significant reduction in intraoperative bleeding remains unclear.

Appropriate monitoring and patient selection are critical elements in avoiding potential complications. Appreciation of the mechanisms (both physiologic and pharmacologic) by which hypotension is achieved is essential to the success of these measures.

Suggested References

Petrozza PH. Induced hypotension. Int Anesthesiol Clin 1990;28:223.

Stoelting RK. Pharmacology and Physiology in Anesthetic Practice. 3rd ed. Philadelphia, Lippincott-Raven, 1998.

Van Aken H, Miller ED. Deliberate hypotension. In Miller RD, ed. Anesthesia. 5th ed. Philadelphia: Churchill Livingstone, 2000:1470–1490.

67
Calcium Channel Blockers

David J. Cook, M.D.

This structurally diverse group of drugs is used to control supraventricular tachyarrhythmias, essential hypertension, angina, and coronary vasospasm. They have also been evaluated in the treatment of cerebral vasospasm and as agents that might provide cerebral protection during ischemia and myocardial protection during coronary bypass.

Mechanism of Action

Calcium channel blockers (CCBs) interfere with Ca^{2+} movement through the plasmalemma in all types of tissues with calcium channels. These (slow) calcium channels in the cell membrane are 100 times more selective for Ca^{2+} than for Na^+ or K^+ and are thought to have an outer voltage-dependent gate and an inner phosphorylation-dependent gate. Also known as calcium entry blockers, they have electrophysiologic effects and alter excitation-contraction coupling (Fig. 67–1).

Electrophysiologic Effects. CCBs are negative chronotropes because the slow Ca^{2+} channel is responsible for depolarization at the sinoatrial (SA) and atrioventricular (AV) nodes. CCBs are negative dromotropes because they slow AV nodal conduction and increase its refractoriness.

Effects on Excitation-Contraction Coupling. CCBs impede Ca^{2+} influx through the plasmalemma and **may** alter intracellular Ca^{2+} movement. They alter myocardial and smooth muscle contraction. Therefore, they are negative inotropes and both arteriodilators and venodilators.

Structural Diversity

CCBs are structurally similar to unrelated compounds:

□ Phenylalkylamine: verapamil.
□ Benzothiazepine: diltiazem.
□ Dihydropyridines: nifedipine, nicardipine, nimodipine, isradipine, amlodipine, felodipine.
□ Diarylaminopropylamine: bepridil.
□ Tertatolol derivative: mibefradil (unique in that it is a "T-type" as opposed to "L-type" Ca^{2+} blocker).

The verapamil molecule has local anesthetic potency exceeding that of procaine; it blocks the fast Na^+ channel. Like the CCBs, calcium channels are heterogeneous. Therefore, CCBs have multiple sites of action and different potencies for each site (Table 67–1).

In Vivo Versus In Vitro Effects

Because CCBs have multiple sites of action with different potencies, their net physiologic effect in intact systems may be very different than in experimental preparations. For example, because these agents are both negative inotropes **and** vasodilators, they may produce no change in cardiac output. Compensatory responses of the autonomic nervous system to vasodilation may offset negative electro-

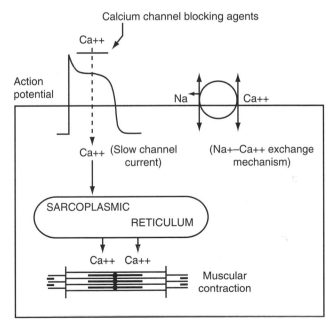

Figure 67–1. Schematic representation of calcium influx during the plateau phase of ventricular depolarization and "calcium-triggered" calcium release from sarcoplasmic reticulum initiating muscular contraction. Calcium channel blocking drugs block Ca^{2+} influx during the plateau phase of the action potential. The Na^+-Ca^{2+} exchange mechanism also regulates cellular Ca^{2+} levels. (From Kates R.)

Table 67–1. Cardiovascular Effects of Calcium Antagonists

	Diltiazem	Verapamil	Dihydropyridines	Bepridil
Coronary vasodilation	Increase	Increase	Increase	Increase
Systemic vasodilation	Increase	Increase	Increase strongly	Increase
Myocardial contraction	Decrease	Decrease strongly	No effect or decrease	No effect or decrease
Myocardial oxygen demand	Decrease	Decrease	Decrease	Decrease
Heart rate	Decrease strongly	Decrease	No effect or increase	Decrease
Atrioventricular nodal conduction	Decrease	Decrease strongly	No effect	No effect or decrease

From Weiner DA.

physiologic or inotropic effects. Because of heterogeneity of the Ca^{2+} channels and the CCBs, their net physiologic effect may differ greatly at high doses versus low doses.

Net pharmacodynamic effect is thus the result of direct tissue effects and reflex responses. Their profiles will be affected by sympathetic tone and the presence of other compounds with cardiovascular activity.

Bepridil, a new type of Ca^{2+} antagonist, has antianginal, antihypertensive, and type 1 antiarrhythmic properties. These type I actions make bepridil contraindicated in patients with conduction system disease. Moreover, bepridil has been associated with torsades de pointes in patients with long QT syndrome. As such, it is used only as a second-line agent.

Interaction with Volatile Agents

Halothane and enflurane are primarily negative inotropes, whereas isoflurane is primarily a vasodilator. In cardiac muscle, the volatile anesthetics profoundly decrease intracellular Ca^{2+} availability, although they may also alter Ca^{2+} binding to regulatory proteins. Ca^{2+} physiology is less well understood in smooth muscle. Thus, volatile agents augment the negative inotropic, dromotropic, and vasodilatory effects of CCBs.

Volatile agents also attenuate sympathetic tone and may significantly impair normally compensatory physiologic responses. These effects are more profound with acute administration and in the presence of impaired left ventricular function, conduction system disorders, autonomic dysfunction, or other pharmacologic agents.

Miscellaneous Effects

CCBs have the potential to impair neuromuscular function and may augment the effects of both depolarizing and nondepolarizing neuromuscular blockers. The mechanism may be through CCB inhibition of Na^+ flux through fast Na^+ channels, the same mechanism thought to be responsible for verapamil's local anesthetic effects. These agents also have antiaggregatory effects on platelets.

Verapamil and nifedipine both decrease lower esophageal sphincter tone and have been used to treat esophageal spasm. Nifedipine has been shown to decrease pulmonary vascular resistance and systemic vascular resistance. It probably impairs hypoxic pulmonary vasoconstriction, especially in the presence of volatile anesthetics. Nimodipine has been approved to treat vasospasm in patients after subarachnoid hemorrhage. CCBs, like nitrates, can significantly increase intracranial pressure.

Suggested References

Jenkins LC, Scoates PJ. Anaesthetic implications of calcium channel blockers. Can J Anesth 1985;32:436.

Kates R. Antianginal drug therapy. In Kaplan JA, ed. Cardiac Anesthesia. 2nd ed. New York: Grune and Stratton, 1987:451.

Royster RL, Zvara DA. Anti-ischemic drug therapy. In Kaplan JA, Reich DL, Konstadt SN, eds. Cardiac Anesthesia. 4th ed. Philadelphia: WB Saunders, 1999:114–123.

Salvador A, Del Pozo E, Carlos R, Baeyens JM. Differential effects of calcium channel blocking agents on pancuronium and suxamethonium-induced neuromuscular blockage. Br J Anaesth 1988;60:495.

Stoelting RK. Calcium Channel Blockers. In Stoelting RK ed. Pharmacology and Physiology in Anesthetic Practice. 3rd ed. Philadelphia: Lippincott-Raven, 1998:344–356.

van Zwieten PA. Protective effects of calcium antagonists in different organs and tissues. Am Heart J 1993;125:566.

Weiner DA. Calcium antagonists in the treatment of ischemic heart disease: Angina pectoris. Coron Artery Dis 1994;5:14–20.

68
Monoamine Oxidase Inhibitors and Anesthesia

Mary B. Jedd, M.D.

Monoamine oxidase (MAO) inhibitors are a heterogeneous group of drugs that prevent deactivation of naturally occurring biologically active amines. MAO inhibitors are used in the treatment of hypertension, narcolepsy, chronic headache, and severe depression unresponsive to tricyclic and other antidepressants. Examples include phenelzine (Nardil), isocarboxazid (Marplan), iproniazid, tranylcypromine (Parnate), pargyline (Eutonyl), clorgyline, and deprenyl. These drugs have the potential for serious adverse drug interactions, especially during anesthesia.

Mechanism of Action

MAO is a general term for a group of mitochondrial enzymes distributed widely throughout the body. Intraneuronal MAO is the main enzyme involved in the oxidative deamination of amine neurotransmitters such as epinephrine, norepinephrine, dopamine, and serotonin. By inhibiting this enzyme, MAO inhibitors increase intraneuronal transmitter pools. On depolarization, an increased amount of neurotransmitter is released into the synaptic cleft, resulting in augmented postsynaptic depolarization and adrenergic stimulation. This is the speculated mechanism of action for the antidepressant effects of MAO inhibitors in the central nervous system.

MAO inhibitors are classified as hydrazine or nonhydrazine derivatives, with further subdivision based on differences in substrate preferences. MAO-A preferentially deaminates dopamine and the neurotransmitters clinically relevant in psychiatric disorders, serotonin and norepinephrine. Theoretically, the use of selective MAO inhibitors for type A could reduce the incidence rate of adverse side effects.

Side Effects

The main side effects are related to inhibition of MAO in the liver and gastrointestinal tract and to altered sympathetic nervous system activity.

Orthostatic Hypotension. Orthostatic hypotension is the most common serious side effect of MAO inhibitor therapy. Orthostatic hypotension can occur with administration of any MAO inhibitor and may reflect accumulation of octopamine, a false neurotransmitter. Octopamine is less active than norepinephrine and results in decreased sympathetic nervous system activity.

Tyramine-Induced Hypertension. Because MAO inhibitors impair the deactivation of tyramine, ingestion of tyramine-containing foods (e.g., some cheeses, chianti wine, chocolate, liver, fava beans, avocados) may result in a hypertensive crisis by evoking the release of endogenous catecholamines present in excessive amounts.

Interaction with Sympathomimetics. MAO inhibitors exaggerate the actions of indirect-acting and, to a lesser extent, direct-acting sympathomimetics. To treat hypotension, a reduced dose (one-third the usual dose) of a direct-acting sympathomimetic such as phenylephrine is recommended.[1]

Interaction with Opioids. Administration of opioids to patients taking MAO inhibitors has resulted in two forms of adverse reactions, excitatory and depressive. The excitatory reaction is thought to be from central serotonergic overactivity manifesting as hypertension, hypotension, tachycardia, diaphoresis, hyperthermia, muscle rigidity, seizures, and coma. Meperidine (Demerol), which blocks neuronal uptake of 5-hydroxytryptamine, has been associated with fatal excitatory reactions. Adverse reactions have also been reported in patients on MAO inhibitors who were given fentanyl,[2] alfentanil, or sufentanil. The depressive form is due to accumulation of free narcotic and comprises respiratory depression, hypotension, and coma. Other opioids may also be associated with this depressive reaction.

Inhibition of Hepatic Enzymes. Inhibition of hepatic enzymes has been proposed as an explanation for the exaggerated depressant effects of opioids, barbiturates, antihistamines, anticholinergics, and tricyclic antidepressants.

Hepatotoxicity. The use of hydrazine-containing compounds has been greatly limited because of their hepatotoxicity.

Management of Anesthesia

Traditionally, discontinuation of MAO inhibitors is recommended at least 14 to 21 days before elective surgery, to allow regeneration of these enzymes (because inhibition of MAO is often irreversible). On the other hand, it has also been suggested that "discontinuation of chronic MAO inhibitor therapy prior to surgery is not necessary."[3] MAO inhibitors are often used as a therapy of last resort in severe psychiatric conditions, and it may be unreasonable to compromise the patient's status by discontinuing them. This is still a point of controversy, and the decision whether to discontinue MAO inhibitors before elective surgery should be guided by the patient's dependence on these drugs. For emergency surgery, or when MAO inhibitor therapy cannot be discontinued, conduct of anesthesia should be adjusted accordingly.

Opioids are best avoided in the preoperative and intraoperative periods and titrated carefully in the postoperative period, with close monitoring for adverse effects. Morphine has been considered the preferred narcotic, and meperidine should be avoided. These patients are excellent candidates for postoperative analgesia with regional block procedures.

Barbiturates and benzodiazepines are acceptable, keeping in mind that central nervous system and respiratory depression may be exaggerated.

Because of the risk of decreased plasma cholinesterase activity (the reason for which is not understood), neuromuscular monitoring should be performed when succinylcholine is used.

Nitrous oxide and volatile agents are acceptable, but preexisting liver disease should be considered when selecting a volatile agent. Requirements for volatile agents are increased in animals, presumably because of accumulation of norepinephrine in the central nervous system. This is a theoretical but unproven concern for humans.

Because undue stimulation of the sympathetic nervous system may be hazardous, ketamine and pancuronium should be avoided.

Selected References

1. Well DG, Bjorksten AR. Monoamine oxidase inhibitors revisited. Can J Anaesth 1989;36:64–74.
2. Noble WH. MAO inhibitors and coronary artery surgery: A patient death. Can J Anaesth 1962;39:1061.
3. El-Ganzouri AR, Ivankovick A, Braverman B, McCarthy R. Monoamine oxidase inhibitors: Should they be discontinued preoperatively? Anesth Analg 1985;64:592–596.

Suggested References

Stack CG, Rogers P, Linter SPR. Monoamine oxidase inhibitors and anaesthesia. A review. Br J Anaesth 1988;60:222.
Stoelting RK. Drugs used for psychopharmacologic therapy. In Stoelting RK, ed. Pharmacology and Physiology in Anesthetic Practice. 3rd ed. Philadelphia: Lippincott-Raven, 1998:364–367.

69
Benzodiazepines

Mary B. Jedd, M.D.

Benzodiazepines cause sedation, anxiolysis, muscle relaxation, and anterograde amnesia and have anticonvulsant effects.[1] They are frequently prescribed for a variety of indications and are useful in the operative and perioperative periods. Benzodiazepines act by facilitating the actions of γ-aminobutyric acid (GABA). Fatigue and drowsiness are common side effects.

Midazolam

Midazolam is a short-acting, water-soluble benzodiazepine with sedative, anxiolytic, amnesic, and anticonvulsant properties. Midazolam is two to three times as potent as diazepam. Midazolam is commonly used for preoperative sedation, conscious sedation during surgery, and induction or supplementation of general anesthesia.

Pharmacology

Midazolam causes practically no local irritation after injection and can be mixed with other drugs commonly used for premedication. Like diazepam, it is highly bound to plasma proteins. Rapid redistribution from the brain to other tissues and rapid metabolism by the liver account for the short duration of action.

Metabolism

Midazolam is hydroxylated in the liver to two hydroxylated derivatives that are excreted by the kidney after conjugation. These metabolites are active, but their clinical significance is not established. Elimination half-life of midazolam is 1 to 4 hours.

Effects on Organ Systems

Cardiovascular. An intravenous midazolam dose of 0.2 mg/kg produces an increase in heart rate and decrease in blood pressure similar to that of an induction dose of thiopental (3 to 4 mg/kg).

Respiratory. Ventilation is depressed by 0.015 mg/kg of midazolam, especially in patients with COPD.[1] Transient apnea may occur, especially when midazolam is given in conjunction with opioids.

Central Nervous System. Administration of midazolam results in dose-related decreases in cerebral blood flow and cerebral oxygen consumption.

Placenta. Midazolam crosses the placenta and enters the fetal circulation. Its effects on the fetus are not known.

Diazepam

Diazepam is a water-insoluble benzodiazepine useful for treatment of seizures, preoperative anxiolysis, intravenous sedation, skeletal muscle relaxation, and induction and maintenance of general anesthesia.

Pharmacology

Because of its insolubility in water, diazepam is dissolved in propylene glycol and sodium benzoate and may cause pain when injected intravenously or intramuscularly. Diazepam is taken up rapidly into the brain because of its high lipid solubility and then redistributed extensively to other tissues. Diazepam is highly protein bound; thus, diseases associated with decreased albumin concentration may increase its effects.

Metabolism

Diazepam is metabolized by hepatic microsomal enzymes producing two main metabolites, desmethyldiazepam and oxazepam. Desmethyldiazepam is slightly less potent than diazepam and is metabolized more slowly, contributing to sustained effects. Elimination half-life ranges from 21 to 37 hours in healthy persons and increases progressively with age and markedly in the presence of cirrhosis. The elimination half-life of desmethyldiazepam is 48 to 96 hours.

Effects on Organ Systems

Cardiovascular. Diazepam given in intravenous doses of 0.3 to 0.5 mg/kg results in mild reductions in blood pressure, peripheral vascular resistance, and cardiac output.[1] Occasionally, hypotension will occur after even small doses of diazepam.

Respiratory. Diazepam causes a depression of the slope of the ventilatory response to CO_2, but the CO_2 response curve is not shifted to the right as it is after opioid administration. Occasionally, small doses of diazepam may result in apnea.

Skeletal Muscle. Diazepam reduces skeletal muscle tone through its action on spinal internuncial neurons.

Anticonvulsant Activity. Diazepam (0.1 mg/kg) abolishes seizure activity in status epilepticus and alcohol withdrawal, although the effect is short-lived. It also increases the threshold for local anesthetic induced seizure activity.

Placenta. Diazepam crosses the placenta easily. An increased risk of congenital malformations has been associated with the use of diazepam during pregnancy.

Tolerance

Abrupt discontinuation of diazepam after prolonged administration of high doses may result in symptoms of withdrawal, including anxiety, hyperexcitability, and convulsions.

Lorazepam

Lorazepam is a relatively long-acting benzodiazepine that is a more potent amnesic than diazepam or midazolam.[2] Its cardiovascular, ventilatory, and muscle relaxant effects resemble those of diazepam and midazolam. Its elimination half-life is 10 to 20 hours. Lorazepam is used clinically for preoperative sedation and anterograde amnesia but is seldom used for induction of anesthesia or intravenous sedation, because of its slow onset.

Other Benzodiazepines

Oxazepam, clonazepam, flurazepam, temazepam, triazolam, and quazepam are benzodiazepines used most commonly to treat insomnia.

Selected References

1. Aston A. Guidelines for the rational use of benzodiazepines: When and what to use. Drugs 1995;48:25–40.
2. Stoelting RK. Benzodiazepines. In Stoelting RK. Pharmacology and Physiology in Anesthetic Practice. 3rd ed. Philadelphia: Lippincott-Raven, 1998:126–139.

Suggested Reference

Reves JG, Glass PSA, Lubarsky DA. Nonbarbiturate intravenous anesthetics. In Miller RD, ed. Anesthesia. 5th ed. Philadelphia: Churchill Livingstone, 2000:228–237.

70
Antiemetic Agents

Thomas J. Christopherson, M.D.

Emesis is a complex reflex coordinated by the vomiting center in the medulla. Stimuli are relayed to this center via several pathways (Fig. 70–1). The chemoreceptor trigger zone (CRTZ) has a high density of dopaminergic receptors that are stimulated by drugs and metabolic disturbances. Impulses from the CRTZ are subsequently relayed to the vomiting center, and a reflex is initiated. Several medullary nuclei are in close approximation to the vomiting center, which accounts for the associated physiologic reactions observed with vomiting (i.e., vasomotor, respiratory, and salivary reactions).

Butyrophenones (Haloperidol [Haldol], Droperidol [Inapsine])

Mechanism of Action. Butyrophenones are powerful antiemetic agents by virtue of their inhibition of dopaminergic receptors in the CRTZ.

Clinical Trials. Numerous trials have demonstrated droperidol to be efficacious in both preventing and treating postoperative nausea and vomiting, not only in the adult population, but also in the pediatric age group undergoing ophthalmic procedures.[1,2]

Side Effects. Intravenous droperidol may result in a prolonged recovery room stay secondary to excessive sedation. Droperidol has also been associated with acute extrapyramidal reactions.

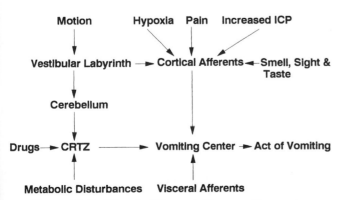

Figure 70–1. Stimuli of the medullary vomiting center.

Metoclopramide (Reglan)

Mechanism of Action. Metoclopramide is a dopaminergic receptor antagonist, eliciting its effect at the vomiting center and the CRTZ. Metoclopramide is also a selective peripheral cholinergic agonist that stimulates upper gastrointestinal motility, thereby enhancing gastric emptying.

Clinical Trials. The efficacy of metoclopramide as an antiemetic has received mixed reviews, ranging from clinical trials describing no nausea or vomiting following oral administration in female patients undergoing laparoscopy[3] to reports of no benefit (in comparison to controls) in decreasing the incidence rate of postoperative nausea and vomiting.[4]

Side Effects. Extrapyramidal reactions, sedation, and diarrhea are potential concerns for patients treated with metoclopramide.

Phenothiazines (Chlorpromazine [Thorazine], Prochlorperazine [Compazine])

Mechanism of Action. Phenothiazines exert antiemetic effects by virtue of their antagonism of the dopaminergic receptors in the CRTZ.

Side Effects. Prominent extrapyramidal reactions are often seen, especially when the piperazine phenothiazines (e.g., Compazine) are used. Sedation, mucosal dryness, and orthostatic hypotension can also occur, especially with the aliphatic phenothiazines (e.g., Thorazine).

Trimethobenzamide (Tigan)

Mechanism of Action. Trimethobenzamide exerts antiemetic effects by inhibiting stimulation of the CRTZ.

Side Effects. Trimethobenzamide has a low incidence rate of adverse reactions.

Domperidone (Motilium)

Mechanism of Action. Domperidone retards nausea and vomiting by increasing lower esophageal sphincter tone and increasing gastric emptying. It also is a dopamine receptor antagonist, but it fails to cross the blood-brain barrier.

Concerns. Domperidone is effective for treating nausea and vomiting associated with gastroenteritis. However, no clinical trials have been able to show its ability to effectively treat postoperative nausea and vomiting, perhaps related to its inability to cross the blood-brain barrier.

Anticholinergic Agents

Mechanism of Action. Anticholinergic agents inhibit nausea and vomiting by reducing the excitability of labyrinth receptors, thus depressing conduction via the vestibular-cerebellar pathways.

Concerns. Clinical trials using transdermal scopolamine have received increasing attention. Although the use of transdermal scopolamine in treating motion sickness has been widely accepted, its ability to treat or prevent postoperative emesis remains uncertain.

Antihistamines (Dimenhydrinate [Dramamine], Meclizine [Antivert])

Mechanism of Action. H_1 antihistamines act similarly to the anticholinergic agents, suppressing transmission of neuronal impulses originating in the labyrinth. They are used primarily to treat or prevent motion sickness.

Serotonin Receptor Antagonist (Ondansetron)

Mechanism of Action. Ondansetron is a selective serotonin 5-HT3–type receptor antagonist.

Clinical Applications. Ondansetron is highly effective in controlling emesis occurring after chemotherapy, somewhat effective in radiation-induced emesis and postoperative emesis, and ineffective in motion sickness.

Conclusion

Postoperative nausea and vomiting are only indications of altered function; they are not diseases. Rational therapy therefore depends on diagnosis of the underlying disorder and may or may not include medications.

Selected References

1. Valanne J, Korttila K. Effect of a small dose of droperidol on nausea, vomiting, and recovery after outpatient enflurane anesthesia. Acta Anaesth Scand 1985;29:359.
2. Lerman J, Eustis S, Smith DR. Effect of droperidol pretreatment on postanesthetic vomiting in children undergoing strabismus surgery. Anesthesiology 1986;65:322–325.
3. Rao TLK, Suseela M, El-Etr AA. Metoclopramide and cimetidine to reduce gastric juice pH volume. Anesth Analg 1984;63:264.
4. Pandit SK, Kothary SP, Pandit UA, et al. Dose-response study of droperidol and metoclopramide as antiemetics for outpatient anesthesia. Anesth Analg 1989;68:798–802.

71
Anti-Aspiration Drugs

Mary B. Weber, M.D.

In an attempt to reduce morbidity and mortality from aspiration pneumonitis, various drugs are used to alter the volume and/or acidity of gastric fluid contents. The most important factor determining the severity of aspiration pneumonitis is the acidity of the aspirate. The greater the acidity, the greater the damage to tracheal mucosa and lung parenchyma. With pH above 2.5, recovery appears to be faster, although the initial physiologic insult may be as severe as pneumonitis caused by aspiration of gastric contents with a pH below 2.5. The volume of aspirate also affects the severity of lung parenchymal damage; damage is more severe if the volume of aspirate is 0.4 mL/kg or more. Several classes of drugs may assist the anesthesiologist in manipulating gastric fluid contents.

Metoclopramide (Reglan)

Metoclopramide is a dopamine antagonist useful for reducing gastric fluid volume by increasing lower esophageal sphincter tone, speeding gastric emptying time, and acting as an antiemetic. It has no known effect on gastric fluid pH. A selective peripheral cholinergic agonist, metoclopramide facilitates the action of acetylcholine on the proximal gastrointestinal (GI) tract, and its gastrokinetic effect is opposed by atropine and opioids. Its effect is variable depending on the basal state of GI motility. Its gastrokinetic effect could be useful before the induction of anesthesia in outpatients, obese patients, trauma patients, parturients, and patients with a full stomach.

Metoclopramide may be given orally or parenterally. After an oral dose of 10 mg, onset of action occurs within 30 to 60 minutes and peak plasma concentrations are achieved in 40 to 120 minutes. Onset of action is 1 to 3 minutes after intravenous administration. Rapid intravenous administration may produce abdominal cramping, which can be prevented by giving it over 3 to 5 minutes. The elimination half-life is 2 to 4 hours. About 85% of the drug is excreted in the urine, either unchanged or as glucoronide or sulfate conjugates.

Metoclopramide blocks dopamine receptors in the central nervous system, thereby inducing secretion of prolactin and creating the possibility of extrapyramidal symptoms from large doses given chronically. Other side effects include sedation, dysphoria, rash, and dry mouth. Metoclopramide should be avoided in the presence of pheochromocytoma or GI obstruction and in patients taking monoamine oxidase inhibitors, tricyclic antidepressants, or other drugs that may cause extrapyramidal symptoms.

Antacids

Antacids increase gastric fluid pH by neutralizing or removing acid from gastric fluid. Antacids consist of magnesium, aluminum, and calcium salts that react with hydrochloric acid. By raising gastric fluid pH, antacids increase gastric motility. Lower esophageal sphincter tone increases after the administration of calcium and magnesium salts.

Disadvantages of **particulate antacids** include incomplete mixing with gastric fluid, making them less effective in increasing the pH of gastric fluid. The aspiration of antacid particles can cause as severe an insult as that resulting from an acidic aspirate. This can lead to the chronic functional and histologic changes associated with a foreign body reaction.

Preparations of particulate antacids include the following:

- Aluminum hydroxide. In contrast to other antacids, this slows gastric emptying and causes constipation.
- Calcium carbonate. Patients with renal disease taking this antacid may develop hypercalcemia.
- Magnesium oxide. Absorption of magnesium may be dangerous in patients with renal disease.
- Sodium bicarbonate. Systemic alkalosis may occur.

Nonparticulate or soluble antacids offer certain advantages. They mix with gastric contents more easily. Aspiration of soluble antacids is associated with faster recovery and is less likely to cause a foreign body reaction. Available preparations include sodium citrate; Bicitra, which contains sodium citrate and citric acid; and Polycitra, which contains sodium citrate, potassium citrate, and citric acid.

Histamine (H₂) Blockers

The H_2-receptor antagonists block histamine-induced secretion of acid by the gastric parietal cells. They reduce the risk of aspiration by raising gastric pH.

Cimetidine (Tagamet)

Cimetidine is used to treat or prevent peptic ulcer disease, especially that associated with excess gastric acid secretion. Administration of cimetidine before the induction of anesthesia increases gastric pH and is used preoperatively to reduce the risk of aspiration pneumonitis. Cimetidine may be given prophylactically along with H_1-receptor antagonists and steroids to patients susceptible to an allergic reaction associated with certain procedures or exposures, such as dye or chymopapain. It may be useful for preventing loss of acid and subsequent alkalosis in patients undergoing prolonged nasogastric suctioning.

Cimetidine may be administered intramuscularly, intravenously, or orally. After an oral dose, cimetidine is absorbed from the small intestine and achieves peak plasma concentrations in 60 to 90 minutes. Cimetidine given intravenously requires 45 to 60 minutes to take effect. Therapeutic effects last for approximately 4 to 7 hours regardless of the route of administration.

Cimetidine produces a large number of side effects. By binding to microsomal cytochrome P-450 enzymes and inhibiting enzyme function and by reducing hepatic blood flow, cimetidine reduces the clearance of many drugs that undergo oxidative degradation. These include lidocaine, propranolol, diazepam, theophylline, caffeine, warfarin anticoagulants, phenobarbital, phenytoin, and others. Benzodiazepines eliminated by glucuronidation are not affected.

Because cimetidine crosses the blood-brain barrier, it can produce central nervous system dysfunction such as agitation, confusion, convulsions, coma, and delayed awakening from anesthesia. Cardiopulmonary changes reflect inhibition of H_2 receptors in other organs. Cardiovascular effects include hypotension from peripheral vasodilation, bradycardia, heart block, and cardiac arrest after rapid intravenous administration to ill patients. Because it blocks H_2-receptor–mediated bronchodilation, cimetidine may predispose to bronchoconstriction in the asthmatic patient.

Prolonged elevation of gastric fluid pH and impaired acid reduction capabilities in the stomach may predispose to overgrowth of other organisms. Other adverse effects include occasional mild increases in serum transaminase or alkaline phosphatase levels, transient serum creatinine elevation, neutropenia, thrombocytopenia, and gynecomastia and impotence from antagonism of androgen receptors.

Ranitidine (Zantac)

Ranitidine, the second H_2-receptor antagonist introduced, has a furan structure and is four to eight times more potent than cimetidine in inhibiting acid secretion. Like the other H_2 blockers, ranitidine does not affect lower esophageal sphincter tone or gastric emptying time. After an oral dose of 150 mg, peak plasma concentrations are achieved in 30 to 60 minutes with a duration of action of about 8 to 12 hours. Ranitidine also may be given parenterally. About one-half of the drug is excreted unchanged by the kidneys, and about one-fourth undergoes hepatic metabolism. The elimination half-life is 2 to 3 hours. Ranitidine is less likely than cimetidine to produce side effects. Because of poor entrance into the central nervous system, it also is less likely to produce central nervous system dysfunction. Although ranitidine does decrease hepatic blood flow, it has much less effect than cimetidine on the metabolism of those drugs metabolized by the cytochrome P-450 system.

Famotidine (Pepcid)

Famotidine (Pepcid) is the most potent highly competitive H_2-receptor antagonist available and has the longest duration of action. After an oral dose of 40 mg, peak plasma concentrations are reached in 2 hours, with a plasma half-life of 3 to 3.5 hours. Famotidine also may be given parenterally. Metabolism and excretion of famotidine are similar to that of other H_2-receptor antagonists, with 60% to 70% excreted unchanged in the urine. Several large studies revealed a prevalence rate of side effects of 1.2% to 2%.

Nizatidine (Axid)

Nizatidine (Axid) is an H_2-receptor antagonist with a potency similar to that of ranitidine. The plasma half-life is 1.5 to 2 hours. About 60% to 65% is excreted unchanged in the urine. A large study revealed no clinically important adverse reactions.

Proton Pump Inhibitors

Gastric acid pump inhibitors consist of a family of substituted benzimidazoles, including omeprazole (Prilosec) and lansoprazole (Prevacid). These drugs are converted to active metabolites that irreversibly inhibit Ht/Kt ATPase, an enzyme on the surface of gastric parietal cells. Gastric acid production is suppressed, thereby increasing gastric pH. Omeprazole 20 mg can be given orally 2 to 4 hours before surgery. The effects can last up to 24 hours.

Suggested References

American Society of Anesthesiologists Task Force on Preoperative Fasting. Practice guidelines for preoperative fasting and the use of pharmacologic agents to reduce the risk of pulmonary aspiration: Application to healthy patients undergoing elective procedures. Anesthesiology 1999;90:896–905.

Goodman, G. The Pharmacologic Basis of Therapeutics. 9th ed. New York, McGraw-Hill, 1995.

Kallar SK, Everett LL. Potential risks and preventive measures for pulmonary aspiration: New concepts in preoperative fasting guidelines. Anesth Analg 1993;77:171–182.

McCammon RL. Prophylaxis for aspiration pneumonitis. Can J Anaesth 1986;33:47.

Moyers JR. Preoperative medication. In Barash PG, Cullen BF, Stoelting RK, eds. Clinical Anesthesia. 3rd ed. Philadelphia: Lippincott-Raven, 1996:519–533.

Pounder R. Histamine H_2-receptor antagonists. Bailliere's Clin Gastroenterol 1988;2:593.

Schunack W. Pharmacology of H_2-receptor antagonists: An overview. J Int Med Res 1989;17:9A–16A.

Stoelting RK. Pharmacology and Physiology in Anesthesia Practice. 3rd ed. Philadelphia, Lippincott-Raven, 1998.

72
Diuretics

Thomas N. Spackman, M.D.

Diuretic medications are commonly used in the treatment of fluid overload conditions, such as congestive heart failure and pulmonary edema. Diuretics are some of the most commonly prescribed medications in this country for the treatment of hypertension. Diuretics are classified on the basis of their site of action in the nephron (Fig. 72–1). Diuresis by definition is "an increase in sodium loss from the kidney."[1]

Mannitol

Mannitol is an osmotic diuretic that causes water to be drawn intravascularly from the tissues. It is excreted unchanged in the urine and produces a greater flow rate through the lumen of the nephron, resulting in reduced efficiency of sodium reabsorption and significant diuresis. The osmotic diuresis can lead to volume depletion and electrolyte imbalances, especially of sodium, potassium, and magnesium. Oral absorption is unreliable. The intravenous (IV) dose range is 0.25 to 1.0 g/kg over 15 to 30 minutes.

In patients with elevated intracranial pressure (ICP), mannitol can decrease ICP within 30 minutes, with maximum effect within 1 to 2 hours and duration of effect of approximately 6 hours. Mannitol is also frequently used in an attempt to prevent acute tubular necrosis and to preserve renal function in aortic or renal artery revascularizations.

Thiazides

Thiazides reduce the reabsorption of sodium and chloride primarily in the distal convoluted tubule and also in part of the cortical ascending limb of the loop of Henle. Water follows the unreabsorbed salt, causing the diuresis. Because the distal convoluted tubule accounts for only 5% or less of the total sodium reabsorption, the diuretic effect is much weaker than that of loop diuretics.

Thiazides are rapidly and effectively absorbed from the gastrointestinal tract. They reach their peak action within a few hours and exert a diuretic effect for up to 12 hours. Thiazides are most commonly used to treat hypertension.

The most common side effects of thiazides (as well as most diuretics) are dehydration and hypokalemia. Because hypokalemia can potentiate digoxin toxicity, this must be monitored in patients on both medications. Side effects unique to thiazides include hypercalcemia and hyperuricemia from decreased renal excretion of calcium and uric acid. Other potential side effects include hyponatremia, hypomagnesemia, metabolic alkalosis, fatigue, lethargy, carbohydrate intolerance, hypersensitivity reactions, purpura, and dermatitis with photosensitivity.

Potassium-Sparing Diuretics

Spironolactone is an aldosterone antagonist. Its site of action is the distal half of the convoluted

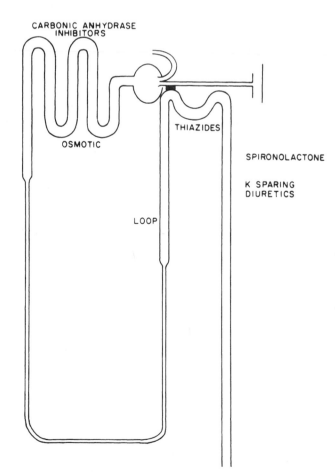

Figure 72–1. Schematic diagram of the nephron, which indicates the sites of action of different diuretics. (From Branch RA.[1])

tubule and the cortical portion of the collecting duct. A sodium diuresis is produced as a result of competitive inhibition of aldosterone that blocks the exchange between sodium and both potassium and hydrogen in the distal tubule and collecting duct. Excessive loss of potassium is prevented. Spironolactone has no effect if aldosterone is absent.

In contrast, **triamterene** and **amiloride** do not depend on the presence of aldosterone, even though they exert a similar action in the nephron. All three of these relatively weak diuretics are more effective when used with a thiazide or loop diuretic, which acts more proximally in the nephron.

Spironolactone is most commonly used in patients with ascites from cirrhosis with secondary hyperaldosteronism. Side effects include dehydration, electrolyte imbalance (possible hyperkalemia in renal impairment), nausea with higher doses, and gynecomastia in men as a result of the steroid structure.

Acetazolamide

Acetazolamide acts in the proximal tubule as a potent inhibitor of carbonic anhydrase, which reduces the supply of hydrogen ions in the proximal and distal tubules. More than 90% of filtered bicarbonate is reabsorbed in the proximal tubule via an exchange with hydrogen. Because sodium is normally reabsorbed in exchange for hydrogen, more sodium and bicarbonate remain within the tubules. A diuresis is produced by the sodium excretion, and the urine is alkaline from the bicarbonate. Acetazolamide is a weak diuretic, because its proximal site of action accounts for only a small percentage of the total filtered sodium absorbed.

Acetazolamide can be administered orally or intravenously. Peak plasma levels occur within a few hours when taken orally. There is no appreciable metabolism, and elimination is usually complete in 24 hours.

Acetazolamide is used to induce an alkaline urine in certain drug overdoses (e.g., salicylates). It is also used to treat glaucoma, acute mountain sickness, and significant metabolic alkalosis.

Side effects common to other diuretics are infrequent, because acetazolamide is a weaker diuretic. Patients on chronic therapy for glaucoma can present with a metabolic acidosis. Large dosages can lead to paresthesias and drowsiness.

Loop Diuretics

Furosemide, bumetanide, ethacrynic acid, piretanide, and **torsemide** are classified as loop diuretics because of their action to inhibit the reabsorption of electrolytes in the thick ascending loop of Henle. They also exert a direct effect on electrolyte transport in the proximal tubule and cause renal cortical vasodilation and increased renal blood flow (RBF). The potent diuresis results in enhanced excretion of Na^+, Cl^-, K^+, H^+, Ca^{2+}, Mg^{2+}, NH_4^-, and HCO_3^-. Cl^- excretion exceeds Na^+ excretion. Excessive losses of K^+, H^+, NH_4^-, and Cl^-, as well as rapid contraction of extracellular fluid volume, may result in metabolic alkalosis.

A temporary but substantial decrease in glomerular filtration rate, along with decreased pulmonary vascular resistance and increased peripheral venous capacitance, occur after IV administration of furosemide in patients with congestive heart failure. This decreases left ventricular filling pressures, an acute action occurring before the onset of diuresis.

All five drugs are rapidly absorbed from the gastrointestinal tract and are excreted mostly in the urine with small amounts metabolized in the liver. After IV administration of furosemide, diuresis occurs within 5 minutes, reaches a maximum within 20 to 60 minutes, and persists for approximately 2 hours.

Too vigorous a diuresis may induce an acute hypotensive episode. Potassium depletion can predispose to digoxin toxicity and prolonged neuromuscular blockade in patients receiving nondepolarizing neuromuscular blocking agents. Hyperuricemia is common. Gastrointestinal disturbance (including bleeding), marrow depression, hepatic dysfunction, rashes, and decreased carbohydrate tolerance (furosemide may interfere with hypoglycemic effect of insulin) also have been reported. Ethacrynic acid and bumetanide have been associated with hearing loss, and ethacrynic acid is associated with a higher incidence rate of gastrointestinal disturbance than furosemide. Congenital abnormalities have been reported in animals; thus, furosemide should be avoided in pregnancy. Patients receiving chronic anticonvulsant therapy have a reduced diuretic response, and it is postulated that renal sensitivity to furosemide is diminished by these drugs. Allergic interstitial nephritis leading to reversible renal failure has been attributed to furosemide. Competition for binding sites on albumin may lead to an increased effect of drugs such as warfarin and clofibrate.

Selected Reference

1. Branch RA. Diuretics. In Wood M, Wood AJJ, eds. Drugs and Anesthesia: Pharmacology for Anesthesiologists. 2nd ed. Baltimore: Williams & Wilkins, 1990:493.

Suggested References

Braunwald E. Heart failure. In Fauci AS, Braunwald E, Isselbacher KJ, et al, eds. Harrison's Principles of Internal Medicine. 14th ed. New York: McGraw-Hill, 1998:1287.
Jackson EK. Diuretics. In Hardman JG, Limbird LE, eds. Goodman and Gilman's The Pharmacological Basis of Therapeutics. 9th ed. New York: McGraw-Hill, 1996:685.
Stoelting RK. Pharmacology and Physiology in Anesthetic Practice. 3rd ed. Philadelphia, Lippincott-Raven, 1998.

73
Bronchodilators

Scott A. Lockwood, M.D.

Three major classes of bronchodilators are used to treat bronchoconstriction: β agonists, methylxanthines, and anticholinergics.

β-Agonists

The effects of sympathomimetics are thought to be mediated by cyclic adenosine monophosphate (cAMP). Selective $β_2$-agonists dilate bronchioles and uterine smooth muscle without affecting the heart via $β_1$ stimulation. These drugs activate adenylate cyclase, which converts ATP to cAMP, which in turn causes bronchodilation. Nonselective β-agonists used for bronchodilation include epinephrine, isoproterenol, and isoetharine (Bronkosol). Selective $β_2$-agonists include albuterol, terbutaline, metaproterenol, and others (Table 73–1). Side effects associated with the nonselective medications include in-

creased heart rate, contractility, and myocardial oxygen consumption. Selective agonists also may produce some cardiac effects, especially if administered subcutaneously or intravenously. Hypokalemia and hyperglycemia may also occur. Chronic use can be associated with tachyphylaxis.

Therapeutic aerosols may be administered either by a metered-dose inhaler (MDI) or as a wet aerosol from a nebulizer containing the medication. Only particles with an aerodynamic diameter of 1 to 5 μm are efficiently deposited in the lower respiratory tract. Only 13% of the output from MDIs and 1% to 5% of the output from nebulizers reaches the lower respiratory tract.

Epinephrine has both α and β properties. A dose of 0.3 to 0.5 mg given subcutaneously is commonly used to treat acute bronchospasm. The effects are rapid, peaking in 5 to 25 minutes, and improvements in pulmonary function tests are seen for up

Table 73–1. Bronchodilators

Drug	Trade Name(s)	Route	Mechanism of Action
β-Agonists			
Isoproterenol 0.05%	Isuprel	Nebulizer	Prototypical β-agonist, significant $β_1$ side effects
Albuterol 0.5%	Ventolin Proventil	MDI/nebulizer	$β_2$-agonist, increase in cAMP
Isoetharine hydrochloride 1%	Bronkosol	MDI/nebulizer	$β_2$-agonist, increase in cAMP
Metaproterenol sulfate 5%	Alupent Metaprel	MDI/nebulizer/oral	$β_2$-agonist, increase in cAMP
Racemic epinephrine 2.25%	Vaponephrine Racepinephrine	Nebulizer	Weak $β_2$ and mild α mucosal vasoconstrictor
Terbutaline 0.1%	Brethine Bricanyl	Nebulizer/IV	$β_2$-agonist
Methylxanthines			
Aminophylline	Somophyllin	Oral/intravenous	Inhibition of cAMP breakdown by phosphodiesterase (questionable)
Theophylline	TheoDur Theolair		Adenosine antagonism
Anticholinergics			
Atropine sulfate 2% or 5%		Nebulizer	Cholinergic blocker, decreased cGMP
Ipratroprium bromide 0.02%	Atrovent	MDI/nebulizer	Cholinergic blocker, decreased cGMP

cGMP, cyclic guanosine monophosphate.
Adapted from Peruzzi WT, Shapiro BA.

to 4 hours. Side effects include increased heart rate, cardiac output, and systolic blood pressure and decreased diastolic blood pressure and systemic vascular resistance.

Isoproterenol (Isuprel) is the most potent β-agonist of the sympathomimetics. It is effective by the intravenous route and/or by inhalation. However, it has essentially been replaced by selective β2-agents.

Albuterol (Ventolin, Proventil) is a selective β2-agonist that promptly reduces airway resistance for 4 to 6 hours when administered as an aerosol. Cardiac effects are unlikely when the dose is below 400 μg.

Terbutaline (Brethine, Bricanyl) is a selective β2-agonist. A dose of 0.25 mg subcutaneously is an alternative treatment for acute severe bronchospasm when the cardiac effects of epinephrine must be avoided. However, when given subcutaneously, terbutaline will have some β1 effects. When administered subcutaneously, terbutaline may cause ventricular arrhythmias in patients anesthetized with halothane.

Metaproterenol (Alupent) is a selective β2-agonist available as an MDI that can also be given orally. The dose is 1.0 to 1.5 mg via inhaler and is effective for 1 to 4 hours.

Methylxanthines

Theophylline is a poorly soluble methylated xanthine found in high concentrations in tea leaves. Methylxanthines inhibit the breakdown of cAMP by phosphodiesterase. **Aminophylline** is the water-soluble salt of theophylline that can be administered orally (3 to 6 mg/kg) or intravenously (loading dose of 5 mg/kg, followed by 0.5 to 1.0 mg·kg^{-1}·h^{-1}). Therapeutic plasma concentrations of theophylline are between 10 and 20 μg/mL, although levels as low as 5 μg/mL have been clinically effective.

Aminophylline works in vitro by inhibiting phosphodiesterase and thereby cAMP breakdown. Aminophylline's in vivo mechanism is less clear. Anti-inflammatory actions on neutrophils that release mediators that cause bronchospasm, sympathetic stimulation, and adenosine antagonism are possible mechanisms. Aminophylline's narrow therapeutic range and potential for arrhythmias have made its use in the perioperative setting controversial. Theophylline is metabolized principally by the liver, and 10% is excreted unchanged in urine. Smokers metabolize the drug faster than nonsmokers. Heart failure, liver disease, and severe respiratory obstruction all slow the metabolism of theophylline and increase the likelihood of toxicity. Metabolism is slowed by cimetidine and β-adrenergic antagonists.

Theophylline improves pulmonary function and resolves obstruction in asthmatic patients, in a dose-dependent manner. The drug decreases pulmonary vascular resistance and increases cardiac output. Cardiac-stimulating effects are still seen in the presence of β blockade, because xanthines are not receptor dependent. Theophylline and caffeine have been shown to decrease the number and duration of apneic episodes in preterm infants.

Side effects are often seen when plasma levels exceed 20 μg/mL. The most frequent complaint is nausea and vomiting. Seizures may result from toxic levels and are likely with plasma concentrations above 40 μg/mL. Tachycardia and other dysrhythmias may occur with high plasma levels. Theophylline facilitates neuromuscular transmission; thus, there may be an increased requirement for nondepolarizing muscle relaxants.

Anticholinergics

Cholinergic mechanisms play a major role in mediating reflex bronchoconstriction, and anticholinergic drugs may be used to reduce these responses. These medications have been found to be somewhat more effective than β-agonists in some patients with chronic bronchitis and emphysema. In the management of asthma, anticholinergic agents are generally less effective than β-agonists, but in acute asthma, a combination of the two types of agents may produce a greater response. **Atropine** can be given by nebulizer. **Ipratropium** bromide (Atrovent) is a quaternary amine delivered by nebulizer or MDI that is associated with little systemic absorption. Viscosity of secretions may be increased, which may hinder the clearance of secretions from the airway.

Antiallergy Agents

These drugs are also frequently used to treat bronchospastic diseases. Cromolyn sodium works through stabilization of mast cell membranes. Various steroid preparations (e.g., beclomethasone dipropionate, dexamethasone, flunisolide, and triamcinolone) are given via MDI for their anti-inflammatory properties.

Suggested References

Gal TJ. Bronchospasm. In Gravenstein N, Kirby RJ, eds. Complications in Anesthesiology. 2nd ed. Philadelphia: Lippincott-Raven 1996:199–210.

NewHousey MT. Control of asthma by aerosols. N Engl J Med 1986;315:870.

Peruzzi WT, Shapiro BA. Respiratory Care. In Murray MJ, Cousin DB, Pearl RG, Prough DS, eds. Critical Care Medicine: Perioperative Management. Philadelphia: Lippincott-Raven, 1997:467–487.

Shapiro BA, Peruzzi WT. Respiratory Care. In Miller RD, ed. Anesthesia. 5th ed. Philadelphia: Churchill Livingstone. 2000:2403–2442.

Stoelting RK. Pharmacology and Physiology in Anesthetic Practice. 3rd ed. Philadelphia, Lippincott-Raven, 1998.

74
Effect of pKa, pH, and Protein Binding

Mary B. Weber, M.D.

pKa and pH

Most drugs, being weak acids or bases, exist in both the ionized and un-ionized forms. The extent of ionization depends on the pH of the solution and its dissociation constant, pKa. The pKa is defined as the pH at which a compound exists as 50% ionized and 50% un-ionized forms. When the pKa is close to the surrounding pH, smaller changes in pH produce greater changes in the degree of ionization. Basic drugs tend to be highly ionized at a low pH, whereas acidic drugs are highly ionized at a high pH. The Henderson-Hasselbalch equation gives the relationship between pH and pKa:

$$pH - pKa = \log [A-]/[HA] \text{ for an acid}$$

$$pH - pKa = \log [B]/[BH^+] \text{ for a base}$$

where $[A^-]$ is ionized acid concentration, $[HA]$ is un-ionized acid, $[B]$ is un-ionized base, and $[BH^+]$ is the concentration of ionized base.

Un-ionized drug molecules generally are lipid soluble and can traverse the lipid component of cell membranes. Therefore, this fraction is more readily absorbed from the gastrointestinal tract, reabsorbed from renal tubules, and subject to hepatic metabolism.

Ion Trapping

When a pH gradient exists across a membrane, the concentration of total drug may be quite different on each side. The un-ionized fraction traverses the membrane freely and equilibrates. But the ionized form, which cannot cross the membrane, is trapped on the side with a pH that favors ionization. This mechanism is known as ion trapping. For example, the un-ionized fraction of local anesthetic crosses the placenta, where it is changed to the ionized fraction in the relatively acidic fetus. The ionized fraction cannot leave the placenta; un-ionized drug continues to enter the fetal circulation, where it is ionized and maintains a gradient across the placenta.

Protein Binding

Drugs exist in the blood in two forms, either dissolved in plasma or bound to proteins. The two main plasma proteins that bind with drugs are albumin and α-1-acid glycoprotein (AAG), although globulins, lipoproteins, and erythrocytes may bind drugs as well.

Protein binding affects drug distribution and action, because generally only the free portion traverses cell membranes and reaches its site of action. By limiting drug excursion into the tissues, extensive protein binding results in a small calculated volume of distribution. Protein binding influences clearance of drug, because it is the unbound fraction that is available for metabolism and clearance by the liver and kidney.

Drug binding is described by the following equation:

$$K_a = \frac{k_1}{k_2} = \frac{[\text{drug-protein complex}]}{[\text{unbound drug}][\text{protein}]}$$

K_a (the equilibrium association constant) describes the affinity of drug–protein binding.

These reactions occur quite rapidly, with half-lives of a few milliseconds, because the complex is maintained by a weak ionic bond. As unbound drug is eliminated, bound drug immediately dissociates to restore equilibrium.

As a general rule, albumin is the major drug that binds protein in the body, attracting mainly acids, whereas AAG binds many basic drugs, including many narcotics, propranolol, verapamil, quinidine, and amide local anesthetics. Certain drugs (e.g., fentanyl, sufentanil) can bind to both proteins.

The degree of protein binding is higher with drugs having higher lipid solubility. Acid-base disturbances affect drug binding, as do plasma concentrations of the drug in question and available sites for binding.

Changes in protein binding have a much greater effect on drugs that are highly protein bound. For example, a decrease in binding from 98% to 94% will triple the fraction of free drug, whereas a decrease in binding from 68% to 64% results in a much smaller percentage increase of free drug.

Factors Affecting Drug Binding

Age and Gender. With advancing age, the plasma concentration of albumin decreases, whereas that of AAG increases. These small changes are not clinically important. Gender-related differences are nonexistent.

Renal Disease. Albumin levels may be decreased with renal disease. In addition, it is thought that renal failure alters the albumin molecule, thereby reducing binding with organic acids. On the other hand, binding of basic drugs with AAG is variable, depending on the type of renal disease.

Hepatic Disease. Because plasma albumin levels frequently are decreased in liver disease, free fractions of drugs that are typically bound to albumin are increased. Free fractions of basic drugs that are normally bound to AAG are unaffected.

Miscellaneous. Because AAG is an acute phase reactant, its plasma concentration is increased in patients experiencing the physiologic stress of surgery, trauma, myocardial infarction, neoplastic disease, or inflammatory disease.

Suggested References

Hudson RJ. Basic principles of clinical pharmacology. In Barash PG, Cullen BF, Stoelting RK, eds. Clinical Anesthesia. Philadelphia: Lippincott-Raven, 1996:221–242.

Stoelting RK. Pharmacology and Physiology in Anesthetic Practice. 3rd ed. Philadelphia, Lippincott-Raven, 1998.

75
Anaphylactic and Anaphylactoid Reactions

Thomas J. Christopherson, M.D.

Anaphylactic and anaphylactoid reactions are acute, potentially fatal events involving the cardiovascular, respiratory, cutaneous, and gastrointestinal systems. Anaphylactic reactions are immunologically mediated. Anaphylactoid reactions produce a similar clinical syndrome but are not immunologically mediated.

Pathophysiology

In anaphylactic reactions, the allergen may be the injected substance itself, a nonenzymatically generated product, or a metabolic product formed in the patient. These allergens bind to immunospecific immunoglobulin E (IgE) antibodies on the surface of mast cells and basophils. This causes the release of histamine and eosinophilic chemotactic factors of anaphylaxis (ECF-A) from storage granules. Other chemical mediators, including leukotrienes, kinins, and prostaglandins, are synthesized and released in response to this cellular activation.[1]

In anaphylactoid reactions, the offending agent works by nonimmunologically activating systems that cause degranulation of mast cells and basophils. The systems that can be activated to cause release of mediators from these cells include the complement, coagulation, fibrinolytic, and kinin-generating systems (Fig. 75–1).

Once these chemical mediators are released, the onset and severity of the anaphylactic (or anaphylactoid) reaction relates to the mediator's specific end-organ effects (Table 75–1).

Etiologic Agents

Commonly used agents that have the potential to initiate anaphylactic and anaphylactoid reactions in the anesthetized patient include muscle relaxants, thiobarbiturates, antibiotics, and local anesthetics.

Muscle Relaxants. Certain muscle relaxants, such as d-tubocurarine, metocurine, atracurium,

and cisatracurium, can produce nonimmunologic histamine release. Life-threatening anaphylactic reactions have been reported with succinylcholine, pancuronium, atracurium, cisatracurium,[2] d-tubocurarine, and gallamine. Cross-reactivity may occur between various relaxants because of their common quaternary ammonium groupings.

Thiobarbiturates. Thiopental is the barbiturate most often implicated in case reports, although anaphylactic and anaphylactoid reactions to metho-

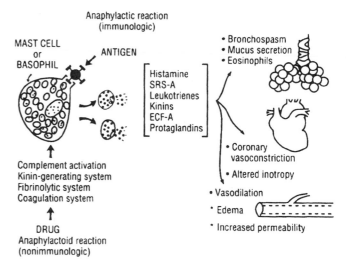

Figure 75–1. A summary of the pathophysiologic changes in anaphylactic and anaphylactoid reactions. (Top) **Anaphylactic reactions.** The allergen enters the body and combines with IgE antibodies on the surface of mast cells and basophils. The mast cells and basophils degranulate, releasing mediators (histamine, slow-reacting substance of anaphylaxis [SRS-A], leukotrienes, kinins, eosinophilic chemotactic factor [ECF-A], prostaglandins, and others). The release of these substances is associated with the signs and symptoms of anaphylaxis: bronchospasm; pharyngeal, glottic, and pulmonary edema; vasodilation; hypotension; decreased cardiac contractility and arrhythmias; subcutaneous edema; and urticaria. (Bottom) **Anaphylactoid reactions.** The offending agent enters the body and works by nonimmunologically activating systems that cause degranulation of mast cells and basophils. When activated, the complement system, the coagulation and fibrinolytic system, and the kinin-generating system can cause release of mediators from basophils and mast cells, resulting in a syndrome that is clinically indistinguishable from anaphylaxis. (From Levy JH.[1])

Table 75–1. Symptoms of Anaphylaxis

System	Signs
Cardiovascular	Diaphoresis
	Hypotension (↓ SVR)
	Tachycardia
	Arrhythmias
	Cardiac arrest
	Pulmonary hypertension
Respiratory	Wheezing
	Coughing
	Acute pulmonary edema
Cutaneous	Facial edema
	Urticaria
	Flushing
Gastrointestinal	Vomiting
	Diarrhea

Table 75–2. Management of Anaphylaxis

1. Stop the suspected causative drug.
2. Maintain ventilation and administer 100% oxygen.
3. Start intravascular volume expansion with 2 to 4 L of crystalloid.
4. Give epinephrine, titrating in 50 to 100 µg IV (0.5 to 1.0 mL of 1:10,000). In severe anaphylaxis doses, more than 500 to 1000 µg might be necessary.
5. Consider secondary therapies:
   • Diphenhydramine (50 to 100 mg)
   • Catecholamine infusions
   • Corticosteroids (0.25 to 1 g hydrocortisone or 1 to 2 g methylprednisolone)
   • Bronchodilators

hexital have also been described. Most of these reactions would appear to be anaphylactoid in nature; IgE-mediated reactions to thiobarbiturates have an incidence of less than 1 in 22,000.

Antibiotics. Penicillin, cephalosporins, and vancomycin are the antibiotics most often implicated in anaphylactic and anaphylactoid reactions. Of all parenteral medications, penicillin has the highest prevalence rate (0.7% to 10%) of allergic reactions. In a study of 152 anaphylactic fatalities following penicillin administration, 70% had received penicillin previously, 33% had previous allergic reactions to penicillin, and 14% had a history of nonpenicillin drug allergies. Patients who are allergic to penicillin have a 2% to 8% prevalence rate of cephalosporin cross-reactivity. The prevalence rate of allergic reactions to cephalosporins in patients not allergic to penicillin has been reported to be 1.7%. When administered rapidly, vancomycin may result in transient histamine release with resultant hypotension and flushing (the so-called "red man syndrome").

Local Anesthetics. Most adverse reactions to local anesthetics are nonallergic, due instead to overdosage or epinephrine-induced effects. True allergy to ester agents is well described, but documented allergic reactions to the amide local anesthetics are rare. Anaphylactic reactions after local anesthetic administration are most likely from methylparaben, a derivative of para-aminobenzoic acid that is used as a preservative in multidose vials, or sulfiting agents, preservatives and antioxidants added to local anesthetic solutions that have vasopressors (e.g., epinephrine) added.[3] Various other parenterally administered agents have been reported to cause anaphylactic or anaphylactoid reactions perioperatively. These include narcotics, mannitol, protamine, radiocontrast dye, chymopa-

pain, methylmethacrylate (bone cement), blood products, and colloid volume expanders.

Therapy

Retrospective studies of anaphylactic shock indicate a 6% mortality, but patients should respond to appropriate therapy instituted immediately.[4] Once the offending agent has been discontinued, maintenance of the patient's airway, administration of 100% oxygen, expansion of the intravascular blood volume, and titration of epinephrine become the mainstay of therapy (Table 75–2).

Retrospective Diagnosis

The diagnosis of anaphylactic and anaphylactoid reactions must be made clinically so that therapy can be instituted immediately. Although histamine's half-life is short, tryptase, another chemical released during mast cell degranulation, remains in the plasma for 3 hours.[5] Methylhistamine, a metabolite of histamine has a 2- to 3-hour half-life and can be detected in the urine. Specific drug sensitivity can be confirmed later by skin prick testing.

Selected References

1. Levy JH. Anaphylactic Reactions in Anesthesia and Intensive Care. Boston, Butterworths, 1986.
2. Levey RH, Roizen MF, Morris JM. Anaphylactic and anaphylactoid reactions: A review. Spine 1986;11:282–289.
3. Toh KW, Deacock SJ, Fawcett WJ. Severe anaphylactic reaction to cisatracurium. Anesth Analg 1999;88:462–464.
4. Beamish D, Brown DT. Adverse response to IV anesthetics. Br J Anaesth 1981;53:55.
5. Simon RA. Adverse reactions to drug additives. J Allergy Clin Immunol 1984;74:623.

Physical Sciences

76
Coronary Circulation and the Myocardial Conduction System

Michael L. Bishop, M.D.

Coronary Circulation

The right and left main coronary arteries arise from ostia located behind the right and left aortic valve cusps near the top of the sinus of Valsalva (Fig. 76–1). The third aortic cusp is named the posterior or noncoronary cusp.

The **left main coronary artery** travels anteriorly and leftward from the left coronary sinus, and after a 2- to 10-mm course between the pulmonary trunk and the left atrium, it divides into the left anterior descending and left circumflex arteries. Occasionally, a diagonal branch is also present.

The **left anterior descending** (LAD) or left interventricular coronary artery is a direct continuation of the left main coronary artery, traveling anterior and caudad, descending in the anterior interventricular groove. This artery terminates in the inferior aspect of the cardiac apex. Branches of this artery include (1) the first diagonal, (2) the first septal perforator, (3) right ventricular branches (inconstant), (4) three to five additional septal perforators, and (5) two to six additional diagonal branches. The LAD provides blood to most of the ventricular septum (anterior two-thirds), the anterior, lateral, and apical walls of the left ventricle, most of the right and left bundle branches, and the anterolateral papillary muscle of the left ventricle. It can provide collaterals to the anterior right ventricle via the circle of Vienssen, to the ventricular septum via septal perforators, and to the posterior descending artery via the distal LAD or a diagonal branch.

The **left circumflex artery** (LCA) travels posteriorly around the heart in the left atrioventricular sulcus. In 85% to 90% of individuals, it terminates

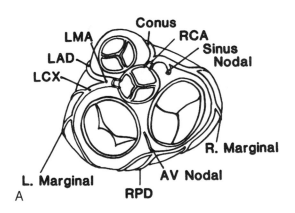

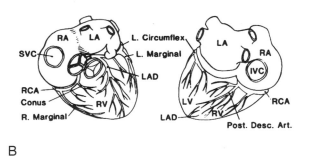

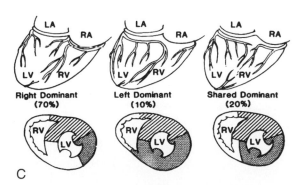

Figure 76–1. Coronary arterial distribution. *A*, The right and circumflex coronary arteries travel in the AV sulcus, adjacent to the tricuspid and mitral valves, respectively (view of base of heart). *B*, The left anterior descending and posterior descending coronary arteries travel in the interventricular sulcus and demarcate the plane of the ventricular septum (superior [left] and inferior [right] views). *C*, Coronary dominance is determined by the origin of the posterior descending branch (white, LAD distribution; dotted, left circumflex coronary artery; striped, RCA). (From Edwards WD.[1])

near the obtuse margin of the left ventricle; in the remaining 10% to 15%, it continues around to the crux of the heart to become the posterior descending artery. Branches include (1) a branch to the sino-atrial (SA) node in 40% to 50% of individuals, (2) a left atrial circumflex branch, (3) an anterolateral marginal, (4) a distal circumflex, (5) posterolateral marginals, and (6) the posterior descending artery, as noted. This artery provides blood to the left atrium, the posterior and lateral left ventricle, the anterolateral papillary muscle of the left ventricle, and the SA node as above. If it continues on as the posterior descending artery (in 10% to 15% of hearts), it also supplies blood to the atrioventricular (AV) node, the proximal bundle branches, the remainder of the inferoposterior left ventricle, the posterior interventricular septum, and the postero-medial papillary muscle of the left ventricle.

The **right coronary artery** (RCA) passes forward to emerge between the pulmonary trunk and the right atrium and then descends in the right atrioventricular sulcus. In most hearts, it turns posteriorly and to the left at the apex of the heart, traveling in the posterior atrioventricular sulcus to terminate as a left ventricular branch or to anastomose with the LCA. Branches include (1) the conus artery, (2) the artery to the SA node (in 50% to 60% of hearts), (3) anterior right ventricular branches, (4) right atrial branches, (5) an acute marginal branch, (6) an artery to the AV node and proximal bundle branches, (7) the posterior descending artery (in 85% to 90% of hearts), and (8) terminal branches to the left atrium and left ventricle. The RCA supplies blood to the SA node (as above), the right ventricle, the crista supraventricularis, and the right atrium. If it provides the posterior descending artery, it also supplies blood to those areas dis-

cussed above. The RCA provides collaterals to the LAD via the conus artery and septal perforators.

The **coronary venous system** consists of three primary systems: (1) the coronary sinus, (2) the anterior right ventricular veins, and (3) the thebesian veins (Fig. 76–2). The **coronary sinus** is located in the posterior atrioventricular groove and receives blood from the great, middle, and small cardiac veins; the posterior veins of the left ventricle; and the left atrial oblique vein of Marshall. The coronary sinus drains blood primarily from the left ventricle and opens into the right atrium. The two to four **anterior right ventricular veins** originate in and drain blood from the right ventricular wall. These veins enter the right atrium directly or enter into a small collecting vein at the base of the right atrium. The **thebesian veins** are tiny venous outlets that drain directly into the cardiac chambers, primarily the right atrium and right ventricle.

Myocardial Conduction System

The **conducting system of the heart** is composed of specially differentiated cardiac muscle fibers that are responsible for initiating and maintaining normal cardiac rhythm as well as ensuring proper coordination between atrial and ventricular contraction. This system comprises the SA node, the AV node, the bundle of His, right and left branch bundles, and Purkinje fibers.

The **SA node** is a horseshoe-shaped structure located in the upper part of the sulcus terminalis of the right atrium (Fig. 76–3). It extends through the atrial wall from epicardium to endocardium. SA nodal fibers have a higher intrinsic rate of depolar-

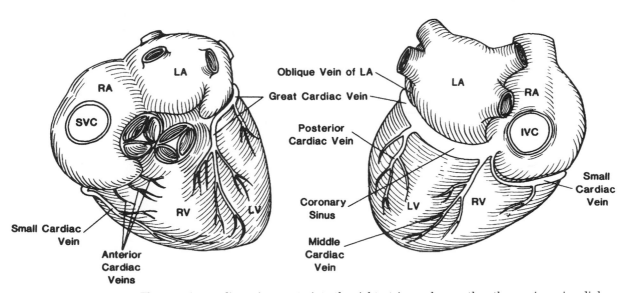

Figure 76–2. Coronary veins. The anterior cardiac veins empty into the right atrium, whereas the other major epicardial coronary veins drain into the coronary sinus. (From Edwards WD.[1])

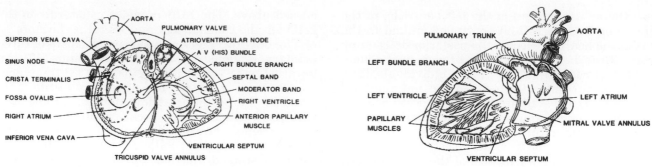

Figure 76–3. Cardiac conduction system. *A,* Right heart. The SA and AV nodes are both right atrial structures. *B,* Left heart. The left bundle branch forms a broad sheet that does not divide into distinct anterior and posterior fascicles. (From Edwards WD.[1])

ization than any other cardiac muscle fibers and act as the pacemaker of the heart. Three internodal pathways facilitate conduction of impulses between the SA and AV nodes: the anterior (Bachman's bundle), middle, and posterior internodal tracts. The **AV node** lies in the medial floor of the right atrium at the base of the atrial septum above the orifice of the coronary sinus. The **bundle of His** begins at the anterior aspect of the AV node and penetrates through the central fibrous body. Here the bundle of His divides into the **left and right branch bundles.** The division straddles the upper border of the muscular ventricular septum, and the bundles run superficially down either side of the septum. About midway to the apex, the left bundle divides into the **anterior superior and posterior inferior fascicles.** These fascicles continue to the base of the papillary muscles of the left ventricle, where they form plexuses of **Purkinje fibers** that distrib-

ute to all portions of the left ventricular myocardium. The **right branch bundle** continues to the anterior papillary muscle of the right ventricle, where it forms a plexus of Purkinje fibers that distribute to all portions of the right ventricular myocardium.

Selected References

1. Edwards WD. Applied anatomy of the heart. In Brandenburg RO, Fuster V, Giuliani ER, et al, eds. Cardiology: Fundamentals and Practice. 2nd ed. St Louis: Mosby-Year Book, 1991:47.

Suggested References

Waller BF, Schlant RC. Anatomy of the heart. In Alexander RW, Schlant RC, Fuster V, eds. Hurst's The Heart. 9th ed. New York: McGraw-Hill, 1998:19.

Williams PL, Warwick R, Dyson M, et al. Gray's Anatomy. 37th ed. New York, Churchill Livingstone, 1989.

77
Cerebral Circulation

Douglas A. Dubbink, M.D.

The brain receives its blood supply from the **internal carotid arteries** (80% of total cerebral flow) and the **vertebrobasilar** system (20% of total cerebral flow). These two systems are connected at the **circle of Willis**, a ring of vessels beneath the hypothalamus (Fig. 77–1). The circle of Willis consists of the anterior communicating artery and the paired anterior cerebral, internal carotid, posterior communicating, and posterior cerebral arteries.

Anterior Circulation

The **internal carotid** artery courses through the carotid canal in the temporal bone, exits anteriorly, and then enters the posterior part of the foramen lacerum, eventually piercing the dural layers of the cavernous sinus. The **carotid siphon** refers to the artery's S-shaped course within the sinus. The first branch is the **ophthalmic artery**, followed by the **posterior communicating artery**, and then the **anterior choroidal artery.** The internal carotid then terminates into the **anterior** and **middle cerebral arteries** (Figs. 77–2, 77–3, and 77–4).

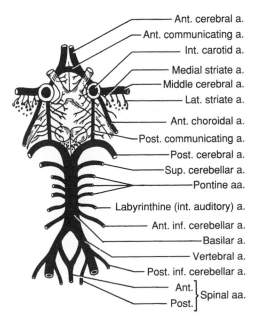

- Ant. cerebral a.
- Ant. communicating a.
- Int. carotid a.
- Medial striate a.
- Middle cerebral a.
- Lat. striate a.
- Ant. choroidal a.
- Post. communicating a.
- Post. cerebral a.
- Sup. cerebellar a.
- Pontine aa.
- Labyrinthine (int. auditory) a.
- Ant. inf. cerebellar a.
- Basilar a.
- Vertebral a.
- Post. inf. cerebellar a.
- Ant.⎫ Spinal aa.
- Post.⎭

Figure 77–1. Diagram of the arterial supply to the brain stem and the constituents of the circle of Willis. (From Pansky B.[1])

Posterior Circulation

The vertebrobasilar system supplies the posterior cerebrum, midbrain, pons, medulla, and cerebellum. The **vertebral arteries** ascend through the transverse process of C6 to C1 before entering the skull through the foramen magnum. Branches of the vertebral arteries include the anterior spinal artery (single), posterior spinal arteries (paired), and the posterior inferior cerebellar artery (see Figs. 77–3 and 77–4).

Venous Drainage of the Head

Diploic veins are endothelial-lined canals draining the skull (Fig. 77–5). There are four main diploic veins on each side, named after the anatomical region being drained: frontal, anterior temporal, posterior temporal, and occipital. **Emissary veins** connect the venous sinuses and diploic veins to the veins on the surface of the skull.

Dural venous sinuses are located between the endosteal and meningeal layers of the dura mater. The sinuses receive blood from the brain, meninges, skull, and scalp.

Clinical Considerations

There are no valves in the dural venous sinuses and in the diploic, emissary, and meningeal veins. This makes the spread of infection from the scalp to inside the intracranial vault possible.

Arterial anastomoses are quite numerous on the surface of the brain, but are relatively rare within the brain parenchyma. Thus, occlusion or rupture of an intraparenchymal artery likely will cause more damage than a similar incident occurring on the brain's surface.

Some 95% of all aneurysms can be found near the circle of Willis at one of the following five sites (see Fig. 77–1):

- Anterior communicating artery (25%).
- Internal carotid artery between posterior communicating and anterior choroidal arteries (22%).

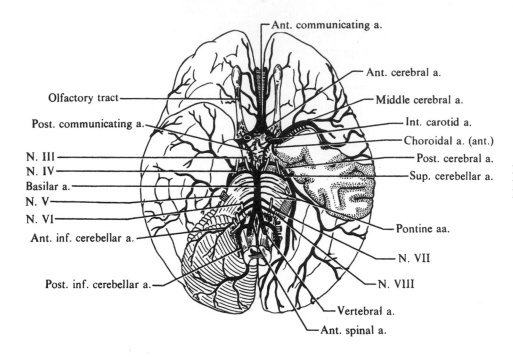

Figure 77–2. Basal view of the arterial supply to the brain. (From Pansky B.[1])

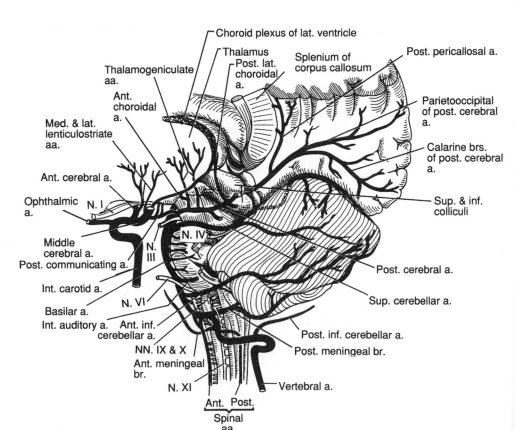

Figure 77–3. Arterial supply to the posterior fossa. (From Pansky B.[1])

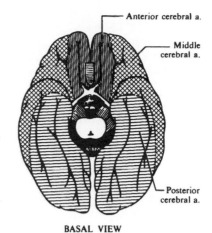

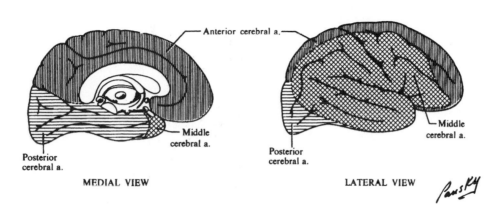

Figure 77–4. Areas of the brain supplied by the anterior, middle, and posterior cerebral arteries. (From Pansky B.[1])

BASAL VIEW

MEDIAL VIEW

LATERAL VIEW

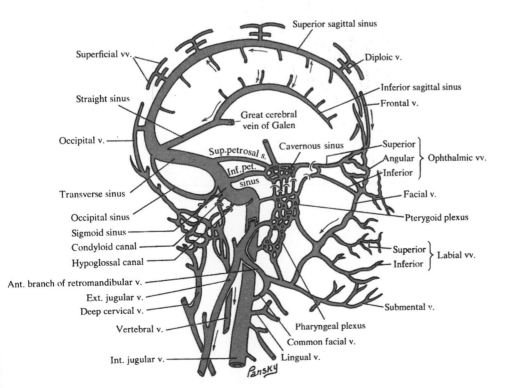

Figure 77–5. Venous drainage of the head. (From Pansky B.[1])

□ Middle cerebral artery (25%).
□ Internal carotid bifurcation (4%).
□ Basilar bifurcation[2] (7%).

Selected References

1. Pansky B. Review of Gross Anatomy. 5th ed. New York, Macmillan, 1984.
2. Fein JM, Flamm ES. Cerebrovascular Surgery. New York, Springer-Verlag, 1985.

Suggested References

Michenfelder JD. Anesthesia and the Brain: Clinical, Functional, Metabolic and Vascular Correlates. New York, Churchill Livingstone, 1988.
Sano K, Asano T, Tamura A. Acute Aneurysm Surgery: Pathophysiology and Management. New York, Springer-Verlag, 1987.

78
Anatomy of the Posterior Fossa

Daniel J. Janik, M.D.

The posterior cranial fossa contains the brain stem, cerebellum, and cranial nerves. Surgical procedures in this fossa include neurosurgical approaches to gliomas, meningiomas, acoustic neuromas, arteriovenous malformations, microvascular decompressions, aneurysm repairs, and otologic operations.

Boundaries

The posterior fossa is bounded in front by the dorsum sellae, the clivus, the posterior aspects of the sphenoid bone, and the basilar part of the occipital bone; behind by the lower part of the occipital squama below the sulci for the transverse sinuses and internal occipital protuberance; laterally by the petrous and mastoid parts of the temporal bones and lateral parts of the occipital bone; and above and behind by the mastoid angles of the parietal bones. It contains all structures caudal to the tentorium cerebelli (Fig. 78–1). The foramen magnum is in the fossa's floor.

Neural Contents

The posterior fossa contains the cerebellum, pons, and medulla oblongata (see Fig. 78–1). The cranial nerves listed below either traverse or are contained within the posterior fossa (Fig 78–2):

- Trochlear nerve (IV).
- Trigeminal nerve (V).
- Abducens nerve (VI).
- Facial nerve (VII).
- Vestibulocochlear nerve (VIII).
- Glossopharyngeal nerve (IX).
- Vagus nerve (X).
- Spinal accessory nerve (XI).
- Hypoglossal nerve (XII).

The fourth ventricle lies between the cerebellum and the brain stem. Multiple cranial nerve nuclei, cardiovascular, and respiratory centers lie close to the anterior floor of the fourth ventricle (see Fig. 78–2).

Venous Contents

The veins of the posterior fossa drain the cerebellum and brain stem and may contribute to intraop-

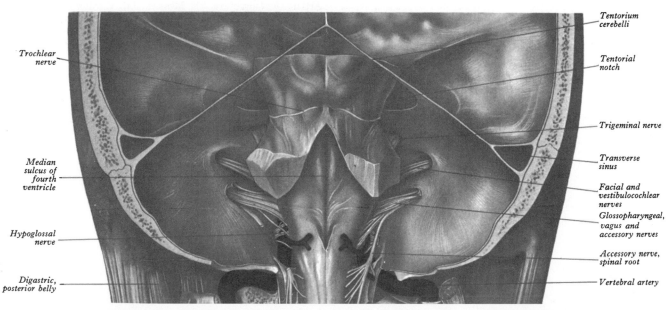

Figure 78–1. The posterior fossa, viewed from posterior in a coronal section with the cerebellar hemispheres removed. (From Williams PL, Warwick R, Dyson M, et al.)

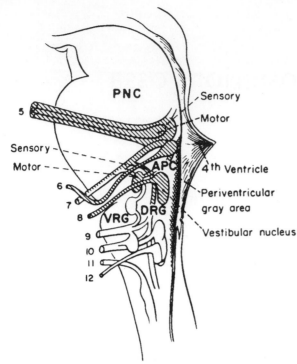

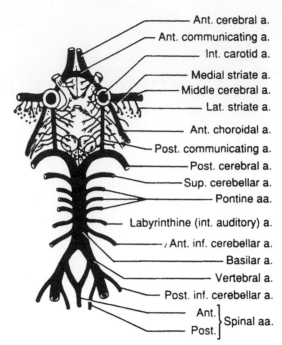

Figure 78–2. General locations of cardiovascular centers *(hatched area)*, respiratory centers *(boldface-lettered areas)*, and cranial nerves *(slanted-line areas)* affected in this case. Respiratory centers are designated by the following abbreviations: PNC, pneumotaxic center; APC, apneustic center; DRG, dorsal respiratory group; VRG, ventral respiratory group. (From Artru AA, Cucchiara RF, Messick JM.)

Figure 78–3. Arterial supply to the brain stem and the constituents of the circle of Willis (From Pansky B.)

erative complications such as hemorrhage, hematoma, or venous air embolism. As seen in Figure 77–5, the major venous structure include:

□ Great cerebral vein of Galen.
□ Petrosal vein.
□ Superior petrosal sinus.
□ Straight sinus.
□ Left and right transverse sinuses.
□ Lateral sinus.
□ Occipital sinus.

Arteries

Arteries arising from the vertebrobasilar system (Fig. 78–3) supply the pons, medulla, and cerebellum (see Figs. 77–2, 77–3, and 78–3). Major arteries include:

□ Left and right vertebral arteries.
□ Basilar artery (formed from vertebrals).
□ Posterior inferior cerebellar artery.
□ Anterior inferior cerebellar artery.
□ Superior cerebellar artery.
□ Labyrinthine (internal auditory) artery.
□ Posterior cerebral artery.

Suggested References

Artru AA, Cucchiara RF, Messick JM. Cardiorespiratory and cranial nerve sequelae of surgical procedures involving the posterior fossa. Anesthesiology 1980;52:83–86.
Pansky B. Review of Gross Anatomy. 5th ed. New York, Macmillan, 1984.
Williams PL, Warwick R, Dyson M, et al. Gray's Anatomy. 37th ed. New York, Churchill Livingstone, 1989.

79
Spinal Cord Anatomy and Blood Supply

Thomas J. Christopherson, M.D.

Anatomy

The **vertebral column** encompasses the spinal cord and comprises 33 vertebrae (7 cervical, 12 thoracic, 5 lumbar, and 4 coccygeal) and 4 curvatures. Anteriorly, the cervical and lumbar curves are convex, whereas in the thoracic and sacral areas, the vertebral column is concave (Fig. 79–1).[1] These vertebral curvatures markedly influence the spread of local anesthetic during spinal anesthesia. The stability and elasticity of the vertebral column is gained via several ligaments (Fig. 79–2):[2]

- The **supraspinal ligament** is a band of longitudinal fibers interconnecting the tips of the spinous processes from the sacrum to C7. It is continuous with the interspinal ligament at all levels and with the ligamentum nuchae cephalad.
- The **interspinal ligament** is a thin, membranous band that unites adjacent spinous processes and extends from the supraspinal ligament posteriorly to the ligamentum flavum anteriorly.
- The **ligamentum flavum** is the "yellow ligament" that connects the laminae of adjacent vertebrae.
- The **longitudinal ligaments** (anterior and posterior) provide vertebral column stability by binding the vertebral bodies.

The **epidural space** surrounds the spinal meninges and contains fat, alveolar tissue, nerve roots, and extensive networks of arteries and vertebral venous plexuses. This space extends from the foramen magnum to the sacral hiatus and is widest in its posterior dimension. L2 is thought to be the widest part of the epidural space, measuring 5 to 6 mm at this level. The epidural space is bounded anteriorly by the posterior longitudinal ligament, laterally by the intervertebral foramina, and posteriorly by the ligamentum flavum.

The **spinal meninges** are three individual membranes that surround the spinal cord:

- The **dura** is the tough, fibroelastic, outermost membrane extending from the foramen magnum superiorly to the lower border of S2 inferiorly, where it becomes pierced by the filum terminales (i.e., the distal end of the **pia mater**).
- The **arachnoid** is the middle membrane that is closely attached to the dura. This layer is very thin and avascular.
- The **pia** is a highly vascular membrane that closely approximates the spinal cord. The space

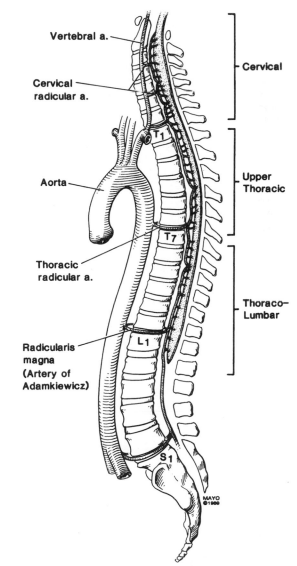

Figure 79–1. A lateral view of the vertebral column, illustrating its curvatures and the line and center of gravity of the body. Blood supply is via radicular arteries, which are variable in location but are shown here at T1, T7, L1, and S1. (From Mahla ME, Horlocker TT.[1])

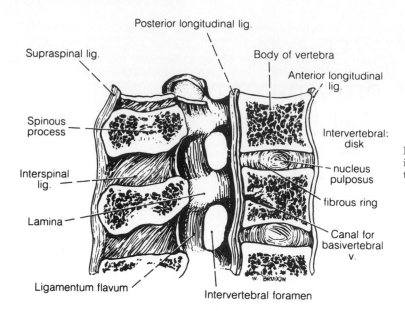

Figure 79–2. A median section of several vertebrae, illustrating the intervertebral disk and the ligaments of the column. (From Woodburne RT.[2])

between the arachnoid and pia is the subarachnoid space. This space contains the spinal nerves and cerebral spinal fluid, as well as numerous delicate trabeculae that intertwine within this space. Lateral extensions of the pia mater, the denticulate ligaments, help support the spinal cord by binding to the dura.

The **spinal cord** begins at the level of the foramen magnum and ends below as the conus medullaris. At birth, the cord extends to L3, but it moves to its adult position at the lower border of L1 by age 1 year.

Blood Supply

The spinal cord is supplied by one **anterior spinal artery** and two **posterior spinal arteries**.

Throughout their length, these three spinal arteries receive contributions from radicular branches of intercostal arteries:[3]

□ The **anterior spinal artery**, which lies in the anterior median sulcus, is formed at the level of the foramen magnum by the union of the two vertebral arteries. Although the anterior spinal artery is often considered a continuous structure, this often is not the case (especially at the level of the thoracic cord). Contributing to the anterior spinal arterial system is a group of 6 to 10 radicular arteries (see Fig. 79–1).[1] In the cervical region, these arteries derive from the cervical branches of the vertebral and ascending cervical arteries. In the superior thoracic cord, contributions arise from the ascending and deep cervical arteries. The radicular arteries augmenting blood flow to the middle and lower thoracic cord are less promi-

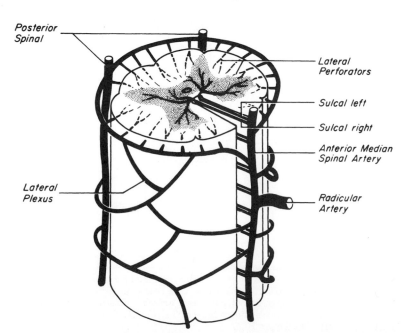

Figure 79–3. Intrinsic arterial supply is to the cord. The central sulcal supply is from the anterior median spinal artery, and the lateral supplies are from anterior and posterior spinal arteries. (From Buchan AM, Barnett HJM.[5])

nent. The lower thoracic and lumbar cord is supplied by the radicularis magna (**artery of Adamkiewicz**). This artery has variable origin along the spinal cord, arising between T5 and T8 in 15% of patients, between T9 and T12 in 60%, and between L1 and L5 in 25%.[4] The lumbosacral cord is supplied by branches of the hypogastric and sacral arteries. Finally, the anterior spinal artery itself gives rise to sulcal vessels that perfuse the anterior two-thirds of the spinal cord (Fig. 79–3).[5]

□ The **posterior spinal arteries** arise from the vertebral or posterior inferior cerebellar arteries and descend as two branches, one anterior and the other posterior to the dorsal nerve root. These arteries are segmentally reinforced with radicular collaterals from the vertebral, cervical, and posterior intercostal arteries, and they provide much better vertical continuity than the anterior spinal arterial system.

□ The peripheral border of the spinal cord receives its blood supply from ventral and dorsal penetrating vessels. Collateral circulation of the peripheral cord is adequate. However, within the spinal cord itself, there are no anastomoses, and the penetrating vessels are essentially end arterioles.

Selected References

1. Mahla ME, Horlocker TT. Vertebral column and spinal cord surgery. In Cucchiara RF, Black S, Michenfelder JD, eds. Clinical Neuroanesthesia. 2nd ed. New York: Churchill Livingstone, 1998:403–448.
2. Woodburne RT. Essentials of Human Anatomy. 8th ed. Oxford, UK, Oxford University Press, 1988.
3. Gillilian L. The arterial supply of the human spinal cord. J Comp Neurol 1958;110:75.
4. Marcus ML, Heistad DD, Ehrhardt JC, Abboud FM. Regulation of total and regional spinal cord flow. Circ Res 1977;41:128–134.
5. Buchan AM, Barnett HJM. Infarction of the spinal cord. In Barnett HJM, Mohr JP, Stein BM Yatsu FM, eds. Stroke Pathophysiology, Diagnosis, and Management. New York: Churchill Livingstone, 1986:707.

80
The Autonomic Nervous System

James D. Hannon, M.D.

The autonomic nervous system has also been called the visceral, the vegetative, or the involuntary nervous system. This self-controlling (autonomous) system comprises nerves, ganglia, and plexuses that innervate the heart, blood vessels, glands, visceral organs, and smooth muscle. It is widely distributed throughout the body and regulates functions that occur without conscious control. However, it does not function in a completely independent fashion; rather, it responds to somatic motor and sensory input.

The autonomic nervous system can be divided functionally into the sympathetic nervous system and the parasympathetic nervous system. Most visceral organs are innervated by both systems, and the moment-to-moment level of activity represents the integration of the influences of the two components. A clear understanding of the anatomy and physiology of the autonomic nervous system is fundamental to the study and practice of anesthesiology. The actions of drugs that affect the heart muscle, smooth muscle, and glandular tissue can be understood and classified according to their modifying or mimicking the actions of neurotransmitters released by this system.

Anatomy

Sympathetic Nervous System. Activation of the sympathetic nervous system produces an expenditure of energy stores (fight or flight response) and occurs in response to stresses that threaten normal homeostasis: physical activity, psychologic stress, blood loss, and disease processes. The arrangement of the main parts of the peripheral autonomic nervous system is illustrated in Fig. 80–1. The sympathetic nervous system is widely distributed throughout the body. The cell bodies that give rise to the preganglionic fibers of the sympathetic nervous system lie in the intermediolateral columns of the thoracolumbar spinal cord from T1 to L2, and the sympathetic nervous system is sometimes referred to as the thoracolumbar nervous system. The axons of these cells are carried in the anterior nerve roots and synapse with neurons lying in sympathetic ganglia found in three locations: paravertebral, prevertebral, and terminal. The paravertebral ganglia

consist of 22 pairs that lie on either side of the vertebral column. The unpaired prevertebral ganglia lie in the abdomen or pelvis near the ventral surface of the vertebral column (celiac, superior mesenteric, and inferior mesenteric). The terminal ganglia lie near the innervated organs (rectum, bladder, and cervical ganglia). They then exit with somatic nerves. The cells of the medulla are embryologically and anatomically analogous to sympathetic ganglia.

Parasympathetic Nervous System. Activation of the parasympathetic nervous system triggers restorative processes that results in the conservation or accumulation of energy stores. The distribution of the parasympathetic nervous system to effector organs is more limited than that of the sympathetic system, as shown in Fig. 80–1. Preganglionic fibers travel all the way to innervated organs; postganglionic cell bodies are located near or within affected organs. The parasympathetic nervous system has fewer postganglionic nerves for each preganglionic fiber and is able to produce discrete, limited effects, in contrast to the diffuse, mass effects characterizing sympathetic nervous system function.

The preganglionic fibers of the parasympathetic nervous system originate in the midbrain, the medulla (cranial), and the sacral part of the spinal cord; it is also referred to as the craniosacral nervous system. Cranial parasympathetic fibers innervate the ciliary, sphenopalatine, sublingual, submaxillary, and otic ganglia. The vagus nerve (X) contains preganglionic fibers that do not synapse until they reach the many small ganglia lying in or on the organs of the thorax and abdomen. These include the heart, intestinal system, lungs, liver, gallbladder, pancreas, and ureters. Other cranial nerves (oculomotor [III], facial [VII], and glossopharyngeal [IX]) and the 2nd, 3rd, and 4th sacral nerves compose the rest of the parasympathetic nervous system. Parasympathetic sacral outflow forms the pelvic nerves. These synapse in ganglia near or within the bladder, rectum, and sexual organs.

Functional Effects
Sympathetic

□ Eyes: contraction of the radial muscle of the iris: mydriasis (α_1); relaxation of the ciliary muscle for far vision (β_2).

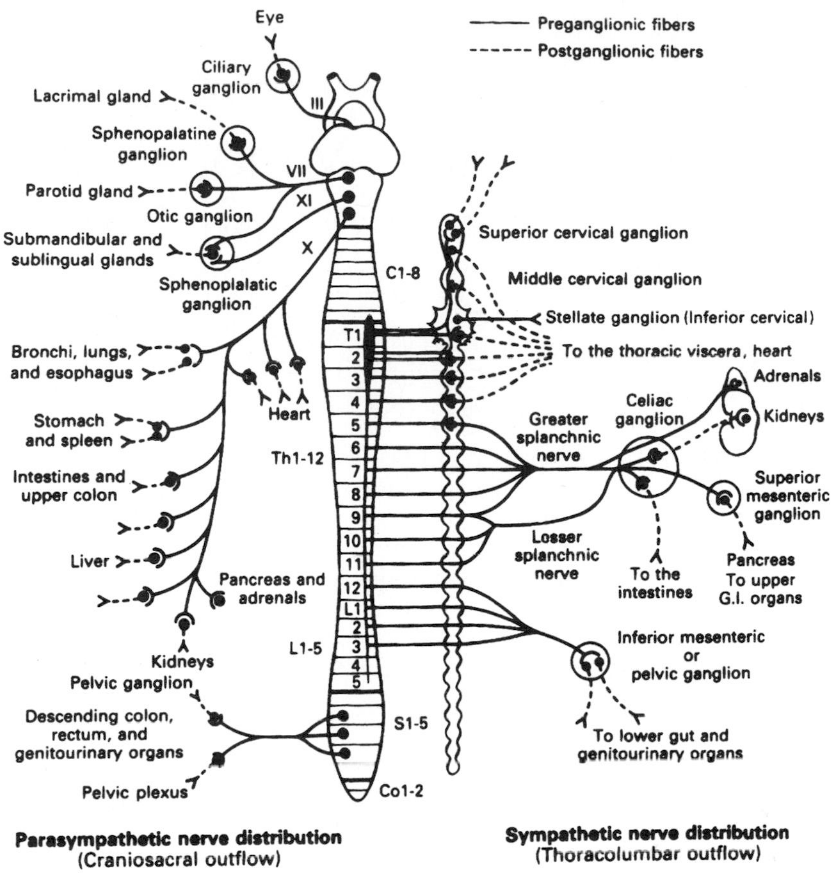

Figure 80–1. Schematic distribution of the craniosacral (parasympathetic) and thoracolumbar (sympathetic) nervous systems. (From Lawson NW, Meyer DJ.[1])

□ Heart: increased inotropism (β_1, β_2), chronotropism (β_1, β_2), conduction velocity (β_1, β_2), coronary vasodilation (β_1), and coronary vasoconstriction (α_1, α_2).

□ Vascular smooth muscle: contraction (α_1, α_2), relaxation (β_2).

□ Kidney: vasoconstriction (α_1, α_2), vasodilation (β_1, β_2).

□ Bronchial smooth muscle: relaxation (β_2).

□ GI smooth muscle: decreased motility and tone (α_1, α_2, β_1, β_2), sphincter contraction (α_1).

□ GU smooth muscle: contraction of trigone and sphincter (α_1), relaxation of detrusor (β_2).

□ Liver: glycogenolysis (α_1, β_2).

□ Adipose tissue: lipolysis (α_1, β_1, β_3).

□ Endocrine pancreas: inhibition of insulin and glucagon release (α_2), stimulation of insulin and glucagon release (β_2).

□ Adrenergic nerve endings: inhibition of transmitter release (α_2).

□ Salivary glands: thick, viscous secretions (α_1).

□ Uterus: pregnant: contraction (α_1), relaxation (β_2); nonpregnant: relaxation (β_2).

□ Sex organs, male: ejaculation (α_1).

Parasympathetic

□ Eyes: contraction of sphincter muscle of iris: miosis.

□ Heart: decreased chronotropism, conduction velocity, and inotropism; coronary constriction.

□ Vascular smooth muscle: dilation of cerebral, pulmonary, skeletal muscle, and skin arterioles.

□ Bronchial smooth muscle: contraction.

□ GI smooth muscle: increased motility and tone, sphincter relaxation, gallbladder contraction.

□ GU smooth muscle: contraction of detrusor, relaxation of trigone and sphincter.

□ Endocrine pancreas: increased insulin and glucagon secretion.

□ Salivary glands: profuse, watery secretions.

□ Sex organs, male: erection.

Selected References

1. Lawson NW, Meyer DJ. Autonomic nervous system: Physiology and pharmacology. In Barash PG, Cullen BF, Stoelting RK (eds). Clinical Anesthesia. 3rd ed. Philadelphia: JB Lippincott, 1997:243.
2. Lefkowitz RJ, Hoffman BB, Taylor P. Neurotransmission: The autonomic and somatic nervous systems. In Hardman JG, Limbird LE, Molinoff PB, Ruddon RW, Gilman AG (eds). Goodman and Gilman's: The Pharmacological Basis of Therapeutics. 9th ed. New York: McGraw-Hill, 1996:105.

Suggested References

Ganong WF. Review of Medical Physiology. 19th ed. Stamford, CT, Appleton and Lange, 1999.

81
Central Venous Cannulation: Anatomy and Complications

Roger E. Hofer, M.D.

Central venous cannulation is an important technique for measuring central venous pressure, providing long-term intravenous nutrition, administering vasoactive drugs, and providing rapid restoration of blood volume after trauma. The four most commonly used veins for central venous access are the basilic (antecubital) vein, subclavian vein, external jugular vein, and internal jugular vein.

Basilic Vein

Cannulation of the basilic vein is achieved via the medial antecubital vein (Fig. 81–1). This technique is associated with relative ease of insertion and a low complication rate (Table 81–1). However, advancement of the catheter via the basilic vein can be time-consuming and unsuccessful, because it is difficult to pass the catheter around the corner at the shoulder to the axillary and subclavian veins. Central venous cannulation via the basilic vein is most commonly used for monitoring central venous pressure when the subclavian and the internal and external veins are unavailable (e.g., sitting craniotomy) or when long-term venous access is needed.

Subclavian Vein

The subclavian vein is a continuation of the axillary vein beginning at the border of the first rib (see

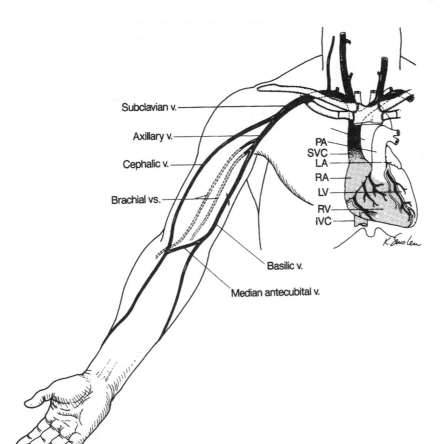

Subclavian v.
Axillary v.
Cephalic v.
Brachial vs.
PA
SVC
LA
RA
LV
RV
IVC
Basilic v.
Median antecubital v.

Figure 81–1. Antecubital approach showing the location of the antecubital veins. Because the vein is cannulated at the basilic vein at the level of the elbow, long central venous catheters are used. (From Liu PL.[1])

Table 81–1. Advantages of Different Approaches to Central Vein Catheterization*

	Basilic Vein	Subclavian Vein	External Jugular Vein	Internal Jugular Vein
Ease of insertion and safety for inexperienced practitioners	1	4	1	3
Complications	1	3	1	2
Ability to insert a central venous or pulmonary artery catheter	4	1	3	1

*In each category, 1 = best, 4 = poorest.
From Stoelting RK, Miller RD.[2]

Fig. 81–1; Fig. 81–2). The subclavian vein has a wide caliber and is held open by surrounding tissue, even in severe circulatory collapse.[3] It may be cannulated through either the supraclavicular or infraclavicular approach. When using the infraclavicular technique, venipuncture is performed inferior to the clavicle. The needle is aimed toward the suprasternal notch and passed between the clavicle and the first rib. Care must be taken to keep the needle tip close to the posterior portion of the clavicle, to reduce the risk of pneumothorax. The infraclavicular approach is the most popular, because it is generally safer to the subclavian vein than other approaches and because it is relatively easy to stabilize the catheter on the anterior chest wall.[2]

The supraclavicular route to the subclavian vein has little to recommend it.[2] It has none of the catheter stability advantages of the infraclavicular approach and has a higher complication rate than the internal jugular approach.[2]

The subclavian approach has a higher incidence of serious complications as compared to the other approaches (see Table 81–1). In addition, this technique requires the most skill and experience for successful cannulation. However, once the subclavian vein is cannulated, insertion of the central venous catheter is completed with relative ease.

Pneumothorax is the most common complication when using this technique. Therefore, after an unsuccessful cannulation attempt, attempts at cannulation of the opposite subclavian vein should be approached with caution because of the risk of producing bilateral pneumothorax.

External Jugular Vein

The external jugular vein (see Fig. 81–2; Fig. 81–3) is usually visible and is relatively easy to cannulate successfully. The complication rate is relatively low, although this technique is felt to be more complicated than the basilic vein approach.[2] It is a safe technique for the patient receiving anticoagulants or has a coagulation problem.

Passage of the central venous catheter using this technique may be met with some difficulty, usually at the junction where the external jugular vein goes

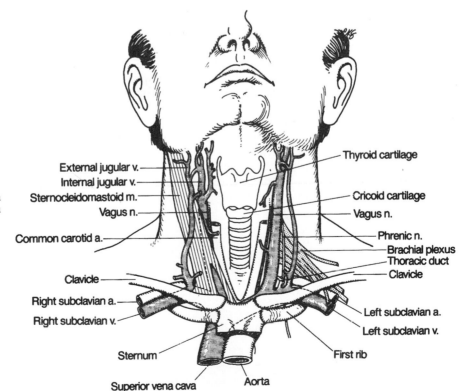

Figure 81–2. Jugular and subclavian vein anatomy: anterior view. (From Liu PL.[1])

External jugular v.
Internal jugular v.
Sternocleidomastoid m.
Vagus n.
Common carotid a.
Clavicle
Right subclavian a.
Right subclavian v.
Sternum
Superior vena cava
Thyroid cartilage
Cricoid cartilage
Vagus n.
Phrenic n.
Brachial plexus
Thoracic duct
Clavicle
Left subclavian a.
Left subclavian v.
First rib
Aorta

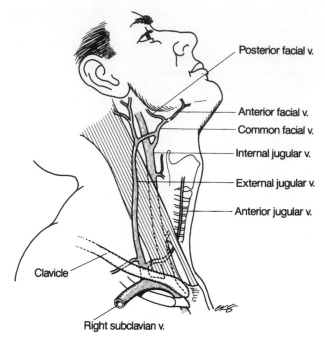

Posterior facial v.

Anterior facial v.
Common facial v.
Internal jugular v.
External jugular v.
Anterior jugular v.

Clavicle

Right subclavian v.

Figure 81–3. The jugular and subclavian vein anatomy is shown in the anterolateral view. The patient is always placed in a 10° to 15° head-down position for all jugular and subclavian central line placements. This position promotes full venous distention. (From Liu PL.[1])

under the clavicle or at the junction of the external jugular vein and the subclavian vein.

Internal Jugular Vein

The internal jugular vein is a favorite site for central venous access among anesthesiologists.[2] It is readily accessible, has a high success rate, and has a relatively low incidence of complications. Although either side may be used, the preferred approach is from the right side. The reasons are the straight access to the superior vena cava, the presence of the thoracic duct on the left, and the fact that the performance of this technique on the right is easier for right-handed operators.[2]

An important landmark is the triangle formed by the sternal and clavicular heads of the sternocleidomastoid muscle and the clavicle (see Fig. 81–3).

Table 81–2. Complications of Central Venous Cannulation

Arterial puncture	Nerve injury
Pneumothorax	Perforation
Hemothorax	Hydro- or hemothorax
Arrhythmias	Hydro- or hemomediastinum
Malposition	Hydro- or hemopericardium
Air embolism	Infection

From Gravenstein N.[4]

With the patient's head turned to the side opposite the site of insertion, the course of the internal jugular vein, and thus the axis of needle insertion, is determined by drawing a line connecting the mastoid process and the medial insertion of the sternocleidomastoid muscle on the clavicle.[2] Venipuncture could be performed at any point along this line; however, the carotid artery lies anterior to the vein high in the neck and the cupola of the lung lies low in the neck (see Fig 81–2). The carotid artery should be palpated before venipuncture to verify that it is medial to the intended puncture site. After puncture though the skin, the needle tip should be directed toward the ipsilateral nipple with the needle at about a 45° angle to the skin.

The most common complication associated with this technique is carotid artery puncture.[2] Careful palpation of the artery during the initial puncture, the use of a small "finder" needle, transducing the pressure in the vessel before insertion of the sheath, and imaging the vessels are techniques used to avoid cannulation of the carotid artery. The most common complications associated with central venous catheter placement are listed in Table 81–2.

Selected References

1. Liu PL. Atlas of basic anesthesia procedures. In Liu PL, ed. Principles and Procedures in Anesthesiology. Philadelphia: JB Lippincott, 1992:379.
2. Stoelting RK, Miller RD. Monitoring. In Stoelting RK, Miller RD, ed. Basics of Anesthesia. 3rd ed. New York: Churchill Livingstone, 1994:201–215.
3. Vender JS, Gilbert HC. Monitoring the anesthetized patient. In Barash PG, Cullen BF, Stoelting RK, eds. Clinical Anesthesia. 3rd ed. Philadelphia: Lippincott-Raven, 1997:621.
4. Gravenstein N. Invasive vascular monitoring. In Gravenstein N, ed. Manual of Complications During Anesthesia. Philadelphia: JB Lippincott, 1991:253.

82
Anatomy of the Larynx

Douglas A. Dubbink, M.D.

Definition

The larynx connects the inferior pharynx with the trachea. Its function is threefold:

- A valve to guard air passages, especially during swallowing.
- Maintenance of a patent airway.
- Vocalization.

Description

The larynx is about 5 cm in length. It lies at the level of C3-6. In cross section at the level of the laryngeal prominence (Adam's apple), the larynx is triangular because of the shape of the thyroid cartilage. At the level of the cricoid cartilage, the larynx becomes more round. The larynx provides the area of greatest resistance to passage of air to the lungs.

Laryngeal Skeleton

The laryngeal skeleton has a total of nine cartilages. **Paired cartilages** include the following:

- Arytenoid: shaped like a three-sided pyramid that articulates with the upper border of the cricoid lamina.
- Corniculate: at apices of arytenoid cartilage in the posterior part of the aryepiglottic folds.
- Cuneiform: in the aryepiglottic folds, not always present.

Unpaired cartilages include the following:

- Thyroid: largest cartilage, comprising two laminae that are fused anteriorly to form the laryngeal prominence.
- Cricoid: ring-shaped, with a posterior part (lamina) and anterior part (arch). The arytenoids articulate with the lateral parts of the superior border of the lamina. Lies at the level of C6 in adults.
- Epiglottic: thin and leaflike, located behind the root of the tongue and in front of the inlet of the larynx. The mucous membrane covering the epiglottis is continued onto the base of the tongue, forming two depressions called the epiglottic valleculae.

Joints, Ligaments, and Membranes of the Larynx

Joints include the following:

- Cricothyroid: articulation between the lateral surfaces of the cricoid cartilage and the inferior horns of the thyroid cartilage.
- Cricoarytenoid: articulation between the bases of the arytenoid cartilage and the upper surface of the cricoid lamina.

Membranes include the following:

- Thyrohyoid membrane: extrinsic ligament connecting the thyroid cartilage to the hyoid bone.

Ligaments include the following:

- Cricothyroid and cricotracheal: connect the cricoid to the thyroid cartilage and first tracheal ring, respectively.
- Vocal ligament: extends from the thyroid cartilage to the arytenoid cartilage.
- Vestibular ligament: extends from the thyroid cartilage to the arytenoid cartilage above the vocal fold.

Interior of the Larynx

There are **three divisions** of the interior of the larynx, as shown in Figs. 82–1 and 82–2:

- Vestibule: above the vestibular folds (false cords).
- Ventricle: between the vestibular folds above and the vocal folds (cords) below.
- Infraglottic cavity: from the vocal folds to the tracheal cavity.

The **vocal folds** consist of vocal ligament, conus elasticus, vocalis muscle fibers, and a covering of mucous membrane. The rima glottidis is the opening between the vocal folds. The glottis comprises the vocal folds, the rima glottidis, and the narrow part of the larynx at the level of the vocal folds.

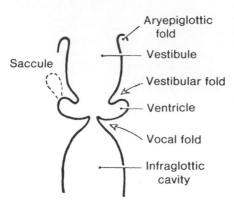

Figure 82–1. Sketch of a coronal section of the larynx showing its compartments: (1) a vestibule, (2) a middle compartment having right and left ventricles, and (3) an infraglottic cavity. (From Moore KL.[1])

The **vestibular folds** are ligaments covered by folds of mucous membrane. They meet during swallowing to prevent aspiration. The rima vestibuli is the space between the false cords.

Innervation

The **superior laryngeal nerve** (Fig. 82–3) is a branch of the vagus nerve (X) and has two terminal branches:

□ Internal laryngeal nerve: purely **sensory,** with fibers from mucosa from the tongue to the vocal folds, including the superior surface of these folds.

□ External laryngeal nerve: purely **motor,** innervates the cricothyroid muscle.

The **recurrent laryngeal nerve** is also a branch of cranial nerve X.

□ It gives branches to all muscles of the larynx, except the cricothyroid.

□ It provides sensory innervation below the vocal cords.

□ Its terminal branch, the inferior laryngeal nerve, has anterior and posterior branches.

Muscles

The **extrinsic muscles** move the larynx as a whole:

□ Depressors: omohyoid, sternohyoid, sternothyroid.

□ Elevators: stylohyoid, digastric, mylohyoid (geniohyoid), and stylopharyngeus.

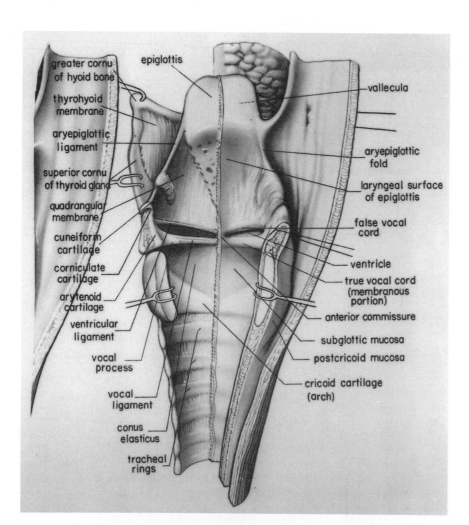

Figure 82–2. Larynx bisected in the posterior midline. Mucosa removed from the left half, showing the relation between mucosal features and underlying ligaments and cartilages. (From Silver CE.[2])

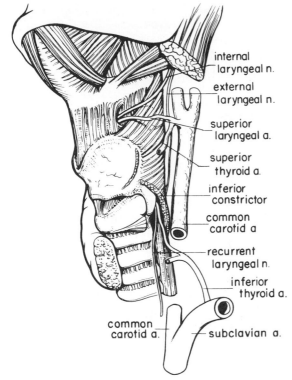

internal laryngeal n.

external laryngeal n.

superior laryngeal a.

superior thyroid a.

inferior constrictor

common carotid a

recurrent laryngeal n.

inferior thyroid a.

common carotid a.

subclavian a.

Figure 82–3. Vessels and nerves of the larynx. (From Silver CE.[2])

The **intrinsic muscles** are considered as functional groups:

- □ Abductors (openers) of vocal cords: open inlet to larynx; include arytenoid muscle, aryepiglottic muscle, transverse arytenoid muscle, oblique arytenoid muscle, and thyroepiglottic muscle.
- □ Closer of vocal folds: lateral cricoarytenoid muscle.

Blood Supply

The **superior laryngeal artery** is a branch of the superior thyroid artery off the external carotid. The **inferior laryngeal artery** is a branch of the inferior thyroid artery off the thyrocervical trunk off the subclavian artery.

Considerations with the Infant Larynx

The infant's larynx is more anterior than the adult's. The cricoid cartilage is at the level of C3-4 in the infant, compared with C4-5 in the adult (see Chapter 162). The infant's epiglottis is relatively longer, stiffer, and further away from the anterior pharyngeal wall. The narrowest point is at the level of the **cricoid cartilage**. The tongue is relatively larger.

Selected References

1. Moore KL. Clinically Oriented Anatomy. 4th ed. Philadelphia, Lippincott Williams & Wilkins, 1999.
2. Silver CE. Surgery for Cancer of the Larynx and Related Structures. 2nd ed. Philadelphia, WB Saunders, 1996.

Suggested References

Eckenhoff J. Some anatomic considerations of the infant larynx influencing endotracheal anesthesia. Anesthesiology 1951;12:401.
Redden RJ. Anatomic considerations in anesthesia. In Hagberg CA, ed. Handbook of Difficult Airway Management. Philadelphia: Churchill Livingstone, 2000:1–13.
Stone DJ, Gal TJ. Airway management. In Miller RD, ed. Anesthesia. 5th ed. Philadelphia: Churchill Livingstone, 2000:1414–1415.

83
Brachial Plexus Anatomy

Douglas A. Dubbink, M.D.

The brachial plexus supplies all of the motor and most of the sensory function to the upper extremity. The intercostobrachial branch of the second intercostal nerve supplies sensation to the skin on the posterior medial aspect of the arm, proximal to the elbow. The skin over the shoulder receives sensory innervation from the descending branches of the cervical plexus (Fig. 83–1).

Roots

The brachial plexus derives from the anterior primary rami of the fifth, sixth, seventh, and eighth cervical nerves and the first thoracic nerve, with variable contributions from the fourth cervical and second thoracic nerves (Fig. 83–2).

Trunks

On leaving the intervertebral foramina, these nerves course anteriolaterally and inferiorly to lie between the anterior and middle scalene muscles. At this point the roots join to form three major trunks named by their relationship to one another vertically: **superior (C5-6), middle (C7), and inferior (C8-T1).**

The phrenic nerve lies in close approximation to the plexus in its position over the anterior scalene muscle, thus explaining its vulnerability to blockade during interscalene techniques. The anterior scalene muscle arises from the anterior tubercles of the cervical vertebrae and passes caudad and laterally to insert onto the scalene tubercle of the first rib. The middle scalene muscle arises from the posterior tubercles of the cervical vertebrae and inserts onto the first rib posteriorly to the subclavian artery, which passes between these two scalene muscles within the subclavian groove. Both the anterior and middle scalene muscles are invested with prevertebral fascia that fuses laterally to enclose the brachial plexus within a fascial sheath at the level of the neck.

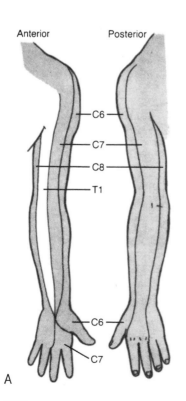

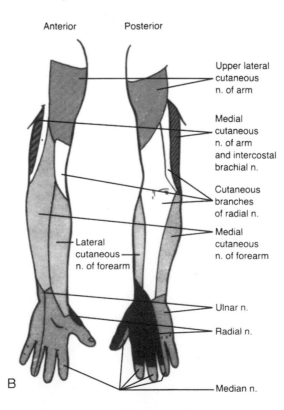

Figure 83–1. *A,* Cutaneous distribution of the cervical roots. *B,* Cutaneous distribution of the peripheral nerves. (From Wedel DJ.[1])

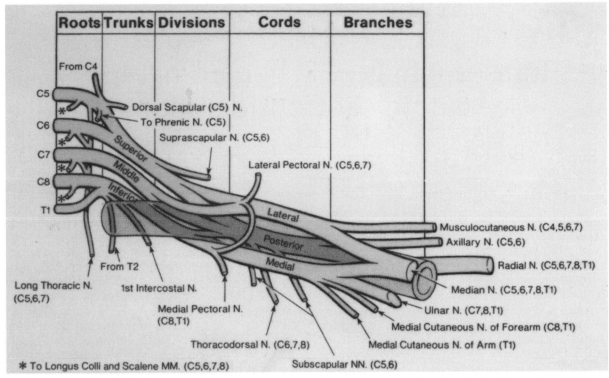

Figure 83–2. Roots, trunks, divisions, cords, and branches of the brachial plexus. Note also the relationship to the subclavian artery. Note that the intercostobrachial nerve is not shown. (From Bridenbaugh LD.[2])

Divisions

The trunks maintain close proximity to one another as they approach the upper surface of the first rib. At this point they leave the interscalene groove to lie cephaloposterior to the subclavian artery as it courses along the first rib. This vertical orientation is in contrast to the inaccurate but common depiction of the trunks of the brachial plexus lying in a horizontal formation along the first rib. At the lateral edge of the rib, each trunk forms an anterior and posterior **division,** which pass below the midportion of the clavicle to enter the axilla through its apex.

Cords

In the axilla, three cords are formed that are named after their relationship to the second segment of the second part of the axillary artery. The **medial cord** is a continuation of the anterior division of the inferior trunk, the **lateral cord** derives from the superior divisions of the superior and middle trunks, and the inferior divisions from all three trunks form the **posterior cord**.

Branches

The three cords divide in the region of the lateral border of the pectoralis minor muscle and form the peripheral nerves of the upper extremity. The lateral cord separates into the **lateral head of the median nerve** and the **musculocutaneous nerve**. The medial cord divides into the **medial head of the median**, the **ulnar,** the **medial antebrachial,** and the **medial brachial cutaneous** nerves. The posterior cord gives rise to the **axillary** and **radial** nerves.

Selected References

1. Wedel DJ. Nerve blocks. In Miller RD, ed. Anesthesia. 5th ed. New York: Churchill Livingstone, 2000:1520–1548.
2. Bridenbaugh LD. The upper extremity: Somatic blockade. In Cousins MJ, Bridenbaugh PO, eds. Neural Blockade and Clinical Anesthesia and Management of Pain. 2nd ed. Philadelphia: JB Lippincott, 1988:387.

Suggested References

McMinn RMH, Hutchings RT. Color Atlas of Human Anatomy. Chicago, Year Book Medical Publishers, 1982.
Winnie AP. Plexus Anesthesia, Perivascular Techniques of Brachial Plexus Block. Philadelphia, WB Saunders, 1983.

84
Transesophageal Echocardiography: Anatomical Considerations

Martin D. Abel, M.D. □ Susanne D. Pfeffer, M.D.

Echocardiography uses ultrasound (frequencies above the audible range) to produce images of the heart and great vessels. Sound waves are absorbed, reflected, and scattered to varying degrees by passage through human tissue. Reflected echoes are produced at boundaries between two inhomogeneous media; for example, the blood–soft-tissue interface. More homogeneous tissues result in greater ultrasound scattering and less reflection.

Biplane transesophageal echocardiography (TEE) probes have two ultrasound transducers mounted at the tip, one aligned horizontally and one vertically, allowing for orthogonal sections of the heart (Table 84–1). A multiplane probe that can be electronically rotated in any plane has recently become available and allows one to optimize the cardiac image, irrespective of the position of the heart in the thorax.

Vocal cord paresis, esophageal perforation, oropharyngeal trauma, aspiration, bronchospasm, and arrhythmias may occur (although the incidence of these complications was extremely low in a multicenter European study of more than 10,000 patients). Of greater concern are those patients with suspected aortic dissection or cardiac disease in which TEE may produce hypertension, tachycardia, and myocardial ischemia.

Anatomic Correlations

Irrespective of the reason for the TEE study, a comprehensive examination has been recommended

Table 84–1. Comparison of Standard and Biplane TEE

Specific Anatomy	Horizontal (Standard) View	Longitudinal (Biplane) View
Right atrium (RA); vena cavae (SVC and IVC)	SVC visible at several levels in short axis. IVC not seen as well but can be viewed as it enters RA. RA is well seen.	SVC and IVC entering RA well seen in long-axis view, facilitating visualization of anomalous connections.
Right ventricle (RV)	Satisfactory images of RV in four-chamber view.	Complements horizontal views of RV.
Tricuspid valve (TV)	TV orifice is oblique to plane of section. Accurate Doppler examination impossible.	TV leaflets and orifice can be visualized. Optimal for viewing RV outflow tract and pulmonary valve.
Pulmonary artery (PA)	Main PA and right PA well visualized. Left PA poorly seen.	Right PA seen in short axis. Left PA well visualized in long-axis views.
Pulmonary veins (PV)	Left upper lobe PV well visualized. Anomalous right PV to SVC connection well seen.	Improves images of all pulmonary veins. Anomalous left PV best seen.
Left atrium (LA)	Excellent images of LA.	Complements horizontal views.
LA appendage (LAA)	Well-seen in basal short-axis views.	Improves ability to rule out thrombus in LAA.
Atrial septum (AS)	Satisfactory images.	Superior views especially of fossa ovalis and of atrial septal defects.
Mitral valve (MV)	Good views of MV allow assessment of MV repair.	Aids visualization of eccentric or multiple regurgitant jets, thrombi, vegetations.
Left ventricle (LV)	LV is foreshortened in four-chamber view—cannot obtain true long axis.	Full LV long-axis obtainable with transgastric views; additional views improve assessment of regional wall motion abnormalities.
Aortic valve and LV outflow tract (LVOT) and ascending aorta	Short-axis view only. Cannot align. Doppler to evaluate pressure gradient. Blind spot in upper ascending aorta.	LVOT extremely well visualized in long axis. Vastly superior visualization of ascending aorta with near elimination of blind spot.

in every patient, preferably before focusing on a specific question or application.[1] It is beyond the scope of this brief description to detail all the anatomical views obtainable with TEE; the reader is referred to other reviews of the subject.[1–4]

Intraoperative Image Orientation

Transducer location and the near field (vertex) of the image sector are at the top of the display; the far field is at the bottom. At a multiplane angle of 0 degrees (horizontal or transverse plane), with the imaging plane directed anteriorly from the esophagus through the heart, the patient's right side appears on the left of the image display (Fig. 84–1).

Standard Horizontal Views

Basal Short-Axis Views. These views are used to visualize the left and right atrium, atrial septum and fossa ovalis, atrial appendages, ascending aorta, aortic valve, proximal coronary arteries, pulmonary veins, main pulmonary artery and its bifurcation, and the vena cavae.

Four-Chamber Views. These are used to visualize the mitral and tricuspid valves and supporting structures, the major cardiac chambers, the left ventricular outflow tract, and the coronary sinus emptying into the right atrium just above the tricuspid valve. By convention, the left ventricle is on the right with its apex at the bottom of the video screen.

Transgastric Short-Axis Views. These are used to assess global and regional left ventricular function at the base, midcavity, and apex of the heart. The left ventricle is to the right of the screen, and the right ventricle is to the left.

Thoracic Aortic Views. These are used to assess the aortic valve, proximal ascending aorta, part of the aortic arch, and descending thoracic aorta. Because the trachea is interposed between the esophagus and the upper ascending aorta and aortic arch, these structures cannot be seen with TEE and constitute a blind spot.

Standard Biplane Longitudinal Views

Primary Longitudinal Views (Fig. 84–2). These images are in the sagittal plane of the thorax but are oblique cuts of the body of the heart because

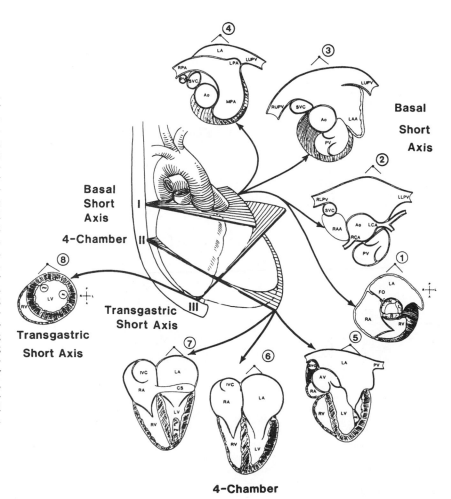

Figure 84–1. Diagram of common scan planes: I, basal short-axis; II, four-chamber (frontal long-axis); III, transgastric short-axis. Resultant tomographic planes of section. Basal short-axis sections: 1, aortic root; 2, coronary arteries; 3, left atrial appendage; and 4, pulmonary artery bifurcation. Four-chamber sections: 5, left ventricular outflow view; 6, four-chamber view; and 7, coronary sinus view. 8, Transgastric short-axis section: ventricular short-axis view. AL, anterolateral papillary muscle; Ao, aorta; AV, aortic valve; CS, coronary sinus; FO, fossa ovalis; IVC, inferior vena cava; L, left coronary cusp; LA, left atrium; LAA, left atrial appendage; LCA, left coronary artery; LLPV, left lower pulmonary vein; LPA, left pulmonary artery; LUPV, left upper pulmonary vein; LV, left ventricle; MPA, main pulmonary artery; N, noncoronary cusp; PM, posteromedial papillary muscles; PV, pulmonary valve or pulmonary vein; R, right coronary cusp, RA, right atrium; RAA, right atrial appendage; RCA, right coronary artery; RLPV, right lower pulmonary vein; RPA, right pulmonary artery; RUPV, right upper pulmonary vein; RV, right ventricle; SVC, superior vena cava. Directional axes: A, anterior; L, left; P, posterior; R, right. (Modified from Seward JB et al.[2])

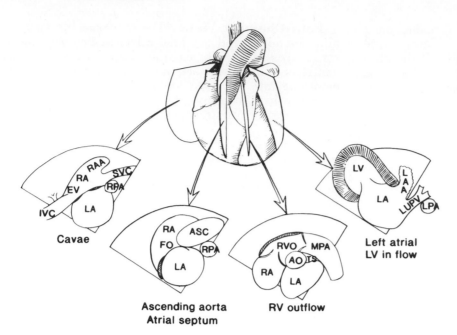

Figure 84–2. Primary longitudinal views in biplanar TEE. With the tip of the endoscope in a neutral long-axis orientation within the esophagus, four views are obtained by rotating the scope from the left to right sides of the heart. Sequentially imaged structures in the sagittal plane (from right to left) are left ventricular-left atrial two-chamber view (section 1), right ventricular outflow long-axis view (section 2), ascending aorta-atrial septal view (section 3), and caval, right atrial, and atrial septal view (section 4). AO, aorta; ASC, ascending aorta; EV, eustachian valve; FO, fossa ovalis; IVC, inferior vena cava; LA, left atrium; LAA, left atrial appendage; LPA, left pulmonary artery; LUPV, left upper pulmonary vein; LV, left ventricle; MPA, main pulmonary artery; RA, right atrium; RAA, right atrial appendage; RPA, right pulmonary artery; RV, right ventricle; RVO, right ventricular outflow; SVC, superior vena cava; TS, transverse sinus. (From Seward JB et al.[3])

of its position in the thorax. With the TEE probe in the neutral position in the esophagus, positioned with the transducer behind the left atrium, four primary tomographic cuts are obtained by clockwise rotation of the shaft from left to right. Section 1 in Fig. 84–2 shows the two-chamber view of the left atrium and left ventricle with the left atrial appendage and left upper pulmonary veins anteriorly. Section 2 shows the long axis view of the right ventricular outflow tract with the pulmonary valve and proximal left pulmonary artery (poorly imaged in the horizontal plane). Section 3 shows the ascending aorta and valve of the fossa ovalis in the atrial septum. Section 4 gives long-axis views of the vena cavae entering the right atrium with the right atrial appendage anteriorly and the atrial septum separating the atria.

Secondary Longitudinal Views. Flexing the tip of the transducer to the left can optimize views of the left ventricular outflow tract (Fig. 84–3).

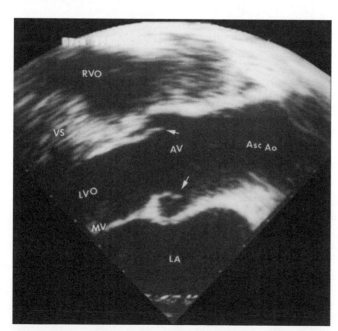

Figure 84–3. View of aortic outflow track. LVO = left ventricular outflow, AV = aortic valve (arrowheads), AscAo = aortic root (ascending aorta), MV = mitral valve, LA = left atrium, VS = ventricular septum, RVO = right ventricular outflow tract. (From Seward JB et al.[3])

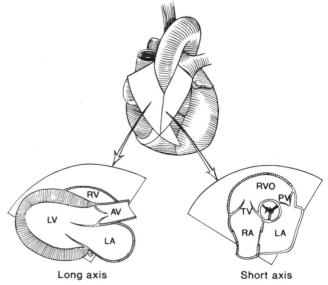

Figure 84–4. Biplanar transesophageal echocardiographic secondary (off-axis) long- and short-axis views in the longitudinal plane. Leftward (lateral flexion) of the tip of the endoscope reorients the longitudinal plane into the long-axis view of the left ventricle (section 5). Rightward (medial) flexion reorients the longitudinal array into the short-axis plane relative to the aortic valve (section 6). AV, aortic valve; PV, pulmonary valve; TV, tricuspid valve; other abbreviations as in Fig. 84–1. (From Seward JB et al.[3])

Rightward flexion produces a basal short-axis view of the heart with the right ventricular inlet and outlet, left atrium, and aortic valve seen in the same image.

Transgastric Longitudinal View (Fig. 84–4). This view is comparable to the parasternal long-axis view and offers the best opportunity to view the complete left ventricular long axis, including the true apex, with TEE. Also, it is likely that an improved estimate of regional wall motion will be obtained by combining images from both horizontal and longitudinal views. In theory, an infinite number of views might be obtained with a multiplane TEE probe. The precise advantages and disadvantages of multiplanar imaging are yet to be determined. Table 84–1 compares standard (horizontal) and biplane (longitudinal) views of the heart and aorta.

Selected References

1. Shanewise JS, Cheung AT, Aronson S, et al. ASE/SCA guidelines for performing a comprehensive intraoperative multiplane transesophageal echocardiography examination: Recommendations of the American Society of Echocardiography council for intraoperative echocardiography and the Society of Cardiovascular Anesthesiologists task force for certification in perioperative transesophageal echocardiography. Anesth Analg 1999;89:870–884.
2. Seward JB, Khandheria BK, Oh JK, et al. Transesophageal echocardiography: Technique, anatomic correlations, implementation, and clinical applications. Mayo Clin Proc 1988;63:649–680.
3. Seward JB, Khandheria BK, Edwards WD, et al. Biplanar transesophageal echocardiography: Anatomic correlations, image orientation, and clinical applications. Mayo Clin Proc 1990;65:1193–1213.
4. Seward JB, Khandheria BK, Freeman WK, et al. Multiplane transesophageal echocardiography: Image orientation, examination technique, anatomic correlations, and clinical applications. Mayo Clin Proc 1993;68:523–551.

85
Transesophageal Echocardiography: Intraoperative Uses

David J. Cook, M.D.

Background

M-mode and two-dimensional (2-D) echocardiography generate images based on changes in the reflected signal as high-frequency sound strikes tissues of different densities. Doppler techniques (pulsed wave, continuous wave, and real time with color flow mapping) are based on the detection of changes in reflected frequency as the sound strikes moving objects. The frequency shift is proportional to the object's speed, and inferences can be made regarding flow dynamics through either mathematical manipulation or by color coding of velocity and direction.

Transesophageal Echocardiography

Transesophageal echocardiography (TEE) can combine 2-D and Doppler techniques. The probe's placement behind the heart provides less distortion in image than transthoracic technique; additionally, the transducer position is more stable, does not interfere with most surgical procedures, and allows for continuous recording.

Intraoperatively, two tomographic planes have been of greatest use (Fig. 85–1). The **short axis at mid-papillary level view** allows an estimate of global left ventricular (LV) function on the basis of ventricular wall thickening, and by estimation of end-diastolic and end-systolic volume differences. This view is of greatest use in assessing regional wall motion.

The **four-chamber view** can assess all chamber sizes, mitral and tricuspid valve function, and septal motion and thickening. It is the view of choice when monitoring for air emboli and is very useful for evaluating intracardiac shunts and atrioventricular (AV) valvular repair.

Intraoperatively, TEE can be used to monitor cardiac function or to make certain specific intraoperative diagnoses. Table 85–1 provides general indi-

cations and contraindications for the use of the technique.

Monitoring

Regional Wall Motion Abnormality. Studies have shown that regional wall motion abnormalities (RWMAs) precede a rise in wedge pressure, electrocardiogram ST-T changes, and the onset of angina when coronary occlusion occurs. The determination of RWMA has been found to be reproducible between trained observers.

Global Ventricular Function. Global ventricular function can be assessed serially by estimation of systolic wall thickening (an indirect indicator of **afterload** as related to wall tension) and through estimation of LV end-diastolic volume (an estimate of preload). Stroke volume can be estimated on the basis of systolic and diastolic dimensions.

Air Embolism. Of all detection methods, TEE has been found to be the most sensitive monitor for the detection of intracardiac air and currently is

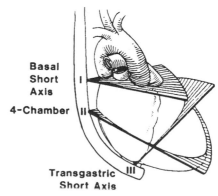

Figure 85–1. Planes of section for TEE. Three primary tomographic planes are obtained. Basal short-axis planes (I) are initially obtained, usually 25 to 30 cm from the transducer tip from the incisors. Four-chamber (frontal) planes (II) are obtained by retroflexion or slight advancement of tip of endoscope (or both) from position I (approximately 30 cm from the incisors). Transgastric short-axis planes (III) are obtained from within the fundus of the stomach, 35 to 40 cm from the incisors. (From Seward JB et al.[1])

Table 85–1. Transsesophageal Echocardiography

Indications	Contraindications
Assessment	**Absolute**
Chamber size	Esophageal pathology: stricture, varices,
Valvular function	scleroderma, esophagitis, or a history
Septal thickness	of esophageal surgery
Intracardiac shunts	**Relative**
Intracardiac masses	Coagulopthy or heparinization
Thoracic aorta	Left atrial myxoma with history of
Myocardial perfusion	embolization
Monitoring	
Global ventricular function	
Regional ventricular function	
Intracardiac contrast	
Venous/paradoxical air	
embolism	

Modified from Thys et al.[2]

the only device for monitoring for paradoxical air embolism.

Intraoperative Diagnosis

□ Intraoperative TEE can detect both early ischemia and air embolism.

□ TEE can quickly provide information as to the cause of intraoperative hypotension, particularly during separation from cardiopulmonary bypass, when ventricular compliance is changing and wedge pressures may not accurately reflect ventricular filling.

□ TEE can effectively determine the adequacy of myectomies and repairs of AV valves or atrial and ventricular septal defects, especially with the use of contrast.

□ TEE can be used to quantitatively evaluate valve area as well as pressure gradients across valves.

□ TEE can be used to evaluate aortic disease and diagnose aortic dissection.

□ Intraoperative TEE can be used to assess an intracardiac mass (e.g., thrombus, myxoma, or vegetation) and observe for embolus.

□ The use of contrast techniques, such as albumin microspheres, may someday play a role in determining the area at risk as well as the adequacy of coronary artery bypass grafting.

Limitations of the Technique

□ The equipment is expensive and bulky, and extensive training is required to eliminate intraobserver variability.

□ The peculiarities of cardiac motion make it difficult to assign frames of reference, and estimates of wall thickening and volume change can be unreliable.

□ Risk for ischemia may be very high after anesthetic induction before the TEE probe is placed.

□ Although qualitative hemodynamic measurements can be made with all TEE units intraoperatively, quantitative statements can be made only with the newer units.

□ The technique samples only limited tomographic sections. These sections may not represent global processes and may miss significant changes in unmonitored sections. The technological improvement of multiplane imaging in the newer units has reduced this limitation.

Potential Associated Risks

Esophageal perforation is a serious complication that has been reported. Transient vocal cord paralysis in the sitting position has been reported in two patients. In these cases, the combination of endotracheal tube, TEE probe, and extreme neck flexion may have exerted pressure on the recurrent laryngeal nerve. Severe postoperative macroglossia has also been reported in a sitting patient monitored with a TEE probe. Minor bleeding and atrial and ventricular arrhythmias have also been documented. Instrumentation of the esophagus may produce bacteremia and increase the risk of endocarditis in patients at risk. Finally, it is important to note that focus on TEE may distract providers from more pressing issues of patient care.

Selected References

1. Seward JB, Khandheria BK, Oh JK, et al. Transsesophageal echocardiography: Technique, anatomic correlations, implementations, and clinical applications. Mayo Clin Proc 1988;63:649.
2. Thys DM, Hillel Z, Konstadt S. Intraoperative echocardiography. Semin Anesth 1989;8:44.

Suggested References

Abel MD, Nishimura RA, Callahan MJ, et al. Evaluation of intraoperative transsesophageal two-dimensional echocardiography. Anesthesiology 1987;66:64.
Cahalan MK, Lurz FC, Schiller NB. Transsesophageal two-dimensional echocardiographic evaluation of anaesthetic effects on left ventricular function. Br J Anaesth 1988;60:995.
Dewhirst WE, Stragand JJ, Fleming BM. Mallory-Weiss tear complicating intraoperative transsesophageal echocardiography in a patient undergoing aortic valve replacement. Anesthesiology 1990;73:777.
Kahn RA, Konstadt SN, Louie EK, et al. Intraoperative echocardiography. In Kaplan JA, Reich DL, Konstadt SN, ed. Cardiac Anesthesia. 4th ed. Philadelphia: WB Saunders, 1999:401–484.
Kuhnert SM, Faust RJ, Berge KH, Piepgras DG. Postoperative macroglossia: Report of a case with rapid resolution after extubation of the trachea. Anesth Analg 1999;88:220–223.
Sanders JS, Cheung AT, Aronson S, et al. ASE/SCA Guidelines for performing a comprehensive intraoperative multiplane transsesophageal echocardiography examination. Anesth Analg 1999;89:870–884.

86
Medical Gas Cylinders: Physics, Handling Safety, Pin Indexing

Scott A. Lockwood, M.D.

Medical gas cylinders are used to store compressed gas. Compressed gas is defined as a gas with a pressure exceeding 40 pounds per square inch (psi) at 70°F; or a gas with a pressure greater than 104 psi at 130°F, or a liquid with a vapor pressure greater than 40 psi at 100°F. Sometimes psi is abbreviated as psig (pounds per square inch on the gauge). Some sources measure pressures in kilopascals (kPa), the Systéme International (SI) units of pressure. Conversion factors for SI units are given in Table 86–1.

Cylinder sizes are designated according to letters, with size A being the smallest. Size E is the cylinder size most commonly used on anesthesia machines. Cylinders are color coded according to the gas the cylinder contains (Table 86–2). In the United States, **green** indicates oxygen; **blue,** nitrous oxide; **gray,** carbon dioxide; **yellow,** air; and **brown,** helium. An international code exists that differs from that used in the United States; therefore, cylinder color should be regarded only as an aid to gas identification.

Content and Pressure

In cylinders containing a nonliquified gas such as oxygen, helium, or air, the pressure in the cylinder declines proportionally as the gas is withdrawn from the cylinder. For example, an E size cylinder contains approximately 660 L of oxygen at a pressure of 1900 psi when full. When this same cylinder is half empty (330 L), the pressure is 950 psi. Therefore, it is possible to calculate how long a given flow

rate can be maintained until a given cylinder is empty (Fig. 86–1).

In contrast, in a cylinder containing a liquified gas such as nitrous oxide, carbon dioxide, or cyclopropane, pressure in the cylinder depends on the **vapor pressure** of the liquid gas and does not indicate the amount of liquified gas remaining in the cylinder. Only when all of the liquid nitrous oxide is vaporized does the pressure start to fall. For example, a full E size nitrous oxide cylinder contains 1590 L at a pressure of 745 psi. This pressure remains constant until all the liquid has vaporized, at which point the pressure starts to drop. At this point, approximately 400 L of nitrous oxide remains in the cylinder (Fig. 86–2). Vaporization of a liquid to a gas absorbs heat from the atmosphere and the liquid in the cylinder. This results in cooling of the liquified gas. Frost can form on the outside of the tank. This decrease in temperature will decrease the vapor pressure of the liquid and result in a slight decrease in pressure measured within the cylinder.

Pin Index Safety System

The pin index safety system was incorporated into most anesthetic equipment produced after 1953

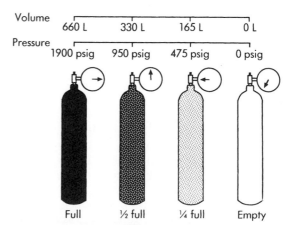

Figure 86–1. Oxygen remains a gas under high pressure. The pressure falls linearly as the gas flows from the cylinder; thus, in contrast to nitrous oxide, for oxygen the pressure always reflects the amount of gas remaining in the cylinder. (From Eichorn JH, Ehrenwerth J.[3])

Table 86–1. Conversion Table for Pressure Units

| | | Conversion Factors | |
		Old to SI (Exact)	SI to Old (Approximate)
SI Unit	Old Unit		
kPa	lbs/sq in	6.894	0.145
kPa	mm Hg	0.133	7.5
kPa	cm H$_2$O	0.0981	10

Adapted from the Association of Anaesthetists of Great Britian and Ireland.[1]

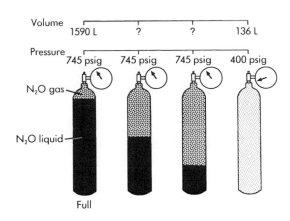

Figure 86–2. At ambient temperature (20°C), nitrous oxide liquifies under high pressure and the pressure of the gas above the liquid remains constant *independent* of how much liquid remains in the cylinder. Only when all of the liquid has evaporated does the pressure start to fall, and then it does so rapidly as the residual gas flows from the cylinder. (From Eichorn JH, Ehrenwerth J.[3])

Table 86–2. Medical Gas Cylinders

| Gas | Color | | 70°F Service Pressure (psi) | State in Cylinder | E Cylinder Capacity (L) |
	U.S.	International			
Oxygen	Green	White	1900–2200	Gas	660
Carbon dioxide	Gray	Gray	838	Liquid <88° F	1590
Nitrous oxide	Blue	Blue	745	Liquid <98° F	1590
Helium	Brown	Brown	1600–2000	Gas	496
Nitrogen	Black	Black	1800–2200	Gas	651
Air	Yellow	White and black	1800	Gas	625

Adapted from Dorsch JA, Dorsch SE.[2]

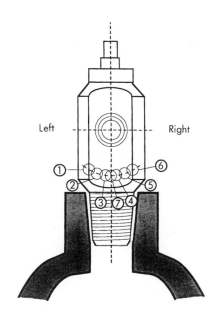

Figure 86–3. Pin index safety system pin location. Perspective shown looking at the placement of holes in the tank. Pins are placed precisely complementary in the tank yoke. Two pins are used to identify each type of gas. Pin positions: air (1–5), cyclopropane (3–6), nitrogen (1–4), nitrous oxide (3–5), oxygen (2–5), helium (4–6; 2–4), carbon dioxide (2–6; 1–6). (From Eichorn JH, Ehrenwerth J.[3])

to prevent the attachment of the wrong gas cylinder to the yoke on an anesthesia machine (which could result in the administration of a hypoxic gas mixture). The pin index system consists of two pins projecting from the cylinder yoke, which correspond to holes drilled into the cylinder valve on the gas cylinder (Fig. 86–3). A yoke that has not been pin indexed may accept any cylinder valve. However, a yoke containing pins will accept only the correct cylinder valve.

Handling Safety

Gas cylinders should be stored in a cool, well-ventilated place, away from open flames. They should never be exposed to temperatures over 130°F. Cylinders should be properly secured and protected to prevent damage. The valve is the most easily damaged component and should be protected by protector caps when not in use. Before use, the valve and pin index holes should be inspected for damage. Any defective cylinder valves should be returned to the supplier. Cylinders with pressures greater than service pressure should not be used. The valve should always be fully open when using a cylinder, to avoid inadequate gas delivery.

Selected References

1. Association of Anaesthetists of Great Britain and Ireland: Système International (SI) conversion tables. Anaesthesia 1976;31:457.
2. Dorsch JA, Dorsch SE. Understanding Anesthesia Equipment. 2nd ed. Baltimore, Williams & Wilkins, 1984.
3. Eichorn JH, Ehrenwerth J. Medical gases: Storage and supply. In Ehrenwerth J, Eisenkraft JB, eds. Anesthesia Equipment: Principles and Applications. St. Louis: Mosby, 1993:3.

Suggested References

Andrews JJ. Delivery Systems for Inhaled Anesthetics. In Barash PG, Cullen BF, Stoelting RK, eds. Clinical Anesthesia. 3rd ed. Philadelphia: Lippincott-Raven, 1997:535–572.

87

Flowmeters: Physics of Gas Flow

Mary M. Rajala, M.D.

The flowmeter assembly is a device that measures, controls, and indicates the flow of gas passing through it. Modern flowmeters, known as variable orifice or Thorpe flowmeters, are vertically placed tempered-glass tapered tubes that have the smallest diameter at the bottom (Fig. 87–1). Gas flow rate into the tube is controlled by a needle valve. Gas enters from the bottom and leaves through the top, elevating an indicator float or bobbin that moves up and down the tapered tube freely, depending on the flow of gas within the tube. The indicator floats at the point of equilibrium where the downward force of gravity on the bobbin is equal to the upward force of the gas flow. It is prevented from leaving the tube by a stop at the top. A scale calibrated specifically for each gas is marked along the side of the tube indicating the gas flow. The higher the float rises in the tube, the greater the gas flow around it.

Rate of gas flow through the flowmeter depends on the change in pressure across the constriction, the circumference around the indicator float, and the physical properties of the gas.

Physical Principles

Pressure Change Across the Constriction. As gas flows around the bobbin, friction between the glass and bobbin is encountered, causing a pressure drop. This change is constant for all positions within the tube and equals the weight of the float divided by its cross-sectional area. Increasing flow will not increase the pressure drop.

Magnitude of the Annular Opening. The space between the float and the wall of the tube forms a channel or annular opening. Gas flow increases directly with increases in the circumference or annular opening. The pressure change across the constriction is balanced by the weight of the float, so that a change in area is accompanied by a corresponding change in lifting force, which is caused by changing the flow of gas.

Physical Properties of the Gas. At low flows, the annular opening or circumference around the float will be narrow. The opening enlarges with increasing flow. At low flows, when the tube is narrow, gas flow varies according to the viscosity of the gas. (**Poiseuille's law** states that the volume of flow in a tube is directly proportional to the pressure drop along the length of the tube, and to the fourth power of the radius of the tube, and is inversely proportional to the length of the tube and the viscosity of the fluid.)

At high flows, the tube is wider, and gas flow becomes a function of the density of the gas (**Graham's law**). Increases in flow allow the float to rise, providing a larger opening for gas flow. The level of the float is related to the size of the annular opening and therefore to flow. Flowmeters are calibrated for use with a specific gas density and viscosity and thus cannot be interchanged.

Effects of Temperature and Pressure

Changes in temperature and pressure alter both the viscosity and density of gases, thereby affecting

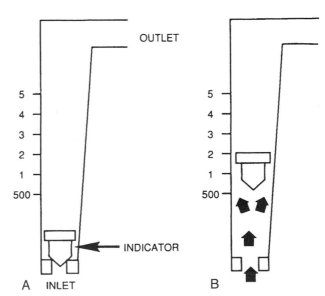

Figure 87–1. Variable orifice flowmeter. Gas enters at the base and flows through the tube, causing the float to rise. The gas passes through the annular opening around the float. The area of this annular space increases with the height of the indicator. Thus the height of the indicator is a measure of gas flow. (From Dorsch JA, Dorsch SE.[1])

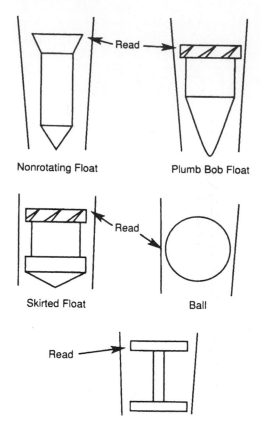

Figure 87–2. Flowmeter indicators. The plumb bob and skirted floats are examples of rotameters, which are kept centered in the tube by constant rotation. The reading is taken at the top. The ball indicator is held centered by rib guides. The reading is taken at the center. The nonrotating float and H float do not rotate and are kept centered by gas flow. (From Dorsch JA, Dorsch SE.[1])

accuracy of the indicator on the flowmeters, which are calibrated at atmospheric pressure (760 mm Hg) and room temperature (20°C). Practically speaking, temperature changes are slight and are not responsible for significant changes. Large fluctuations in temperature, however, will make calibrations inaccurate.

As altitude increases, barometric pressure decreases, resulting in increased flow. At low flow rates, flow is laminar and dependent on gas viscosity, a property independent of altitude. However, at high flow rates, flow becomes turbulent, and flow becomes a function of density, a property that *is* influenced by altitude. The resulting decrease in density will increase the actual flow rate, so the flowmeter will read lower than the actual flow rate. At pressures below 630 mm Hg, the delivered flow rate will exceed the set flow rate by 9% to 20%. At increased pressure, as in a hyperbaric chamber, the reverse is seen, with the delivered flow rate slightly less than the set flow rate.

Types of Indicators

The indicator float or bobbin is generally made of aluminum, nickel, sapphire, or glass. Numerous styles are in use, including the free-spinning, rotameter ball float, nonrotating float, and H float (Fig. 87–2). These are designed so that gas flowing through the tube keeps the float in the center of the tube and allows the float to spin freely (for types that rotate), maintaining the central position, reducing friction, and improving accuracy. Deviations of the tube from a vertical position cause the float to strike the side of the tube.

Arrangement of Flowmeters

Two flowmeter tubes for the same gas may be arranged in series or in parallel for finer control of gas flow. Modern machines have a series arrangement, using only one valve for each gas. Normal flow is from bottom to top and from left to right. An oxygen analyzer must be used to determine whether a hypoxic mixture exists.

Hypoxia can result from poor sequencing of flowmeters (Fig. 87–3). When the oxygen flowmeter is upstream, a leak in the system will cause oxygen to leak out before being added to other gases, a potentially dangerous situation. It is safer to have oxygen as the most downstream gas. In the United States and Canada, the standard is for the oxygen

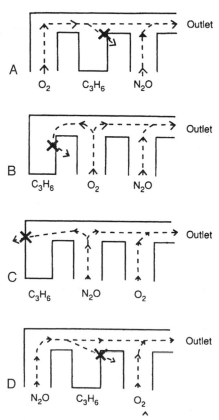

Figure 87–3. Flowmeter sequence. A and B, With the oxygen flowmeter upstream, a potentially dangerous situation arises if a leak should occur. C and D, With the oxygen entering downstream from the other gases, a safer situation is achieved. (From Eger et al.[3])

flowmeter to occupy the right-hand location nearest the normal outlet and downstream from all other gases. Some machines are manufactured with pin indexing of the flowmeter module as a safety feature. In some units, all flowmeters are serviced as a unit, preventing transposition of the rotameter tubes. Some newer models have incorporated identical flowmeter tubes that are entirely interchangeable, relying instead on exterior scales that are etched. Other new trends include electronic flow controls. Servicing flowmeters or dissembling the anesthesia machine should be performed only by qualified personnel.

Hypoxia can also result from human error on older machines. To prevent this, modern machines have mandatory minimum oxygen flows, mechanical or pneumatic linkages between oxygen and nitrous oxide flow control valves, and alarms to prevent administration of hypoxic mixtures.

Problems

Inaccuracy. Error increases inversely with rate of flow and may become clinically significant (up to 70%) at flows below 1 L/min. Between 1 and 5 L/min flow, delivered flow is within 5% of set flow. Flowmeters are calibrated to the lowest accurate point on the scale. Flows extrapolated below the first mark on the scale are not accurate. Low-flow tubes arranged in series allow greater accuracy when low gas flow is desired. It is important to measure oxygen concentration during low flow to avoid a hypoxic mixture caused by flowmeter inaccuracy.

Back Pressure. If pressure at the common outlet increases, then the gas above the float is compressed and the pressure above the indicator rises, forcing the float down and causing the flowmeter to read lower than the actual gas flow rate.

Improper Alignment. Inaccuracy may result from improper alignment of the floats in the flowmeter tube, leading to an asymmetric circumference of the channel around the float.

Improper Sequence. A 1998 report described a case where rotameter tubes for carbon dioxide and nitrous oxide were transposed after servicing. The anesthesiologist recognized the problem after the gas flows were turned on, when the calibration for nitrous oxide was incorrect in scale, color, and labeling, and was able to compensate by using 100% oxygen and volatile agent.

Static Electricity. Inaccuracy may result from static electricity causing the float to stick to the side of the tube. The electrostatic charges are negligible as long as the float rotates freely. Moisture or anti-static spray applied to the outside of the tube will successfully remove charges. More technical approaches are required to remove charges from within the tube.

Hidden Floats. The float may adhere to the stop at the top of the tube even if no gas is flowing. If the stops are broken or are not replaced after cleaning, the float may disappear from view. Dirt particles, frequent components of compressed air, can cause to flow to stick and create inaccurate gas flow readings; excessive pressure buildup inside the tube can lead to explosion.

Selected References

1. Dorsch JA, Dorsch SE. Understanding anesthesia equipment. 4th ed. Baltimore, Williams & Wilkins, 1999:75–120.
2. Andrews JJ. Inhaled Anesthetic Delivery Systems. In Miller RD, ed. Anesthesia. 5th ed. Philadelphia: Churchill Livingstone, 2000:174–206.
3. Eger EI, Hylton RR, Irwin RH, Guadagni N. Anesthetic flow meter sequence: A cause for hypoxia. Anesthesiology 1963;24:396–397.
4. Walmsley AJ, Holloway J. Transposition of rotameter tubes. Br J Anesth 1998;80:124–125.
5. Walmsley AJ, Cooke R. Transposition of rotameter tubes. Br J Anesth 1998;80:698–699.

Suggested References

Andrews JJ. Delivery systems for inhaled anesthetics. In Barash PG, Cullen BF, Stoelting RK, eds. Clinical Anesthesia. 3rd ed. Philadelphia: Lippincott-Raven, 1997:535–572.

88
Vaporizers

Jerry A. Dorsch, M.D.

The vapor pressures of most anesthetic agents at room temperature are much greater than the partial pressure required to produce anesthesia (Table 88–1). To produce clinically useful concentrations, a vaporizer must bring about dilution of the saturated vapor. The total gas flow from the flowmeters goes through the vaporizer, picks up a predictable amount of vapor, then flows to the common gas outlet. A single calibrated knob or dial on the vaporizer is used to control agent concentration.

Concentration-Calibrated Vaporizers

All vaporizers in common use today in developed countries are calibrated by the output concentration, expressed in volume percent. This is known as a concentration-calibrated (or variable bypass, direct-reading, dial-controlled, automatic plenum, percentage-type or tec-type vaporizer, vaporizer chamber bypass arrangement) vaporizer. The standard requires that all vaporizers at the anesthesia workstation be concentration calibrated.

Concentration calibration can be accomplished by splitting the flow of gas that passes through the vaporizer. Some gas passes through the vaporizing chamber (the part of the vaporizer containing the liquid anesthetic agent), and the remainder goes through a bypass to the vaporizer outlet (Fig. 88–1). The ratio of bypass gas to gas going to the vaporizing chamber is called the *splitting ratio* and depends on the resistances in the two pathways. This in turn depends on the variable (adjustable) orifice. This orifice may be in the inlet to the vaporizing chamber, but in most modern vaporizers it is in the outlet. The splitting ratio may also depend on the total flow to the vaporizer.

Another method of controlling the outlet concentration is to direct a measured flow of carrier gas through the vaporizing chamber. This method is used in one type of electronic vaporizer. Unlike the old Copper Kettle and Vernitrol vaporizers, which had a separate flowmeter to measure the carrier gas and required calculations to determine the output concentration, the flow of carrier gas is determined by a computer. This allows sufficient carrier gas to flow through the vaporizing chamber to achieve the concentration set on the vaporizer. The flow depends on the concentration determined by a gas monitor.

In many concentration-calibrated vaporizers, the composition of the carrier gas affects vaporizer output (vaporizer aberrance). Most vaporizers are calibrated using oxygen as the carrier gas. Usually, little change in output occurs if air is substituted for oxygen. Addition of nitrous oxide to the carrier gas typically results in both temporary and long-lasting effects on vaporizer output. The temporary effect is usually reduced vapor concentration. The duration of this effect depends on the gas flow rate and on the volume of liquid in the vaporizer. The longer-term effect may be increased or decreased output concentration, depending on the construction of the vaporizer. With most vaporizers, output decreases as fresh gas flow increases, because of incomplete saturation in the vaporizing chamber.

At low barometric pressure (higher altitudes), variable-bypass concentration-calibrated vaporizers will deliver approximately the same anesthetic partial pressure but increased concentrations as measured in volume percent. At high barometric pressure (as in a hyperbaric chamber), these vaporizers deliver decreased anesthetic output, measured as volume percent because vapor pressure of the agent is affected only by temperature and not by ambient pressure; the partial pressure and clinical effects remain relatively unchanged.

Vaporization Methods

Flow Over. In a flow-over vaporizer, carrier gas passes over the surface of the liquid. Increasing the area of the carrier gas-liquid interface can enhance the efficiency of vaporization. This can be done us-

Table 88–1. Vapor Pressure of Anesthetics at 20°C

Halothane	243 mm Hg
Enflurane	175 mm Hg
Isoflurane	239 mm Hg
Sevoflurane	160 mm Hg
Desflurane	664 mm Hg

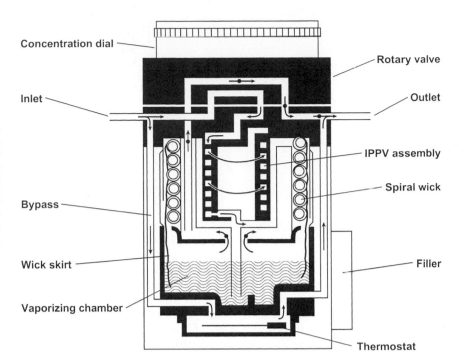

Figure 88–1. Schematic of concentration-calibrated variable bypass design of the Ohmeda Tec 5 vaporizer. The bimetallic strip thermostat at the bottom decreases gas flow through the bypass as temperature decreases. Gas flowing through the vaporizing chamber passes through the rotary valve, then through the helical intermittent positive pressure ventilation assembly, then past the spiral wick. (From Dorsch JA, Dorsch SE.[1])

ing baffles or spiral tracks to lengthen the pathway of the gas over the liquid. Another method is to use wicks with their bases in the liquid. The liquid moves up the wicks by capillary action.

Bubble Through. Another way to increase contact between the carrier gas and the volatile liquid is to bubble the gas through the liquid. The gas may break up into small bubbles, further increasing the gas-liquid interface.

Injection. Some vaporizers control the vapor concentration by injecting a known amount of liquid anesthetic (from a reservoir in the vaporizer or from the bottle of agent) into a known volume of gas.

Temperature Compensation

When a liquid is vaporized, energy in the form of heat is lost. As the temperature of the liquid decreases, so does the vapor pressure. Three methods have been employed to maintain a constant vapor output with fluctuations in liquid anesthetic temperature.

Thermostatic Compensation. Most concentration-calibrated vaporizers compensate for changes in vapor pressure with temperature by altering the flow of carrier gas through the vaporizing chamber. This is accomplished by altering the splitting ratio. In mechanical vaporizers, a thermostatic element performs this function by increasing resistance to the bypass flow of gas, forcing more flow through the vaporizing chamber as the vaporizer cools. In electronic vaporizers, gas flow is controlled

by a computer that alters the flow of carrier gas through the vaporizing chamber to maintain the output concentration needed to deliver the set concentration.

Supplied Heat. An electric heater can be used to supply heat to a vaporizer and maintain it at a constant temperature.

Desflurane Tec 6. Because of desflurane's high vapor pressure at room temperature, the vaporizer for this agent requires unique features. The drug's low boiling point (22.8°C) would make the volume of gas delivered by either a measured-flow or a variable-bypass vaporizer unpredictable. The Ohmeda Tec 6 vaporizer warms and pressurizes liquid desflurane to 1500 mm Hg. To adjust for changes in the relative pressures of gaseous desflurane and diluent gas flow in the device, it controls release of the gas with variable resistance controlled automatically by a differential pressure transducer.

Selected References

1. Dorsch JA, Dorsch SE. Vaporizers (anesthetic agent delivery devices). In Understanding Anesthesia Equipment. 4th ed. Baltimore: Williams and Wilkins, 1999:121–181.

Suggested References

Andrews JJ. Delivery Systems for Inhaled Anesthetics. In Barash PG, Cullen BF, Stoelting RK, eds. Clinical Anesthesia. 3rd ed. Philadelphia: Lippincott-Raven, 1997:535–572.
Andrews JJ, Johnston RV, Jr. The new Tec 6 desflurane vaporizer. Anesth Analg 1993;76:1338–1341.

89
Closed-Circuit Anesthesia

Theresia L. Lee, M.D.

Closed-circuit anesthesia (or closed-system anesthesia) is a type of low-flow anesthesia in which the fresh gas inflow is equivalent to the uptake of anesthetic gases and oxygen and the relief valve on the anesthesia circle is closed. A standard anesthesia machine may be used for closed-circuit anesthesia if it has an accurate flowmeter that can register flows as low as 100 mL/minute. Use of a reliable oxygen analyzer and carbon dioxide monitor is essential. Respiratory gas analysis via mass spectrometry facilitates this technique, but additional gas must be added to the circle to compensate for that removed through the mass spectrometer capillary tube.

If the standard circle system used has a mechanism for bypassing the absorber, it should be removed so that the bypass is not inadvertently opened. The system should be free of leaks. A ventilator with bellows that rise during expiration will detect leaks more readily than one with bellows that descend during expiration. Anesthetic gases may be added to the circle via syringe injection of liquid volatile anesthetic into the expiratory limb, in-circle vaporizers, or out-of-system vaporizers.

Induction with low-flow anesthesia is difficult for two reasons. If low fresh gas inflow is used during induction, then excretion of nitrogen will dilute the gases present in the system. Although this is not a problem if oxygen alone is used, hypoxia may result if both nitrous oxide and oxygen make up the fresh gas inflow. Furthermore, the presence of nitrogen may decrease the concentration of nitrous oxide enough to allow patient awareness. Second, maximal uptake of the volatile agent during this period makes it difficult to predict dosage, and inadequate or excessive concentrations could frequently develop in the circle. To circumvent these problems, denitrogenation and anesthetic induction are usually first done with high-flow anesthesia. Low-flow anesthesia is then initiated after adequate anesthetic concentrations have been established.

Maintenance of Anesthesia

During maintenance of anesthesia, it is important to note the concentration of oxygen, especially when nitrous oxide is included in the fresh gas inflow. Over time, decreased tissue uptake of nitrous oxide can result in decreased alveolar concentrations of oxygen. This can lead to hypoxia if the gas inflow of nitrous oxide is not decreased. Similarly, the concentration of inhaled volatile anesthetic is influenced by the concentration present in the exhaled gases, which reflects tissue uptake of the anesthetic. Initially, tissue uptake is maximal. Over time, decreased tissue uptake will reduce the required inflow of the anesthetic.

The volume of anesthetic gas derived from each mL of liquid can be derived from Table 89–1. Knowing this, closed-circuit anesthesia could be performed without the use of a vaporizer, injecting measured volumes of liquid anesthetics into the anesthetic circuit at the proper time. In clinical practice, most will choose low or moderate flow rates to avoid the necessity of these calculations and to facilitate rapid changes in inspired anesthetic concentration.

The nitrous oxide and oxygen ratio must be maintained at an acceptable oxygen concentration. Constant circle volume can be achieved by a constant bag position at end-tidal volume. If a ventilator with upright bellows is used, constant volume will be maintained if the fresh gas flow is adjusted so that the bellows height is about 100 to 200 mL below the top at end tidal volume.

If rapid changes in anesthetic concentrations or oxygen concentration are necessary, fresh gas flow should be increased (e.g., to increase or decrease anesthetic level). It is recommended that high flows

Table 89–1. Useful Values for Inhalational Anesthetics

Gas	MAC (%)	Blood-Gas Partition Coefficient	Vapor Pressure (20°C) (mm Hg)	mL Vapor/ mL Liquid (37°C)
Halothane	0.75	2.4	243	240
Enflurane	1.7	1.9	175	210
Isoflurane	1.14	1.5	239	206
Desflurane	6.4	0.45	664	
Sevoflurane	2.0	0.65	160	
Nitrous oxide	101	0.47	37,845 (732 psi)	

Modified from Lowe HJ and Ernst EA[1] and other sources.

be used for 1 to 2 minutes every hour to eliminate buildup of nitrogen, carbon monoxide, and anesthetic metabolites in the system.

Emergence

Recovery from anesthesia using low-flow techniques occurs very slowly. In most instances, high flows are needed to clear the nitrous oxide and other volatile anesthetics quickly.

Advantages of Closed-Circuit Anesthesia

Closed-circuit anesthesia has the following advantages:
- □ Reduction of operating room pollution.
- □ Conservation of moisture and heat.
- □ Gradual changes of anesthetic depth.
- □ Economy in the use of anesthetics.

Disadvantages of Closed-Circuit Anesthesia

Closed-circuit anesthesia has the following disadvantages:

- □ Inability to quickly alter inspired concentrations.
- □ Increased danger of hypercarbia when low flows are used.
- □ More attention required to constantly adjust anesthetic fresh gas flows, which could divert attention from other aspects of patient care.
- □ Possible accumulation of high concentrations of undesired gases and vapors in the system.

Selected References

1. Lowe HJ, Ernst EA. The Quantitative Practice of Anesthesia: Use of Closed Circuit. Baltimore, Williams & Wilkins, 1981:178.

Suggested References

Andrews J. Delivery systems for inhaled anesthetics. In Barash PG, Cullen BF, Stoelting RK, eds. Clinical Anesthesia. 3rd ed. Philadelphia: Lippincott-Raven, 1997:535–562.

Dorsch JA, Dorsch SE. Understanding Anesthesia Equipment. 4th ed. Baltimore, Williams & Wilkins, 1999.

Eger EI II. Uptake and distribution. In Miller RD, ed. Anesthesia. 5th ed. New York: Churchill Livingstone, 2000:74–951.

90
Carbon Dioxide Absorption

John M. Van Erdewyk, M.D.

Scientists first began experimenting with substances capable of absorbing carbon dioxide (CO_2) in the early 1900s. Progress was made during World War I, when chemical warfare stimulated research to eliminate CO_2 from the closed breathing system of the gas mask. Today, CO_2 absorption is used daily to remove CO_2 from semiclosed or closed anesthetic circuits. **Soda lime** was one of the first substances used for this purpose and, although many refinements have been made since, the basic ingredients remain unchanged.

Carbon Dioxide Absorbers

An ideal CO_2 absorber would have the following characteristics: low cost, efficiency, ease of handling, lack of toxicity when used with common anesthetics, and low resistance to air flow. **Soda lime** and **baralyme** are the two most common CO_2 absorbers in use today. Both chemically neutralize CO_2 (an acid after combining with water to form carbonic acid) by reaction with a base.

Soda lime has the following composition: 4% sodium hydroxide, 1% potassium hydroxide, 14% to 19% water, 0.2% silica, and approximately 80% calcium hydroxide. The following chemical reactions take place to neutralize CO_2 through formation of calcium carbonate, giving off water and heat:

$$CO_2 + H_2O \leftrightarrow H_2CO_3$$

$$H_2CO_3 + 2\,NaOH(KOH) \leftrightarrow Na_2CO_3(K_2CO_3) + 2\,H_2O + heat$$

$$Na_2CO_3(K_2CO_3) + Ca(OH)_2 \leftrightarrow CaCO_3 + 2\,NaOH(KOH)$$

Baralyme is composed of 20% barium hydroxide and 80% calcium hydroxide. The reaction of CO_2 with baralyme is as follows:

$$Ba(OH)_2 \cdot 8\,H_2O + CO_2 \leftrightarrow BaCO_3 + 9H_2O + heat$$

$$9H_2O + 9CO_2 \leftrightarrow 9H_2CO_3$$

$$9H_2CO_3 + 9Ca(OH)_2 \leftrightarrow CaCO_3 + 18H_2O + heat$$

Unlike baralyme, **soda lime** contains silica. Silica is added to increase the hardness of the granules and minimize the formation of alkaline dust, which can cause airway irritation if inhaled. Baralyme does not require silica because barium hydroxide is inherently harder than sodium hydroxide.

Baralyme does not contain water as an ingredient, because its water is derived from the bound water of crystallization in the octahydrate salt of the barium hydroxide. Thus baralyme gives more reliable performances in a dry environment, whereas soda lime may react more erratically.

Efficiency of Absorption

The maximum amount of CO_2 that can be absorbed is approximately 26 L of CO_2 per 100 g of absorbent. However, in practical use, much less is actually absorbed due to factors such as channeling of gas flow around the granules, canister design, moisture content, and the endpoint used to detect exhaustion of the granules. In a dual-chambered canister, 18 to 20 L of CO_2 is absorbed per 100 g of absorbent, and 10 to 15 L CO_2 is absorbed in a single-chambered canister.

For the greatest efficiency of absorption, the patient's entire tidal volume should be accommodated within the void space of the container. Therefore, a properly packed canister should contain approximately one-half of its volume in granules and one-half as intergranular space.

The greater the **surface area** available for CO_2 absorption, the greater the absorptive ability. However, as granule size decreases (surface area increases), the resistance to air flow through the canister increases. A compromise has been reached in a granule size of 4 to 8 mesh, which allows good CO_2 absorption with an acceptable resistance to flow.

Channeling is the preferential passage of exhaled gases through the canister via the pathways of least resistance. Excessive channeling will bypass much of the granule bulk and decrease the efficiency of CO_2 absorption. Proper canister design with screens and baffles plus proper packing helps decrease channeling (Fig. 90–1).

An ideal water content is needed for optimal CO_2 absorption. Too much water reduces the surface

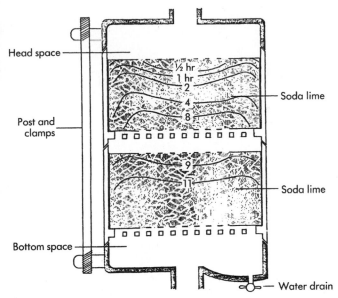

Figure 90–1. Modern "jumbo" canister. Originated by Elam and Brown, these transparent twin-chambered canisters are now supplied by all producers. Permanently mounted with a vertical gas-flow axis, they eliminate dusting, channeling, and packing problems. Used as intended, with the exhausted canister changed only when the second half is exhausted, they use the absorptive capacity of soda lime fully, as shown by the lines illustrating patterns of exhaustion. Drop-in, prepacked containers add convenience. The nearly standard shape is 8 cm high and 15 cm in diameter. Because water of condensation may collect at the bottom, forming a caustic lye solution with the dust, a drain valve is an important component. Convenience of opening, closing, and sealing varies with design; but most now have a single-action clamp mechanism. The casting for the top and bottom should be resistant to alkaline corrosion and may incorporate other components of the breathing circuit (e.g., bag mount, inflow site, and valve housing). (From Smith TC.[1])

area available for absorption and too little water retards the formation of carbonic acid, especially with soda lime. If there is too little water, the granules will also absorb halothane and thereby prolong induction.

Soda lime and baralyme contain ethyl violet, a pH-sensitive dye that changes color as the granules near exhaustion and carbonic acid accumulates.

Sevoflurane is unstable in soda lime. Although other modern anesthetic gases are stable in soda lime and no toxic products are produced, soda lime is incompatible with trichloroethylene. The combination produces phosgene, a pulmonary irritant and a neurotoxin.

Benefits

CO_2 absorption is cost-effective because it allows lower gas flows and use of less volatile agents when using a semiclosed or a closed circuit to deliver anesthesia. The use of lower gas flows decreases pollution in the operating room. In addition, the CO_2 absorber generates both heat and water, which help warm and humidify inspired gases.

Selected References

1. Smith TC. Anesthesia breathing systems. In Ehrenwerth J, Eisenkraft JB, eds. Anesthesia Equipment: Principles and Applications. St. Louis: Mosby, 1993:89.

Suggested References

Andrews JJ. Delivery Systems for Inhaled Anesthetics. In Barash PG, Cullen BF, Stoelting RK, eds. Clinical Anesthesia. 3rd ed. Philadelphia: Lippincott-Raven, 1997:552–553.
Andrews JJ. Inhaled Anesthetic Delivery Systems. In Miller RD, ed. Anesthesia. 5th ed. Philadelphia: Churchill Livingstone, 2000:193–194.

91
Causes of Carbon Dioxide Retention in Anesthetic Breathing Systems

Theresia L. Lee, M.D.

Carbon dioxide (CO_2) is produced by cellular metabolism and eliminated through the lungs. However, hypercarbia can occur with otherwise adequate ventilation if CO_2 is present in the inspired gases.

CO_2 Absorption

CO_2 is chemically neutralized by soda lime or baralyme in the anesthesia circle system. The CO_2 absorber's function depends on canister design, moisture content, absorbent particle size, and the degree of channeling of gas within the canister. Hypercarbia can occur if the absorbent becomes exhausted or if the anesthetic gases are allowed to bypass the absorbent (see Chapter 90).

Rebreathing

Even when the valves on the anesthesia circle are functioning properly, some rebreathing occurs. Dead space exists in the circle system between the Y-piece and the patient. This contributes slightly to hypercarbia by adding apparatus dead space to the patient's physiologic dead space. A normal apparatus will increase V_D/V_T from 33% to 46% in an intubated patient and to 64% in patients ventilated by mask. This leads to varying amounts of rebreathing. Rebreathing gases from the anatomic dead space or from the alveoli results in warmer gases saturated with water vapor. However, alveolar gases consist of 5% to 6% CO_2. Therefore, rebreathing alveolar gases where CO_2 has not been removed will cause hypercarbia.

The Mapleson breathing circuits (Fig. 91–1), listed in order of increasing rebreathing, are:

□ Spontaneous ventilation: Mapleson A < D < C < B.
□ Controlled ventilation: Mapleson D < B < C < A.

No rebreathing of exhaled gases will occur if the fresh gas inflow is adequate. Different Mapleson circuits have different fresh gas inflow require-

ments to prevent rebreathing (Table 91–1). A low fresh gas flow in systems without CO_2 absorption will result in rebreathing and hypercarbia.

The Bain system is a modification of the Mapleson D system. It delivers fresh gas flow to the patient via a small tube fixed inside a larger expiratory tube. With the Bain system, hypercarbia will occur if the inner tube becomes kinked, has a leak,

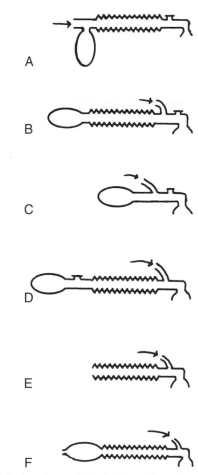

Figure 91–1. Mapleson classification of breathing circuits. Components include a reservoir bag, corrugated tubing, adjustable pressure limiting valve, fresh gas inlet, and patient connection. They lack carbon dioxide absorbers, unidirectional valves, and separate inspiratory and expiratory limbs. (Adapted from Mapleson WW[1] by Dorsch JA, Dorsch SE.[2])

Table 91–1. Minimum Fresh Gas Flow Requirement to Prevent Rebreathing of Exhaled Gases

	Minimum Fresh Gas Inflow
Mapleson circuit A	Patient's alveolar ventilation
Mapleson circuit B	2 × patient's minute ventilation
Mapleson circuit C	2 × patient's minute ventilation
Mapleson circuit D	2 × patient's minute ventilation
Brain system	
Controlled ventilation	70 mL/kg
Spontaneous ventilation	3 × patient's minute ventilation
Mapleson circuit E	
Ayre's T-piece	3 × patient's minute ventilation
Jackson–Rees (modification of Ayre's T-piece)	2 × patient's minute ventilation

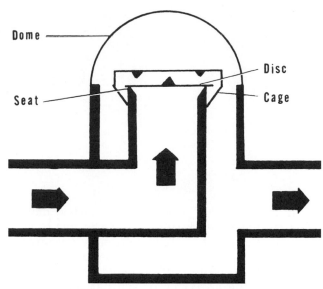

Figure 91–2. Unidirectional valve in closed position. Gas flowing into the valve raises the disc from its seat, stopping further retrograde flow. The guide (cage) prevents lateral or vertical displacement of the disc. The transparent dome allows observation of disc movement. (From Dorsch JA, Dorsch SE.[2])

is absent, or becomes dislodged and does not extend to the patient port, or if fresh gas flow is too low.

Rebreathing can occur in a circle system if the valves are incompetent or absent, or if a nonrebreathing valve allows a significant back leak of exhaled gases or is assembled improperly (Fig. 91–2).

Low tidal volume, wasted ventilation because of distention of system components, compression of gases in the system, inappropriate adjustment of the pop-off valve, leaks in the anesthesia machine, and/or disconnections can lead to hypoventilation and result in hypoxia and hypercarbia.

Monitoring vital signs, observing chest motion, and using a precordial or esophageal stethoscope are important means of detecting inadequate ventilation. End-tidal CO_2 monitoring, measurement of exhaled volumes, and blood gas analysis serve as invaluable clinical tools. In addition to elevated expired CO_2 levels, capnography will detect malfunctioning valves on the anesthesia circle by displaying an elevation of the inspired CO_2 level and a waveform that does not return to baseline.

Selected References

1. Mapleson WW. The elimination of rebreathing in various semiclosed anesthetic systems. Br J Anesth 1954;26:323–332.
2. Dorsch JA, Dorsch SE. Understanding Anesthesia Equipment. 4th ed. Baltimore, Williams & Wilkins, 1999.

Suggested References

Andrews JJ. Inhaled anesthetic delivery systems. In Miller RD, ed. Anesthesia. 5th ed. Philadelphia: Churchill Livingstone, 2000:174–206.

Smith TC. Anesthesia breathing systems. In Ehrenwerth J, Eisenkraft JB, eds. Anesthesia Equipment: Principles and Applications. St. Louis: Mosby, 1993:89.

92
Capnography

Eric A. Bedell, M.D.

The measurement of respiratory carbon dioxide (CO_2) concentration during anesthesia has become a standard of practice that is strongly encouraged by the American Society of Anesthesiologists.[1] CO_2 monitoring is used to confirm endotracheal intubation, follow the adequacy of ventilation, and estimate arterial partial pressure of CO_2 ($PaCO_2$). Capnometry (from the Greek *metrein*, to measure) is the measurement of CO_2 concentration in a gas sample, while capnography (from the Greek *graphein*, to write) is the visual representation of the relative or absolute concentration of CO_2 in the sample.

Sampling Methods

Gas samples to be evaluated are obtained either by removing a sample from the circuit, called **side-stream sampling**, or by having the total volume pass through the sensing device, called **direct flow-through**. Side-stream sampling withdraws gas (usually 50 to 150 mL/min) via a sampling tube from near the endotracheal tube and transports it to a distant device for evaluation. Side-stream systems allow for unobtrusive sampling near the patient, but are prone to gas leaks, sample tube occlusion, and moisture problems. Direct flow devices are usually located at the endotracheal tube and analyze all gas flow into and out of the endotracheal tube. These systems (e.g., Siemens Sirecurst 300 and FEF end-tidal CO_2 detector) tend to be large, bulky, and inappropriate for use in some situations and may add significant deadspace when used in small pediatric patients. The Siemens system also uses a heated sensor that is fragile and has been associated with thermal skin burns. For these reasons, side-stream sampling remains the most common sampling method in the operating room.

CO_2 Measurement

The actual measurement of CO_2 is done by three general methods, each of which has its own particular strengths and weaknesses.

Infrared Absorption. Differential infrared absorption between the gas sample and a reference allows for rapid, reliable, and durable CO_2 measurement. While used most commonly with side-stream sampling, it also is used with flow-through devices (Siemens Sirecurst 300). Major drawbacks when used with side-stream sampling include continuous withdrawal of gas from the respiratory system, propensity to leak or occlude, and sensitivity to water accumulation.

Mass Spectrometry. Gas is continuously withdrawn through capillary lines from a T-piece in each patient's circuit. A switching device directs gas from each patient into the mass spectrometer where the sample is **ionized**, then exposed to a **magnetic field** in a **vacuum** chamber, where the ionized molecules in the gas are separated by **mass-charge ratio**. Collectors in the vacuum chamber determine the concentration of each specific gas component. This system allows for analysis of multiple gases and is very accurate and stable. The system is also large and expensive, with common practice constraints requiring a central unit servicing multiple users, leading to delay times. The system may also be damaged by water or drugs taken up by the system (i.e., β-agonist inhaled agents).

Colorimetric Detection. Hydration of CO_2 leads to hydrogen ion liberation and acidification of a pH-sensitive medium and subsequent color change. This is the basis for colorimetric CO_2 detection. The FEF CO_2 detector (FEF end-tidal CO_2

Table 92–1. Increased $P_{ET}CO_2$

Causes	$PaCO_2$ to $P_{ET}CO_2$ Gradient
Rebreathing (CO_2 absorber failure, circle system failure, increased circuit dead space)	Normal
Hypoventilation	Normal
Increased cardiac output	Normal
Increased CO_2 production (hyperthermia, malignant hyperthermia, shivering, convulsions, bicarbonate administration, tourniquet release)	Normal
Right-to-left cardiac shunt	Increased
Endobronchial intubation?	Increased

Adapted from Dorsch A, Dorsch S.[2]

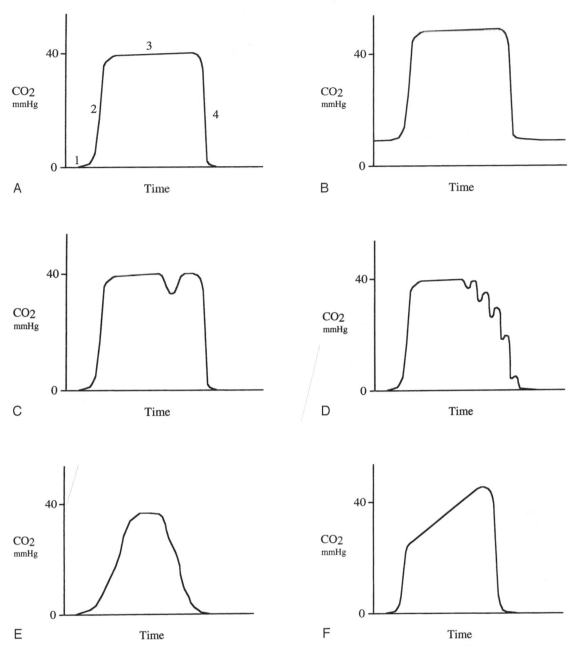

Figure 92–1. Common capnograms: (A) normal pattern; (B) rebreathing with elevated baseline; (C) diaphragmatic movement or breathing, also called "curare notch"; (D) cardiac oscillations; (E) obstruction or sample contamination; and (F) bronchospasm or obstructive pulmonary disease.

detector, Fenen, Inc., New York, NY) uses a flow-through device that attaches to the endotracheal tube. It rapidly changes color in the presence of CO_2 (purple to yellow) and back to the original color after the removal of CO_2. The device is portable and easy to use, fits standard endotracheal tubes, and requires no other equipment. The CO_2 differentiation is crude, however, with color ranges of purple ($CO_2 \leq 2.3$ torr), purple-yellow (CO_2 3.7 to 7.6 torr), and yellow ($CO_2 \geq 15.2$ torr).[3] This device is best used to confirm presence or absence of expired CO_2 to rule out esophageal intubation. It is commonly used for resuscitation and in remote sites when endotracheal intubation is required (i.e., emergency room, intensive care unit, etc.).

Capnometry and Capnography

In most situations, the expired CO_2 end-tidal ($P_{ET}CO_2$) closely follows the $PaCO_2$, with gradients of less than 5 torr. Deadspace ventilation leads to some dilution of expired CO_2, making $P_{ET}CO_2$ lower than $PaCO_2$. With increases in deadspace ventilation, the gradient will increase. Factors affecting $P_{ET}CO_2$ and the $PaCO_2$-to-$P_{ET}CO_2$ are given in Tables 92–1 and 92–2. Evaluation of the CO_2 waveform (capnography) is also very important. The common waveform [Fig. 92–1A] comprises a baseline CO_2 (1), a rapid increase in CO_2 during exhalation (2), a flat or slightly upsloping plateau (as dis-

Table 92–2. Decreased $P_{ET}CO_2$

Causes	$PaCO_2$ to $P_{ET}CO_2$ Gradient
Increased dead space ventilation (thrombotic/air pulmonary embolism, bronchospasm)	Increased
Hyperventilation	Normal
Esophageal intubation	Increased
Decreased CO_2 production	Normal
Decreased cardiac output	Increased
Sample contamination (disconnection, cuff leak, sample tube leak)	Increased

Adapted from Dorsch A, Dorsch S.[2]

tal alveoli are emptied) (3), and a rapid loss of CO_2 as the next inspiration occurs (4). Abnormalities of all components are possible, with Figure 92–1 (B)–(F) giving some of the most common.

Selected References

1. ASA Standards for basic intra-operative monitoring. In American Society of Anesthesiologists, 2000 Directory of Members. Park Ridge, IL, American Society of Anesthesiologists, 2000:477.
2. Dorsch A, Dorsch S. Understanding Anesthesia Equipment. 4th ed. Baltimore, Williams & Wilkins, 1999.
3. Goldberg J, Rawle P, Zehnder J, Sladen R. Colorimetric end-tidal carbon dioxide monitoring for tracheal intubation. Anesth Analg 1990;70:191–194.

Suggested References

Gravenstein JS, Paulus DA, Hayes TJ. Capnography in Clinical Practice. Boston, Butterworths, 1989.
Knill RL. Practical CO_2 monitoring in anaesthesia. Can J Anaesth 1993;40:R40.

93
Disconnect Monitors

Glenn E. Woodworth, M.D.

Major anesthesia morbidity and mortality is often related to problems with the airway and ventilation. The most common critical incident is disconnection of the breathing circuit during mechanical ventilation.[1] The average anesthesia circuit contains approximately 10 connections that can disconnect. The most common disconnection site is at the Y-piece.

Numerous procedures and mechanical aids have been introduced over the last several years to reduce the risk of serious injury due to disconnections. Risk-reduction measures have focused on three general areas: (1) secure locking of mated components, (2) use of disconnect monitors and alarms for detection, and (3) education.[2]

Disconnects cannot be prevented completely; therefore, monitoring for such an event is essential. All alarms should be checked and enabled whenever possible. Some, but not all, disconnect alarms are automatically activated and deactivated when the ventilator is turned on and off. However, even with all of the currently available monitors in use, under certain circumstances a disconnect or partial disconnect may be missed. Disconnect alarms can be classified into four categories:

- Pressure monitors.
- Respiratory volume monitors.
- CO_2 monitors.
- Miscellaneous.

Pressure Monitors

Pressure monitors are designed to monitor pressures within the breathing system. An alarm condition is registered if the maximum inspiratory pressure does not exceed a set threshold within a predetermined time (usually 15 seconds). This aspect of the pressure monitor is not enabled during spontaneous respiration. Certain conditions can cause a disconnect, yet fail to trigger the pressure monitor. This is especially likely if the tube disconnects from the 15-mm connector (a site of high resistance). A similar situation occurs if the disconnection is partially obstructed and generates a resistance; for example, if the circuit is disconnected at the Y-piece and is obstructed by bed sheets. Factors that influence alarm effectiveness include the disconnection site, pressure sensor site, threshold alarm limit, inspiratory flow rate, and resistance within the disconnected circuit. Because of these types of problems, once ventilator use has been initiated, the airway pressures should be verified to be within the expected limits. If the threshold pressure alarm is adjustable, then it should be set approximately 5 cm of H_2O below the peak inspiratory pressure.[3] In addition to disconnections of the breathing circuit, a low-pressure alarm may signify other problems in the breathing circuit or anesthesia machine that can lead to inadequate ventilation.

The pressure monitor may also be used to detect subatmospheric, high, or continuing pressure conditions. The pressure sensor is usually located just proximal to the inspiratory valve, to minimize moisture within the sensing line and provide ready access.

Respiratory Volume Monitors

The respiratory volume monitor normally resides in the expiratory limb of the breathing circuit. Its function is to measure the exhaled tidal volume, respiratory rate, minute volume, and flow direction. Several different types of volume meters are available.[4] Many include electronic analysis and alarms under conditions of low rate, low volume, or reverse flow. These monitors are useful during spontaneous respiration as well as mechanical ventilation.

Like pressure alarms, volume alarms can fail to signal during a disconnect. A common example occurs when using a ventilator with bellows that descend during exhalation (e.g., descending or hanging bellows). During expiration, in the presence of a disconnect, descent of the bellows due to gravity may entrain room air and generate a flow within the circuit. A false-negative alarm may also occur even if the breathing circuit is totally obstructed. The compliance of the breathing circuit and compression of gas during an inspiratory cycle may yield an "exhaled volume" that can exceed alarm limits. In addition, during spontaneous respiration, a disconnect on the machine side of either directional valve will go undetected, depending on the location of the volume meter. A frequent criticism of these monitors is that **flow in the expiratory limb does not guarantee gas exchange**.

CO₂ Monitors

CO_2 monitors not only allow titration of ventilation, but also can serve as disconnect monitors. CO_2 is monitored by mass spectrometry, infrared absorption, or Raman scattering. A change in CO_2 concentration or absence of CO_2 in the exhaled gas can implicate various ventilatory problems, including a disconnect. The CO_2 monitor is probably the best monitor for evaluating the adequacy of ventilation. Capnography is discussed in Chapter 92.

Miscellaneous Monitors

□ The esophageal stethoscope is an excellent monitor for detecting disconnects. Breath sounds should be monitored continuously. A disconnect can be picked up immediately. Observation of chest wall excursion may also be helpful.
□ Pulse oximeters offer a late warning of disconnections that lead to hypoxemia.
□ Observation of the ventilator bellows may detect a disconnect. Ascending bellows will collapse with a loss of pressure within the breathing circuit, whereas descending bellows will descend normally due to gravity during expiration and appear to be functioning normally.
□ Occasionally, an oxygen analyzer will detect oxygen concentrations within the breathing circuit that are lower than expected in the presence of a disconnect.

Selected References

1. Cooper JB, Newboer RS, Kitz RJ. An analysis of major error and equipment failures in anesthesia management: Considerations for prevention and detection. Anesthesiology 1984;60:34–42.
2. Schreiber P. Safety Guidelines for Anesthesia Systems. North American Drager, Boston, Merchants Press, 1985.
3. Dorsch JA, Dorsch SE. The breathing system: General principles, common components, and classification. In Dorsch JA, Dorsch SE, eds. Understanding Anesthesia Equipment. Baltimore: Williams & Williams, 1999:183–206.
4. Raemer DB. Monitoring ventilation. In Ehrenwerth J, Eisenkraft JB, eds. Anesthesia Equipment: Principles and Applications. St. Louis: Mosby, 1993:221.

Suggested References

Eichorn JH. Risk management. In Benumoff JL, Saidman LJ, eds. Anesthesia and Perioperative Complications. St. Louis: Mosby, 1992:648.
Raphael DT. The low-pressure alarm condition: Safety considerations and the anesthesiologist's response. Anesthesia Patient Safety Foundation Newsletter 1999;13:33–40.

94
Pulse Oximetry

Michael L. Bishop, M.D.

Technology

Oximetry is the measurement of oxyhemoglobin concentration (O_2Hb) based on the Lambert-Beer Law. **Fractional oximetry (SaO_2)** is defined as O_2Hb divided by total hemoglobin. Total hemoglobin is calculated as the sum of O_2Hb, deoxyhemoglobin (Hb), methemoglobin (MetHb), and carboxyhemoglobin (COHb). In contrast, **functional oximetry (SpO_2)** is defined as O_2Hb divided by the sum of O_2Hb and Hb. In clinical practice, SaO_2 is estimated using a pulse oximeter to calculate SpO_2.

$$SaO_2 = O_2Hb/(O_2Hb + Hb + MetHb + COHb)$$

$$SpO_2 = O_2Hb/(O_2Hb + Hb)$$

Deoxyhemoglobin absorbs more light in the red band (600 to 750 nm) than O_2Hb, whereas O_2Hb absorbs more light in the infrared band (850 to 1000 nm) than Hb. The pulse oximeter probe contains two light-emitting diodes (LEDs) that emit light at specific wavelengths, one in the red band and one in the infrared band. Typical wavelengths are 660 nm and 940 nm. When the probe is placed on an appendage, the light emitted from the LEDs is transmitted through the intervening blood and tissue and is detected by sensors built into the probe. The amount of transmitted light is sensed several hundred times per second to allow precise estimation of the peak and trough of each pulse waveform. At the trough, light is absorbed by the intervening arterial, capillary, and venous blood, as well as by the intervening tissue. At the peak, additional light is absorbed in both the red and infrared bands by an additional quantity of purely arterial blood, the pulse volume. The pulse amplitude accounts for 1% to 5% of the total signal. The resulting red:infrared ratio is then used to calculate SpO_2 by using an algorithm built into the software of the pulse oximeter. Isolation and measurement of the pulsatile component allows individuals to act as their own controls, and thus eliminates potential problems with interindividual differences in baseline light absorbance. The "calibration curve" used to calculate SpO_2 was derived from studies of healthy volunteers.

The pulse search process initiated with application of the probe to the subject includes sequential trials of various intensities of light to find one strong enough to transmit through the tissue without overloading the sensors.

Accuracy

Pulse oximeters have generally been found to be accurate to within 5% of in vitro oximeters in the range of 70% to 100%. The most widely used "gold standard" for comparison is the IL282 co-oximeter. Studies have often found ear probes to be slightly more accurate than finger probes. In discussing the accuracy of pulse oximeters, the terms bias and precision are used. Bias is the mean value of ($SaO_2 - SpO_2$). Precision is the standard deviation of the bias.

There are two potential problems with pulse oximeter accuracy below values of 70%. First, as stated previously, pulse oximeters have been calibrated using studies of healthy volunteers (Olympic athletes in one case). Therefore, it is unlikely that much data have been collected for calibration. Second, the absorption spectrum of deoxygenated Hb is maximally steep at 600 nm. Therefore, any slight variance in the light emitted from the 660-nm LED has significant potential to introduce measurement error into the system. Since decreasing oxygen saturation leads to an increasing proportion of deoxyhemoglobin, there is the potential for increasing inaccuracy as SpO_2 decreases. These potential problems are unlikely to be of much clinical significance. For example, it is unlikely that a treatment decision would be based on whether SpO_2 is 50% versus 60% at a given time. Some studies have reported poor accuracy of pulse oximeters at SpO_2 values of less than 70%.

Response Time

Most pulse oximeters average pulse data over 5 to 8 seconds before displaying a value. Some oximeters allow for an override of this lag by providing for a shortened averaging interval or allowing a beat-by-beat display. Response time is also related to probe location. Desaturation response times range from 7.2 to 19.8 seconds for ear probes, from 19.5 to 35.1 seconds for finger probes, and from 41.0 to 72.6 seconds for toe probes.

Low-Amplitude States

Pulse oximeters depend on a pulsatile waveform to calculate SpO_2; therefore, under conditions of low or absent pulse amplitude, the pulse oximeter may not accurately reflect arterial oxygen saturation. This situation could present clinically during cardiac arrest, proximal sphygmomanometer cuff inflation, tourniquet application, hypovolemia, hypothermia, vasoconstriction, or cardiac bypass. In addition, pulse oximeters are more sensitive to movement artifact during low–pulse-amplitude states.

The earlobe appears to be the least sensitive area to pulse signal loss. There has been some question of pulse oximeter accuracy in the face of an arrhythmia in which not all electrocardiographic (ECG) complexes translate into a good peripheral pulsatile waveform, creating a pulse deficit between the ECG and the pulse oximeter. But Wong et al[1] found no relationship between pulse deficit and bias. These investigators suggested that a noise-free pulsatile plethysmogram was of paramount importance.

Dyshemoglobins

Because pulse oximeters use only two wavelengths of light, they can accurately measure only two species of hemoglobin—O_2Hb and Hb. The presence of a third or fourth species of hemoglobin (e.g., MetHb or COHb) can interfere with accurate measurement by causing changes in the absorbance of light in the critical red and infrared regions.

Carboxyhemoglobin is interpreted by the pulse oximeter as a mixture of approximately 90% O_2Hb and 10% Hb. Thus, at high levels of COHb, the pulse oximeter will overestimate true SaO_2. This is of potential importance in patients with recent carbon monoxide exposure (e.g., house fire or cigarette smoking).

Methemoglobin is formed when the heme iron is oxidized from the ferrous (Fe^{2+}) to the ferric (Fe^{3+}) state. Methemoglobin is very dark and tends to absorb equal amounts of red and infrared light, resulting a red:infrared ratio of 1. When extrapolated on the calibration curve, a ratio of 1 corresponds to a saturation of 85%. Thus, as MetHb increases, SpO_2 approaches 85% regardless of the true level of O_2Hb. Drugs capable of causing methemoglobinemia (defined as greater than 1% MetHb) include nitrates, nitrites, chlorates, nitrobenzenes, antimalarial agents, amyl nitrate, nitroglycerin, sodium nitroprusside, and local anesthetics. High levels of MetHb may cause symptoms from diminished oxygen-carrying capacity as well as a leftward shift in the oxyhemoglobin dissociation curve.

Little has been published on the effect of sickle and other abnormal hemoglobins on the accuracy of pulse oximetry. Keifer et al[2] cited a case involving a patient with homozygous sickle hemoglobin in whom SpO_2 values were "widely discrepant" from SaO_2 as measured by an in vitro oximeter. They found differences in the absorption spectra of Hb S and Hb A, especially the oxygenated forms. They could not rule out irreversible denaturation of a portion of the Hb S sample as the cause of their results, however.

Dyes and Pigments

Scheller et al[3] studied the effect of three intravenously administered dyes on SpO_2 as measured via toe and finger probes. They found that injection of 5 mL of 1% methylene blue produced a large and consistent spurious decrease in SpO_2. The lowest reading seen was $SpO_2 = 1\%$ (median = 65%). Readings remained below baseline for 1 to 2 minutes. Injection of 5 mL of 0.25% indocyanine green caused a SpO_2 decrease to 93% at a finger probe and to 84% at a toe probe. The duration of these changes was 10 to 70 seconds. Injection of 5 mL of 0.8% indigo carmine produced the smallest changes, with a transient SpO_2 reading of 92% at the toe probe only. In general, the latency from injection to observation of changes was 30 to 45 seconds.

The presence of elevated serum bilirubin per se does not affect the accuracy of SpO_2. If the bilirubin is the result of hemolysis, then the CO also produced could cause spurious elevation of SpO_2.

Ambient Light

Inaccurate SpO_2 readings have been reported due to surgical lamps, fluorescent light, infrared light, and fiberoptic surgical units.

Skin Pigment

Rarely, pulse oximetry is not possible in deeply pigmented individuals because of a failure of LED light transmission.

Electrocautery

Electrocautery results in decreased SpO_2 readings from interference caused by wide-spectrum radio frequency emissions at the pulse oximeter probe.

Motion Artifact

Repetitive and persistent motion artifact of any kind will tend to cause the SpO$_2$ to approximate 85%.

Fingernail Polish

The presence of fingernail polish may cause a decrease in SpO$_2$, although this effect is not constant and may be related to the number of layers of polish present. Synthetic nails may also result in a decreased SpO$_2$.

Complications of Pulse Oximetry

Generally only minor complications have been reported, including mild skin erosions and blistering, tanning of the skin with prolonged continuous use, and ischemic skin necrosis.

Selected References

1. Wong DH, Tremper KK, Davidson J, et al. Pulse oximetry is accurate in patients with dysrhythmias and a pulse deficit. Anesthesiology 1989;70:1024–1025.
2. Keifer JC, Russell GB, Snider MT. Pulse oximetry inaccuracy with sickle hemoglobin. Is it due to different absorption spectra? Anesthesiology 1989;71:A370.
3. Scheller MS, Unger RJ, Kelner MJ. Effects of intravenously administered dyes on pulse oximetry readings. Anesthesiology 1986;65:550–552.

Suggested References

Szocik JF, Barker SJ, Tremper KK. Fundamental principles of monitoring instrumentation. In Miller RD, ed. Anesthesia. 5th ed. Philadelphia: Churchill Livingstone, 2000:1053–1077.

95
Hyperbaric Oxygen Therapy

Neil G. Feinglass, M.D. □ Timothy S. J. Shine, M.D.

Hyperbaric oxygen (HBO) is the application of oxygen in an environment where the barometric pressure is greater than 1 atmosphere (ATM). Note that 1 ATM absolute is equivalent to a gauge pressure of 0 (see Table 95–1). Thus, if a regulator is registering a pressure of 1 ATM, such a pressure is in reality 2 ATM absolute. The exposure to increased gas pressures can occur in several situations, such as with breathing compressed gas mixtures while diving (scuba), working in underground tunnels (caisson workers), or in a medical facility (hyperbaric chamber). In each case, the gases follow fundamental gas laws that are predictable and reproducible:

□ **Boyle's law:** A volume of gas is inversely proportional to pressure at a constant temperature

$$PV = K$$

where P is absolute pressure, V is volume, and K is a constant.
□ **Gay-Lussac's law:** At a constant volume, pressure is proportional to absolute temperature.
□ **Charles' law:** At a constant pressure, volume will vary directly with the absolute temperature.
□ **Dalton's law:** The total pressure of a mixture of gases is equal to the sum of the partial pressures of the component gases.
□ **Henry's law:** At constant temperature, the amount of gas dissolved in a liquid is proportional to the partial pressure of the gas.

In clinical medicine the solution of interest is blood and oxygen; specifically, the driving pressure of oxygen into solution in blood (partial pressure, PaO_2). Note that it is the partial pressure of oxygen, not the percentage of oxygen, that is important (Ta-

ble 95–2). As the PaO_2 increases in blood, the saturation of hemoglobin approaches 100% (PaO_2 100). Above this level, all additional oxygen-carrying capacity of blood comes from oxygen dissolved in the plasma. HBO can increase oxygen transport in the face of severe anemia or hypoperfusion. In addition, application of increased barometric pressure can reduce intravascular air bubbles in patients with decompression sickness, improving perfusion and increasing the removal of nitrogen from the blood (Fig. 95–1).

In practice, HBO's effectiveness for some purported indications has been hard to prove in controlled studies examining outcome. It has earned the dubious distinction of being labeled a "therapy in search of diseases."[4] Table 95–3 lists conditions for which HBO therapy has been used.

Table 95–1. Units of Pressure

1 ATM aboslute =	14.7 lb/sq in (psi)
	29.9 in Hg
	34 feet fresh water (ffw)
	33 feet salt water (fsw)
	1.033 kg/cm²
	1.013 bars
	760 mm Hg

Modified from Sommers LH.[2]

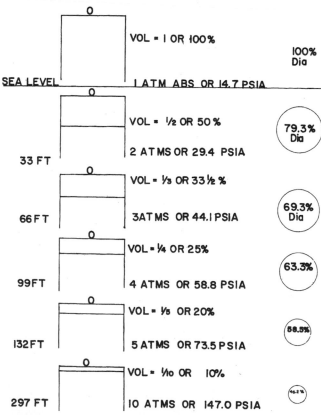

Figure 95–1. Gas volume and bubble size as a function of depth: Boyle's law. (From Somers LH.[2])

Table 95–2. Expected Gas Tensions and Arterial Blood Oxygen Content at Various Ambient Pressures in a Normal Individual (Hb = 14 g/dL)

ATM	F$_{I}$O$_2$	Inspired PO$_2$ (mm Hg)	P$_A$O$_2$ (mm Hg)	PaO$_2$ (mm Hg)	CaO$_2$ (Total) (mL/dL)	CaO$_2$ (Dissolved) (mL/dL)	PaCO$_2$ (mm Hg)
1	0.21	150	102	87	18.7	0.3	40
1	1.0	713	673	572	21.2	1.7	40
2	1.0	1,473	1,433	1,218	23.1	3.7	40
3	1.0	2,233	2,193	1,864	25.1	5.6	40
6	0.21	898	848	>750	21.8	2.3	40

Modified from Moon RE, Comporese EM.[3]

Effects of Hyperbaric Oxygen

Pulmonary. High P$_{O_2}$ is thought to overcome the scavenging system for free radicals, resulting in the formation of superoxides, hydrogen peroxide, and hydroxyl radicals. Pulmonary oxygen toxicity can cause retrosternal burning, coughing, and fibrosis. This toxicity is duration and Pa$_{O_2}$ dependent and is cumulative. Most HBO chambers reduce this effect by introducing air breaks between oxygen treatment periods.

Central Nervous System Effects. HBO causes a decrease in cerebral blood flow with increasing P$_{O_2}$. This is reported to decrease intracranial pressure and edema formation in patients with central nervous system (CNS) disorders. CNS toxicity becomes manifest breathing 100% oxygen at 2 ATM (3 ATM absolute). Common signs and symptoms include nausea, facial numbness, facial twitching, unpleasant taste or smell, finally progressing to full tonic/clonic seizure activity.

Cardiovascular Effects. A Pa$_{O_2}$ above 1500 torr causes an increase in systemic vascular resistance and the development of hypertension and bradycardia. Flow to the periphery is reduced; however, total oxygen delivery to these sites is markedly increased. Diffusion of oxygen away from the vascular bed is greatly enhanced. This mechanism underlies most of the indications for HBO use in situations of tissue hypoxia.

Air-Containing Cavities. Sinuses, the middle ear, and noncommunicating bullae may be affected by the application of pressure. This may result in potential harm to the patient. Endotracheal tube cuffs and intravenous drip chambers are also similarly affected. Most mechanical ventilators are not accurate in hyperbaric environments.

Anesthetic Management in a Hyperbaric Chamber

The production of anesthesia by volatile agents depends on the partial pressure of those agents in the body, not on the concentration in the lung. If 1.1% isoflurane (about 8 mm Hg) produces anesthesia at 1 ATM, then the same effect will be produced by 0.33% isoflurane at 3 ATM, because the alveolar and brain partial pressure of the drug will still be 8 mm Hg.

The effect of increasing pressure on copper kettle, flow-through–type vaporizers is to decrease anesthetic concentration in the gas leaving the vaporizer. But nearly the same partial pressure of agent is produced, so that clinical changes are imperceptible.

Slightly increased partial pressures are produced from flow-over, agent-specific vaporizers because of increased gas density. Gas density also causes rotameter flowmeters to read falsely high under hyperbaric conditions. Gas cylinders should function normally.

Inhalation anesthetic agents are not easily used in a hyperbaric chamber because of cumbersome

Table 95–3. Indications for Hyperbaric Oxygen Therapy

Diseases in which scientific evidence supports HBO therapy as effective
 Primary therapy
  Arterial gas embolism
  Decompression sickness
  Exceptional blood-loss anemia
  Severe carbon monoxide poisoning
 Adjunctive therapy
  Clostridial myonecrosis
  Compromised skin grafts and flaps
  Osteoradionecrosis prevention
Diseases for which scientific evidence suggests HBO therapy may be helpful
 Primary therapy
  Less severe carbon monoxide poisoning
 Adjunctive therapy
  Acute traumatic ischemic injury
  Osteoradionecrosis
  Refractory osteomyelitis
  Selected problem wounds
  Radiation-induced soft-tissue injury
Diseases for which scientific evidence does not support the use of HBO therapy, but for which it may be helpful
 Adjunctive therapy
  Necrotizing fasciitis
  Thermal burns

Adapted from Tibbles PM, Edelsberg JS.[5]

equipment, increased fire risk, increased oxygen toxicity from high inspired oxygen concentrations, and pollution of the chamber with anesthetic gases. The use of nitrous oxide would aggravate decompression air emboli. Intravenous anesthesia is frequently chosen for simplicity. Regional anesthesia may also be used.

Other anesthesia equipment may not function normally. Cuffs on endotracheal tubes and intravenous and bladder catheters should be filled with fluid. Air-filled cuffs will undergo large volume changes with changes in pressure. Pressure-operated ventilators should be used, because electrically operated ventilators carry the potential for fire hazard. Petroleum-based lubricants must be avoided.

Selected References

1. Kizer KW. Diving medicine. Emerg Med Clin North Am 1984;2:513.
2. Somers LH. Diving physics. In Bove AA, ed. Diving Medicine. 3rd ed. Philadelphia: WB Saunders, 1997:15–25.
3. Moon RE, Camporesi EM. Respiratory monitoring. In Miller RD, ed. Anesthesia. 5th ed. Philadelphia: Churchill Livingstone, 2000:1255–1296.
4. Gabb G, Robin ED. Hyperbaric oxygen: A therapy in search of diseases. Chest 1987;92:1074.
5. Tibbles PM, Edelsberg JS. Hyperbaric-oxygen therapy. New Eng J Med 1996;334:1642–1648.

96
Direct Arterial Pressure Monitoring

Kevin P. Ronan, M.D.

Arterial catheters are indicated for hemodynamic monitoring and blood gas determination in critically ill patients and those undergoing major surgery. The beat-to-beat visual arterial pressure wave and numerical pressure display enables prompt identification of trends or changes in blood pressure that could potentially be missed with noninvasive blood pressure monitoring. The most frequently used cannulation site is the radial artery. Other sites include the femoral, brachial, axillary, dorsalis pedis, and ulnar arteries. The most important complications of invasive pressure monitoring include air embolism, thrombosis, infection, and hemorrhage (from a disconnected arterial pressure line).

Equipment

The mechanical coupling of the patient to the monitoring device consists of the arterial catheter, pressure tubing, a continuous-flush device, and the pressure transducers.

Mechanism

An electronic system for measuring arterial or any other intravascular pressure comprises four components:

- **Mechanical coupling** is achieved by connecting fluid-filled tubing to the intravascular space. The mechanical motion of fluid in that tubing is converted into electrical signals by a mechanoelectrical transducer.
- The **pressure transducer,** or strain gauge, converts mechanical motion of fluid in the tubing into electrical signals. Most modern pressure transducers include a diaphragm that forms the base of a fluid-filled plastic dome. This plastic dome is connected to the mechanical coupling tube and usually a stopcock. Pressure of fluid on the tubing moves the diaphragm in the dome. Sensing elements connected to the diaphragm convert its movement into an electrical signal. The electrical signal consists of very small voltages proportional to the pressure that distorts the diaphragm. Pressure transducer diaphragms must be made of very light, stiff metal so they can monitor rapid transient changes in pressure. Although capacitance and inductance transducers have been used, most vary resistance across a Wheatstone bridge to convert mechanical changes to electrical changes.
- The **amplifier and processing unit** amplifies the small electrical signals generated by the pressure transducer.
- The **display** presents the processed signal to the observer through an oscilloscope, digital readout, or galvanometer.

System Setup

The measuring system must be zeroed. Zeroing the transducer provides a reference point. The most common reference point is atmospheric pressure. The transducer is zeroed by opening the stopcock to the atmosphere and indicating to the monitor that this is the zero reference pressure. It is important to remember that the weight of the column of fluid within the tubing exerts a pressure on the transducer diaphragm; therefore, the transducer is usually placed at the level of the right atrium or the midaxillary line. For a sitting patient, the arterial transducer is placed at the level of the brain.

Physics

With Fourier analysis, any waveform can be described by the summation of sinusoidal waves with varying frequencies and amplitudes. These waveforms are the **fundamental** waveform and the **sine waves** whose frequencies are multiples of the fundamental frequency (harmonics).

Left ventricular ejection initiates a pressure wave that is propagated down the aorta and its branches with a transmission velocity considerably greater than that of the actual forward movement of the blood itself. The transmission velocity varies inversely with the capacitance of the vessels. As the wave travels towards the periphery, it becomes progressively more distorted. Distortion of the wave occurs with (1) damping of high-frequency components secondary to the viscoelastic properties of the arterial walls, and (2) augmentation and narrowing of the systolic portion of the wave caused by reflection of waves at branching points, tapering of the arteries, resonance, and changes in transmission velocity. In young people, the systolic pressure in a large peripheral artery is commonly 10 mm Hg higher than the aortic pressure. The diastolic pressure is not affected as much. The mean pressure is the least sensitive to artifacts within the system and is usually lower in the periphery secondary to the loss of pressure across the arterial resistance.

When the catheter tip is facing the flow of blood, some of the **kinetic energy** of the flowing blood is converted into potential energy (pressure). This partially accounts for direct invasive blood pressure measurements that are higher than simultaneous noninvasive measurements.

For the measuring system to provide an accurate depiction of the measured waveform, it must have an appropriate **natural frequency** and **damping**. Problems within the system usually are due to problems with the mechanical connection system; that is, the catheter, fluid-filled tubing, and stopcock.

When the rapidity of pressure changes approaches the resonant peak frequency, the fluid-filled tubing is unable to accurately convey the original waveform. Each measuring system has a natural frequency about which it can oscillate. This frequency is proportional to the stiffness of the tubing and diaphragm and the cross-sectional area of the catheter and is inversely proportional to the catheter length and fluid density. If the frequency of the harmonics of the pressure wave being measured (25 Hz for blood pressure waves) approaches the natural frequency of the system, then it will distort the measurements by excessive amplification (ringing or resonance). It is not uncommon for a hyperresonant system to overestimate the systolic pressure by 25% and underestimate the diastolic pressure by 10% (Fig. 96–1). The mean pressure is not affected. To optimize the frequency response of the system, short, wide, and stiff tubing should be used. The natural frequency of a system can be estimated measured by introducing a square wave and measuring the frequency of the oscillations produced.

Artifacts

Damping prevents a system from overshoot or oscillating after responding to a change, particularly at frequencies close to the natural frequency of the system. Overdamping reduces the frequency response and yields a sluggish system that can underestimate the systolic pressure and overestimate the diastolic pressure. A complex formula relating the amplitude of successive oscillations is used to calculate a **damping coefficient**. An optimally damped system has a coefficient between 0.6 and 0.7. Blood clots, air bubbles in the tubing, and kinked catheters are common causes of an overdamped waveform. The combination of the natural frequency of a system and damping determines how accurately the system records pressures. Systems with low natural frequencies that are either overdamped or underdamped will tend to be inaccurate.

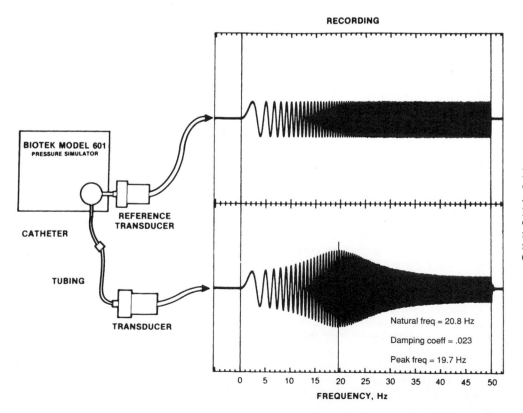

Natural freq = 20.8 Hz

Damping coeff = .023

Peak freq = 19.7 Hz

Figure 96–1. A waveform of increasing frequency is applied. As the frequency of the wave approaches the natural frequency of the system, the system resonates and distorts the measurement (lower transducer). (From Gardner RM.[1])

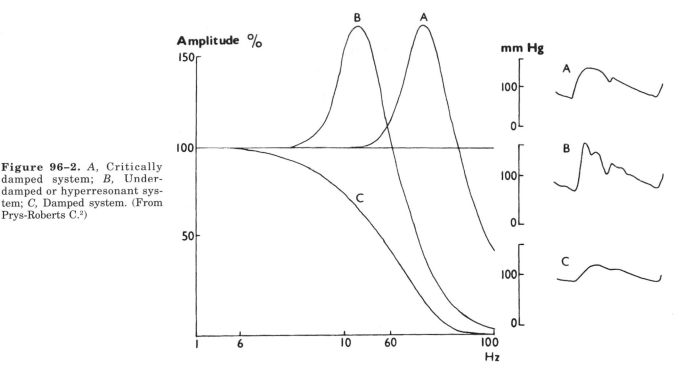

Figure 96–2. *A,* Critically damped system; *B,* Underdamped or hyperresonant system; *C,* Damped system. (From Prys-Roberts C.[2])

Hyperresonance or an **underdamped system** arises when long connecting lines (more than 1.4 m long) or small tubing (smaller than 1.5 mm internal diameter) are used, or when the intravascular catheter occludes the vessel (e.g., an 18-gauge cannula in a radial artery). The system then can resonate at high frequencies, which produces exaggerated peaks and troughs in the pressure waveform (Fig. 96–2). This will lead to falsely high systolic pressure and falsely low diastolic pressure.

Whip is usually seen in intracardiac catheters. In this effect, the tip of the catheter is free and begins to oscillate in a whip-like fashion because of cardiac motion. The column of fluid in the measuring system then begins to oscillate. This can result in false high or low readings, depending on whether the oscillations are in phase or out of phase with the pulsation.

To avoid artifacts, the following steps are advised:

□ Choose the appropriate-size cannula for the intended vessel (20 gauge for radial and brachial arteries, 18 gauge for axillary and femoral arteries).

□ Choose connecting tubing that is rigid, has an internal diameter of 1.5 to 3.0 mm, and ideally has a maximum length of 120 cm.

□ Use only one stopcock per line. Keep tubing, stopcock, and domes free of bubbles and clots. Avoid kinks in the tubing.

□ Keep the entire mechanical coupling system flushed with heparinized saline. A continuous flushing system is preferred, at 1 to 3 mL/hr (1 unit of heparin/mL of saline).

□ Use a transducer with the highest possible frequency response. This will allow a faithful reproduction of rapid transient pressure changes.

□ Check for improper zeroing and drift. Readjust after changes in patient position.

Selected References

1. Gardner RM. Direct blood pressure measurement—Dynamic response requirements. Anesthesiology 1981;54:227–236.
2. Prys-Roberts C. Invasive monitoring of the circulation. In Saidman LJ, Smith NT, eds. Monitoring in Anesthesia. Stoneham, MA: Butterworths, 1984:79.

Suggested References

Gardner RM, Hollingsworth KW. Optimizing ECG and pressure monitoring. Crit Care Med 1986;14:651.
Lake CL. Monitoring of arterial pressure. In Lake CL, ed. Clinical Monitoring. Philadelphia: WB Saunders, 1990:115.
Reich DL, Moskowitz DM, Kaplan JA. Hemodynamic monitoring. In Kaplan JA, ed. Cardiac Anesthesia. 4th ed. Philadelphia: WB Saunders, 1999:321.
Szocik JF, Barker SJ, Tremper KK. Fundamental principles of monitoring instrumentation. In Miller RD, ed. Anesthesia. 5th ed. New York: Churchill Livingstone, 2000:1053–1086.

97
Pitfalls of Pulmonary Artery Pressure Monitoring

Theresia L. Lee, M.D.

Although associated with significant risks, the pulmonary artery catheter (PAC) is an important option for monitoring left ventricular function. However, it is imperative that the hemodynamic data obtained be accurately interpreted in the presence of physiologic changes and therapeutic maneuvers.

PAC Complications

Insertion of a PAC may lead to various complications. Mark et al[1] have classified these complications as being secondary to catheter insertion, to the presence of the catheter, or to misinterpretation of findings (Table 97–1). These complications are in addition to the complications of cannulating a central vein. Air embolism can occur during placement of the catheter. The risk is higher with a PAC than with central venous line placement because of the PAC's large lumen (8 Fr). Air embolism can also occur from balloon rupture or during cardiac output determinations. Caution is especially important in patients with right-to-left intracardiac shunts.

Transient arrhythmias occur commonly during catheter placement and are generally benign. Arrhythmias occur (1) from trauma to the right bundle leading to right bundle branch block or complete heart block in patients with left bundle branch block, (2) because of direct irritation of the heart, (3) if the balloon is not inflated until the catheter tip has reached the right ventricle, or (4) if knotting or coiling occurs. Therefore, it is vital to monitor the electrocardiogram continuously during PAC placement and to inflate the balloon as soon as the tip passes the introducer (approximately 20 cm). Premature ventricular contractions may be suppressed by lidocaine.

Pulmonary artery rupture is rare but can occur if the balloon is overinflated or continuously inflated. The balloon should be inflated slowly using a minimal amount of air to obtain a wedge. Pulmonary artery rupture is frequently fatal and is more common in patients with pulmonary hypertension.

Pulmonary infarction is usually caused by prolonged balloon inflation and occasionally by migration of catheter clots. Thrombi can form on PACs,

but this is less common with heparin-bonded catheters. Thromboembolism of aseptic valve vegetations and mural thrombosis are very rare.

Infections range from minor site infections to thrombophlebitis, sepsis, and endocarditis. Sterile technique should be followed and appropriately timed catheter replacements made if prolonged monitoring is required. Infectious complications have led some to seriously question whether the benefits of PACs outweigh the risks.

Coils, kinks, and knots may be prevented by avoiding insertion of excessive lengths of the catheter (see Table 97–2). The pulmonary artery tracing should be seen within 15 cm of the right ventricle,

Table 97–1. Complications of Pulmonary Artery Pressure Monitoring

Complications of central venous line placement
Catheterization
  Catheter shearing
  Guidewire embolization
  Arrhythmias
    Supraventricular arrhythmias, atrial fibrillation
    Ventricular arrhythmias, ventricular tachycardia, ventricular fibrillation
    Right bundle branch block
    Complete heart block
  Air embolism
Catheter residence (late complications)
  Mechanical problems
    Catheter entrapment
    Catheter coiling, knotting
    Catheter tip migration
    Introducer sheath problems
    Balloon rupture
  Thrombosis, pulmonary embolism
  Thrombocytopenia
  Pulmonary infarction
  Infection
    Sepsis
    Endocarditis/valvular damage
  Structural damage
    Delayed vascular injury or fistula
    Cardiac perforation
    Endocardium, tricuspid valve, pulmonic valve
    Pulmonary artery
      Rupture
      Pseudoaneurysm
Misinterpretation and misuse

Adapted from Mark JB, Slaughter TF, Reves JG.[1]

Table 97–2. Distance from Access Site to Right Ventricle

Access Site	Distance to Right Ventricle (cm)
Right internal jugular vein	35
Right subclavian vein	35
Left internal jugular vein	45
Femoral vein	50
Right antecubital vein	60
Left antecubital vein	70

and the pulmonary capillary wedge pressure (PCWP) tracing should be seen within another 5 to 10 cm.

Balloon rupture is usually the result of improper technique. Inflation should be done slowly using a minimal amount of air. Deflation should be passive (i.e., disconnect the syringe and let the balloon empty by itself). Although the amount of air released from a rupture is minimal, this may be devastating in patients with a right-to-left shunt. CO_2 may be used to inflate the balloon in these patients in the event that rupture occurs.

The PAC may be difficult to float in patients with pulmonary hypertension, enlarged right ventricle, or tricuspid regurgitation. If peripheral veins are used, venospasm may prevent catheter passage.

PAC Interpretation Problems

Once the catheter is in place, the equipment must be calibrated and the transducer leveled with the right atrium. Damping may occur with clot formation over the catheter tip, air bubbles, or the tip against the pulmonary artery wall. Fling or catheter whip results from cardiac contractions causing catheter motion. Harmonic resonance is from high-frequency components of the pressure wave signals matching the resonating frequency of the fluid-filled monitoring system. The resonating frequency can be altered by changing the length of the tubing or using tubing of a different material.

During spontaneous respiration, negative and positive pressure artifacts may be transmitted to the PAC during inspiration and exhalation, respectively. During mechanical ventilation, positive pressure artifacts may be seen. Factors affecting the degree of artifact interference include lung and chest wall compliance, position of the PAC, and use of positive end-expiratory pressure (PEEP).

Preload, the length of the myocardial fiber at end diastole, is determined by left ventricular end-diastolic volume (LVEDV) and ventricular compliance. Left ventricular end-diastolic pressure (LVEDP) has been used to estimate preload but may be inaccurate with changes in compliance. Factors that decrease compliance include myocardial ischemia, restrictive cardiomyopathy, right-to-left interventricular septal shift, aortic stenosis, cardiac tamponade, effusion, myocardial fibrosis, inotropic drugs, and hypertension. Factors that increase compliance include vasodilators, congestive myopathies, left-to-right interventricular septal shift, mitral regurgitation, and aortic regurgitation.

Left atrial pressure is generally a good approximation of LVEDP. In the case of mitral stenosis, left atrial pressure is greater than LVEDP. In patients with mitral regurgitation, systole causes retrograde flow and left atrial pressure is greater than LVEDP, as evidenced by a large V wave on the PCWP tracing.

Aortic regurgitation and premature closure of the mitral valve leads to LVEDP greater than left atrial pressure because of retrograde flow from the aorta into the ventricle.

A decrease in left ventricular compliance also decreases the accuracy of using left atrial pressure to approximate LVEDP. With decreased left ventricular compliance, atrial contraction causes a greater increase in LVEDP than left atrial pressure. In this instance, the A wave of the PCWP tracing best reflects LVEDP, assuming that there is no pulmonary vascular obstruction or valvular heart disease.

In a normal patient, the pulmonary circulation has a low resistance, and thus the gradient between pulmonary artery pressure (PAP) and LVEDP is low. Therefore, the PCWP or pulmonary artery diastolic pressure (PAD) correlates well with the LVEDP. However, patients with acute respiratory failure, chronic obstructive pulmonary disease, hypoxia, or pulmonary emboli can have increased pulmonary vascular resistance. Increased heart rate also alters the relationship between PAD and PCWP.

Another factor that alters proper interpretation of the PCWP is PAC tip location. The lung is categorized into three zones:

□ Zone 1: PAP < alveolar pressure (P_A) > pulmonary venous pressure (PVP).
□ Zone 2: PAP > P_A > PVP.
□ Zone 3: PAP > P_A < PVP.

Accuracy of PCWP measurement depends on an open fluid channel between the catheter tip and the left atrium, which occurs only in Zone 3. Placement of the catheter tip in supine patients usually occurs in this zone. PEEP and hypovolemia can alter the usual pressure relationships even in Zone 3.

Selected References

1. Mark JB, Slaughter TF, Reves JG. Cardiovascular monitoring. In Miller RD, ed. Anesthesia. 5th ed. Philadelphia: Churchill Livingstone, 2000:1117–1206.

Suggested References

Bedford RF. Complications of invasive cardiovascular monitoring. In Gravenstein N, Kirby RR, eds. Complications in Anesthesiology. 2nd ed. Philadelphia: Lippincott-Raven, 1996:93.

Layon AJ. The pulmonary artery catheter: Nonexistential entity or occasionally useful tool? Chest 1999;115:859–862.

Tuman KF, Gilbert GC, Ivankovich AD. Pitfalls in interpretation of pulmonary artery catheter data. J Cardiothorac Anesth 1989;3:625.

98
Effect of Cardiac Function on Central Venous Pressure

Kevin P. Ronan, M.D.

The central venous pressure (CVP) is anatomically defined as that pressure of blood measured in the vena cava at the junction with the right atrium. CVP catheters are easy to place, and the pressures are easy to interpret. If the factors affecting the CVP and its limitations are understood, it is a useful monitor.

Central Venous Pressure

The CVP reflects right heart function and is not a reliable indicator of left ventricular performance. The pulmonary artery catheter is a more reliable monitor for left-sided pressures and performance (Fig. 98–1). The CVP reflects right atrial (RA) pressure, which reflects changes in right ventricular end-diastolic pressure. The CVP only secondarily reflects changes in pulmonary venous and left-sided pressures.

The CVP can help assess venous return to the right atrium, intravascular blood volume, and right ventricular function. If right-sided preload decreases, the CVP decreases. A decreased CVP usually correlates with decreased blood volume, but serial measurements, trends, and changes in response to therapy must be monitored. It is possible to have a patient develop pulmonary edema with a normal CVP.

Inspiratory and expiratory values in healthy individuals are normally -2 and $+4$ cm H_2O, respectively; 10 to 12 cm H_2O is usually the upper limit of normal for acutely ill patients. Although CVP can be measured with a water manometer, it is more commonly now measured in mm Hg; the conversion factor for this unit is 1.3 cm H_2O = 1 mm Hg. Many

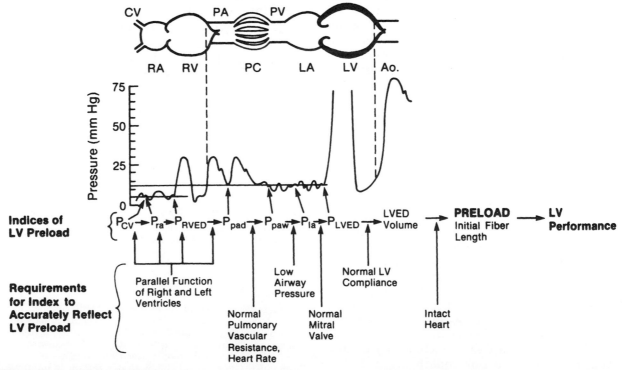

Figure 98–1. Indices of left ventricular preload, listing requirements for accurate prediction of preload. (From Benumof JL.[1])

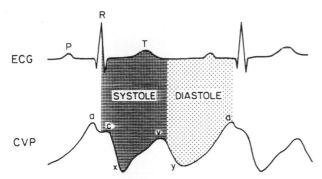

Figure 98–2. The normal CVP waveform. Systolic events include the C wave, X descent, and V wave; diastolic events include the Y descent and A wave. The ECG trace serves as a useful marker to discern the components of the CVP trace. Mechanical pressure events in the RA are always delayed relative to the electrical events on the ECG. (From Mark JB.[2])

factors affect CVP, including cardiac performance, blood volume, vascular tone, increased intra-abdominal or intrathoracic pressures, and vasopressor therapy.

An elevated CVP secondary to right ventricular failure most commonly results from left ventricular failure. Less commonly, right ventricular failure with elevated CVP occurs secondary to pulmonary hypertension, pulmonary emboli, or respiratory failure.

CVP Trace

The normal venous tracing has three positive waves (A, C, and V) and two negative deflections (X and Y) (see Fig. 98–2).[2]

□ The A wave is produced by RA contraction and begins before the first heart sound. The A wave is absent in atrial fibrillation and is inconsistent in the presence of various heart blocks. Large A waves are present with resistance to RA emptying (tricuspid stenosis, right ventricular hypertrophy, pulmonary stenosis, and pulmonary hypertension). Giant A waves (cannon) occur when the RA contracts against a closed tricuspid valve.

□ The C wave is produced by bulging of the tricuspid valve into the RA during the onset of ventricular contraction. The C wave occurs after the first heart sound and the QRS complex.

□ The X descent results from an atrial relaxation and downward displacement of the tricuspid valve during ventricular systole. In tricuspid regurgitation, the X descent disappears, and a large V wave is seen.

□ The V wave is formed by RA filling with a closed tricuspid valve.

□ The Y descent occurs with opening of the tricuspid valve and blood flow into the right ventricle.

Selected References

1. Benumof JL. Anesthesia for Thoracic Surgery. Philadelphia, WB Saunders, 1987.
2. Mark JB. Central venous pressure monitoring: Clinical insights beyond the numbers. J Cardiothorac Vasc Anesth 1991;5:163.

Suggested References

Mark JB, Slaughter TF, Reves JG. Cardiovascular monitoring. In Miller RD, ed. Anesthesia. 5th ed. Philadelphia: Churchill Livingstone, 2000:1117–1206.

Vender JS, Porembka DT. Hemodynamic assessment in the critically ill patient. In Murray MJ, Cousin DB, Pearl RG, et al, eds. Critical Care Medicine: Perioperative Management. Philadelphia: Lippincott-Raven, 1997:85–98.

99
Factors Affecting
Thermodilution Cardiac Output

Kevin P. Ronan, M.D.

The thermodilution technique for measuring cardiac output using a pulmonary artery catheter is the method of choice in the clinical setting. The technique is similar to the dye dilution technique, except that a cooled dextrose solution is used as the indicator. Excellent correlation of the thermodilution and dye dilution techniques has been demonstrated.

Technique

The pulmonary artery catheter thermistor records the decrease in temperature as an electrical resistance change. Because the current is small in the thermistor, it does not significantly heat the blood (Fig. 99–1). Cardiac output is proportional to the difference between the baseline and injectate temperatures divided by the area under the temperature change curve (as per the Fick principle).

The theory and calculation of the thermodilution technique assume several conditions:

□ Complete mixing of the indicator with blood.
□ A constant flow rate.
□ Flow of the indicator solution past the thermistor only once.
□ Injecting the indicator solution as a bolus.

Calibration numbers or computation constants must first be entered into the thermodilution computer. This constant is a correction factor for the increase in injectate temperature through the catheter, injectate volume, and the area lost by cutoff of the curve at 30% of peak.

Factors Affecting Thermodilution Techniques

Patient variables affecting thermodilution cardiac outputs include the following:

□ Motion or change in position can alter venous return to the heart.
□ Right-sided valvular disease or tricuspid or pulmonic insufficiency can reduce the reliability because of recirculation of blood.
□ Left-to-right intracardiac shunts will produce falsely elevated cardiac outputs.
□ Arrhythmias can significantly alter cardiac output, especially premature ventricular contractions.
□ Pulmonary artery temperature variation occurs because of right ventricular surface cooling from the overlying lung during panting, deep spontaneous respirations, and with Valsalva maneuvers.
□ Right ventricular output decreases during inspiration and reaches a plateau after increasing during expiration (Fig. 99–2).
□ A change in the hemodynamic state will cause variability in cardiac outputs.

Injectate factors affecting thermodilution cardiac output include the following:

□ The area under the thermodilution curve is proportionately smaller if the syringe volume is less than 10 mL (volume entered in the computer). This will cause an overestimation of the cardiac output. An error of 0.5 mL in the injectate volume will cause a 5% to 10% error in measurement.

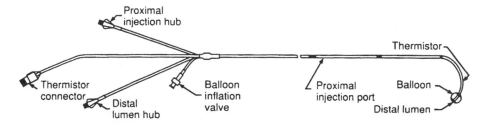

Figure 99–1. Four-lumen pulmonary artery balloon catheter designed to obtain hemodynamic pressures and to determine cardiac output by thermodilution technique. (Drawing courtesy of Edwards Laboratories, Santa Ana, CA.) (From Spackman TN, Rorie DK.[1])

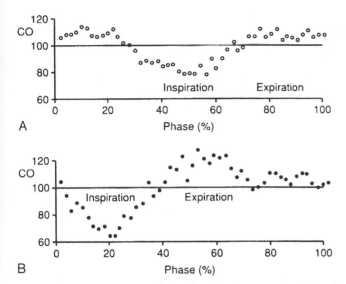

Figure 99–2. Alterations in left side of the heart output *(A)* and right side of the heart output *(B)* during a single respiratory cycle. Flow decreases during inspiration and increases and reaches a plateau during expiration. For this reason, thermodilution outputs should be determined at end-expiration. (From Jansen JRC, Schreuder JJ, Bogaard JM.[2])

□ Injection rates must be consistent and the injection completed within 4 seconds or less. If the injection takes longer than 4 seconds, the computer constants will be affected.

□ Inaccurate injectate temperature monitoring is a source of inaccuracy.

Thermistor factors affecting thermodilution cardiac outputs include the following:

□ A partly wedged or completely wedged catheter will reduce flow past the thermistor, producing unreliable cardiac outputs. The thermistor should also be located in the center of the flowing blood. Only if there is an undamped pulmonary artery waveform should one assume acceptable thermistor position.

□ A distance of 20 cm between the injectate port and the thermistor is needed for adequate injectate and blood mixing. A catheter looped in the right ventricle will provide an improper thermistor position.

□ Septal defects within the catheter between the proximal and distal lumens will decrease the cardiac outputs, because the injectate will engage near the thermistor.

□ Catheter thrombi will produce errors proportional to the size of the thrombus, underestimating flow as thrombus size increases.

Rapid volume infusions or electrocautery can lead to incorrect measurements. Inconsistent clinical technical performance, equipment malfunction, use of improper constants, or incorrect setup of the pulmonary artery catheter and cardiac output injectate tubing can all produce incorrect cardiac outputs.

Selected References

1. Spackman TN, Rorie DK. Monitoring during cardiovascular surgery. In Tarhan S, ed. Cardiovascular Anesthesia and Postoperative Care. 2nd ed. Chicago: Year Book Medical Publishers, 1989:81–103.
2. Jansen JRC, Schreuder JJ, Bogaard JM. Thermodilution technique for assessment of cardiac output during artificial ventilation. J Appl Physiol 1981;51:584.

Suggested References

Mark JB, Slaughter TF, Reves JG. Cardiovascular monitoring. In Miller RD, ed. Anesthesia. 5th ed. Philadelphia: Churchill Livingstone, 2000:1117–1206.
Reich DL, Moskowitz DM, Kaplan JA. Hemodynamic monitoring. In Kaplan JA, ed. Cardiac Anesthesia. 4th ed. Philadelphia: WB Saunders, 1999:321.

100
Hemodynamic Monitoring for Patients with COPD

Mary M. Rajala, M.D.

In patients with cardiopulmonary disease, an elevated central venous pressure (CVP) is an unreliable indicator of left ventricular (LV) function and in fact may vary inversely with pulmonary capillary wedge pressure (PCWP). Pulmonary artery (PA) catheterization is clinically useful in circumstances involving hemodynamic instability and when it is desirable to obtain measurements of LV function and determine intracardiac pressures, mixed venous oxygenation, and cardiac output. It is not uncommon for a patient who has significant pulmonary disease to require PA catheterization. The technique remains useful given a knowledge of factors that alter the validity of data obtained and the potential complications.

Background

The information derived from PA catheterization is based on several assumptions. These include that wedging of the catheter into the PA will obstruct flow and that the resulting static column of fluid between the wedged catheter tip and the left atrium will reflect pressures beyond the pulmonary circulation. The tip must be properly located below the level of the left atrium in zone 3 (Fig. 100–1). These conditions are generally met without difficulty. In the absence of pulmonary disease, PCWP is 1 to 4 mm Hg less than pulmonary artery diastolic pressure (PADP) and correlates with left atrial pressure (LAP) over a range of 5 to 25 mm Hg. Disease states may affect various portions of the continuous chamber, creating gradients (Fig. 100–2), diminishing accuracy and making interpretation of all downstream measurements difficult.

Chronic Obstructive Pulmonary Disease

In chronic obstructive pulmonary disease (COPD), there is airway obstruction and loss of elastic recoil leading to air trapping, increases in compliance and pulmonary vascular resistance (PVR), and subsequent right-sided heart failure and elevated CVP, independent of LV function. There is decreased LV compliance from shifting of the intraventricular septum as a result of fluid overload in the right ventricle. Marked variations in intrathoracic pressures are seen, along with similar variations in PCWP. PVR increases directly with the severity of lung disease and correlates with oxygen desaturation and acidosis. Increased PVR and diastolic pressure differences across the pulmonary vascular bed result in increased PA pressures. As PVR increases, there is obstruction to blood flow, the gradient between PADP and PCWP increases, and PADP cannot be assumed to correlate with pulmonary artery wedge pressure (PAWP) and left ventricular end-diastolic pressure (LVEDP). PADP will reflect LV pressures and PCWP provided that there are no severe pulmonary vascular changes. If a patient has COPD but an insignificant gradient,

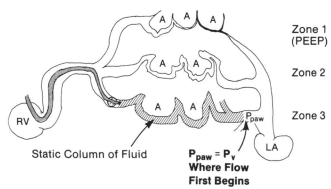

Figure 100–1. Mechanism by which PAWP records left atrial pressure. When the balloon on the pulmonary artery catheter is inflated, a static column of fluid is created distal to the catheter tip, which serves as an extension of the catheter over to the venous side of the pulmonary circulation. Consequently, PAWP is a pulmonary venous pressure. Because there is virtually no pressure gradient between the pulmonary veins and the left atrium, PAWP is regarded as equal to left atrial pressure. Because the pulmonary veins are continuously collapsed in zone 1 and intermittently collapsed in zone 2, the PAWP may not accurately reflect left atrial pressure in these regions of the lung. (From Benumof JL.[1])

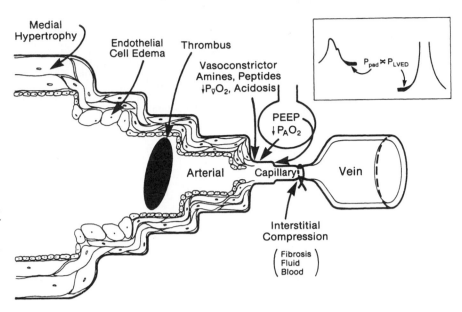

Figure 100–2. Causes of increased PVR during acute and chronic respiratory failure are multiple. In an anatomical progression from the arterial to the venous side of the pulmonary circulation, the causes of increased PVR include medial hypertrophy, endothelial cell edema, pulmonary thromboembolism, and arteriolar constriction by vasoactive amines, peptides, or decreased mixed venous oxygen tension (↓ PVo₂). PEEP can compress the pulmonary capillaries. Increased interstitial hydrostatic pressure because of transudated fluid and blood, which can later fibrose, can compress the venous side of the pulmonary capillaries. All these causes of increased PVR will create a PADP-to-LVEDP gradient (see inset). (From Benumof JL.[1])

there is close agreement between PAWP and PADP, and PADP can then be used to estimate LV function and to avoid frequent balloon inflation and associated complications. Expiration, generally a passive process, becomes active in COPD, as stored elastic forces are lost and cannot overcome the airway resistance. Intrathoracic pressure then increases throughout the lungs. Despite these changes, as long as the increased resistance is proximal to the point of PCWP measurement, there is a correlation between PCWP and LAP and LVEDP, even when disease is severe. PCWP may then be used to follow trends in LV filling pressures.

Air trapping in COPD can cause intrinsic PEEP (and loss of zone 3 conditions) and thereby artifactually increase PCWP even in the presence of low LVEDP by transmitting pressure to the pulmonary vasculature or by increasing the intrathoracic pressures and decreasing venous return. If lungs are noncompliant or PEEP levels are low to moderate, then this pressure will not be transmitted, and PCWP will correlate with LAP and LVEDP. Spontaneous ventilation or intermittent mandatory ventilation promotes normal venous return and normal pulmonary venous pressure. If PEEP is greater than or equal to 10 mm Hg, and particularly if it exceeds 15 to 20 mm Hg, or if there is low LAP in the face of PEEP, the correlation decreases. When PVR increases, PADP also increases, and the relationship between PADP and PCWP is altered and cannot be assumed to correlate with PCWP or LVEDP.

Risks

Although PA catheterization is more useful than CVP monitoring, it has more associated risks when used in the setting of COPD. Pneumothorax oc-

curring from catheter insertion may be fatal in COPD patients. Pulmonary hypertension increases the likelihood of PA rupture. Therefore, it is more important to avoid prolonged wedging or overinflation of the balloon. In addition, it may be more difficult to obtain a wedged position.

Other Monitoring

Despite pitfalls of PA pressure measurements in COPD, other parameters obtained with a PA catheter are helpful in guiding patient management. Central access is needed when large blood loss and fluid shifts are anticipated along with rapid fluid administration, for the injection of vasoactive drugs, for possible venous air embolism, and to assess adequacy of tissue oxygenation, volume status, and LV performance. Because CVP monitoring cannot reliably provide all of this, a PA catheter is often useful in patients with COPD. PA catheterization is often indicated in patients with pulmonary disease undergoing major surgery who have FEV₁ to FVC ratios below 60%, coexisting cardiac disease, PaO₂ less than 55 mm Hg on room air, maximum voluntary ventilation less than 50% predicted, an anticipated need for PEEP, or interstitial edema on the chest radiograph. Cardiac output and mixed venous oxygen saturation information are useful in guiding fluid, inotrope, and ventilatory management.

Arterial blood pressure monitoring is useful in patients with COPD who are undergoing major or prolonged surgery or open chest procedures; whose condition is ASA III or greater; in cases where large fluid shifts, blood loss and transfusion, or changes in blood pressure, preload or afterload, or contractility are anticipated; or where frequent blood gas monitoring is desirable perioperatively, as in patients who are expected to require prolonged mechanical ventilation.

Selected References

1. Benumof JL. Anesthesia for Thoracic Surgery. Philadelphia, WB Saunders, 1995.

Suggested References

Tuman KF, Gilbert GC, Ivankovich AD. Pitfalls in interpretation of pulmonary artery catheter data. J Cardiothorac Anesth 1989;3:625.

Vender JS. Pulmonary artery catheter monitoring. Anesthesiol Clin N Am 1988;6:743.

101
Line Isolation Monitors: Leakage Currents

John K. Erie, M.D.

The human body is not very tolerant of electrical current. As little as 50 microamperes (μA) passing through the heart can cause ventricular fibrillation. Because every operating room has many devices that use electricity, line isolation monitors have been developed to detect leakage currents.

Isolation Transformers

To increase operating room safety, electricity is isolated from the main power source by isolation transformers. Although the line source is made grounded by the electrical provider, the secondary circuit is intentionally not grounded. In such an ungrounded circuit, both conductors must be contacted to cause a shock. When only one conductor is contacted, no electrical current will pass through the body (Fig. 101–1).

Line Isolation Monitors

Line isolation monitors were developed to detect short circuits (or leakage currents). They monitor the isolation of the transformer from ground, and thus are also called ground fault detectors. The line isolation monitor reads approximately 0 A (no leakage current) when current is unable to make a complete path. (Small "leakage currents" are present that slightly degrade the isolation of the system.) However, if the ungrounded side of the electric circuit becomes grounded due to a short, touching the circuit allows the current to make a complete path, causing an electrical shock. The severity of the shock depends on the amount of current and the duration. In the context of electrical safety in the operating room, electrical shock is divided into two categories, macroshock and microshock (Table 101–1).

Figure 101–1. Even though a person is grounded, no shock is received on contacting one wire of an isolated circuit. (From Bruner JMR, Leonard PF.[1])

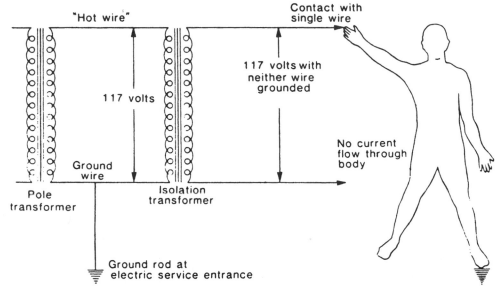

Table 101–1. Effects of 60-Hz AC on an Average Human for a 1-Second Duration of Contact

Current	Effect
Macroshock	
1 mA (0.001 A)	Threshold of perception.
5 mA (0.005 A)	Accepted as maximum harmless current intensity.
10–20 mA (0.01–0.02 A)	"Let-go" current before sustained muscle contraction.
50 mA (0.05 A)	Pain, possible fainting, mechanical injury; heart and respiratory functions continue.
100–300 mA (0.1–0.3 A)	Ventricular fibrillation will start, but respiratory center remains intact.
6000 mA (6 A)	Sustained myocardial contractions, followed by normal heart rhythm; temporary respiratory paralysis; burns if current density is high.
Microshock	
100 μA (0.1 mA)	Ventricular fibrillation.
10 μA (0.01 mA)	Recommended maximum allowable 60-Hz leakage current.

From Pashayan AG, Ehrenwerth J.[2]

□ Macroshock refers to the application of large amounts of current to tissue at locations remote from the heart, such as skin.

□ Microshock refers to the application of small currents directly to the heart, such as occurs with pacemakers.

Line isolation monitors are usually set at 2 to 4 mA and thus do not warn of leakage currents in the microshock range (50 μA). Because of this, additional precautions should be taken with equipment that is in direct contact with the heart, such as central venous pressure monitors and intracardiac electrocardiogram monitoring during right atrial catheter placement.

The sounding of a line isolation alarm means that one side of the secondary circuit has been grounded. At this time, the electrical equipment that triggered the alarm should be shut off, unplugged, and repaired. If the source of the alarm is not clear, electrical devices in the room can be turned off one at a time until the faulty device is identified.

Selected References

1. Bruner JMR, Leonard PF. Electricity, Safety and the Patient. Chicago, Year Book Medical Publishers, 1989.
2. Pashayan AG, Ehrenwerth J. Lasers and electrical safety in the operating room. In Ehrenwerth J, Eisenkraft JB, eds. Anesthesia Equipment: Principles and Applications. St. Louis: Mosby, 1993:436.

102
Microshock Hazards

Michael E. Johnson, M.D., Ph.D.

Quantitative Aspects

Externally applied 60-Hz current induces ventricular fibrillation (VF) at 100 mA, while the same current applied through a ventricular catheter can induce VF at 50 μA. The national code requires less than 10 μA maximum permissible leakage through electrodes or catheters that contact the heart.

Electrocardiograph Monitor Protection

A standard line isolation monitor (LIM) in the operating room gives a warning only when leakage current from a device is greater than 2 mA. Thus it provides little protection against microshock. For example, an electrocardiograph (ECG) monitor used to assist in the placement of a central line (e.g., a right atrial catheter) advanced into the ventricle could have an internal fault that would deliver a shock of 500 μA (0.5 mA) and induce VF without ever setting off the LIM. Thus, ECG monitors isolate the monitoring electrodes from the monitors' power circuits by an isolation transformer and should also be tested periodically for microampere leakage currents. Some ECG monitors translate the electrical ECG signal into light with a photodiode and transmit it optically to the ECG monitor, providing greater electrical isolation and protection.

Protective Factors

In practice, several factors act to reduce the risk of VF from microshock. There is less danger if the catheter is floating free in the ventricle instead of being lodged in the ventricular wall. There is less danger if the catheter tip is in the atrium (where it requires greater than 3 mA to induce VF in dogs with atrial catheters).

A pressure transducer prevents current proximal to the transducer from flowing down the catheter into the patient by its plastic diaphragm. The diaphragm provides electrical isolation between the catheter hydraulic system and the body of the transducer. There is also additional insulation between the transducer's case and its diaphragm.

An electrically conductive catheter filled with saline is safer than a nonconductive catheter because the conductive catheter allows an externally applied current to leak through its wall before reaching the catheter tip. This advantage is negated by the presence of a conductive guidewire that allows current to reach the catheter tip more quickly before it can leak through the catheter walls.

Static Electricity

Static electricity transmitted from physician fingertip to external end of a right ventricular pacemaker in dogs can initiate preventricular contractions and, rarely, VF. This is preventable by wearing conductive operating room "booties" and by wearing rubber gloves whenever direct contact with the external ends of a pacing catheter is necessary.

Incidence of Microshock Injury

A 1972 study by Bruner and colleagues (cited by Hill[1]) reported 55 electrical accidents with 3 episodes of VF over 3.5 years at Massachusetts General Hospital. **None** of these accidents involved microshock to the heart. A recent case report described a patient in whom VF may have been triggered by electrosurgical cautery stimulating the myocardial leads of a permanent pacemaker.

Selected References
1. Hill DW. Physics Applied to Anaesthesia. 4th ed. Boston, Butterworths, 1980.

Suggested References
Aggarwal A, Farber NE, Kotter GS, et al. Electrosurgery induced ventricular filtration during pacemaker replacement—A unique mechanism. J Clin Monit 1996;12:339–342.
Lipton MJ, Ream AK, Hyndman BH. A conductive catheter to improve patient safety during cardiac catheterization. Circulation 1978;58:1190.
Litt L. Electrical safety in the operating room. In Miller RD, ed. Anesthesia. 5th ed. Philadelphia: Churchill Livingstone, 2000:2691–2700.
McCarty RJ, Glasser SP. The arrhythmogenic effect of static electricity on the dog heart. Am Heart J 1977;93:496.

103
Laser Combustion

Gregory A. Nuttall, M.D.

Ignition Hazard: Laser Surgery

The laser (*l*ight *a*mplification by *s*timulated *e*mission of *r*adiation) is an intense source of electromagnetic radiation. Most medical lasers use light of wavelengths in the visible and infrared parts of the spectrum. These wavelengths, when absorbed, produce heat in biological and nonbiological material. There are differences in the power density, energy flux (rate of energy delivery), and depth of penetration of the various laser beams; their effects on tissues are also affected by tissue factors (Fig. 103–1). Endotracheal (ET) tubes differ greatly. Predominantly two types of lasers are used within the airway: the CO_2 laser and the neodymium-yttrium aluminum garnet (Nd-YAG) laser.

The CO_2 laser is strongly absorbed by water, blood, and biological tissues. It has the shallowest penetration of the medical lasers, and edema formation is minimal. It primarily vaporizes cells (see Fig. 103–1). The CO_2 laser is especially well suited as a cutting tool and is used predominantly in the upper airway to excise a variety of benign and malignant lesions. The CO_2 laser provides good hemostasis of small blood vessels, minimal postoperative edema, and good healing with little scar formation.

The Nd-YAG laser is absorbed mostly by pig-

ments. It has the greatest tissue penetration of the medical lasers, and scattering in tissue is strong. The Nd-YAG is also one of the most powerful of the medical lasers. The result of these properties is that large areas of tissue edema are produced, which makes this laser a very effective coagulator. The Nd-YAG usually is applied to the tracheobronchial tree to secure hemostasis (especially from larger vessels) and in the palliative treatment of obstructive tracheobronchial neoplasms. If a laser beam strikes an ET tube, ignition may occur. The probability of ignition depends on the following:

- The type of ET tube. Studies by Patel and Hicks[2] and Meyers[3] have shown that PVC ET tubes are more likely to ignite than red rubber ET tubes.
- The wattage of the laser beam.
- The duration of exposure of the tube to the beam.
- The gas mixture in the ET tube. Reduced concentrations of oxygen and nitrous oxide were shown to reduce the risk of ignition.

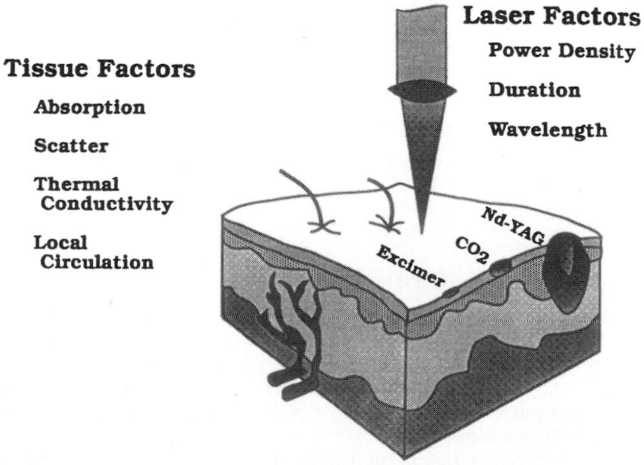

Prevention

ET tubes can be protected by wrapping them with copper, aluminum, or other metal tapes. Wrapping reduces tube flexibility and increases tube external diameter. Moreover, the wrapping may detach in the airway, and the rough surface of the tape may be traumatic and may make intubation more difficult. Other types of ET tubes have been developed specifically for laser surgery (Table 103–1). These tubes have their own problems (e.g., high cost, large diameter). Alternatives include jet ventilation via surgical laryngoscopy and intermittent extubation.

Because oxygen and N_2O support combustion, the lowest FIO_2 that will maintain adequate oxygenation should be used. Air is substituted for N_2O to decrease the risk of an ET tube fire.

Thermal Injury and Response

ET tube fires can burn with intensity, and a laser-ignited explosion can cause thermal and chemical injury. The thermal injury results from direct

Tissue Factors

Absorption

Scatter

Thermal Conductivity

Local Circulation

Laser Factors

Power Density

Duration

Wavelength

Nd-YAG

Excimer

CO_2

Figure 103–1. Different wavelengths of laser light cause different patterns of tissue destruction. The actual destructive effect of laser light on tissue depends on both laser parameters and tissue factors. (From Rampil IJ.[1])

Table 103–1. Advantages and Disadvantages of Commercially Available Laser-Resistant Tracheal Tubes

Description of Resistant Tube	Applicable Laser	Advantages	Disadvantages
Aluminum/silicone spiral with self-inflating foam cuff (Fome-Cuf, Bivona, Inc., Gary, IN)	CO_2	Atraumatic external surface; cuff maintains seal even if punctured by laser; nonflammable inner surface.	Contains flammable material (silicone); cuff difficult to deflate if punctured.
Airtight, stainless steel, corrugated spiral with PVC tip and double cuff (Laser Flex, Mallinckrodt, St. Louis, MO)	CO_2, KTP	Tube maintains shape well; double cuff maintains seal after proximal cuff puncture; body of tube is nonflammable; noncuffed version available.	Cuffed version contains flammable material (PVC); tubes are thick walled; metal may reflect beam onto nontargeted tissue.
Silicone tubes wrapped with aluminum and Teflon, with methylene blue in cuff (Laser-Shield, Xomed, Inc., Jacksonville, FL)	CO_2, KTP	Wrapping protects flammable material and is smoother than manual tape wrapping; methylene blue aids in detection of cuff perforation.	Contains flammable material (silicone); single cuff is vulnerable to laser damage.

From Pashayan AG, Ehrenwerth J.[4]

exposure to the flame; the severity of the burn depends on the duration of exposure and the heat intensity. Inhalation of smoke may produce a chemical burn resulting in acute respiratory failure secondary to bronchospasm, intra-alveolar hemorrhage, edema, or loss of surfactant. PVC tubes release hydrogen chloride when burned, which produces a severe pneumonitis. Carbon monoxide is a decomposition product of burning red rubber ET tubes.

Table 103–2. Response to Fires During Laser Operations on the Airway

Steps	Measure
Immediate	
First	Disconnect oxygen source at the Y-piece and remove burning objects from the airway.
Second	Irrigate the site with water if the fire is still smoldering.
Third	Ventilate the patient by mask or reintubate the trachea and ventilate with as low an F_{IO_2} as possible.
Secondary	
Fourth	Evaluate the extent of injury by bronchoscopy and laryngoscopy.
Fifth	Reintubate the trachea or perform a tracheostomy if needed.
Sixth	Monitor with oximetry, arterial blood gas analysis, or both, and chest radiograms for at least 24 hours.
Seventh	Use ventilatory support, steroids, and antibiotics as needed.

From Pashayan AG, Ehrenwerth J.[4]

If the ET tube ignites (Table 103–2), the tube should be immediately removed and the source of oxygen and N_2O should be disconnected. The area should be flushed with sterile water or normal saline. The patient should be reintubated with a new ET tube and ventilated with 100% oxygen. Bronchoscopy should be performed to assess the extent of injury and remove any foreign bodies, and the large airways should be lavaged to remove carbonaceous deposits. Prolonged intubation and ventilatory assistance may be required. Prophylactic steroid and antibiotic treatment is controversial.

Selected References

1. Rampil IJ. Anesthetic considerations for laser surgery. Anesth Analg 1992;74:424–435.
2. Patel KF, Hicks JN. Prevention of fire hazards associated with the use of CO_2 lasers. Anesth Analg 1981;60:885–888.
3. Meyers A. Complications of CO_2 laser surgery of the larynx. Ann Otol Rhinol Laryngol 1981;90:132.
4. Pashayan AG, Ehrenwerth J. Lasers and electrical safety in the operating room. In Ehrenwerth J, Eisenkraft JB, eds. Anesthesia Equipment: Principles and Applications. St. Louis: Mosby, 1993:436.

Suggested References

Rampil IJ. Anesthesia for laser surgery. In Miller RD, ed. Anesthesia. 5th ed. Philadelphia: Churchill Livingstone, 2000:2199–2212.
Sosis M, Dillon F. What is the safest foil tape for endotracheal tube protection during Nd-YAG laser surgery? A comparative study. Anesthesiology 1990;72:553–555.

104
Physics and Physiology of Neuromuscular Monitoring

Michael D. Taylor, M.D.

Neuromuscular monitoring is used routinely to determine adequacy of neuromuscular blockade intraoperatively and adequacy of relaxant reversal postoperatively. Head lift is a sensitive clinical test of neuromuscular function in conscious patients. If more than 33% of a patient's neuromuscular junction receptors are still occupied by relaxant, sustained head lift will be impossible. A normal tidal volume can be present when 80% of receptors are blocked. Although patients with partial blockade may have adequate ventilation, airway reflexes are impaired and perceived weakness can be a frightening symptom.

The reaction of individual muscle fibers to a motor nerve stimulus is an all-or-none phenomenon. The responses of the muscle as a whole depend on the number of fibers blocked. Because of this, any stimulus to the nerve used to monitor neuromuscular function must be maximal. Generally, stimuli are 20% to 25% supramaximal.

Nerve Stimulators

Important characteristics for optimal function of nerve stimulators include operation by battery, the ability to deliver multiple stimulus patterns (i.e., single-twitch, train-of-four, tetanus, double-burst), the ability to generate 60 to 80 mA of current, and the capacity to deliver a wave impulse 0.2 to 0.3 msec long (Table 104–1).

The impulse should be monophasic and rectangular (square wave) with an optimal duration of 0.1 to 0.3 msec. (Longer than 0.5 msec may stimulate the muscle directly or lead to repetitive firing.) Various types of electrodes may be used with nerve stimulators, including rubber electrodes (impedance increases with age), pregelled silver/silver chloride electrodes, and coated needle electrodes. The site for nerve stimulation may vary; the ulnar nerve is the most common choice. Other possible sites include the median, posterior tibial, common peroneal, and facial nerves.

Patterns of Nerve Stimulation

Single-twitch stimulations (Fig. 104–1) are single supramaximal stimuli at frequencies ranging from 1.0 to 0.1 Hz. The response depends on the frequency of the stimulus. Rates greater than 0.15 Hz may lead to a gradual decrease in the response, reaching a plateau at a lower level. Results obtained at differing frequencies cannot be compared, and this mode of stimulation cannot be compared with train-of-four stimulation. Except for a faster onset with depolarizing relaxants, no significant difference in single-twitch results exists between depolarizing and nondepolarizing blockade.

Tetanic stimulation involves the rapid delivery of supramaximal stimuli at 30, 50, or 100 Hz. Normally (in the absence of block), muscle response to 50-Hz tetanic stimulation for 5 seconds is sustained. That is, there is continued maximal contraction and no fade. If postsynaptic receptors are blocked by a nondepolarizing relaxant, **fade** occurs. There is a decrease in twitch height, but no fade occurs with depolarizing block unless phase II block is present. Fade depends on the frequency and length of stimulation, and these factors must be held constant for

Table 104–1. Desirable Features of a Nerve Stimulator

Essential
- Square-wave impulse, <0.5 msec duration.
- Ability to maintain selected current for duration of impulse (i.e., constant current, variable voltage).
- Battery power.
- Multiple patterns of stimulation: single-twitch, train-of-four, double-burst, tetanus, post-tetanic count.

Optional
- Rheostat for adjustable current output.
- Polarity output indicator.
- Ability to calculate and display fade ratio and/or percent depression of single-twitch amplitude from control value.
- High-output (up to 80 to 100 mA) and low-output (<5 mA) sockets.
- Audible signal with each stimulus delivered.
- Alarm for excessive impedance, lead disconnect, low battery.
- Battery charge indicator.

From Brull SJ, Silverman DG.[1]

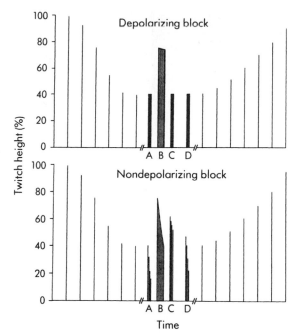

Figure 104–1. Patterns of block. During depolarizing block, there is a progressive decrease of single-twitch height but no fade in response to rapid stimulation [TOF (A) or tetanus (B)], and there is no post-tetanic facilitation of neuromuscular transmission (C and D). During nondepolarizing block, in addition to decline in single-twitch height, there is fade in response to TOF (A) and tetanus (B), and facilitation of subsequent (post-tetanic) neuromuscular transmission (C and D). (From Brull SJ, Silverman DG.[1])

comparison. **Post-tetanic facilitation** can be seen after tetanic stimulation when partial blockade with a nondepolarizing relaxant is present. Post-tetanic facilitation does not occur after succinylcholine. Tetanic stimulation can be painful to a conscious person.

The **train-of-four (TOF)** involves four supramaximal stimuli applied every 0.5 second. The amplitude of the fourth response divided by the amplitude of the first response is known as the TOF ratio. During a nondepolarizing block, the TOF ratio decreases. The degree of blockade may be directly estimated from the TOF ratio without a preoperative control value. When the TOF ratio is greater than 0.7, single-twitch height should be normal. Depolarizing blockade does not lead to a decrease (or fade) in the TOF ratio. If fade occurs following administration of a depolarizing relaxant alone, phase II block should be suspected.

In **post-tetanic count stimulation (PTC)**, a tetanic stimulation (i.e., 50 Hz for 5 seconds) is applied, and the response is observed to single-twitch stimulation at 1 Hz starting 3 seconds after the tetanic stimulation. The number of single-

twitch responses measured is the value of PTC. This technique allows quantification of neuromuscular blockade, even when no response to single-twitch or TOF can be elicited. Although the PTC depends primarily on the degree of neuromuscular block, it also depends on (1) the frequency and duration of tetanic stimulation, (2) the length of time between the tetanic stimulation and the first post-tetanic stimulus, (3) the frequency of the single-twitch stimulation, and (4) the length of single-twitch stimulation before the tetanic stimulation. Because antagonism of neuromuscular blockade may develop, tetanic stimulation should not be given more frequently than every 6 minutes.

Double-burst stimulation (DBS) involves two short bursts of 50-Hz stimulation separated by 750 msec. The duration of each square wave impulse is 0.2 msec. The most common pattern is three impulses in each burst, designated as DBS 3,3. Nonparalyzed muscle demonstrates equal responses to both bursts. During nondepolarizing blockade, the second response is decreased. The ratio of the second to first impulses in DBS correlates well with the TOF ratio. The chief advantage to DBS is that the responses may be easier to evaluate by tactile means.

Recording Devices

Several means are available for evaluating muscular response to nerve stimulation. The most common method is visual or tactile assessment. Recording devices include (1) mechanomyography (isometric measurement of evoked tension after a preload of 200 to 300 g is applied to the thumb, as measured by a force-displacement transducer), (2) electromyography (measurement of evoked electromyographic responses), and (3) measurement of acceleration by a piezoelectric transducer (accelerometry).

Selected References

1. Brull SJ, Silverman DG. Neuromuscular block monitoring. In Ehrenwerth J, Eisenkraft JB, eds. Anesthesia Equipment: Principles and Applications. St. Louis: Mosby, 1993:297.

Suggested References

Bevan DR, Donati F. Muscle relaxants. In Barash PG, Cullen BF, Stoelting RK, eds. Clinical Anesthesia. 3rd ed. Philadelphia: Lippincott-Raven, 1997:400–402.
Savarese JJ, Caldwell JE, Lien CA, et al. Pharmacology of muscle relaxants and their antagonists. In Miller RD, ed. Anesthesia. 5th ed. Philadelphia: Churchill Livingstone, 2000:412–490.

Clinical Sciences

105

Preemptive Analgesia and Perioperative Pain Control

Beth A. Elliott, M.D.

In recent years, considerable time and effort has been directed toward improving perioperative pain control. The concept of preempting pain by instituting antinociceptive therapies before the nociceptive stimulus occurs has captured the attention of many investigators and clinicians alike. Despite the interest in proving or disproving the ability to achieve preemptive analgesia, confusion, misunderstanding, and misapplication of the concept continue.

Simply defined, preemptive analgesia is an antinociceptive modality that prevents the establishment of central hyperexcitability that follows a nociceptive stimulus. This is not as easy to determine or measure as many studies presume. Reduction of postoperative pain medication requirements and lower scores on visual analog scales for pain will perhaps indicate the possibility of a preemptive effect, but by themselves they do not reliably confirm a preemptive effect from any given intervention.

Pain Theory

It is generally accepted that tissue injury produces a biphasic response whereby both peripheral and central nervous sensitization occur. **Peripheral sensitization** results from the local release of excitatory neurotransmitters and chemical mediators of the inflammatory response (substance P, prostaglandins, leukotrienes, bradykinin, serotonin, and histamine). This leads to an exaggerated response to further physical stimulation of the injured area.

This second phase, or **central sensitization**, occurs as a result of the continued barrage of afferent traffic from the site of injury and activation of excitatory amino acid NMDA receptors in the spinal cord. This leads to an amplification of afferent nociceptive input by expansion of receptive fields within the CNS, a decrease in threshold of dorsal horn neurons, and enhancement of dorsal horn responses to repetitive C-fiber input. This central hypersensitivity is responsible for the establishment of the zone of hypersensitivity surrounding the area of injury and for the persistent duration of hypersensitivity within the area of injury itself. Once established, central sensitization may decrease the effectiveness of pain relief modalities targeting the initial area of injury (Fig. 105–1).

A good deal of the evidence supporting this theory comes from laboratory studies using animal models. In a rat model, local anesthetics, central neuraxial opioids, and NSAIDs have all been shown to significantly reduce secondary hyperexcitability when administered before rather than after formalin injection into the forepaw.

One of the problems with direct application of these findings to the clinical situation is that unlike many experimental models that use a short-lived nociceptive stimulus, continued afferent stimulation from a surgical wound persists during the period of wound healing, allowing central sensitization even in the postoperative period. A single "preemptive" intervention may well reduce the amount of pain experienced postoperatively, but due to its short duration, is usually ineffective in preventing the hypersensitivity second phase of the pain response. Animal studies using a sustained nociceptive stimulus (carrageenan injection) failed to show any preemptive effects. This underscores the belief that unless the treatment/intervention is effective for the entire duration of the noxious stimulus, central sensitization can still occur.

Many clinical studies evaluating the value of preemptive analgesic modalities have been inconclusive, in part because of the difficulty in providing an effective antinociceptive intervention that covers the entire postoperative period. A compounding predicament with clinical application of preemptive analgesic modalities is the responsibility we have to our patients to provide humane care, adequate pain relief, and anxiolysis in the perioperative period. This can minimize differences between study groups and lead to negative findings.

Role of Regional Anesthesia

Local anesthetic infiltration of surgical wounds has some potential in providing preemptive analge-

A POST-SURGICAL AFFERENT INPUT

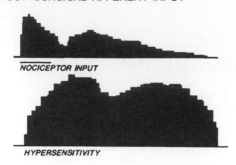

B PRE-SURGICAL ANALGESIA

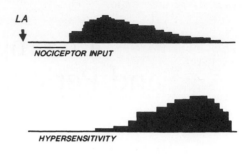

C POST-SURGICAL ANALGESIA

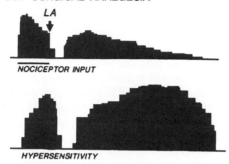

D PRE- and POST-SURGICAL ANALGESIA

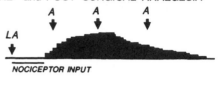

Figure 105–1. Model illustrating why single-treatment preemptive analgesia may be insufficient for the management of postoperative pain. *A,* Surgery leads to a nociceptive input not only during the surgery itself (solid line beneath the drawing of nociceptor input represents the duration of surgery), but also postoperatively as a result of the inflammatory response to the damaged tissue. This secondary wave of input can sustain the hypersensitivity state. *B,* Regional anesthesia administered for the duration of the surgery, although eliminating the first phase of nociceptive input, and thus preempting the first stage of postsurgical hypersensitivity will not prevent the initiation of central sensitization in response to the second "inflammatory" phase, although *(C)* it might have a greater relative effect than a single postoperative treatment. *D,* The optimum form of treatment may be one that acts continuously both on the first intraoperative phase (e.g., regional anesthesia or preoperative opioids) and on the afferent activity generated postoperatively (e.g., nonsteroidal antiinflammatory drugs or opioids). LA, local anesthesia. (From Woolf CJ, Chong MS.[1])

sia. In addition to blocking neuronal transmission from the surgical site, local anesthetics may reduce neurogenic inflammation by blocking the axon reflex and sympathetic efferents. Local anesthetics have also been shown to have effects on nonneuronal aspects of the inflammatory response. Antimicrobial activity of local anesthetics, inhibition of leukocyte migration to the surgical site, and metabolic activation at the surgical site may have implications in terms of outcome and wound healing that are well beyond the scope of investigations regarding effects on analgesia.

Preoperative local anesthetic administration, by either local tissue infiltration or nerve block, has proven to be effective in reducing postoperative pain in patients undergoing surgery under general anesthesia. This has been demonstrated in a variety of surgical settings including tonsillectomy, inguinal hernia, cholecystectomy, and dental extractions. There is some evidence to suggest that continuous infusion of local anesthetics may be of greater benefit than single dose administration.

Local infiltration and peripheral nerve blocks seem to be more efficacious than central neuraxial anesthetic techniques in reducing postoperative pain. In one study, patients undergoing inguinal herniorrhaphy under spinal anesthesia had less postoperative pain than those who received general anesthesia alone, but the effect was less pronounced than that seen with general anesthesia plus local infiltration. Yet another study evaluated the efficacy of ilioinguinal/iliohypogastric nerve block with 10 mL 0.5% bupivacaine as an adjunct to spinal anesthesia for inguinal herniorrhaphy. They found significant differences in pain at 3, 6, 24, and 48 hours after surgery. Similar results have been found in patients undergoing total knee arthroplasty under spinal anesthesia either with or without femoral nerve block.

The differences found in these studies should not surprise practitioners who routinely use regional anesthetic techniques in their clinical practice. The profundity of conduction blockade would be expected to be greatest where the local anesthetic is placed on or near peripheral nerves. Epidural and spinal blockade may not provide complete conduction blockade, thereby potentially allowing some degree of central sensitization to occur. This is not to diminish the effectiveness of epidural or spinal anesthesia in reducing postoperative pain. There are many clinical situations where local infiltration/ nerve block is not technically feasible. In these circumstances, epidural anesthesia can be quite effective in reducing postoperative pain.

A recent study of patients undergoing radical retropubic prostatectomy found significant reductions in long-term pain relief and increased activity levels in patients whose epidurals were injected with local anesthetics and narcotics pre-incision versus at the time of closure. The combination of local anesthetics and narcotics for perioperative epidural infusions may be superior to narcotics alone. Another study looking at patients having partial colectomy, found significantly better pain relief and return of bowel function 1.5 days earlier in those patients whose epidural infusion included both narcotics and local anesthetic rather than narcotic alone.

Current investigations are focusing on other receptor populations within the spinal cord where the roles of alpha-2 agonists, N-methyl-D-aspartate (NMDA) antagonists, and GABA agonists have yet to be clearly defined.

Although the goal of providing a true preemptive analgesic intervention may be elusive or even impractical in many clinical circumstances, the goal of providing a relatively pain-free postoperative period for surgical patients is not unrealistic. Modification of the pain response can occur at several different levels—the site of the injury itself with local anesthetic infiltration or administration of systemic NSAIDs, peripheral neural blockade, and central neuraxial administration of local anesthetics and narcotics. There remain many questions regarding the timing and duration of antinociceptive interventions, optimal combinations and doses of agents, patient selection, and cost-effectiveness.

Selected Reference

1. Woolf CJ, Chong MS. Preemptive analgesia: Treating postoperative pain by preventing the establishment of central sensitization. Anesth Analg 1993;77:362–379.

Suggested References

Allen HW, Liu SS, Ware PD, Nairn CS, Owens BD. Peripheral nerve blocks improve analgesia after total knee replacement surgery. Anesth Analg 1998;87:93–97.

Bugedo GJ, Dagnino JA, Carcamo CR, Munoz HR, Mertens RA. Preoperative percutaneous ilioinguinal and iliohypogastric nerve block with 0.5% bupivacaine for post-herniorrhaphy pain management in adults. Reg Anesth 1990;15:130–133.

Carr D. Preempting the memory of pain. JAMA 1999;279:1114–1115.

Gottschalk A, Smith DS, Jobes DR, et al. Preemptive epidural analgesia and recovery from radical prostatectomy. JAMA 1999;279:1076–1082.

Kehlet H. Acute pain control and accelerated postoperative surgical recovery. Surg Clin North Am 1999;79:431–443.

Kissin I. Preemptive analgesia: Why its effect is not always obvious. Anesthesiology 1996;84:1015–1019.

106
Patient-Controlled Analgesia

Martin L. DeRuyter, M.D.

In 1973, Marks and Sachar reported that nearly three-fourths of hospitalized patients receiving parenterally administered narcotics for moderate to severe pain failed to receive adequate analgesia.[1] Other investigators have similarly concluded that some patients receive less than 25% of the pain medications they require. When patients receive parenterally administered analgesics intramuscularly every 3 to 4 hours, the concentration meets or exceeds the minimal analgesic concentration only 35% of the time (Fig. 106–1).

There are many reasons for this undertreatment, including the following:

- Physicians' concerns about overdosing patients.
- Physicians' concerns about the addictive nature of narcotics.
- Psychological issues for patients (e.g., that the patient may be considered "weak" if pain medications are requested).
- Screening by the nursing staff to decide whether the patient "needs" this medication.
- Time interval required by the nursing staff to prepare the injection.
- Pain inappropriately treated with sedation rather than analgesics.

Patient-Controlled Analgesia

In 1968, Sechzer first described patient-controlled analgesia (PCA) with intermittent intravenous (IV) doses of narcotic analgesics.[3] "On-demand" analgesia, the self-administration of preset doses of (typically narcotic) analgesia allowed patients to titrate their own pain control against the amount of sedation.

The patient activates the pump by pressing a button, a preset amount of narcotic is delivered, and a lockout interval is activated, ensuring that another dose cannot be delivered too quickly. Additional features include a maximum dose limit, the capability to provide a basal infusion, and the ability to provide a loading dose. Usual doses are listed in Table 106–1.

Advantages of PCA include the following:

- Superior pain relief with less medication (Fig. 106–2).
- Less daytime sedation.
- Decreased delay between requests for analgesics and their administration.
- Less inappropriate "screening" by nursing staff.
- Improved postoperative pulmonary function.
- Fewer postoperative pulmonary complications.
- Accommodation for diurnal changes in drug requirements and a wider range of analgesic needs.
- Less potential for overdose when small doses per activation are prescribed.
- Improved continuous incremental titration.
- High patient acceptance.
- Improved sleep patterns.

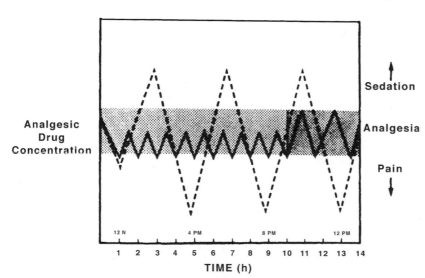

Figure 106–1. Relationship among dose interval, analgesic drug concentration, and clinical effects in a comparison of a PCA system (solid lines) and conventional IM therapy (dashed lines). (From White PF.[2])

Table 106–1. PCA Narcotic Doses

Drug	Concentration (mg/mL)	Bolus (mg)	Lockout (min)	Basal* (mg/hr)	4-hr Limit (mL)
Morphine	1	1–2 (0.4–5.0)	6–10 (0–99)	0.5 (0.5–2.0)	20 (20–30)
Meperidine	10	10 (5–30)	6 (5–15)	5 (5–20)	10 (8–15)

*Basal infusion capability is not available on all pumps.

□ Earlier postoperative mobilization.

Disadvantages of PCA include the following:

□ Patient factors: Requires mental alertness, the physical ability to push the button, and the ability to understand the concept of PCA and to follow instructions.
□ Hypovolemic patients are at increased risk of narcotic-induced respiratory depression.
□ Patients with significant liver, renal, or pulmonary disease should be treated with caution.

□ Narcotic addiction is considered a contradiction by some.
□ Pruritus may be more common with PCA than with intramuscular (IM) narcotics but is significantly less common than with epidural administration.
□ Cost is higher than conventional methods because of special equipment, setup, and training of nursing staff.
□ Complications: Cases of respiratory arrest with PCA have been attributed to faulty equipment, combined IM and IV narcotics, and hypovolemia.

Selected References

1. Marks RM, Sachar EJ. Undertreatment of medical inpatients with narcotic analgesia. Ann Int Med 1973;78:173.
2. White PF. Use of patient-controlled analgesia for management of acute pain. JAMA 1988;259:243.
3. Sechzer PH. Objective measurement of pain. Anesthesiology 1968;29:209–210.
4. Tewes PA, Taylor DR, Bourke DL. Postoperative pain management. In Breslow MJ, Miller CF, Rogers M, eds. Perioperative Management. St. Louis: Mosby, 1990:164.

Suggested References

Ready LB. Acute perioperative pain. In Miller RD, ed. Anesthesia. 5th ed. Philadelphia: Churchill Livingstone, 2000:2323–2350.
Smythe M. Patient-controlled analgesia: A review. Pharmacotherapy 1992;12:132.

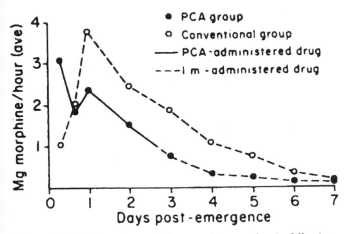

Figure 106–2. Requirements for morphine analgesia following gastric bypass surgery in 10 patients managed with PCA and in 9 patients given 8 to 12 mg morphine IM every 4 to 6 hours on an as-needed basis. (From Tewes PA, Taylor DR, Bourke DL.[4])

107
Epidural Steroid Injection

Lawrence J. Winikur, M.D.

About 80% of the population is affected by back pain at some point in life. Chronic back pain is the third leading cause of disability, with 4% of the population affected. Billions of dollars are spent for the treatment of back pain in the United States alone. Nerve block techniques are often requested in the evaluation and/or treatment of acute and chronic pain conditions. An example of this is the use of lumbar epidural steroid injections in the management of chronic back pain.

Rationale

The practice was introduced at a time when intra-articular injection of steroids was performed on patients with rheumatoid arthritis. Most investigators have proposed an anti-inflammatory role for epidural steroids. The target appears to be neural and perineural inflammation, although this is only presumptive. The perceived advantage of epidural steroids is that the drug is delivered in full dose directly to the site of the inflammation.

Route of Administration

Steroids have been injected into the epidural space by the caudal, lumbar, thoracic, and cervical routes. The advantage of the caudal route is the decreased risk of dural puncture. Disadvantages include the need for large injected volumes in order to reach the target level and the greater degree of technical difficulty. Lumbar epidural injection is most often used; cervical and thoracic epidural injections carry the risk of potential injury to the spinal cord or high spinal block if the subarachnoid space is punctured.

Agents Used

A number of different agents and volumes have been reported in the literature. These have included steroid alone or steroid mixed with or followed by local anesthetic or normal saline. Early studies used hydrocortisone or prednisolone as the steroid. More recent trials use betamethasone, triamcinolone, and dexamethasone. Methylprednisolone or triamcinolone are most frequently used now in doses of 40 to 80 mg. However, the dose-response relationship has not been determined.

Number of Injections

Although four, five, or more injections have been reported at daily to weekly intervals, the most recent literature shows that there is no clinical evidence to justify proceeding beyond three injections if no benefit has been received. After an initial injection, epidural steroids can be repeated up to two times if there is partial improvement. If there is no response after the first injection, a second injection should be performed to ensure proper placement of the steroids. Some practitioners recommend the use of fluoroscopy to confirm correct placement.

Complications

No deleterious effects on neural or perineural tissue have been found with epidural steroid administration. Technical complications include dural puncture, with a prevalence rate of 2%. Enigmatic complications such as headache (2%) and temporary exacerbations of sciatic pain (1.3%) have been reported. Other complications include those caused by intercurrent injection of local anesthetics: local anesthetic allergy, hypotension, and accidental spinal anesthesia. Clinical studies have shown that epidural steroids do depress plasma cortisol levels for as long as 12 weeks, but clinical manifestations rarely appear (1%). Arachnoiditis is a potential complication if Depo-steroids are accidentally injected intrathecally. Epidural abscess and epidural hematoma are rare complications.

Efficacy

Although the principle indications for the use of epidural steroid injections have been symptoms of either chronic or acute back pain, neck pain, shoulder pain, or sciatica, the criteria used for selection of patients have varied. Some trials report an immediate success rate ranging from 25% to 89%, and others report rates between 35% and 86% at review between 6 weeks and 5 years, with an average overall success rate of 45% as defined as those patients being able to return to work. Retrospective studies reveal better results in certain types of patients, for example, those who had not undergone previous surgery, and those with acute radicular pain. One study found that complete relief was obtained in 77% of patients who had symptoms less than 2 weeks, with response rates decreasing to 72%, 60%, and 43% for patients with histories of 4, 6, and longer than 6 weeks, respectively. Other studies and reviews have questioned the efficacy of epidural steroids.

Summary

□ Certain populations of patients may benefit from epidural steroid injections.

□ Overall long-term success rate is 30% to 45%.
□ Best results obtained in early or acute cases.
□ Best performed in patients without previous surgery.
□ Best results are obtained in discogenic, radicular pain.
□ Worst results are obtained in the "failed back."

Suggested References

Cuckler JM, Bernini PA, Wiesel SW, et al. The use of epidural steroids in the treatment of lumbar radicular pain. A prospective, randomized, double-blind study. J Bone Joint Surg 1985:67:63–66.

Ferrante FM, Wilson SP, Iacobo O, et al. Clinical classification as a predictor of therapeutic outcome after cervical epidural steroid injection. Spine 1993;18:730–736.

Flor H, Turk DC. Etiological theories and treatments for chronic back pain. Pain 1984;19:105;209–221.

Kepes ER, Duncalf D. Treatment of backache with spinal injections of local anesthetics, spinal and systemic steroids. A review. Pain 1985;22:33–47.

Nelson DA. Intraspinal therapy using methylprednisolone acetate. Twenty-three years of clinical controversy. Spine 1993;18:278–286.

Rowlingson JC. Epidural analgesic techniques in the management of cervical pain. Anesth Analg 1986;5:938–942.

108
Pain Therapy for Patients with Cancer

Pamela Vick, M.D. □ Tim J. Lamer, M.D.

Patients with malignancies should know that they no longer need to fear a death preceded by prolonged or agonizing suffering from cancer.

Cancer Pain Mechanisms

Cancer pain may result from one or a combination of several mechanisms (Table 108–1). Somatic or nociceptive pain originates from skin, muscle, or bone. Nociceptive pain is mediated by somatic afferent fibers (A delta and C). Visceral pain originates from solid or hollow visceral organs and is mediated by visceral nociceptive afferent fibers that travel along with visceral sympathetic efferent fibers. Sympathetically mediated pain may occur after a nerve or limb injury; this is a diffuse burning pain of the affected extremity, associated with allodynia, hyperpathia, sudomotor dysfunction, and signs of impaired blood flow regulation to the extremity. This pain is believed to be mediated, at least in part, by sympathetic efferents. Neuropathic pain typically is a sharp lancinating pain. Neuropathic and sympathetically mediated pain are generally poorly responsive to opioid therapy. One or more of these mechanisms may contribute to a patient's pain problem and may occur as a result of the tumor itself, radiation therapy, chemotherapy, or surgery. Cancer patients can also suffer from pain secondary to nonmalignant causes, such as herniated nucleus pulposis, spinal stenosis, or myofascial pain syndrome.

Medical Therapy

The World Health Organization has well-established and validated guidelines for the treatment of cancer pain. It progresses in a stepwise approach. The analgesic ladder comprises several steps in conjunction with adjuvant therapy. The general approach is to begin with nonopioid agents and progress to stronger agents as indicated by the patient's clinical condition (Table 108–2).

Adjuvant analgesics include heterocyclic antidepressants (e.g., amitriptyline, desipramine), anticonvulsant medications (e.g., gabapentin, clonazepam, carbamazepine), topical agents (e.g., capsaicin, local anesthetics), and nonsteroidal anti-inflammatory medications (e.g., ibuprofen), anxiolytics, and corticosteroids. This approach is effective in 70% to 90% of patients with cancer related pain. The remaining patients will require more aggressive interventional pain management techniques.

Interventional Therapy

Interventional pain management techniques include injection therapy, neurolytic blocks, spinal analgesia, and neuroaugmentation (Tables 108–3, 108–4, and 108–5). Neurolytic blocks with phenol, ethanol, or radiofrequency techniques are most ap-

Table 108–1. Pain Mechanism Examples

Pain Mechanisms	Examples
Somatic (nociceptive)	Acute postoperative pain, bone fracture, aseptic necrosis, tumor infiltration of bone/joints.
Sympathetic	Complex regional pain syndrome, nerve injury after trauma or radiation.
Visceral	Obstruction of hollow viscus, stretching of liver capsule.
Neuropathic	Vinca alkaloid induced neuropathy, brachial or lumbar plexopathy, phantom limb pain.

Table 108–2. WHO Analgesic Ladder

⌐→ Interventional techniques (e.g., neuraxial catheter, ablative procedures)
Potent oral opioids (moderate to severe pain)[2]
⌐→ (e.g., morphine, hydromorphone, fentanyl patch, oxycodone)
+ or − nonopioid or adjuvant[1]
Weak opioid for mild to moderate pain[2]
⌐→ (e.g., codeine, hydrocodone, propoxyphene, tramidol)
+ or − nonopioid or adjuvant[1]
Nonopioid[2]
(e.g., acetylsalicyclic acid, acetaminophen, nonsteroidal anti-inflammatory drugs)
+ or − adjuvant[1]

[1]Adjuvant agents (e.g., antidepressants, anxiolytics, anticonvulsants).
[2]Nonneurolytic blocks may be helpful in conjunction with other treatment.

Table 108–3. Interventional Techniques for Relief of Cancer Pain

Parenteral administration of opioids Intravenous or subcutaneous infusions Patient-controlled analgesia Spinal analgesia Epidural or intrathecal opioids Epidural or intrathecal local anesthetics Epidural or intrathecal clonidine Combinations	Injection techniques Joint and trigger point injections Nonneurolytic and neurolytic nerve blocks Neurosurgical treatment Neuroaugmentation procedures (e.g., spinal cord stimulator, intrathecal pumps) Neuroablative procedures (e.g., neurectomy, cordotomy, rhizotomy) Neurostimulation

propriate for regional or localized pain in patients with a relatively limited life span (less than 6 months). Examples of neurolytic procedures are outlined in Table 108–5.

Spinal analgesia is indicated for more diffuse pain that is unresponsive to more conservative techniques. Spinal opioids are very effective for somatic pain and are less effective for neuropathic pain. Spinal local anesthetics and clonidine are more effective for neuropathic pain. Combinations or mixtures can be used when more than one mechanism is involved.

The choice of epidural versus intrathecal spinal analgesia is dictated by the pain problem and the patient's prognosis. Intrathecal therapy with a totally implanted pump and catheter is indicated for patients with intractable pain and an anticipated life span of more than 3 months. Epidural analgesia is indicated in patients with an expected life span of less than 3 months.

If survival is anticipated to be less than 3 months, even more aggressive procedures can be considered. These may include neuroablative surgical procedures (e.g., rhizotomy, cordotomy).

Table 108–6 outlines possible approaches to some common cancer pain syndromes. It is important to keep in mind that surgical, radiation, and chemotherapy approaches may also reduce the patient's pain. It is often preferable to await the results of

Table 108–4. Neurolytic Nerve Blocks

Type or Pain	Type of Block
Perineal	Sacral nerve
Chest and abdominal wall	Intercostal or paravertebral nerves
Complex regional pain syndrome	Neurolytic sympathetic block
Visceral pelvic	Hypogastric plexus
Facial	Trigeminal nerve and its divisions
Visceral upper abdominal pain	Celiac plexus or splanchnic nerve block

Table 108–5. Potential Complications of Invasive Procedures

Procedures	Possible Side Effects and Complications
Neurolytic blocks (e.g., radiofrequency denervation, hypobaric vs. hyperbaric spinal, celiac plexus, or hypogastric blocks)	Sensorimotor impairment Sympathetic or parasympathetic impairment Postural hypotension Bowel or bladder dysfunction Pain recurrence Deafferentiation pain Pneumothorax (celiac block)
Spinal opioids with/without catheter	Respiratory depression Pruritis Urinary retention Nausea and vomiting
Spinal clonidine	Hypotension Sedation
Spinal local anesthetic	Sympathetic blockade (hypotension, urinary retention) Exaggerated spread (high block) Motor block
Neurosurgical procedures (e.g., cordotomy, neurectomy)	Bladder dysfunction Motor weakness Deafferentiation pain Respiratory dysfunction (cervical cordotomy)
Spinal axis catheters	Catheter break or leak Catheter obstruction Infection (cellulitis, meningitis, epidural abscess) CSF leak

Table 108–6. Common Pain Syndromes and Therapeutic Interventions

Pain Problem	Intervention
Myofascial pain	Myofascial injection of corticosteroid or local anesthetic, physical modalities, exercise
Postsurgical neuroma	Injection of corticosteroid in neuroma, adjuvant pharmacologic agents, radiofrequency lesion of neuroma
Complex regional pain syndrome	Series of anesthetic sympathetic blocks, spinal cord stimulators, spinal analgesia
Lumbar/brachial plexus pain	Perineural injection of local anesthetic, corticosteroid, or neurolytic block (phenol or ethanol)
Postherpetic neuralgia	Sympathetic or epidural blocks, topical therapy, adjuvant analgesic agents (gabapentin, amitriptyline)
Chest wall pain	Interpleural analgesia, intercostal blocks, spinal analgesia
Perineal pain	Sacral nerve blocks, neurolytic subarachnoid block, spinal analgesia

such treatments before resorting to high-risk ablative procedures.

Other Approaches

Physicians should be aware that therapies besides medication and procedures are often effective. Relaxation training, massage, therapeutic exercise, heat, ice, electrical stimulation, counseling, and orthotic devices can be very useful in the appropriate circumstances. A multidisciplinary or team approach to cancer pain management with participation from oncologists, nurses, psychologists, and pain management specialists will be likely to produce the most appropriate treatment program.

Suggested References

Caraceni A. Clinicopathologic correlates of common pain syndromes. Hematol Oncol Clin North Am 1996;10:57–78.

Cherny NI, Foley KM. Nonopioid and opioid analgesic pharmacotherapy of cancer pain. Hematol Oncol Clin North Am 1996;10:79–102.

Lamer TJ. Treatment of cancer-related pain: When orally administered medications fail. Mayo Clin Proc 1994;69:473–480.

Stevens RA, Stotz A. Neurolytic blocks for management of oncologic pain. Cancer Res Ther Cont 1999;9:345–353.

109
Neuraxial Opioids

Paul E. Carns, M.D.

Opioids were first introduced into the central neuraxis in 1979.[1, 2] Since that time, epidurally and intrathecally administered opioids have been used for both acute and chronic pain control.

The clinical benefits of epidural and intrathecal opioids include[3]:

- Excellent analgesia.
- Earlier ambulation.
- Reduced risk of deep venous thrombosis.
- Better postoperative pulmonary function.
- Earlier extubation.
- Reduced likelihood of respiratory infections.
- Blunted surgical stress response.
- Reduced minimal alveolar concentration (MAC) of inhalation agents.
- Absence of motor, sensory, or autonomic blockade.

The sites of action are the opioid receptors found mainly within the substantia gelatinosa layer in the dorsolateral horn of the spinal cord. When activated, these receptors inhibit the release of excitatory nociceptive neurotransmitters within the spinal cord.

Lipid solubility of each opioid, determined by the **octanol/water partition coefficient**, is the most critical pharmacokinetic property to consider when administering doses near the neuraxis. Table 109–1 lists the octanol/water partition coefficients of commonly used opioids.

Hydrophilic opioids (those with low octanol/water partition coefficients) have a high degree of solubility within the cerebrospinal fluid (CSF), permitting significant cephalad spread. Therefore, thoracic analgesia may be accomplished when either epidural or intrathecal doses are administered at the lumbar level. The epidural or intrathecal dose of morphine is significantly less than that required to achieve an equianalgesic effect through intravenous (IV) administration.[4, 5]

Hydrophilic opioids, used epidurally (see Table 109–2), have a slow onset and prolonged duration of action. An initial epidural bolus dose is required, which may be followed by a continuous infusion through an epidural catheter. Because of the slow onset of action, they are less suitable for patient-controlled epidural analgesia (PCEA). When hydrophilic opioids are used intrathecally, there is a more rapid onset of action and very low doses are required, resulting in less systemic toxicity. Effective analgesia may be seen for up to 24 hours. This method is less expensive because no catheter is used.

Lipophilic opioids (those with a high octanol/water partition coefficient) have a rapid onset and a much shorter duration of action. When used epidurally (see Table 109–2), these drugs are rapidly taken up by epidural fat and redistributed into the systemic circulation, resulting in poor bioavailability to the spinal cord. Neuraxial doses of lipophilic opioids needed to achieve equianalgesic effect are nearly equal to intravenous doses. Plasma levels attained with equal doses of epidural and intravenous infu-

Table 109–1. Octanol/Water Partition Coefficients of Common Opioids

Drug	Octanol/Water Partition Coefficient
Morphine	1.4
Hydromorphone	2
Meperidine	39
Alfentanil	145
Fentanyl	813
Sufentanil	1778

Table 109–2. Clinical Pharmacology of Epidural Opioids

Properties	Advantages	Disadvantages
Hydrophilic opioids		
Slow onset		Delayed onset of analgesia
Long duration	Prolonged single-dose analgesia	Unpredictable duration
High CSF solubility	Minimal dose compared with IV administration	Higher incidence of side effects
Extensive CSF spread	Thoracic analgesia with lumbar administration	Delayed respiratory depression
Lipophilic opioids		
Rapid onset	Rapid analgesia	
Short duration	Decreased side effects	Brief single-dose analgesia
Low CSF solubility	Ideal for continuous infusion or PCEA	Systemic absorption
Minimal CSF spread		Limited thoracic analgesia with lumbar administration

Modified from Grass JA.[11]

sions of fentanyl are nearly identical, suggesting a significant systemic mode of action.[6, 7] Low CSF solubility permits only a limited amount of cephalad spread. Doses must be placed near the corresponding dermatomal level of the insult. Therefore, lumbar administration of a lipophilic opioid would be a poor choice for thoracic analgesia. Side effects are generally fewer,[8, 9] with a lower incidence rate of delayed respiratory depression.[10] These drugs are ideal for continuous infusions and PCEA dosing.

Side effects after neuraxial administration of opioids are dose dependent and are generally similar when used either epidurally or intrathecally. They include respiratory depression with somnolence, pruritus, nausea and vomiting, and urinary retention.

Epidural doses of hydrophilic opioids (morphine) produce a biphasic respiratory depression pattern. A portion of the initial bolus dose is absorbed systemically, accounting for the initial phase, and usually occurs within 2 hours of the bolus dose. Remaining drug within the CSF slowly spreads rostrally, producing a second phase as it reaches the brain stem 6 to 12 hours later. Intrathecal doses of morphine produce only a uniphasic pattern of respiratory depression. Effective intrathecal morphine doses are very low compared with the larger epidural doses and early respiratory depression is not seen. The slow rostral spread of drug deposited directly within the CSF is responsible for the delayed respiratory depression pattern seen 6 to 12 hours later. Somnolence usually precedes the onset of significant respiratory depression. Patients should be closely monitored for the 24-hour period following a neuraxial dose of morphine.

Generalized pruritus is the most common and least dangerous side effect seen with neuraxial opioids. It is thought to not be secondary to histamine release—rather, it is more likely to be brain stem—mediated. Treatment includes dilute naloxone infusions and low-dose mixed agonist/antagonist opioids (nalbuphine). Antihistamines may also be beneficial for the sedation they may provide. Pruritus is more commonly seen in parturients.

Nausea and vomiting are common complications of neuraxial opioid administration. They also commonly occur with parenteral opioid use.[12] Reversible causes, such as hypotension, must be initially ruled out and corrected. Rostral spread of opioids directly stimulates the medullary vomiting center. Treatment options include butyrophenones (droperidol), phenothiazines (prochlorperazine), 5-HT$_3$ antagonists (ondansetron), and antihistamines. Prochlorperazine may cause significant drowsiness, however, which may hinder evaluation of somnolence secondary to the opioid effects.

Opioids may reduce the sacral parasympathetic outflow, resulting in urinary retention. Although this may be reversed by direct antagonism with naloxone, the doses required are often high and may also result in reversal of analgesia. Placement of an indwelling urinary catheter should be considered.

Selected References

1. Behar M, Magora F, Olshwang D, et al. Epidural morphine in the treatment of pain. Lancet 1979;1:527–529.
2. Wang JK, Nauss LA, Thomas JE. Pain relief by intrathecally applied morphine in man. Anesthesiology 1979;50:149–151.
3. Gwirtz KH. Intrathecal analgesia. Problems Anesthesia 1998;10:71–79.
4. Kilbride MJ, Senagore AJ, Mazier WP, et al. Epidural analgesia. Surg Gynecol Obstet 1992;174:137–140.
5. Lauretti GR, Hood DD, Eisenach JC, et al. A multi-center study of intrathecal neostigmine for analgesia following vaginal hysterectomy. Anesthesiology 1998;89:913–918.
6. Loper Ka, Ready LB, Downey M, et al. Epidural and intravenous fentanyl infusions are clinically equivalent after knee surgery. Anesth Analg 1990;70:72–75.
7. Ellis DJ, Millar WL, Reisner LS. A randomized double-blind comparison of epidural versus intravenous fentanyl infusion for analgesia after cesarean section. Anesthesiology 1990;72:981–986.
8. White MJ, Berghausen EJ, Dumont SW, et al. Side effects during continuous epidural infusions of morphine and fentanyl. Can J Anaesth 1992;39:576–582.
9. Fisher RL, Lubenow TR, Liceaga A, et al. Comparison of continuous epidural infusion of fentanyl-bupivacaine and morphine-bupivacaine in management of post-operative pain. Anesth Analg 1988;67:559–563.
10. Etches-Randler AN, Daley MD. Respiratory depression and spinal opioids. Can J Anaesth 1989;36:936–941.
11. Grass JA. Epidural analgesia. Problems Anesthesia 1998;10:45–70.
12. Gregg R. Spinal analgesia management of postoperative pain. Anesthesiol Clin North Am 1989;7:79–100.

110
Celiac Plexus Block

David P. Martin, M.D., Ph.D.

Indications

The celiac plexus provides sensory innervation and sympathetic outflow to most of the upper abdominal viscera. Neurolytic blockade of the celiac plexus is most commonly used to control pain caused by pancreatic cancer, although it can be useful for malignancies of the gastrointestinal tract from the lower esophageal sphincter to the splenic flexure, as well as the liver, spleen, and kidneys. Although potentially long lasting, neurolytic celiac plexus block is not "permanent," because the nerves regenerate in 3 to 6 months. The block can be repeated in such circumstances, but many patients with pancreatic cancer do not outlive the effective duration of neurolytic celiac plexus block.

Temporary diagnostic blockade of the celiac plexus can be used to differentiate visceral pain from somatic pain. Visceral pain is poorly localized and can be referred to somatic areas. For example, pancreatic pain often presents as epigastric tenderness radiating to the back. In addition to its neurolytic and diagnostic uses, celiac plexus injection with local anesthetics and corticosteroids is sometimes used to treat chronic pancreatitis.

Anatomy

The celiac plexus is primarily a sympathetic nervous system structure that lies anterior to the aorta near the celiac arterial trunk (Fig. 110–1). Preganglionic sympathetic fibers originate at T5-12 and combine to form the splanchnic nerves. The splanchnic nerves cross the crura of the diaphragm before joining the vagus nerve to form the celiac plexus anterior to the aorta. The vertebral level of the plexus varies from T12 to L2, and most approaches to the block are directed at the T12-L1 level.

Effective visceral pain relief can be achieved by either blocking the splanchnic nerves before they pierce the diaphragm or blocking the nerves and ganglia anterior to the diaphragmatic crura. The splanchnic nerve block (retrocrural) is also termed the "classical" celiac plexus block, as opposed to "true" blockade of the plexus and ganglia (intercrural).

Procedure

Several approaches to the celiac plexus have been described, but the most common is performed with the patient in the prone position with a pillow under the hips. Landmarks are identified and marked on the skin surface, indicating the 12th ribs and the thoracolumbar spinous processes. Needles are inserted bilaterally at a site approximately 7.5 cm lateral to midline at a point 2 cm inferior to the 12th rib. The initial pass is directed to contact the L1 vertebral body at an angle approximately 45 degrees from the sagittal plane (Fig. 110–2). The path of the needle is roughly parallel to the inferior

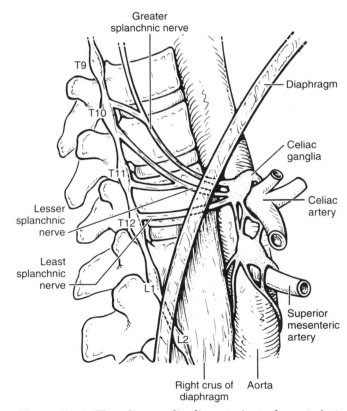

Figure 110–1. The celiac ganglion lies anterior to the aorta just superior to the celiac artery. It receives preganglionic fibers from the splanchnic nerves. Visceral analgesia can be achieved by blocking the splanchnic nerves before they pierce the diaphragm, or by blocking the plexus and ganglion anterior to the diaphragmatic crura. (From Stanton-Hicks MB.[1])

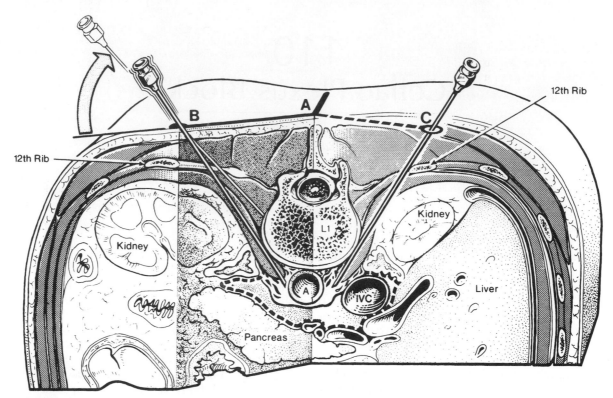

Figure 110–2. The needle is inserted approximately 7.5 cm lateral to the midline along a path inferior to the 12th rib. The initial needle path is at a 45-degree angle from the sagittal plane to contact the vertebral body of L1. The needle is then withdrawn and redirected to pass anterolateral to L1. (From Kopacz DJ, Thompson GE.[2])

border of the 12th rib, directed toward the middle of the L1 vertebral body. After noting the depth at which bone was contacted, the needle is withdrawn to skin level and redirected more steeply so that it passes just lateral to the L1 body, and then advanced an additional 1 to 2 cm. Ideal positioning is anterolateral to the body of the L1 vertebra.

Once the needle is placed, careful aspiration is performed to exclude vascular or intrathecal position. Proper drug distribution can be confirmed with the injection of radiocontrast dye under fluoroscopy. Ensure that the injectant is not within the psoas muscle, which could result in blockade of the lumbar plexus. Bupivacaine, 0.25 to 0.5%, is a reasonable choice for the diagnostic nerve block. Typically, 10 to 15 mL is injected on each side. For neurolytic procedures, 50 to 100% alcohol is the most common choice. Typically, 10 mL is injected on each side. Triamcinolone, 40 to 80 mg in 10 mL of local anesthetic, is reasonable for the treatment of pancreatitis.

Expected Side Effects

The procedure itself can cause local soreness and bruising. These symptoms are usually transient and can be treated with ice. Psoas spasm is not uncommon after neurolytic celiac plexus block, and can be minimized by preventing the escape of neurolytic

agent through the needle tract. Psoas spasm often responds well to an injection of ketorolac.

Interruption of sympathetic innervation to the viscera can blunt normal postural hemodynamic reflexes, resulting in orthostatic hypotension. Patients should be cautioned that they may feel lightheaded on standing. The sympathectomy can also cause increased gastrointestinal motility and possibly diarrhea. However, the effect of sympatholysis on intestinal motility can be beneficial in counteracting the constipation caused by opiates. Finally, celiac plexus block may mask early presenting symptoms of other intra-abdominal pathology such as cholecystitis or gastric ulceration.

Complications

As with any injection, sterile technique should be observed to minimize the risk of infection. Because of the close proximity of the celiac plexus to the aorta, vascular injury is possible, which can result in hematoma, aortic dissection, or distal ischemia. Intravascular injection of local anesthetic can cause mental status changes, seizures, or possible hemodynamic collapse.

Unintentional intrathecal or epidural spread can cause spinal nerve block. The spread of neurolytic agent to unintended nerve or vascular structures introduces the risk of permanent neurologic injury, including paralysis. Therefore, careful neurologic evaluation after local anesthetic injection is essential before injecting the neurolytic agent. Despite these risks, celiac plexus block is relatively safe when performed by experienced physicians.

Selected References

1. Stanton-Hicks MB. Lumbar sympathetic nerve block and neurolysis. In Waldman SD, Winnie AP, eds. Interventional Pain Management. Philadelphia: WB Saunders, 1996:353–359.
2. Kopacz DJ, Thompson GE. Celiac and hypogastric plexus, intercostal, interpleural, and peripheral neural blockade of the thorax and abdomen. In Cousins MJ, Bridenbaugh PO, eds. Neural blockade in Clinical Anesthesia and Management of Pain. 3rd ed. Philadelphia: JB Lippincott, 1998:451–485.

Suggested References

Brown DL. Celiac plexus block. In Brown DL, ed. Atlas of Regional Anesthesia. 2nd ed. Philadelphia: WB Saunders, 1999:283–291.

Lamer TJ. Sympathetic nerve blocks. In Brown DL, ed. Regional Anesthesia and Analgesia. Philadelphia: WB Saunders, 1996:357–384.

Wong GY, Brown, DL. Celiac Plexus Block for Cancer Pain. Techniques Reg Anesth Pain Manage 1997;1:18–26.

111
Lumbar Sympathetic Block

Jerald O. Van Beck, M.D.

The sympathetic chain and ganglia in the lumbar region lie anterolateral to the vertebral column inside a fascial sheath between the psoas muscle and the vertebral column. Ganglia send branches to the aortic and hypogastric plexuses. Gray rami communicans pass to nerves of the lumbar plexus. The second, third, and fourth lumbar ganglia control sympathetic impulses to the legs (Fig. 111–1).

Indications

Lumbar sympathetic blockade can be used for diagnostic, prognostic, and therapeutic purposes. With local anesthetics, it can predict the utility of surgical lumbar sympathectomy, or can provide short-term therapeutic benefit for **circulatory insufficiency** in the lower extremities from conditions such as arteriosclerotic disease, arterial embolism, thromboangiitis, Raynaud's phenomenon, frostbite, or postvascular surgery. Lumbar sympathetic blockade can also be used to treat **select urogenital pain** such as in renal colic, parturition, or herpes zoster. Use for labor analgesia requires a bilateral blockade and provides effective analgesia for stage 1, but not stage 2, of labor. Compared to continuous labor epidural analgesia, the procedure is technically more difficult, and resolution of the

block may occur during labor; however, it may be less likely to prolong labor, because there is no motor loss.

Neurolytic lumbar sympathetic blockade, using phenol with contrast medium under fluoroscopic guidance, has been used for long-term treatment of lower extremity arterial insufficiency and **chronic pain syndromes**. Conditions such as phantom limb pain, amputation stump pain, reflex sympathetic dystrophy, and postherpetic neuralgia may respond. The procedure's advantages over other techniques include its relative ease of performance compared to surgical sympathectomy and the sparing of motor nerves.

Technique

The patient is placed in the lateral or prone position, and the lumbar region is prepped and draped. The procedure generally takes less than 30 minutes and should cause minimal discomfort to the patient.

Mandle Technique with Two Needles. Mark the spinous processes of L2 to L4. Place a skin wheal 8 to 10 cm off midline with local anesthetic at the L2 level, then infiltrate to the transverse process. Insert a 20-gauge, 12-cm needle to the transverse process, and then redirect medially to-

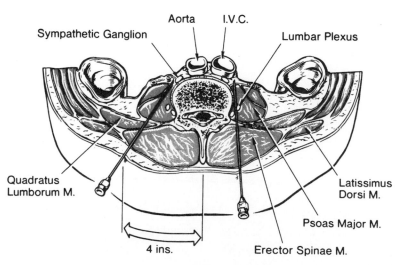

Figure 111–1. Lumbar sympathetic block. Note that insertion of the needle 10 cm from the midline enables the needle to reach the anterolateral angle of the vertebral body. Insertion of needle closer to the midline takes the needle path close to the somatic nerve roots and lateral sympathetic chain. (From Cherry DA, Rao DM.[1])

ward the vertebral body 45 degrees to the coronal plane between the transverse processes (Fig. 111–2). Advance the needle with the bevel toward the vertebral body until contact is made, and then adjust position to slide off the vertebral body 1 cm. Position can be verified by loss of resistance and negative aspiration for cerebrospinal fluid, blood, or urine. Movement of the needle with normal respiration indicates lateral positioning in the diaphragmatic crus. Radiographic screening with contrast injection is recommended to ensure proper needle positioning, especially for neurolytic blocks. Alternatively, ultrasonography has also been used effectively, sparing the patient and physician radiation exposure.[3] Repeat the procedure at the L4 level. Catheters can be placed if an 18-gauge needle is used.

Acute pain and diagnostic blocks are done with local anesthetics, including lidocaine 0.5 or 1% or bupivacaine 0.25% up to 30 mL per side. For neurolytic blocks, phenol 7 to 10% in aqueous radiographic contrast medium is injected under direct radiographic visualization, 1 to 2 mL per location. Alcohol 50% to 100% has been used in the past, but was associated with high incidence of neuralgia.

Technique of Bryce-Smith. A skin wheal is raised three fingerbreadths lateral to the tip of the spinous process of L3. A 20-gauge, 12-cm needle is introduced at 70 degrees to the coronal plane and advanced toward the vertebral body (Fig. 111–3). When the needle reaches the vertebral body, 15 to 20 mL of local anesthetic is deposited that tracks forward to sympathetic chain. Never use this technique with neurolytic agents. A somatic blockade frequently occurs, so it is not indicated for the diagnosis of pain syndromes.

Complications

Neuritis of the genitofemoral nerve or L1 neuralgia is the most common untoward reaction after neurolytic sympathetectomy, occurring in 5% to 10% of cases. This manifests as burning groin pain and typically lasts 2 to 5 weeks. Other complications include kidney perforation, subcapsular hematoma, Horner's syndrome, somatic nerve damage, subarachnoid injection, intravascular injection, perforation of a disk, stricture of the ureter (after neuro-

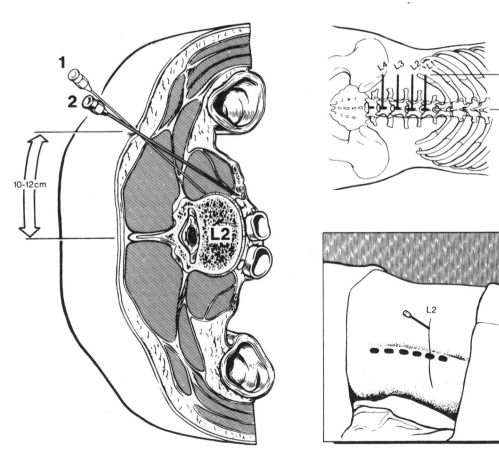

Figure 111–2. Mandle technique of lumbar sympathetic block. Note the location of skin marks for L1 and L4 spinous processes, which then permit identification of L2-3. A line is drawn through the center of the spinous processes; this will lie below the transverse process of that vertebra. Needle insertion is at the lateral margin of the erector spinae muscle (approximately 10 to 12 cm from midline). If it is desired to check the depth of the transverse process, the needle must be angled cephalad. Otherwise the needle is inserted approximately 45 degrees toward the vertebral body until this structure is located. Then the needle is angled more steeply until it slips just past the vertebral body and through the psoas fascia. A single needle can be used instead of two or three needles; however, an increased volume must be injected. (From Löfström JB, Cousins MJ.[2])

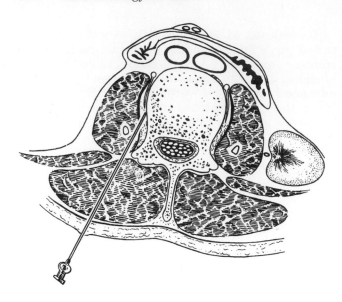

Figure 111–3. Alternative (Bryce-Smith) technique for local anesthetic lumbar sympathetic block. (From Löfström JB, Cousins MJ.[2])

lytic injection), infection, ejaculatory failure, and chronic back pain.

lumbar sympathetic and celiac plexus block: A new technique. Reg Anesth 1992;17:43–46.

Selected References

1. Cherry DA, Rao DM. Lumbar sympathetic and coeliac plexus blocks—an anatomical study in cadavers. Br J Anaesth 1982;54:1037–1039.
2. Löfström JB, Cousins MJ. Sympathetic neural blockade of upper and lower extremity. In Cousins MJ, Bridenbaugh PO, eds. Neural Blockade in Clinical Anesthesia and Management of Pain. 2nd ed. New York: JB Lippincott, 1988:461.
3. Kirvela O, Svedstrom E, Lundbom N. Ultrasonic guidance of

Suggested References

Wheatley JK, Motamedi F, Hammonds WD. Page kidney resulting from massive subcapsular hematoma. Complication of lumbar sympathetic nerve block. Urology 1984;24:361–363.
Wills MH, Korbon GA, Arasi R. Horner's syndrome resulting from a Lumbar sympathetic block. Anesthesiology 1988;68:613–614.
Zenz M, Panhaus C, Niesel HC, et al. Regional Anesthesia. Chicago, Year Book Medical, 1988.

112
Reflex Sympathetic Dystrophy

Pamela Jensen Bundy, M.D.

Terminology

Numerous labels have been given to the syndrome first recognized in 1864 consisting of burning pain, skin hypersensitivity (including allodynia: pain produced by normally non-noxious stimuli), vasomotor and sudomotor instability, and dystrophic changes that may respond to sympathetic denervation. Terms now commonly accepted include:

- **Complex regional pain syndrome (CRPS)**, a neuropathic pain syndrome associated with sympathetic nervous system dysfunction
- **Reflex sympathetic dystrophy (RSD) (CRPS type I)**, a syndrome occurring after minor trauma without specific nerve injury such as sprain, fracture, surgery, or even in the absence of a remarkable trauma history
- **Causalgia (CRPS type II)**, occurring after major nerve injury, usually
- **Sympathetically mediated pain (SMP)**, a global term defining pain that responds to sympathetic blockade. It may be a component of the pain of RSD, causalgia, or other neuropathic pain, such as postherpetic neuralgia.

Stages

Symptoms begin a few hours to a few weeks after the initial insult, with each stage varying in length from weeks to years.

- **Stage I (acute).** Burning or aching pain is present out of proportion to the initial injury. Pain increases with emotion, physical contact, and dependence of affected limb. The temperature and color of the limb are unstable, edema is usually present, and sweating and tremor may be present. A three-phase bone scan may show increased periarticular uptake in the late phase. The limb is usually held in a protective posture. Hair and nail growth may be accelerated.
- **Stage II (dystrophic).** The affected tissue becomes indurated, cool, hyperhydrotic, hairless, and cyanotic and may appear mottled (livedo reticularis). Joints become stiff or immobile, and muscles lose strength and endurance. Pain is constant and exacerbated by any stimulus. Nails become cracked, brittle, or ridged. Radiography shows diffuse osteoporosis. Changes are similar to those of disuse of any cause.
- **Stage III (atrophic).** Irreversible tissue damage occurs. Skin becomes thin and shiny with thickened fascia and contractures. Pain spreads proximally and can spread outside the initial nerve distribution to other extremities. Bony demineralization and ankylosis are seen on radiographs. Cases may resolve spontaneously but tend to recur. Anxiety leads to sympathetic discharge and worsening pain. Many patients develop emotional disorders secondary to intractable pain, but if treated, these psychiatric problems resolve.

Pathophysiology

Many theories on the mechanism of RSD have been postulated, but none explain all of the manifestations of the syndrome. In 1986, Roberts put forth a hypothesis that covered most aspects of RSD.[1] He speculated that a peripheral trauma first activates unmyelinated C-nociceptors that synapse on wide dynamic range (WDR) neurons in the spinal cord that are multiceptive neurons, part of the central nociceptive pathway. These WDR neurons become increasingly sensitized over time, becoming more responsive to all subsequent input. Over time, WDRs respond to input from A-fiber mechanoreceptors, leading to allodynia, the perception of pain from a non-noxious stimulus. Sympathetic efferents in the periphery or in a neuroma at the damage site synapse on the A-mechanoreceptors, leading to SMP. The slow spread of pain over time probably results from a neuronally mediated spread of sensitization to WDR neurons outside the injury site. Because SMP is diagnosed only in 5% of trauma cases, Roberts[1] hypothesized that in most individuals the sensitization of WDRs subsides with healing, but some may be genetically predispositioned to it. In addition, SMP may have a higher incidence than reported.

Diagnosis

SMP is a clinical diagnosis without absolute criteria, although burning pain, allodynia, blood flow regulation disturbances, and sudomotor problems are hallmarks. Pain reduction in response to peripheral or central sympathetic blockade is characteristic of SMP. SMP may represent a variable component (0% to 100%) of the pain of RSD. A history of trauma is important but not essential for the diagnosis of RSD. At the examination, one should note edema, decreased mobility, allodynia, skin and hair changes, hyperhidrosis, and temperature changes in the skin. Supportive evidence can be gained from laboratory tests. The quantitative sudomotor axon reflex test (QSART) measuring sweat response to acetylcholine will be positive in most RSD patients. Three-phase technetium bone scanning shows increased periarticular uptake on delayed images. Demineralization and osteoporosis are shown on plain radiographs. Of most importance for guiding therapy by sympathetic interventions is alleviation of symptoms by sympathetic blockade.

Treatment

The key to symptom relief is early intervention with mobilization and strengthening of affected limbs as well as sympathetic blockade, if indicated. If treatment is started late, results are universally poor. Sympathetic blocks of various types have been used. Stellate ganglion blocks often provide relief of upper extremity symptoms but may need to be repeated frequently. Of equal efficacy for upper extremity symptoms are regional intravenous blocks with bretylium, guanethidine,* or reserpine. Reserpine reduces reuptake of catecholamines, whereas guanethidine displaces norepinephrine from intraneuronal storage granules, as does bretylium.

These blocks can also be performed on the lower extremity. Epidural clonidine has also been evaluated as a therapy for refractory reflex sympathetic dystrophy.[2] Lumbar sympathetic blocks are also used for lower extremity symptoms, as are paravertebral sympathetic ganglionic blockade or ablation with phenol.

---

*Guanethidine for parenteral use has been withdrawn by the FDA in the United States.

Oral pharmacologic sympathectomy has also been reported, using prazosin, phenoxybenzamine, or guanethadine. Surgical sympathectomy is another option, although recurrence of symptoms is common. Less successful modalities include steroids, transcutaneous electrical nerve simulation units, nonsteroidal anti-inflammatory drugs, calcium channel blockers, and acupuncture. Physical therapy modalities may be more effective if they can be performed with partial analgesia; for example, with axillary plexus or epidural blockade (i.e., with 0.125% bupivacaine).

Prognosis

Prognosis varies within all treatment modalities, hinging on time to treatment after trauma. Mobilization remains the key ingredient for success. With early intervention, treatment success ranges from 25% to 90%.

Selected References

1. Roberts WJ. A hypothesis on the physiological basis for causalgia and related pains. Pain 1986;24:297.
2. Rauck RL, Eisenach JC, Jackson K, et al. Epidural clonidine treatment for refractory reflex sympathetic dystrophy. Anesthesiology 1993;79:1163.

Suggested References

Harden RN. A clinical approach to complex regional pain syndrome. Clin J Pain 2000;16:S26–32.
Hord AH, Rooks MD, Stephens BO, et al. Intravenous regional bretylium and lidocaine for treatment of reflex sympathetic dystrophy: A randomized, double-blind study. Anesth Analg 1992;74:818.
Kemler MA, Barendse GA, van Kleef M, et al. Pain relief in complex regional pain syndrome due to spinal cord stimulation does not depend on vasodilation. Anesthesiology 2000;92:1653–1660.
Schwartzman RJ. New treatments for reflex sympathetic dystrophy. New Engl J Med 2000;343:654–656.
Stanton-Hicks M. Complex regional pain syndrome (type I, RSD; type II, causalgia): Controversies. Clin J Pain 2000;16:S33–40.
Wilson PR: Sympathetically maintained pain: Diagnosis, measurement and efficacy of treatment. In Stanton-Hicks M, Raj P, eds. Pain and the Sympathetic Nervous System. Boston: Kluwer Academic, 1990:91.

113
Postherpetic Neuralgia

Christopher Powers, M.D.

Postherpetic neuralgia (PHN) is a potentially devastating sequelae of acute herpes zoster (AHZ). Interestingly, AHZ is itself a sequelae of the usually benign (and painless) childhood infection varicella (chickenpox). Despite the innocent initial viral infection, the pain of PHN can be excruciating and intractable, leading some patients to contemplate suicide.

Although the exact time is debated, PHN is most commonly defined as pain in the area affected by herpes zoster at least 1 month after the crusting of the lesions. Because the distinction between AHZ and PHN pain occasionally blurs, some have advocated addressing the entity as one, calling it zoster-associated pain (Z-aP).

The overall incidence of AHZ and PHN is shown in Fig. 113–1. Major risk factors for the development of PHN include age, cancer, lymphoproliferative disorders, diabetes, immunosuppression, and perhaps the duration and severity of pain associated with AHZ. Fig. 113–1 clearly shows the importance of age in the development of PHN, where 50% of the elderly experience pain that persists for more than 1 year.

Pathophysiology

After the initial infection by varicella zoster, the virus is not eradicated from the body but remains dormant in the cell bodies of sensory afferent nerves. AHZ results when the dormant virus reactivates. The cause of this reactivation is not fully understood but likely involves impairment of the cellular immune system.

This reactivation typically is unilateral and involves either a single thoracic dermatome or the ophthalmic division of the trigeminal nerve. Lumbar, cervical, and sacral involvement is unusual. The viral reactivation is accompanied by inflammation, necrosis, and eventual atrophy within the dorsal root ganglion (DRG). The characteristic dermatomal distribution of cutaneous infectious vesicular lesions results from the transport of the reactivated virus down the peripheral sensory nerve to the skin. Resolution of the AHZ is heralded by the crusting of lesions.

Pain

PHN is a purely neuropathic pain. But the exact pathogenesis of the pain remains unclear. It is likely that changes within the peripheral and central nervous systems play a major role. Peripheral mechanisms may include axonal damage with subsequent abnormal regrowth and neuroma formation. Central mechanisms may include abnormal sensory processing or modulation within the spinal cord or higher centers. The peripheral and central components are not necessarily separate. Increases in afferent input to the cord from abnormal periph-

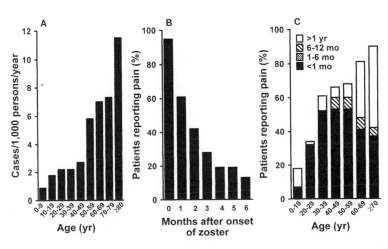

Figure 113–1. Annual incidence rate of herpes zoster and proportion of patients with PHN. *A,* The annual incidence of herpes zoster per 1000 persons in a general medical practice. *B,* The percentage of patients with pain persisting after the onset of the zoster-associated rash. Data are from the placebo group in one large, double-blind treatment study. *C,* The proportion of patients with postherpetic neuralgia according to age.(Adapted from Kost R, Straus S.[1])

eral nerves can induce a hyperexcitable state (wind up) in the CNS, where even nonpainful stimuli are transmitted and perceived as pain. In addition, there is a selective loss of large afferent fibers in the affected nerve, resulting in a relative increase in small fiber input to the spinal cord. Because the large fibers are believed to play a role in inhibiting small fiber input (**gate control theory**), this can also lead to increased pain perception.

Clinically, the aforementioned nervous system changes are evidenced by paresthesias, allodynia, hyperpathia, and other abnormal sensations in the distribution of the previously affected dermatome. Patients often describe a constant burning, stabbing, or squeezing pain with a lancinating component. In addition, patients note a marked allodynia to light touch, in some cases so severe that the patient refuses to wear loose clothing over the affected area. There can also be associated hypopigmentation and scarring of the skin in the affected area.

Therapy

Therapy for PHN ideally begins before diagnosis with early aggressive treatment of AHZ and its associated pain. Unfortunately, the literature is confusing and contradictory regarding optimal therapy or prevention of PHN. Current trends include attempts at prevention by treating AHZ with antiviral agents, analgesics, and possibly oral steroids. No study has convincingly shown a reproducible effective prevention strategy. However, the common thread of most preventive studies has been that aggressive control of the pain of AHZ is believed to be of benefit to the patient.

Treatment of PHN is subject to individual physician and specialty bias. A suggested treatment protocol is given in Table 113–1. A recent study suggests that gabapentin should be a first-line medication for the treatment of PHN, with a gradual dosage increase up to as much as 3600 mg/day divided three times a day. Other therapies to be considered include epidural steroid injections, oral antiarrhythmics, and intrathecal drug delivery systems.

Table 113–1. Postherpetic Neuralgia

Treatment Suggestions for Postherpetic Neuralgia

Antidepressants, amitriptyline, or nortriptyline 10–25 mg and titrate upward to effect over several weeks. Usually 50–100 mg is a sufficient dose.

Anticonvulsants, particularly for a lancinating component of pain. Phenytoin, carbamazepine, and gabapentin are three easily prescribed choices.

A sympathectomy should be considered in patients deemed appropriate for regional anesthesia, particularly with pain lasting less than 1 year.

Enrollment in an interdisciplinary pain management program may be considered.

Narcotic analgesics, particularly in refractory long-standing pain. Methadone and time-released morphine or oxycodone preparations (long-lasting narcotics) have been best used and studied. Start with bid dosing and titrate slowly. Side effects usually subside with time or, if necessary, with a change to a different narcotic.

Counterirritant techniques (TENS, vapocoolants) and topical preparations (EMLA, aspirin, and chloroform or capsaicin) are worth trying because of their simplicity and absence of major side effects.

Spinal column stimulation should be considered before any neurolytic block or neurosurgical procedure is undertaken.

Adapted from Hetherington R.[2]

All aspects of the patient's life can be affected by PHN. The affective component of the pain and the patient's coping skills should be addressed in conjunction with other therapies. Given the complexities of this disease, it should not be surprising that multiple modalities are often required and even then the pain may persist or recur.

Selected References

1. Kost R, Straus S. Postherpetic neuralgia: Pathogenesis, treatment, and prevention. New Engl J Med 1996;335:32–42.
2. Hetherington R. Herpes zoster and postherpetic neuralgia. In Ashburn M, Rice L, eds. Management of Pain. New York: Churchill Livingstone, 1998:351–362.

Suggested Reading

Rowbotham M, Harden N, Stacey B, et al. Gabapentin for the treatment of postherpetic neuralgia. JAMA 1998;280:1837–1842.
Satterthwaite J. Post-herpetic neuralgia. In Tollison C, Satterthwaite J, Tollison J, eds. Handbook of Pain Management. Baltimore: Williams & Wilkins, 1994:503–522.

114
Stellate Ganglion Block

Glenn E. Woodworth, M.D.

Indications

Indications for stellate ganglion block include **circulatory insufficiency in the arm** resulting from traumatic or embolic occlusion, postreimplantation, postembolectomy vasospasm, or arteriopathy; **pain** caused by reflex sympathetic dystrophy, herpes zoster, neoplasm, phantom limb pain, Paget's disease, or lesions in the central nervous system; and **other** symptoms, such as hyperhidrosis, Sudeck's atrophy, tinnitus, and sympathetically maintained pain in the upper extremity, head, or neck.

Anatomy

The peripheral sympathetic nervous system arises from the intermediolateral column of the spinal cord. The efferent preganglionic fibers pass out of the spinal cord via the ventral roots from T1 to L2. The fibers then enter the sympathetic chain through the white rami communicans. The preganglionic fibers may travel for a variable distance within the sympathetic chain before synapsing in ganglia or exiting the chain to synapse in peripheral ganglia.

In the cervical region, the sympathetic chain lies along the anterolateral aspect of the vertebral bodies. It lies in a fascial space bounded posteriorly by the prevertebral muscles and anteriorly by the carotid sheath. The nerve fibers in the cervicothoracic chain originate from preganglionic sympathetic fibers from T1 to T6 and visceral afferent fibers from the head, neck, and upper extremity. These fibers are distributed to the brain, meninges, eye, ear, glands, skin, and vessels of the head, neck, upper extremity, and some thoracic viscera. As the fibers pass up the sympathetic chain, they form several ganglia. The first thoracic and inferior cervical ganglia lie in close proximity and are often fused to form the stellate ganglion. This ganglia is oval and about 1 inch long by 0.5 inch wide. It lies within the fascial space described earlier. It is bounded posteriorly by the neck of the first rib and the transverse process of C7, and anteriorly by the dome of the pleura, the carotid sheath, and the vertebral artery. The medial boundary is the vertebral column. It is important to note that some thoracic preganglionic sympathetic fibers may bypass the stellate ganglion.

Technique

Although posterior and anterior approaches have been described, a paratracheal route is used most frequently. The patient is instructed to lie supine with the head supported by a pillow. The head is kept in the midline in slight extension. The mouth should be slightly open to relax the neck muscles. The stellate ganglion can be blocked at the level of C6 or C7, but because of the risk of pleural puncture, the approach to the fascial space is often made slightly superior to the ganglion at the level of C6 (Chassaignac's tubercle) (Fig. 114–1). Two fingerbreadths (1.5 to 2 cm) above the clavicular head, the trachea, sternocleidomastoid muscle, and carotid sheath are palpated (approximately at the level of the cricoid cartilage). Two fingers press gently down onto the lateral edge of the transverse process of C6 (the most readily palpable cervical

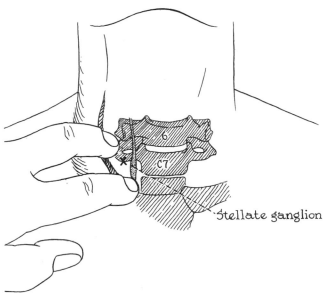

Figure 114–1. Landmarks for injection of the stellate ganglion at the level of C7. (From Adriani J.[1])

anterior tubercle) while simultaneously drawing the contents of the carotid sheath laterally (Fig. 114–2). A 1.5- to 3-inch, 23- or 25-gauge B-bevel needle is inserted just lateral to the trachea after skin infiltration with a local anesthetic. The transverse process of C6 should be encountered between the two palpating fingers at a depth of 1.5 to 2 cm. The needle is withdrawn 2 mm to place it in the correct fascial plane, and 8 to 10 mL of local anesthetic is injected incrementally after careful aspiration. A 0.5-mL test dose is recommended to rule out a vertebral artery injection. A generalized seizure can occur with as little as 0.5 mL of local anesthetic injected into the vertebral artery. If blockage of the sympathetic supply to the upper extremity is desired, the patient is placed in a 30-degree head-up position to encourage diffusion of the local anesthetic to the upper thoracic ganglia. In addition, a larger volume of local anesthetic may be necessary. Position of the needle and spread of solution may be confirmed by fluoroscopy.

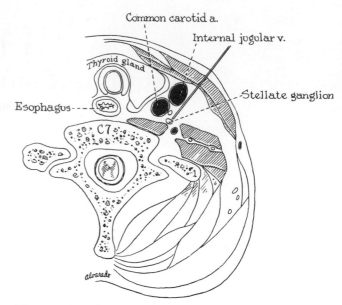

Figure 114–2. Cross-section of the neck at the level of the body of the seventh cervical vertebra. The carotid bundle is retracted laterally for the stellate ganglion block. Note the proximity of the vertebral artery (immediately posterior to the stellate ganglion). (From Adriani J.[1])

Signs of a Successful Block

□ Horner's syndrome (ptosis, miosis, enophthalmos).
□ Ipsilateral nasal congestion.
□ Flushing of the conjunctiva and skin.
□ Temperature increase in the ipsilateral arm and hand.

Common Side Effects and Complications

□ Sensation of "a lump in the throat."
□ Temporary hoarseness and dysphagia because of recurrent laryngeal block (a 60% prevalence rate).
□ Unpleasant effects of Horner's syndrome.
□ Hematoma.

Uncommon Complications

□ Brachial plexus block (rare).
□ Phrenic nerve block.
□ Epidural or subarachnoid block.
□ Pneumothorax (1% prevalence rate).
□ Osteitis of the transverse process or vertebral body.

□ Cardioaccelerator nerve block with hypotension or bradycardia.
□ Puncture of esophagus.
□ Puncture of intervertebral disc.

Potentially Severe Complications

□ Vertebral artery injection causing loss of consciousness and seizure.
□ Intradural injection causing total spinal.
□ Osteomyelitis of the vertebral body or discitis.

Selected Reference

1. Adriani J. Labat's Regional Anesthesia: Techniques and Clinical Applications. Philadelphia, WB Saunders, 1967.

Suggested References

Katz J. Atlas of Regional Anesthesia. Norwalk, CT, Appleton-Century-Crofts, 1985.
Lofstrom J, Cousins M. Sympathetic neural blockade of upper and lower extremity. In Cousins M, Bridenbaugh P, eds. Neural Blockade in Clinical Anesthesia and Management of Pain. 2nd ed. Philadelphia: JB Lippincott, 1988.

115
Postoperative Headache

Michael E. Johnson, M.D., Ph.D.

Postdural puncture headache (PDPHA, spinal headache, postural headache) may occur after diagnostic lumbar puncture, spinal anesthesia, myelography, or intraoperative spinal drainage. The classic PDPHA results from cerebrospinal fluid (CSF) leakage and decreased intracranial pressure (ICP). Other causes of headache after dural puncture are much rarer, but must be considered because they are generally more serious than the classic PDPHA. These include subdural hematoma, pneumocephalus, meningitis, and any cause of increased ICP. Postural headaches can also occur spontaneously.

The classic presentation of PDPHA involves onset 1 to 2 days after dural puncture (more severe if onset sooner); postural component (worse sitting or upright, relieved supine); and occipital or frontal localization, radiating down the posterior neck. Rarely (less than 1% with severe headache), auditory and visual disturbances may also occur.

Prevention of PDPHA

A prospective randomized study of cesarean section patients found a greater incidence of PDPHA in patients kept on bed rest for 24 hours than in those mobilized at 6 hours postoperatively. A decreased incidence is associated with the use of a smaller needle, with injection with the needle bevel oriented parallel to the longitudinal axis of the dural fibers (i.e., caudal to cephalad), with a paramedian instead of a midline approach, and with a lower concentration of glucose in the local anesthetic solution. Additionally, pencil-point needles have been reported to decrease the incidence of PDPHA.

A preoperative history of any of the following increases the risk of PDPHA: young age, female gender, pregnancy, history of motion sickness, or history of previous spinal headache.

Treatment of PDPHA

Most cases of PDPHA resolve spontaneously, and a 24-hour trial of symptomatic therapy (analgesics, hydration to increase CSF production, and bed rest) is often adequate. Intravenous caffeine (500 mg) in conjunction with hydration has been reported to improve PDPHA in 80% of patients, perhaps through its vasomotor effects. The usefulness of caffeine therapy is limited by its side effects (similar to theophylline) and by the fact that it is less effective than the epidural blood patch.

A persistent significant headache is treated with an epidural blood patch: 10 to 20 mL of autologous blood drawn aseptically from the patient's antecubital vein is injected into the epidural space near the site of the original dural puncture. Headache relief is immediate in approximately 90% of these patients. Potential side effects include mild back pain and fever. The epidural blood patch may be repeated if necessary, but persistence of headache after two epidural blood patches strongly suggests a different headache etiology than PDPHA. A thorough evaluation is merited to rule out other serious causes of headache that require therapy (e.g., hematoma, tumor, meningitis).

Headache After Inhalation Anesthetics

There is a 10% to 30% prevalence of headache after minor surgery under general anesthesia. It occurs less commonly after major surgery than after minor surgery; major postoperative pain at the surgical site probably distracts the patient from noticing headache. The incidence of postoperative headaches is higher in patients who drink coffee or other caffeinated beverages on a daily basis, and intravenous caffeine can be useful in treating these headaches in some patients. Preoperative headaches are a predictor of postoperative headaches associated with general anesthesia. There is a greater incidence of headache with isoflurane than with halothane or enflurane for minor gynecological surgery. Treatment of headache after general anesthesia is symptomatic with analgesics or caffeinated beverages in patients who can take oral fluids.

Headache After Vaginal Delivery

Besides PDPHA, there is also a postpartum cervical myofascial pain syndrome. This is associated with a long second stage of labor and prolonged pushing. It is similar to PDPHA in some respects with next-day onset and involvement of the occiput, neck, and shoulder girdle. However, this pain does not change with posture, is associated with marked point tenderness of affected muscles, and responds well to physical therapy.

Headache After Carotid Endarterectomy

In one series, 24 of 50 patients reported headaches, ranging in character from nonspecific diffuse to severe hemicranial headache. The mechanism is postulated to relate to injury to the carotid vessel or sheath. Treatment is symptomatic.

Suggested References

Bridenbaugh PO, Greene NM, Brull SJ. Spinal (subarachnoid) neural blockade. In Cousins MJ, Bridenbaugh PO, eds. Neural blockade. Philadelphia: Lippincott-Raven, 1998:203–241.

Flaatten H, Rodt S, Rosland J, et al. Postoperative headache in young patients after spinal anaesthesia. Anaesthesia 1987;42:202.

Hubbell SL, Thomas M. Postpartum cervical myofascial pain syndrome: Review of four patients. Obstet Gynecol 1985;65:56S.

Kuntz DK, Kokmen E, Stevens JC, et al. Post-lumbar puncture headaches: Experience in 501 consecutive procedures. Neurology 1992;42:1884.

Lambert DH, Huiley RJ, Hertwig L, et al. Role of needle gauge and tip configuration in the production of lumbar puncture headache. Reg Anesth 1997;22:66–72.

Mazze RI, Fujinaga M. Postdural puncture headache after continuous spinal anesthesia with 18-gauge and 20-gauge needles. Reg Anesth (US) 1993;18:47.

Messert B, Black JA. Cluster headache, hemicrania, and other head pains: Morbidity of carotid endarterectomy. Stroke 1978;9:559.

Poukkula E. The problem of post-spinal headache. Ann Chir Gynaecol 1984;73:139.

Roderick L, Moore DC, Artru AA. Pneumocephalus with headache during spinal anesthesia. Anesthesiology 1985;62:690.

Rudehill A, Gordon E, Rahn T. Subdural haematoma. A rare but life-threatening complication after spinal anaesthesia. Acta Anaesthesiol Scand 1983;27:376.

Thornberry EA, Thomas TA. Posture and post-spinal headache. A controlled trial in 80 obstetric patients. Br J Anaesth 1988;60:195.

Tracey JA, Holland AJC, Unger L. Morbidity in minor gynaecological surgery: A comparison of halothane, enflurane, and isoflurane. Br J Anaesth 1982;54:1213.

Weber JG, Ereth MH, Danielson DR. Perioperative ingestion of caffeine and postoperative headache. Mayo Clin Proc 1993;68:842.

116
Local Anesthetics: Mechanisms of Action

Michael J. Joyner, M.D.

Sensory nerve impulses are propagated from peripheral receptors to the central nervous system by depolarization of axon membranes and subsequent transmitter release at a synapse(s). Local anesthetics work by preventing membrane depolarization.

Resting Membrane Potential

The resting membrane potential of most nerve cells is -60 to -90 mV. This occurs because the cells (at rest) are more permeable to K^+ ions and because the concentration of K^+ is approximately 30 times greater inside the cell than outside.

Depolarization

When the nerve is active, Na^+ channels in the membrane are triggered to open and the Na^+ permeability increases so the membrane potential becomes less negative. If the membrane potential increases enough, additional Na^+ channels open, and a wave of depolarization is propagated along the length of the axon.

Local Anesthetic Action

Local anesthetics prevent the opening of the Na^+ channels and prevent the membrane potential from increasing sufficiently (to threshold) to open the additional Na^+ channels. It is unclear whether local anesthetics act by simply plugging the Na^+ channels or whether they prevent channel opening. Both mechanisms are possible.

Local Anesthetic Structure

These molecules are tertiary amines (weak bases). Their pKa ranges between 7.5 and 9.5, so that at pH 7.4, most of the drug is in the charged (ionized) form. The importance of this point is that the uncharged (conjugated) base form of most agents is more lipid soluble and can therefore reach the site of action (the cell membrane) more rapidly where it can become ionized and act to interfere with Na^+ channels (Table 116–1). Additionally, a high lipid solubility is thought to increase the potency and duration of the drug effect since it ensures that the drug will remain on or at the site of action for a longer period.

Properties of Axons

The so-called cable properties of axons and the presence or absence of myelin can affect the ability of anesthetics to block nerve impulses. In general, the greater the axon diameter, the longer (spatially) it takes for the membrane potential to decay. This means that a greater length of larger fibers must be exposed to the drug to establish a successful block. Myelin enhances this effect. This explains why it is usually possible to obtain good sensory and sympathetic blocks (i.e., small unmyelinated fibers) with only marginal effects on the motor system (large myelinated fibers).

Table 116–1. Effect of pH on Local Anesthetic Base Dissociation

Agent	PK$_a$	Percentage of Total Drug in Base Form		
		pH 7.0	pH 7.4	pH 7.8
Benzocaine	3.5	100	100	100
Mepivacaine	7.6	20	39	61
Lidocaine	7.9	11	24	44
Etidocaine	7.7	17	33	56
Bupivacaine	8.1	7	17	33
Tetracaine	8.6	6	14	28
Procaine	8.9	1	3	7
2-Chloroprocaine	9.1	0.8	2	5

From Carpenter RL, Mackey DC.[1]

Selected References

1. Carpenter RL, Mackey DC. Local anesthetics. In Barash P, Cullen B, Stoeling R, eds. Clinical Anesthesia. 3rd ed. Philadelphia: JB Lippincott, 1997:413–442.

Suggested References

Butterworth JF IV, Strichartz GR. Molecular mechanism of local anesthesia: A review. Anesthesiology 1990;72:711–734.

Strichartz GR. Neural physiology and local anesthetic action. In Cousins MJ, Bridenbaugh PO, eds. Neural Blockade in Clinical Anesthesia and Management. 3rd ed. Philadelphia: JB Lippincott, 1998:35–54.

Tucker GT, Mather LE. Properties, absorption, and disposition of local anesthetic agents. In Cousins MJ, Bridenbaugh PO, eds. Neural Blockade in Clinical Anesthesia and Management. 3rd ed. Philadelphia: JB Lippincott, 1998:55–961.

117

Local Anesthetic Pharmacology

Terese T. Horlocker, M.D.

Local anesthetics consist of three major chemical moieties (Fig. 117–1):

□ Lipophilic aromatic ring.
□ Hydrophilic tertiary amine.
□ Ester or amide linkage.

Changes in the amine or ring chemical structure result in marked alterations in lipid/aqueous solubility, potency, and protein binding. Local anesthetics are classified into two major groups based on the linkage between the lipophilic and hydrophilic components: amino esters and amino amides. The major differences between the esters and amides are metabolism (pseudocholinesterase versus liver) and allergic potential (ester greater than amide). The most commonly used local anesthetics and their physiochemical properties are described in Table 117–1.

Physiochemical Properties

Local anesthetics are weak bases with pKa values greater than 7.4. Because the free bases are poorly water soluble, they are dispersed as hydrochloride salts. The resulting solutions are acidic with pH values of 4 to 7.

In solution, the local anesthetics exist in equilibrium as ionized and nonionized forms (Fig. 117–2). Nonionized (lipid-soluble) base crosses axonal membranes. Ionized (water-soluble) cation is responsible for neural blockade.

□ Potency is related to lipid solubility.
□ Duration of action is related to protein binding.

Speed of onset is related to pKa. (Note, however, that the rapid onset of procaine and 2-chloroprocaine blockade [pKa ≈ 9] is because of a high solution concentration and thus a greater diffusion gradient.)

Physiologic Disposition

The local anesthetic drugs are absorbed after injection of the local anesthetic at the site of administration. Only small amounts are excreted unchanged in the urine, and very little metabolism occurs at the site of injection.

Esters

Ester local anesthetics are metabolized by **pseudocholinesterase** (plasma cholinesterase) and partially by red cell esterases. Hydrolysis occurs at the ester linkage and yields an alcohol and *para*-aminobenzoic acid (or a PABA derivative). Because ester local anesthetics are metabolized by pseudocholinesterase, toxicity and duration of blockade may be prolonged in patients with liver disease, in neonates, or in atypical cholinesterase carriers (Table 117–2).

Chloroprocaine is hydrolyzed four times faster than procaine, and procaine is hydrolyzed four times faster than tetracaine.

Amides

Amide local anesthetics are metabolized by the liver. Three main routes of biotransformation have been identified: aromatic hydroxylation, N-dealkylation, and amide hydrolysis.

Clearance of these agents varies in the following order: bupivacaine < mepivacaine < lidocaine < etidocaine < prilocaine.

Liver disease affects metabolism of amide local anesthetics while having minimal effects on ester-linked compounds. In severe cirrhosis, the half-life

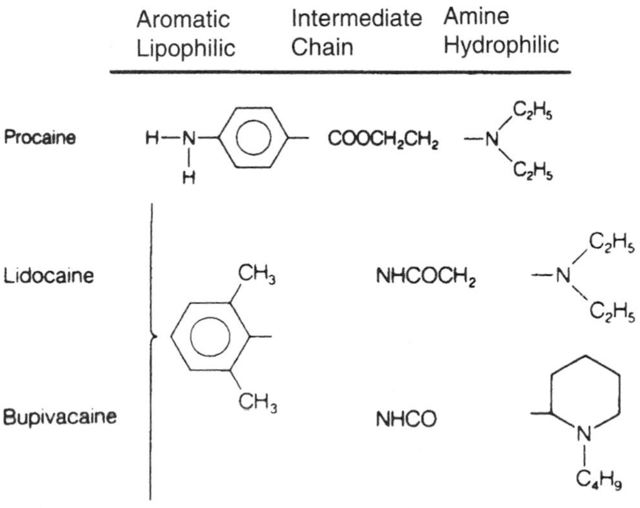

Figure 117–1. Chemical configuration of procaine, lidocaine, and bupivacaine.

285

Table 117–1. Physicochemical Properties of Local Anesthetics

	Physicochemical Properties			Biologic Properties					
Agent	pKa* (25°C)	Partition Coefficient†	Percent Protein Binding	Equieffective§ Anesthetic Concentration	Approximate Anesthetic Duration (min)§	Onset	Recommended Maximum Single Dose (mg)	Comments	pH of Plain Solutions‡
Procaine	9.05	0.02	5.8#	2	50	Fast	1000	Used mainly for infiltration and differential spinal	5–6.5
Chloroprocaine	8.97	0.14	?	2	45	Fast	800 (1000 with epinephrine)	Intrathecal injection may be associated with sensory/ motor deficits	2.7–4
Tetracaine	8.46	4.1	76.6#	0.25	175	Fast	20	Use is primarily limited to spinal and topical anesthesia	4.5–6.5
Lidocaine	7.91	2.9	64¶	1	100	Fast	500 with epinephrine	Most versatile agent	6.5
Mepivacaine	7.76	0.8	77¶	1	100	Fast	500 with epinephrine	Duration of plain solutions longer than lidocaine without epinephrine	4.5
Bupivacaine	8.16	27.5	96¶	0.25	175	Fast	175 (225 with epinephrine)	Lower concentrations provide differential sensory/motor block. Ventricular arrhythmias and sudden cardiovascular collapse reported following rapid i.v. injection	4.5–6
Etidocaine	7.7	141	94¶	0.25	200	Fast	400 with epinephrine	Profound motor block useful for surgical anesthesia but not for obstetrical analgesia	4.5

*pH corresponds to 50% ionization.
†N-heptane/pH 7.4 buffer.
§Data derived from rat sciatic nerve-blocking procedure.
‡Epinephrine-containing solutions have a pH of 1 to 1.5 units lower than plain solutions.
#Nerve-homogenate binding.
¶Plasma protein binding.
Data from Covino BG and Wildsmith JAW[1] and Tucker GT and Mather LE.[2]

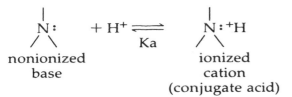

Figure 117–2. Local anesthetic substructure. (From O'Brien JE.[3])

and volume of distribution of lidocaine are increased, while clearance is decreased because of decreased enzyme activity and shunting.

Liver enzyme-inducing agents, such as barbiturates, increase the systemic clearance of amide local anesthetics.

Clinical Use of Local Anesthetics

Esters

□ **Benzocaine.** Almost insoluble in water. Limited to topical applications as in orotracheal administration.

□ **Cocaine.** Topical use only, usually for anesthesia of nasal mucosa for intubation or surgery. Safe dose is 3 mg/kg (150 to 200 mg). Sensitizes myocardium to catecholamines. CNS toxicity is initially excitatory with euphoria, then eventual depression. Cardiovascular side effects can be life-threatening.

□ **Procaine.** Used mainly for skin infiltration and spinal blocks because of its low potency, slow onset, and short duration of action in peripheral nerve blocks.

□ **Chloroprocaine.** Rapid onset, low toxicity make it ideal for labor and delivery. Used for infiltration, axillary, and epidural blocks, but usually intrathecal injection is avoided because of the possibility of prolonged deficits.

□ **Tetracaine.** Tetracaine remains a popular drug for spinal anesthesia because of its rapid onset, dense block, and long duration (4 to 6 hours with epinephrine). Tetracaine can also be used topically, although, toxic reactions have been reported because of the rapid uptake.

Amides

□ **Lidocaine.** Lidocaine is the most commonly used local anesthetic because of its potency, rapid on-

Table 117–2. Half-Life of Chloroprocaine

	Half-Life (sec) (Mean ± SD)
Mothers (n = 7)	20.9 ± 5.8
Umbilical cords (n = 7)	42.6 ± 11.2
Male controls (n = 6)	20.6 ± 4.1
Female controls (n = 5)	25.2 ± 3.7
Homozygous-atypical cholinesterase carriers (n = 10)	106.0 ± 45.0

From O'Brien JE, et al.[3]

set, moderate duration of action, and versatility. It can be used for infiltration as well as peripheral and central nerve blocks in concentrations ranging from 0.5% to 2.0%.

□ **Mepivacaine.** Can be used in the same manner as lidocaine. Duration of action is somewhat longer in the epidural space.

□ **Bupivacaine.** Valued for its long duration in peripheral nerve and epidural blockade. Also popular as an intrathecal agent. Whereas duration of intrathecal blockade is similar to tetracaine, many believe it is more predictable.

□ **Etidocaine.** Etidocaine, although having a similar duration of action to bupivacaine, has a much shorter onset of anesthesia due to its greater lipid solubility. The amount of motor block is also more profound than that seen with bupivacaine, producing a block more suited to prolonged surgical procedures requiring muscle relaxation.

Selected References

1. Covino BG, Wildsmith JAW. Clinical pharmacology of local anesthetic agents. In Cousins MJ, Bridenbaugh PO, eds. Neural Blockade in Clinical Anesthesia and Management of Pain. 3rd ed. Philadelphia: JB Lippincott, 1998:97–128.
2. Tucker GT, Mather LE. Properties, absorption, and disposition of local anesthetic agents. In Cousins MJ, Bridenbaugh PO, eds. Neural Blockade in Clinical Anesthesia and Management of Pain. 3rd ed. Philadelphia: JB Lippincott, 1998:55–96.
3. O'Brien JE, Abbey V, Hinsvark O, et al. Metabolism and measurement of chloroprocaine, an ester-type anesthetic. J Pharm Sci 1979;68:75–78.

Suggested References

Bromage PR. Choice of local anesthetics in obstetrics. In Shnider SM, Levinson G, eds. Anesthesia for Obstetrics. 3rd ed. Baltimore: Williams & Wilkins, 1993:83.
Butterworth JF IV, Strichartz GR. Molecular mechanism of local anesthesia: A review. Anesthesiology 1990;72:711–734.

118
Toxicity of Local Anesthetics

Terese T. Horlocker, M.D.

Most episodes of local anesthetic toxicity result from high blood levels of local anesthetic caused by either accidental intravascular injection or increased uptake from perivascular areas, such as the epidural space or axillary sheath.

Prevention and treatment of local anesthetic toxicity is dependent on the injection of an appropriate volume and concentration of local anesthetic, knowledge of the pharmacologic properties of these drugs, and increased vigilance for the early detection of toxic reactions.

Factors Influencing Blood Levels of Local Anesthetic

The site of injection, choice of drug, dose of local anesthetic, addition of vasoconstrictors, and metabolism determine blood levels of local anesthetic.

Site of Injection. Absorption of local anesthetic is dependent on the blood supply at the site of injection. High perfusion favors high uptake and blood levels. In general, the blood levels after various nerve blocks are:

Intercostal > caudal > epidural > brachial plexus > sciatic > spinal

Choice of Local Anesthetic. Local anesthetics with a high degree of tissue binding (etidocaine and bupivacaine) or a large volume of distribution (prilocaine) will have lower blood levels.

Dose of Local Anesthetic. The relationship between total dose of local anesthetic and peak plasma concentration is linear.

Addition of Vasoconstrictors. The actual effect of the addition of epinephrine or phenylephrine is dependent on the sensitivity of the vasculature at the injection site and also the vasoconstrictive or dilating properties of the specific local anesthetic. In general, the addition of vasoconstrictors lowers the peak blood level and increases the time to peak blood level of local anesthetics.

Metabolism. Because little metabolism of local anesthetics occurs at the site of injection, absorption and delivery to the site of metabolism (for amides, the liver; for esters, the plasma) is necessary for local anesthetic metabolism to occur.

Systemic Toxicity

Most toxic reactions to local anesthetics involve the central nervous system (CNS). Severe reactions also involving the cardiovascular system are less frequent, but more difficult to treat.

Central Nervous System Toxicity. CNS toxicity is proportional to local anesthetic potency. More potent, longer-acting drugs tend to be more toxic.

The signs and symptoms of lidocaine-induced CNS toxicity are shown in Fig. 118–1. Initial symptoms are excitatory, resulting from a selective blockade of the inhibitory pathways. Eventual CNS depression and collapse develop as blood levels increase.

The convulsive threshold is decreased by 50% in the presence of hypercarbia. An increase in Pa_{CO_2} increases cerebral blood flow, and a decrease in pH results in decreased protein binding (more free drug is available).

Cardiovascular System Toxicity. All local anesthetics cause a dose-dependent depression in myocardial contractility and also exhibit vasodilating properties (with the exception of cocaine, a vasoconstrictor).

Myocardial depression is proportional to local an-

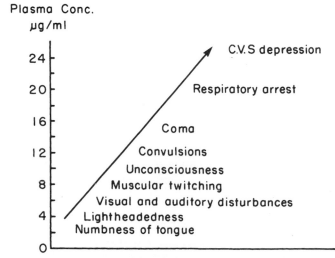

Figure 118–1. Relationship of signs and symptoms of local anesthetic toxicity to plasma concentration of lidocaine. CVS, cardiovascular system. (From Covino BG.)

esthetic potency. Bupivacaine has also been associated with ventricular dysrhythmias, perhaps due to unidirectional conduction blockade resulting in a reentrant pathway.

Allergy to Local Anesthetics

True allergies to amide local anesthetics are extremely rare. Metabolism of ester local anesthetics (Chap. 117) yields para-aminobenzoic acid (PABA), which is a known allergen. A patient who is allergic to PABA should be assumed to be allergic to ester local anesthetics. Methylparaben, a preservative in both ester and amide local anesthetic solutions, is also metabolized to PABA and may cause allergic reactions.

Neural Toxicity

Chloroprocaine has been implicated in the prolonged sensory and motor deficits of at least nine patients. When these reactions occurred, available preparations of chloroprocaine contained 0.2% sodium bisulfite and had a pH of 3.0. Studies have shown that although chloroprocaine itself is not neurotoxic, large amounts of chloroprocaine in the presence of sodium bisulfite and a low pH may cause neurotoxicity. Lidocaine and other local anesthetics also may cause neurotoxicity when administered in high concentrations.[2]

Methemoglobinemia

Methemoglobin may be formed after administration of large doses of prilocaine. In general, doses of about 600 mg are required before clinically significant methemoglobinemia occurs. Usual clinical effects are mild but may be of greater importance in patients with cardiac or respiratory compromise. Methemoglobinemia may be treated by intravenous administration of methylene blue.

Diagnosis, Prevention, and Treatment of Toxic Reactions

Most toxic reactions to local anesthetics can be prevented through safe performance of neural blockade, including careful selection of local anesthetic dose and concentration. Use of a test-dose and incremental injections with intermittent aspiration decrease the risk of systemic toxicity during epidural anesthesia. Recommended maximum single doses for local anesthetics are listed in Table 117–1.

Patients should be closely monitored for signs of intravascular injection (i.e., increased blood pressure and heart rate in the presence of epinephrine) or signs of CNS toxicity. The judicious use of a benzodiazepine will raise the seizure threshold.

Treatment of local anesthetic toxic reactions is similar to the management of other medical emergencies, focusing on ensuring adequate airway, breathing, and circulation. An airway should be established and 100% oxygen administered. Hypoxia and hypercarbia must be avoided. If convulsions occur, a small amount of a short-acting barbiturate (thiopental 50 to 100 mg) will rapidly terminate the seizure without causing cardiovascular compromise. Should intubation be required to secure the airway, succinylcholine may be administered. Although the tonic-clonic motions are inhibited in a patient given a neuromuscular relaxant, seizure activity may still be present electroencephalographically.

Most toxic reactions are limited to the CNS. Cardiovascular collapse with refractory ventricular fibrillation may occur, especially with bupivacaine. Sustained cardiopulmonary resuscitation and repeated cardioversion may be necessary. High doses of epinephrine are often required for circulatory support. Ventricular dysrhythmias should be treated with bretylium instead of lidocaine.

Cauda Equina Syndrome

Prolonged neurologic injury with pain, motor paralysis, and sensory changes is a rare complication of spinal anesthesia. Although preservatives or other contaminants administered with the drug have been cited as the cause of this complication in rare reports, neural toxicity has been described following injection of high concentrations and doses of certain local anesthetics, including chloroprocaine and lidocaine. A number of cases were reported in the 1990s after the use of microcatheters for continuous spinal anesthesia with high-dose lidocaine, presumably because this catheter placement allowed a high concentration of the drug to "streamline" and accumulate near sacral nerve roots.

Transient Neurologic Symptoms

Pollock and others have described a significant incidence (10% to 30%) of transient neurologic symptoms (TNS) after spinal anesthesia with normal doses of lidocaine. Severe pain radiating down both legs is the most commonly described symptom. Associated factors include surgical position (specifically lithotomy), early ambulation, and obesity. This poses a special problem when spinal anesthesia is chosen for short procedures, because there are few alternatives for outpatient regional anesthesia. Alternatives to lidocaine include procaine, mepivacaine (which has also been associated with TNS), very-low-dose lidocaine (25 mg) with fentanyl (25 μg), and very-low-dose bupivacaine (4 to 7 mg) with fentanyl (10 to 25 μg).

Selected References

1. Covino BG, Wildsmith JAW. Clinical pharmacology of local anesthetic agents. In Cousins MJ, Bridenbaugh PO, eds. Neural Blockade. 3rd ed. Philadelphia: Lippincott-Raven, 1998:107.
2. Hodgson PS, Neal JM, Pollock JE, et al. The neurotoxicity of drugs given intrathecally (review). Anesth Analg 1999;88:797–809.

Suggested References

Covino BG. Pharmacology of local anaesthetic agents. Br J Anaesth 1986;58:701.
Drasner K. Models for local anesthetic toxicity from continuous spinal anesthesia. Reg Anesth 1993;18:434–438.
Freedman JM, Li D, Drasner K, et al. Transient neurologic symptoms after spinal anesthesia. An epidemiologic study of 1863 patients. Anesthesiology 1998;89:633–641.
Lambert DH, Hurley RJ. Cauda equina syndrome and continuous spinal anesthesia. Anesth Analg 1991;72:817–819.
Pollock JE, Neal JM, Stephenson CA, et al. Prospective study of the incidence of transient radicular irritation in patients undergoing spinal anesthesia. Anesthesiology 1996;84:1361–1367.
Pollock JE, Liu SS, Neal JM, et al. Is transient radiating back pain caused by a concentration-dependent neurotoxicity of spinal lidocaine? Anesthesiology 1999;90:445–450.
Reiz S, Nath S. Cardiotoxicity of local anaesthetic agents. Br J Anaesth 1986;58:736.
Reynolds F. Adverse effects of local anaesthetics. Br J Anaesth 1987;59:78.
Rigler ML, Drasner K, Krejcie TC, et al. Cauda equina syndrome after continuous spinal anesthesia. Anesth Analg 1991;72:275–281.
Schneider M, Ettlin T, Kaufmann M, et al. Transient neurologic toxicity after hyperbaric subarachnoid anesthesia with 5% lidocaine. Anesth Analg 1993;76:1154–1157.

119
Local Anesthetic Preservatives

Michael L. Bishop, M.D.

Many local anesthetics contain preservatives or antioxidants. Some of these agents have been associated with neurotoxicity.

Antimicrobial Agents

Multiple-dose vials of commercially prepared local anesthetic solutions contain up to 0.1% methylparaben as an antimicrobial agent. Methylparaben is effective in the prevention of contamination by gram-positive bacteria and fungi but has limited efficacy against gram-negative bacteria. This preservative has a chemical structure similar to that of para-aminobenzoic acid (PABA), sulfonamide antibiotics, and ester-type local anesthetics. All three of these classes of drugs are potential allergens. In sensitive individuals, exposure to methylparaben may result in anaphylactoid symptoms, cutaneous lesions, urticaria, and/or edema. The safety of intrathecal methylparaben has been questioned, but risk appears to be minimal in the small doses associated with spinal administration of local anesthetics.

Antioxidants and Stabilizers

Commercially prepared ester-type local anesthetic solutions and epinephrine-containing amide-type local anesthetic solutions may contain one or more antioxidant and/or stabilizing agents. These include sodium metabisulfite, acetone sodium bisulfite, ascorbic acid, citric acid, disodium ethylenediaminetetraacetate (EDTA), and monothioglycerol. These compounds are added to local anesthetics to prolong shelf life and enhance the ability to withstand autoclaving. Although most of these innocuous chemicals are used commonly in the food and wine industries, sodium metabisulfite has two potentially serious toxicities.

Sulfiting agents can cause serious allergic reactions in sensitive individuals, including anaphylactic symptoms such as hypotension and bronchospasm. Known asthmatic patients have an increased risk of allergic reactions to these agents. However, symptoms may occur in nonasthmatic individuals as well. Since these agents are common in commercially prepared foods, most individuals will have received sensitizing doses before any metabisulfite-containing local anesthetic solution is administered.

Sodium metabisulfite also has neurotoxic potential. In the early 1980s, case reports appeared describing prolonged spinal cord neurotoxicity following inadvertent subarachnoid injection of large volumes of 0.2% metabisulfite-containing chloroprocaine solutions. Initially, there was concern regarding the neurotoxicity of chloroprocaine; however, subsequent investigations showed that the etiologic factor was the large volume of highly acidic metabisulfite injected (pH 3). It is currently recommended that local anesthetic solutions used for subarachnoid and epidural injection have a maximum concentration of 0.1% metabisulfite and a pH above 4.5. Peripheral nerves appear to be less sensitive to the neurotoxic effects of metabisulfite.

Because of toxicity concerns, EDTA was introduced as a substitute for metabisulfite. However, tetracaine solutions may still contain acetone sodium bisulfite at a pH of 3.2 to 6. Preservative agents contained in commercially prepared local anesthetic solutions are listed in Table 119-1.

Table 119–1. Preservatives Contained in Local Anesthetic Solutions

Preservatives
Methylparaben
Antioxidants
Sodium metabisulfite
Monothioglycerol
Stabilizers
Edetate calcium disodium
Chelating Agents
Disodium EDTA dihydrate

Suggested References

Cousins MJ, Bridenbaugh PO. Neural Blockade in Clinical Anesthesia and Management of Pain. Philadelphia, Lippincott-Raven, 1998.

Gissen AJ, Datta S, Lambert D. The chloroprocaine controversy. Is chloroprocaine neurotoxic? Reg Anesth 1984;9:135.

Hodgson PS, Neal JM, Pollock JE, et al. The neurotoxicity of drugs given intrathecally (spinal). Anesth Analg 1999;88:797–809.

Ravindrin RS, Bond VK, Tasch MD, et al. Prolonged neural blockade following regional analgesia with 2-chloroprocaine. Anesth Analg 1980;59:447.

Wang BC, Hillamn DE, Spielholz NI, et al. Chronic neurologic deficits and nesacaine-CE: An effect of the anesthetic, 2-chloroprocaine or the antioxidant sodium bisulfite? Anesth Analg 1984;63:445.

120
Cocaine Pharmacology

David R. Becker, M.D.

The alkaloid extract from the leaves of the *Erythoxylon coca* bush, cocaine was the first local anesthetic introduced. It was used for ophthalmologic procedures by Carl Koller in 1884. William Halsted and Richard Hall later used it for regional blocks in the face and arm. The dangers of cocaine were reported in the medical literature only 7 years after its introduction, yet 100 years later illicit use of cocaine became a widespread health problem in the United States.[1,2]

Pharmacology

Cocaine is an **ester** of benzoic acid with the chemical name of benzoylmethylecgonine. It is similar to other ester local anesthetics in that it contains an aromatic residue, an ester link, and a terminal tertiary amine (Fig. 120–1). Cocaine is prepared either as the alkaloid base, soluble in organic solvents, or as a hydrochloride salt that is soluble in water. It can be used topically in 1% to 10% solutions. The **maximum dose** should not exceed **3 mg/kg**. Cocaine is well absorbed across mucous membranes and is taken up quickly into systemic circulation with a half-life of approximately 1 hour. It undergoes rapid hydrolysis by plasma and liver cholinesterases and is excreted by the kidney. Cocaine metabolism is slowed by liver disease and **atypical plasma cholinesterase**.

Actions

Local Anesthetic Actions. Local anesthetic actions are mediated by cocaine's ability to block the flux of sodium ions across the neuronal cell membrane. Systemically, cocaine inhibits the reuptake of norepinephrine, causing stimulation of the sympathetic nervous system.

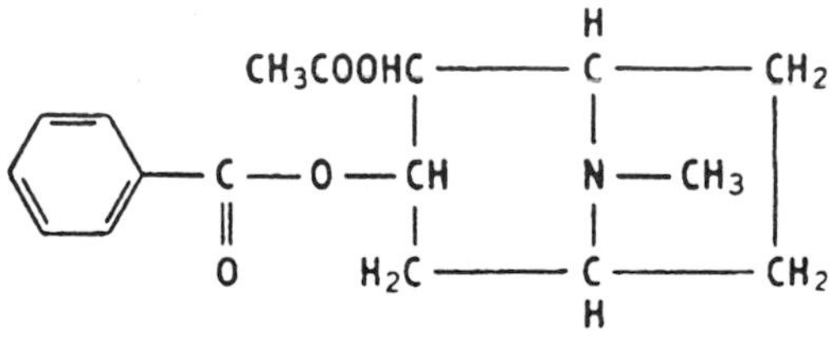

Central Nervous System Action. Initially, cocaine is stimulatory, with euphoria and excitation progressing to tremors, seizures, and occasionally emesis. Its brief behavioral stimulation is intense, with euphoria and arousal, making it a potent behavioral enforcer.[3] At higher doses it is a convulsant. It also can lead to stroke, subarachnoid hemorrhage, and rupture of cerebral aneurysms. Cocaine may cause central anticholinergic syndrome.

Cardiovascular Action. At low doses, cocaine is often characterized by bradycardia secondary to central vagal stimulation. Moderate doses show the characteristic elevations in blood pressure and heart rate, as well as arrhythmias, mydriasis, hyperglycemia, hyperthermia, and myocardial ischemia.

Cocaine use is a risk factor for myocardial infarction, pulmonary edema, ruptured aortic aneurysm, infective endocarditis, vascular thrombosis, myocarditis, and dilated cardiomyopathy. Cardiotoxicity and death can occur after all routes of abuse. First-time users have developed myocardial infarction, and deaths have been reported among this group.[2]

Anesthetic Uses and Considerations

Cocaine's main use is in **topical anesthesia** and **vasoconstriction** in nasal procedures; 2 mL of a 10% solution on cotton pledgets is applied to the area of the nasociliary nerve and sphenopalatine ganglion (Fig. 120–2). An alternative form is a 5% spray and a 10% paste applied similarly. Because of the difficulty in controlling the dose and the toxic side effects, other mixtures have been advocated. Lidocaine (1%) and 0.5% phenylephrine are as efficacious in dilating nasal passage as 5% cocaine.

Cocaine has also been used for topical anesthesia during awake intubations, but 0.05% oxymetazoline

Figure 120–1. Chemical structure of cocaine.

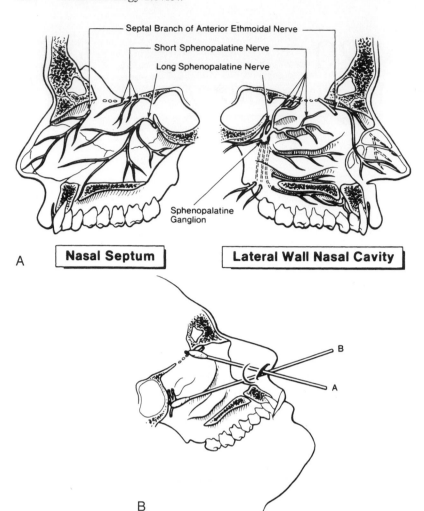

Septal Branch of Anterior Ethmoidal Nerve

Short Sphenopalatine Nerve

Long Sphenopalatine Nerve

Sphenopalatine Ganglion

Nasal Septum

A

Lateral Wall Nasal Cavity

B

B

A

B

Figure 120–2. Nerve supply of the nasal septum and the lateral wall of the nasal cavity. Pledgets of cotton wool are soaked in local anesthetic and inserted as shown to contact branches of the anterior ethmoidal nerve (A) and the sphenopalatine ganglion and nerves (B). Note that pledget A is inserted parallel with the line of the external nose until it reaches the superior extent of the nasal cavity. Pledget B is inserted about 20 degrees to 30 degrees with the horizontal line through the floor of the nose to reach the region of the sphenopalatine foramen. (From Murphy TM.[6])

may prevent epistaxis better than 10% cocaine during nasotracheal intubations. Ocular use is limited by corneal damage, which can result from the effects of vasoconstriction. Cocaine may potentiate the action of muscle relaxants either by reducing the acetylcholine content of quanta or by decreasing the sensitivity of the postjunctional membrane. It is contradicted in patients with hypertension or in those taking guanethidine, reserpine, tricyclic antidepressants, or monoamine oxidase inhibitors. Concurrent administration of catecholamines or sympathomimetics should be done cautiously.

Cocaine abuse by pregnant women can lead to multiple obstetric complications, including placental abruption, precipitate delivery, preterm labor, and stillbirth.[4] The absence of prenatal care is the most important predictor of cocaine abuse in mothers in labor. Hypertension and tachycardia are more frequent; cocaine-induced thrombocytopenia has also been reported and could increase the risks of regional anesthesia. Ester local anesthetics may compete with cocaine for metabolism by plasma cholinesterase, prolonging the effects of both drugs.

Management of Toxic Side Effects

Systemic toxicity is treated by administering supplemental oxygen, a neuromuscular blocking agent to ease manual ventilation, and barbiturates or benzodiazepines to reduce central nervous system excitement. Gay and Loper have warned against the use of pure β-blockers, which may cause unopposed α-stimulation and hypertension.[5]

Selected References

1. Fleming JA, Byck R, Barash PG. Pharmacology and therapeutic applications of cocaine. Anesthesiology 1990;73:518–531.
2. Cregler LL. Cocaine: The newest risk factor for cardiovascular disease. Clin Cardiol 1991;14:449.
3. Musto DF. Opium, cocaine and marijuana in American history. Sci Am 1991;265:40–47.
4. Kain ZN, Rimar S, and Barash PG. Cocaine abuse in the parturient and effects on the fetus and neonate. Anesth Analg 1993;77:835–845.
5. Gay GR, Loper KA. The use of labetalol in the management of cocaine crisis. Ann Emerg Med 1998;17:282.
6. Murphy TM. Somatic blockade of the head and neck. In Cousins MJ, Bridenbaugh PO, eds. Neural Blockade in Clinical Anesthesia and Management of Pain. 2nd ed. Philadelphia: JB Lippincott, 1988:539.

121
Spinal Anesthesia

John C. McMichan, M.B.B.S., Ph.D.

The physiologic effects of spinal anesthesia depend on the level of anesthesia, which itself depends on the volume of solution injected into the subarachnoid space, the concentration of the agent in the solution, the speed of injection of the solution, the site of injection, the specific gravity of the solution, the position of the patient, barbotage, the presence of increased intra-abdominal pressure, and the height of the patient.

The interruption of spinal cord function begins caudally and proceeds in a cephalic direction. Autonomic function is lost before sensory function, which is lost before motor function. Motor function requires the highest drug concentration as the heavy myelinated fibers are the most resistant to block and the first to which function returns. The level of autonomic block is two or more dermatomes cephalic to the level of skin analgesia, whereas the level of motor block lies two to three segments caudal to the level of skin analgesia.

Spinal anesthesia can be classified as follows:

☐ Saddle block: sensory anesthesia involving the lower lumbar and sacral segments.
☐ Low spinal: level of skin anesthesia at the T10 dermatome.
☐ Midspinal: sensory level at the costal margin (T6 segment).
☐ High spinal: sensory level at or above the T4 dermatome.

The level of anesthesia ascends the spinal cord as the concentration of the solution, the volume of the solution, the speed of injection of the solution, and intra-abdominal and intrathoracic pressure are increased. The tall patient requires more drug to achieve a high level. Injection at the L4-5 space produces a lower level than a similar injection at the L2-3 space.

Pharmacologic Agents

Among the commonly used agents are lidocaine, bupivacaine, and tetracaine. Of these, lidocaine has the quickest onset and the shortest duration and thus is favored for short surgical procedures. Popular and without specific complications for more than 50 years, lidocaine has fallen into some disfavor. In 1991, reports of low back pain following lidocaine spinal anesthesia appeared.[1] At first, these transient neurologic symptoms (TNS) were thought to be linked to the high concentration of the drug delivered by microcatheters into the CSF surrounding the lumbar nerves during continuous spinal anesthesia. But after the catheters were removed from clinical practice, the reports continued. Despite lower concentrations of the agent and dilution with CSF, symptoms are reported in 13% to 36% of patients receiving a lidocaine spinal, especially for procedures performed in the lithotomy position. The back pain lasts for about 48 hours and no permanent sequelae have been recorded. It would be wise to inform patients of the risk of transient neurologic symptoms before administering a lidocaine spinal anesthetic.

Needle Choice

Needle size has long been known to correlate with the incidence of postdural puncture headache (PDPH). Pencil-point needles (e.g., Sprotte's, Whitacre's) have been shown to produce PDPH less frequently than cutting needles (e.g., Quincke's).

Physiological Effects of Spinal Anesthesia

Cardiovascular. The sympathetic nervous system is blocked in proportion to the height of the anesthesia level obtained. Total sympathetic block can be expected from high spinal anesthesia. In normal nonmedicated volunteers, this produces a 15% to 20% decrease in mean arterial pressure, central venous pressure, and total peripheral resistance (Fig. 121–1). Minimal reductions in cardiac output, cardiac rate, and stroke volume usually occur. Compensatory vasoconstriction occurs above the level of the block.

In a 2001 review, Pollard noted an increased incidence of cardiac arrests in patients undergoing spinal anesthesia in several large studies.[3] The incidence rate was higher (0.07% to 0.15%) than that of patients undergoing noncardiac surgery in other series (0.03%) and higher than the rate reported

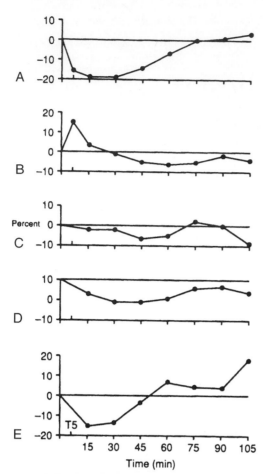

Figure 121–1. Effect of high (T5) spinal anesthesia on renal function. *A,* Mean arterial pressure. *B,* Cardiac output. *C,* Effective renal plasma flow. *D,* Glomerular filtration rate. *E,* Renal vascular resistance. (Modified from Kennedy WF Jr.[2])

during epidural anesthesia (0.01%). Respiratory depression from sedation was not implicated; prospective studies have shown no link between sedation and cardiac arrest during spinal anesthesia. Postulated mechanisms include the sympathetic blockade and decreased venous return that accompany high spinals. Associated risk factors for bradycardia (below 50 beats/min) during spinal anesthesia include:

□ Baseline heart rate below 60 beats/min.
□ ASA physical status I.
□ Use of β-blocking drugs.
□ Sensory level above T6.
□ Age under 50 years.
□ Prolonged PR interval.

Aggressive pharmacologic therapy with atropine, ephedrine, and IV fluids is recommended for any bradycardia or hypotension noted during spinal anesthesia.

If hypotension (arterial pressure less than 25% of the preanesthesia level) occurs, the following steps should be taken:

□ Increase circulating volume with 500 to 1000 mL of crystalloid solution.

□ Place the patient in a mild head-down position to improve venous return.
□ Vasoconstrictors may be used to increase cardiac output and peripheral resistance prophylactically or when hypotension occurs. Ephedrine is the drug of choice, especially in obstetric patients because of its lack of effect on uterine blood flow.

Renal and Genitourinary. Spinal anesthesia alters renal function by interrupting autonomic control of the kidney and by decreasing renal blood flow secondary to arterial hypotension. In normal subjects, in the absence of surgery, high spinal anesthesia reduces glomerular filtration rate and effective renal flow by 5% to 10%. These changes are of little clinical significance in the normotensive, normovolemic patient. In contrast to the anal sphincter, the urinary sphincters are not relaxed. On emergence from spinal anesthesia, the bladder is last to regain function and urinary retention is not uncommon (S2 and S3). Paralysis of the nervi erigentes (S2 and S3) produces penile flaccidity and engorgement.

Hepatic Blood Flow. In the absence of surgical procedures, high spinal anesthesia decreases hepatic blood flow in parallel with the decrease in mean arterial pressure. This change cannot be related to perioperative hepatic dysfunction.

Cerebral Blood Flow. CBF is maintained during spinal anesthesia. A decrease in arterial pressure produces a decrease in cerebral vascular resistance through autoregulation. But if mean arterial pressure is less than about 60 mm Hg (higher in the presence of hypertension or arteriosclerotic disease), cerebral blood flow will decrease, cerebral hypoxia will occur, and nausea and vomiting will follow. A moderate degree of head-down positioning should be used to increase mean cerebral arterial pressure during hypotensive episodes.

Gastrointestinal. After sympathetic blockade, the parasympathetic activity is unopposed. Intestinal sphincters are relaxed. The bowel is contracted, and peristalsis is increased. Nausea and vomiting can result from increased gastric motility. Visceral pain produced by surgical activity in the upper abdomen sends impulses via the unblocked vagal fibers to higher centers.

Endocrine. The adrenal response to surgical stress is either absent or delayed. There is no increase in plasma steroid levels or decrease in eosinophil levels. The level of aldosterone remains unchanged. The catecholamine response to surgery is abolished.

Respiratory. The effects of high spinal anesthesia are more marked on parameters of exhalation than on those of inhalation. Resting ventilation is not impaired as long as phrenic nerve innervation is intact. If all thoracic spinal nerve roots are blocked, inspiratory capacity is decreased by 20% and expiratory reserve volume is decreased to zero. There are no significant alterations in blood gas measurements. The ability to cough effectively is markedly reduced. A saddle block has no effect on respiratory function. Patients should receive an oxygen supplement during spinal anesthesia for prolonged procedures, because airway closure, atelectasis, and hypoxia can occur.

Total spinal or high spinal results when the local anesthetic agent effect is high in the CNS. Apnea and hypotension occur, possibly from hypoperfusion of the brain stem. Immediate ventilation with a bag and mask or an endotracheal tube and measures taken to treat the hypotension can be life-saving. Agents such as midazolam should be administered to ensure amnesia.

Selected References

1. Pollock J, Neal J, Stephenson C, et al. Prospective study of the incidence of transient radicular irritation in patients undergoing spinal anesthesia. Anesthesiology 1996;84:1361–1367.
2. Kennedy WF Jr. Effects of spinal and peridural blocks on renal and hepatic function. In Bonica JJ, ed. Regional Anesthesia: Recent Advances and Current Status. Vol. 2. Philadelphia: FA Davis, 1969:112.
3. Pollard JB. Cardiac arrest during spinal anesthesia: common mechanisms and strategies for prevention. Anesth Analg 2001;92:252–256.

Suggested References

Cousins MJ, Bridenbaugh PO, eds. Neural Blockade in Clinical Anesthesia and Management of Pain. 2nd ed. Philadelphia, JB Lippincott, 1988.

Greene NM, Brull SJ. Physiology of Spinal Anesthesia. 4th ed. Baltimore, Williams & Wilkins, 1993.

Liu SS, McDonald SB. Current issues in spinal anesthesia. Anesthesiology 2001;94:888–906.

Vallejo MC, Mandell GL, Sabo DP, et al. Postdural puncture headache: A randomized comparison of five spinal needles in obstetric patients. Anesth Analg 2000;91:916–920.

122
Epidural Anesthesia

Terese T. Horlocker, M.D.

Epidural anesthesia has clinical applications in three main areas: surgery, obstetrics, and chronic pain relief.

Applied Anatomy of the Epidural Space

The epidural space is a potential space surrounding the spinal meninges and containing fat, nerve roots, and vascular plexi. The anatomy of the spine, ligaments, meninges, and spinal cord blood flow are described in detail in Chapter 79. Knowledge of surface anatomy (Fig. 122–1) and key anatomic features of the cervical, thoracic, and lumbar spinal regions (Table 122–1) are critical to the performance of safe and reliable epidural needle placement.

Identification of the Epidural Space

The epidural space is identified by the passage of the needle from an area of high resistance (ligamentum flavum) to an area of low resistance (epidural space). After the needle is positioned in the ligamentum flavum, a syringe with a freely movable plunger is attached and continuous pressure is applied to the plunger. If the needle is positioned correctly in the ligament, the syringe should not inject when pressure is applied to the plunger. As the needle passes into the epidural space, a sudden loss of resistance in the plunger will be felt, and the air or fluid will easily inject. At this point, a flexible synthetic catheter may be threaded 3 to 4 cm through the needle into the epidural space to allow repeated and incremental injections. A **test dose** of 3 mL of local anesthetic solution containing 1:200,000 epinephrine is then injected and the patient observed for signs of intravascular injection.

Selection and Dose of Local Anesthetic

All segments of the spinal canal from the base of the skull to the sacral hiatus are accessible to epi-

dural injection. Epidural anesthesia, either alone or in combination with general anesthesia, may be adapted to almost any surgical procedure below the chin. Assessment of the dermatomal sensory level enables the anesthesiologist to determine approximate level of sympathectomy and anticipate the resulting hemodynamic effects (Table 122–2).

The major sites of action of epidurally injected local anesthetics are the spinal nerve roots, where the dura is relatively thin. Only a small amount of

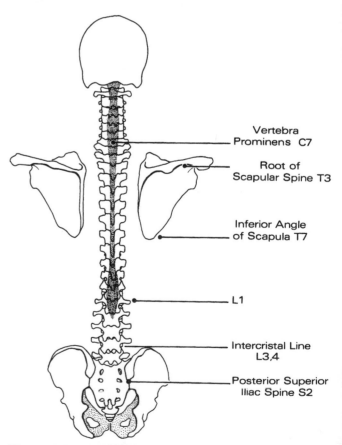

Vertebra Prominens C7

Root of Scapular Spine T3

Inferior Angle of Scapula T7

L1

Intercristal Line L3,4

Posterior Superior Iliac Spine S2

Figure 122–1. Surface anatomy and landmarks for epidural blockade. Termination of the spinal cord is at L1 in adults. The dural sac terminates at S2. Needle placement between C7 and T1 is different because of the narrow epidural space. Between T1 and T7, a paramedian approach is recommended to bypass angled spinous processes. Below T7, needle placement becomes progressively similar to that for L2-3. (From Bromage PR.[1])

Table 122–1. Anatomic Features of Cervical, Thoracic, and Lumbar Spine Regions

Lumbar Spine
The epidural space is widest (5–6 mm).
Needle insertion below L1 (in adults) avoids the spinal cord.
The ligamentum flavum is thickest in the midline in the lumbar area.
The spinous processes have only slight downward angulation.
The epidural veins are prominent in lateral portion of epidural space.

Thoracic Spine
The epidural space is 3–5 mm in the midline, narrow laterally.
The ligamentum flavum is thick, but less so than in the midlumbar region.
The spinous processes have extreme downward angulation; the paramedian approach is recommended.

Cervical Spine
The epidural space is narrow, only 2 mm at C3-6.
The ligamentum flavum is thin.
The spinous process at C7 is almost horizontal.

α-receptors located in the central nervous system, where they can modulate central pain processing. The role of α_2-agonists such as clonidine in prolonging and intensifying anesthetic blocks has been clearly delineated.[3]

Complications

Accidental Dural Puncture. The appearance of cerebrospinal fluid through either the needle or catheter signifies dural puncture. Should this occur, the epidural anesthetic may be converted to a spinal, or an epidural may be attempted again at a different interspace. The risk of postdural puncture headache is increased because of the large needle size.

Intravascular Injection. Preinjection aspiration of epidural catheters and the use of a 3- to 4-mL test dose of local anesthetic with epinephrine decrease the risk of intravascular injection of a large volume of anesthetic. Epidural catheters can "migrate" intravascularly hours after initial placement in the epidural space.

Hypotension. The hemodynamic effects of epidural blockade are similar to those of spinal blockade and are described in Chapter 121. The degree of hypotension is dependent on the level of sympathectomy (including possible involvement of the cardioaccelerator fibers) and the patient's volume status.

High Spinal. Inadvertent intrathecal injection of an "epidural" dose of local anesthetic results in a high spinal block. The use of a test dose before injection of the initial local anesthetic bolus, incremental injections, and aspiration of the catheter before reinjection aid detection of an intrathecally placed catheter and reduce the risk of a high or total spinal.

Epidural Abscess and Hematoma. Epidural abscess and hematoma are extremely rare complications of epidural blockade. Epidural anesthesia is generally avoided in patients who are grossly septic, have a localized infection at the site of needle placement, or are therapeutically anticoagulated. Patients with epidural abscess or hematoma usually present with new-onset radicular back pain that may progress to paraplegia if not diagnosed and treated promptly.

local anesthetic actually diffuses across the dura into the subarachnoid space.

A local anesthetic should be selected on the basis of speed of onset, degree of motor blockade required, and duration of the surgical procedure (Table 122–3).

Local anesthetic dose may be calculated by the following formula: dose = 1 to 1.5 mL of local anesthetic per segment blocked. The dose may need to be significantly reduced in parturients and in obese and elderly patients. In these situations, incremental doses are advised. A second dose of approximately 50% of the initial dose will maintain the original level of anesthesia if injected when the blockade has regressed one or two dermatomes (see Table 122–3).

Addition of epinephrine can prolong the duration of lidocaine nerve block by up to 50%. Less dramatic results are usually observed for bupivacaine and etidocaine. Addition of vasoconstrictors reduces blood flow in the richly vascularized epidural space. This reduces systemic absorption, and because more of the drug remains in proximity to the nerve, the onset of block is quicker and the duration of action longer. Confirmation of this concept comes from studies demonstrating that the peak plasma levels of various agents are lower when epinephrine is present.

The vasoconstrictors normally used also act on

Table 122–2. Sensory Level of Epidural Blockade Required for Surgical Procedures

Cutaneous Landmark	Segmental Level	Type of Surgery	Significance
Fifth finger	C8		All cardioaccelerator fibers (T1-4) blocked
Nipple line	T4-5	Upper abdominal surgery	Possibility of cardioaccelerator blockade
Tip of xiphoid	T6	Lower abdominal surgery	Splanchnics (T5-L1) blocked
Umbilicus	T10	Hip surgery	Sympathetic blockade to lower extremities
Lateral aspect of foot	S1		No lumbar sympathectomy
Perineum	S2-4	Hemorrhoidectomy	

Table 122–3. Clinical Effects of Local Anesthetic Solutions Commonly Used for Epidural Blockade

Drug	Time Spread to ± Four Segments ± 1 SD (min)	Approximate Time to Two-Segment Regression ± 2 SD* (min)	Recommended "Top-Up" Time from Initial Dose* (min)
Lidocaine, 2%	15 ± 5	100 ± 40	60
Prilocaine, 2%–3%	15 ± 4	100 ± 40	60
Chloroprocaine, 2%–3%	12 ± 5	60 ± 15	45
Mepivacaine, 2%	15 ± 5	120 ± 150	60
Bupivacaine, 0.5%–0.75%	18 ± 10	200 ± 80	120
Ropivicaine, 0.75%–1%	20.5 ± 7.9	177 ± 49	120
Etidocaine, 1%–1.5%	10 ± 5	200 ± 80	120

*Note that top-up time is based on duration − 2 SD, which encompasses the likely duration in 95% of the population. In a conscious, cooperative patient, an alternative is to use frequent checks of segmental level to indicate the need to "top-up." All solutions contain 1:200,000 epinephrine. From Cousins MJ, Veering BT.[2]

Selected References

1. Bromage PR. Anatomy. In Epidural Analgesia. Philadelphia: WB Saunders, 1978:8.
2. Cousins MJ, Veering BT. Epidural neural blockade. In Cousins MJ, Bridenbaugh PO, eds. Neural Blockade. 3rd ed. Philadelphia: Lippincott-Raven, 1998:289.
3. Eisenach JC, De Kock M, Klimscha W. α_2-adrenergic agonists for regional anesthesia: A clinical review of clonidine (1984–1995). Anesthesiology 1996;85:655–674.

123
Combined Spinal-Epidural Blockade

Christopher J. Jankowski, M.D.

Combined spinal-epidural (CSE) blockade was first described in 1937 and has become more popular since the early 1980s. It combines the advantages of each of its component techniques. It provides the rapid onset, reliability, and minimal drug toxicity associated with subarachnoid blocks (SABs) with the flexibility of dosing, duration, and analgesic level control of an indwelling epidural catheter.[1, 2] CSE is used primarily for obstetrical analgesia and anesthesia, but its use has been described for a variety of applications, including general surgery, orthopedic and trauma surgery of the lower limb, urologic surgery, and gynecologic surgery.

Applied Anatomy

The essence of CSE is placement of a catheter into the epidural space along with single-shot administration of intrathecal anesthetics/analgesics. The applied anatomy of CSE is the same as that for subarachnoid and epidural blockade. As with all of regional anesthesia, detailed working knowledge of the appropriate surface anatomy and underlying structures is essential.

Indications

CSE is indicated in patients in whom a neuraxial technique is indicated and it is necessary to combine the rapid onset of analgesia achieved with spinal anesthesia with the ability to provide prolonged analgesia, as is usually done with a continuous epidural catheter technique.

Contraindications

Contraindications for CSE are the same as those for all neuraxial blocks (Table 123–1).

Equipment

Traditional spinal and epidural needles can be used via a needle-through-needle technique or by performing separate passes either in the same or different interspaces. When using a needle-through-needle technique, the spinal needle must be longer than the epidural needle to allow dural puncture. The tip of the spinal needle should project 13 to 17 mm beyond the tip of the epidural needle. Specially designed CSE kits include a guide for the spinal needle alongside the outer wall of the epidural needle or incorporated into the epidural needle wall. These kits make it possible to place an epidural catheter before administering intrathecal drugs. They may make spinal needle placement easier, because the tip of the spinal needle does not have to negotiate the curve at the end of a Hustead or Tuohy needle, and may reduce the risk of damage to the spinal needle. These kits are available from various manufacturers.

Technique

The performance of CSE is somewhat more challenging than either spinal or epidural blockade. Several techniques have been described (see Fig. 181–3). These include using separate interspaces for the spinal and epidural portions of the block, using double-catheter techniques, and making separate passes with the spinal and epidural needles in a single interspace. Each of these techniques has deficiencies, and thus they are used infrequently.

Table 123–1. Absolute and Relative Contraindications to Neuraxial Anesthesia/Analgesia

Absolute	Relative
Patient refusal	Preexisting neurologic disease
Bacteremia/sepsis	
Increased intercranial pressure	Severe psychiatric disease or dementia
Infection at needle insertion site	Aortic stenosis
	Left ventricular outflow tract obstruction
Shock or severe hypovolemia	Various congenital heart conditions (absolute contraindication if severe)
Coagulopathy or therapeutic anticoagulation (see Chap. 124)	Deformities or previous surgery of the spinal column

The most commonly used technique is the double-needle technique using a single interspace. A needle-through-needle technique may be used with traditional spinal and epidural needles. Likewise, commercially available CSE kits may be used. As with all neuraxial blocks, strict aseptic technique is necessary. A skin wheal of local anesthetic is injected into a lumbar interspace. After deep infiltration with local anesthetic, an epidural needle is inserted into the ligamentum flavum. Loss of resistance with saline is used to identify the epidural space. A long spinal needle is advanced through the epidural needle into the subarachnoid space. Following the aspiration of cerebrospinal fluid (CSF), the intrathecal anesthetic/analgesic is injected and the spinal needle is removed. Finally, an epidural catheter is advanced through the epidural needle. After negative aspiration, the catheter is secured to the patient's back with tape.

The epidural catheter can be inserted before the spinal needle is introduced if a CSE kit is used. This practice has disadvantages, however. The direction of the epidural catheter is unpredictable. In theory, the subsequently placed spinal needle could damage the epidural catheter. In addition, the catheter could make it difficult to advance the spinal needle into the subarachnoid space.

Epidural Test Doses

The timing of the epidural test dose is controversial. When the SAB is in place, it may be difficult to detect an intrathecal catheter with a test dose. Injection of a test dose into an intrathecal catheter may cause unwanted extension of the existing SAB (high spinal). Furthermore, an early test dose does not guarantee a properly placed epidural catheter, because the catheter could migrate after the test dose but before it is loaded. However, it may not be convenient to wait until the spinal block has worn off before administering a test dose. Most authorities continue to recommend the use of test doses to confirm catheter position.

Complications

Potential complications of CSE are the same as those of spinal and epidural blockade. Besides postdural puncture headache, these include total spinal, hypotension, bradycardia, meningitis, spinal abscess and hematoma, intravascular injection, intrathecal catheter migration, and nerve injury.

Postdural Puncture Headache

The incidence of postdural puncture headache may be lower with CSE than with other neuraxial techniques. There are several possible reasons for this. First, small-gauge spinal needles are used. Also, the epidural needle acts as an introducer for the spinal needle, allowing easy dural puncture and avoiding multiple punctures. Infusing local anesthetics and opioids through the epidural catheter decreases CSF leakage via increases in epidural pressure. Finally, with needle-through-needle techniques, the epidural needle causes the spinal needle to be deflected as it enters the subarachnoid space. The holes in the dura and subarachnoid are less likely to overlap, and the risk of CSF leakage is decreased.

Selected References

1. Albright GA, Forster RM. The safety and efficacy of combined spinal and epidural analgesia/anesthesia (6,002 blocks) in a community hospital. Reg Anesth Pain Med 1999;24:117–125.
2. Rawal N, et al. Combined spinal-epidural technique. Reg Anesth 1997;22:406–423.

Suggested References

Eisenach JC. Combined spinal-epidural analgesia in obstetrics. Anesthesiology 1999;299–302.

Felsby S, Juelsgaard P. Combined spinal and epidural anesthesia. Anesth Analg 1995;80:821–826.

Tsen LC, Thue B, Datta S, et al. Is combined spinal-epidural analgesia associated with more rapid cervical dilation in nulliparous patients when compared with conventional epidural analgesia? Anesthesiology 1999;91:920–925.

124
Neuraxial Anesthesia and Anticoagulation

Terese T. Horlocker, M.D.

The actual incidence of neurologic dysfunction resulting from hemorrhagic complications associated with neuraxial blockade is unknown; however, the incidence cited in the literature is estimated at less than 1 in 150,000 inductions of epidural anesthesia and less than 1 in 220,000 inductions of spinal anesthesia.[1] Vandermeulen et al[2] reported 61 cases of spinal hematoma associated with epidural or spinal anesthesia. In 42 of the 61 patients (68%), the spinal hematomas associated with central neural blockade occurred in patients with evidence of hemostatic abnormality. Regional technique also influenced risk. A spinal anesthetic was implicated in 15 patients. The remaining 46 patients received an epidural anesthetic, including 32 patients with an indwelling catheter. In 15 of these 32 patients, the spinal hematoma occurred immediately after the epidural catheter was removed. Neurologic outcome was partial or good in only 38% of patients, and tended to occur in patients who underwent laminectomy within 8 hours of being diagnosed with spinal hematoma.

Intravenous and Subcutaneous Standard Heparin

Several large studies have documented the safety of short-term intravenous heparinization in patients undergoing neuraxial anesthesia, provided that the heparin activity is closely monitored, indwelling catheters are removed at a time when circulating heparin levels are relatively low, and patients with a preexisting coagulation disorder are excluded. Conversely, traumatic needle placement, initiation of anticoagulation within 1 hour of needle insertion or concomitant aspirin therapy have been identified as risk factors in the development of spinal hematoma in patients receiving anticoagulant therapy.

Low-dose subcutaneous standard (unfractionated) heparin is administered for thromboprophylaxis in patients undergoing major thoracoabdominal surgery. Despite the widespread use of subcutaneous heparin thromboprophylaxis, only a few cases of spinal hematoma have been associated with neuraxial blockade in the presence of low-dose heparin.[2]

The concurrent use of medications that affect other components of the clotting mechanisms may increase the risk of bleeding complications for patients receiving standard heparin. These medications include antiplatelet medications, low molecular weight heparin (LMWH), and oral anticoagulants.[3]

Intravenous heparin administration should be delayed for 1 hour after needle placement. Indwelling catheters should be removed 1 hour before a subsequent heparin administration or 2 to 4 hours after the last heparin dose. Evaluation of the patient's coagulation status may be appropriate before catheter removal if the patient has demonstrated enhanced response or is receiving high doses of heparin. Although a bloody or difficult needle placement may increase risk, no data support mandatory cancellation of a case should this occur. Prolonged therapeutic anticoagulation appears to increase the risk of spinal hematoma formation, especially if combined with other anticoagulants or thrombolytics. Therefore, neuraxial blocks should be avoided in this clinical setting. If systematic anticoagulation therapy is begun with an epidural catheter in place, catheter removal should be delayed for 2 to 4 hours after discontinuation of heparin and after evaluation of coagulation status.[3]

There is no contradiction to the use of neuraxial techniques along with subcutaneous standard heparin therapy. The risk of neuraxial bleeding may be reduced by delaying the heparin injection until after the block and may be increased in debilitated patients or after prolonged therapy.[3]

Low Molecular Weight Heparin

LMWH was introduced for thromboprophylaxis following knee or hip arthroplasty. Extensive clinical testing and use of LMWH in Europe over the last 10 years has suggested no increased risk of spinal hematoma in patients undergoing neuraxial anesthesia while receiving LMWH thromboprophylaxis perioperatively. However, in the first 5 years after LMWH was released for general use in the United States in May 1993, more than 40 cases of spinal hematoma associated with neuraxial anesthesia administered in the presence of perioperative LMWH prophylaxis were reported.[4] Many of these events occurred when LMWH was administered intraoperatively or early postoperatively to patients undergoing continuous epidural anesthesia and analgesia. Concomitant antiplatelet therapy was present in several cases. The apparent difference in incidence in Europe compared to the United States may be a result of differences in dose and dosage schedule. Timing of catheter removal may also have an impact. Although the actual frequency of spinal hematoma in patients receiving enoxaparin while undergoing spinal or epidural anesthesia is difficult to determine, the incidence has been estimated to be 1 in 3,100 continuous epidural anesthetics and 1 in 41,000 spinal anesthetics.

Monitoring the anti-Xa level is not predictive of the risk of bleeding, and thus is not helpful in the management of patients undergoing neuraxial blocks.[4] Antiplatelet or oral anticoagulant medications administered in combination with LMWH may increase the risk of spinal hematoma.[4]

A single-dose spinal anesthetic may be the safest neuraxial technique in patients receiving preoperative LMWH. In these patients, needle placement should be done at least 10 to 12 hours after the LMWH dose. This is consistent with European regimens, where the first dose is administered 12 hours preoperatively. Patients receiving higher "treatment" doses of LMWH (e.g., enoxaparin 1 mg/kg twice daily) will require longer delays (24 hours). Neuraxial techniques should be avoided in patients receiving a dose of LMWH 2 hours preoperatively (i.e., general surgery patients), because needle placement occurs during peak anticoagulant activity.[4]

Patients with postoperative initiation of LMWH thromboprophylaxis may safely undergo single-dose and continuous catheter techniques. The first dose of LMWH should be administered no earlier than 24 hours postoperatively. In addition, it is recommended that indwelling catheters be removed before initiation of LMWH thromboprophylaxis.[4] The decision to implement LMWH therapy in the presence of an indwelling catheter must be made with care. Extreme vigilance of the patient's neurologic status is warranted. If epidural analgesia is anticipated to continue for more than 24 hours, LMWH administration may be delayed, or an alternate method of thromboprophylaxis may be selected (e.g., external pneumatic compression), based on the risk profile for the individual patient. These decisions should be made preoperatively to allow optimal management of both postoperative analgesia and thromboprophylaxis.[4]

For any LMWH prophylaxis regimen, timing of catheter removal is of paramount importance. Catheter removal should be delayed for at least 10 to 12 hours after a dose of LMWH. Subsequent dosing should be withheld for at least 2 hours after catheter removal.[4]

Oral Anticoagulants

Little data exist regarding the risk of spinal hematoma in patients with indwelling epidural catheters receiving anticoagulation with warfarin. Importantly, most clinicians recommend that except in extraordinary circumstances, spinal or epidural needle/catheter placement and removal should not be performed in fully anticoagulated patients.[5] Although neuraxial anesthesia, including postoperative epidural analgesia, may be safely performed in patients anticoagulated perioperatively with warfarin, the optimal duration of indwelling catheter use and the timing of its removal remain controversial. Variable patient response to warfarin anticoagulation is also well documented; a prothrombin time (PT) and corresponding international normalized ratio (INR) must be assessed daily to guide therapy.

Anesthetic management of patients anticoagulated perioperatively with warfarin depends on dosage and timing of initiation of therapy. PT and INR in patients on chronic oral anticoagulation will take 3 to 5 days to normalize after discontinuation of anticoagulant therapy. It is recommended that documentation of the patient's normal coagulation status be achieved before implementation of the neuraxial block.[5]

Often, the first dose of warfarin is administered the night before surgery. For these patients, the PT and INR should be checked before the neuraxial block if the first dose was given more than 24 hours earlier, or if a second dose of oral anticoagulant was administered. Patients receiving low-dose warfarin therapy during epidural analgesia should have their PT and INR monitored on a daily basis, and checked before catheter removal if the initial dose of warfarin was administered more than 36 hours beforehand. Initial studies evaluating the safety of epidural analgesia in association with oral anticoagulation used low-dose warfarin, with mean daily doses of approximately 5 mg. Higher-dose warfarin therapy may require more intensive monitoring of coagulation status. Reduced doses of warfarin should be given to patients who are likely to have an enhanced response to the drug. An INR greater than 3 should prompt the physician to withhold or reduce the warfarin dose in patients with indwelling neuraxial catheters. There is no definitive recommendation for removal of neuraxial catheters in patients with therapeutic levels of anticoagulation during a neuraxial catheter infusion. Caution must be exercised in making decisions about removing or maintaining these catheters.[5]

Table 124–1. Pharmacologic Activities of Anticoagulants, Antiplatelet Agents, and Thrombolytics

| Agent | Effect on Coagulation Variables | | Time to Peak Effect | Time to Normal Hemostasis After Discontinuation | Comments |
	PT	APTT			
Intravenous heparin	↑	↑↑↑	Minutes	4–6 hr	Monitor ACT and APTT, delay heparinization for 1 hour after needle placement.
Subcutaneous heparin	↑	↑↑	40–50 min	4–6 hr	APTT may remain normal; anti-Xa activity reflects degree of anticoagulation.
Low molecular weight heparin	—	—	3–5 hr	12+ hr	Anti-Xa activity not monitored. Use with caution in patients receiving epidural analgesia.
Warfarin	↑↑↑	↑	4–6 days (less with loading dose)	4–6 days	Monitor PT in patients with indwelling catheters.
Antiplatelet agents					
Aspirin	—	—	Hours	5–8 days	Bleeding time is not a reliable predictor of platelet function.
Other NSAIDs	—	—		1–3 days	
Thrombolytic agents	↑	↑	Minutes	1–2 days	Usually heparinized in addition. Monitor closely.
rt-PA					
Streptokinase	↑	↑			

PT = Prothrombin time; APTT = Activated partial thromboplastin time; ACT = Activated clotting time; ↑ = Clinically insignificant increase; ↑↑ = Possibly clinically significant increase; ↑↑↑ = Clinically significant increase; NSAID = Nonsteroidal anti-inflammatory drug; rt-PA = Recombinant tissue plasminogen activator.
From Horlocker and Wedel.[7]

Antiplatelet Medications

Antiplatelet medications are seldom used as primary agents of thromboprophylaxis. Although Vandermeulen et al[2] implicated antiplatelet therapy in 3 of the 61 cases of spinal hematoma occurring after spinal or epidural anesthesia, several large studies have demonstrated the relative safety of neuraxial blockade in both obstetric and surgical patients receiving these medications.

Ticlopidine and clopidogrel are also platelet aggregation inhibitors. These agents interfere with platelet-fibrinogen binding and subsequent platelet-platelet interactions. The effect is irreversible for the life of the platelet. Ticlopidine and clopidogel have no effect on platelet cyclooxygenase, acting independently of aspirin. However, these medications have not been tested in combination. The risk of spinal hematoma in patients receiving ticlopidine and clopidogel is unknown.

Antiplatelet drugs by themselves appear to represent no added significant risk for the development of spinal hematoma in patients having epidural or spinal anesthesia. However, the concurrent use of medications that affect other components of the clotting mechanisms, such as oral anticoagulants, standard heparin, and LMWH, may increase the risk of bleeding complications for patients receiving antiplatelet agents. Assessment of platelet function before performance of neuraxial block is not recommended.[6]

In summary, the decision to perform spinal or epidural anesthesia/analgesia and the timing of catheter removal in a patient receiving anticoagulants perioperatively should be made on an individual basis, weighing the definite (albeit small) risk of spinal hematoma with the benefits of regional anesthesia for a specific patient. The patient's coagulation status should be optimized at the time of spinal or epidural needle/catheter placement, and the level of anticoagulation must be carefully monitored during the period of epidural catheterization[7] (Table 124–1).

It is important to note that patients respond with variable sensitivities to anticoagulant medications. Indwelling catheters should not be removed in the presence of therapeutic anticoagulation, as this appears to significantly increase the risk of spinal hematoma. Patients should be closely monitored in the perioperative period for early signs of cord compression, such as severe back pain, progression of numbness or weakness, and bowel and bladder dysfunction. A delay in diagnosis may lead to irreversible cord ischemia. Significant neurologic recovery is unlikely if surgery is postponed more than 8 hours.[2]

Selected References

1. Tryba M. Epidural regional anesthesia and low molecular heparin: Pro. Anästh Intensivmed Notfallmed Schmerzther 1993;28:179–181.
2. Vandermeulen EP, Van Aken H, Vermylen J. Anticoagulants and spinal-epidural anesthesia. Anesth Analg 1994;79:1165–1177.
3. Liu SS, Mulroy MF. Neuraxial anesthesia and analgesia in the presence of standard heparin. Reg Anesth Pain Med 1998;23:157–163.

4. Horlocker TT, Wedel DJ. Neuraxial block and low molecular weight heparin: Balancing perioperative analgesia and thromboprophylaxis. Reg Anesth Pain Med 1998;23:164–177.

5. Enneking KF, Benzon HT. Oral anticoagulants and regional anesthesia: A perspective. Reg Anesth Pain Med 1998;23:140–145.

6. Urmey WF, Rowlingson JC. Do antiplatelet agents contribute to the development of perioperative spinal hematoma? Reg Anesth Pain Med 1998;23:146–151.

7. Horlocker TT, Wedel DJ. Anticoagulation and neuraxial block: Historical perspective, anesthetic implications, and risk management. Reg Anesth Pain Med 1998;23:129–134.

125
Upper Extremity Blocks

Denise J. Wedel, M.D.

Successful neural blockade of the upper extremity requires extensive anatomic knowledge of the brachial plexus from its origin as the roots emerge from the intervertebral foramina to its eventual termination in the distal peripheral nerves of the hand. Also important is a knowledge of the side effects and complications of peripheral nerve blocks in the upper extremity, as well as the clinical application of available local anesthetics for these blocks. Finally, one must not underestimate the role of appropriate sedation during placement of the block and during the surgical procedure.

Interscalene Block

The interscalene approach to the brachial plexus is best suited to surgery on the shoulder where a block of the cervical plexus is also desirable. Blockade of the inferior trunk (C8-T1) is often incomplete, requiring supplementation at the ulnar nerve for adequate surgical anesthesia in that distribution. Advantages of this block include technical ease because of easily palpated landmarks and the ability to perform the block with the arm in any position, which is especially important for cases involving upper extremity trauma or other painful conditions. Use of a nerve stimulator or elicitation of paresthesias is recommended with this technique to place the local anesthetic solution accurately.

Side Effects and Complications. Nerve damage or neuritis can occur secondary to needle trauma or pharmacologic toxicity, but is uncommon and usually self-limited. Local anesthetic toxicity as a result of intravascular injection should be guarded against by careful aspiration and incremental injection. The phrenic nerve is blocked in up to 100% of interscalene blocks, probably because of its anatomic proximity on the anterior surface of the anterior scalene muscle.[1] The patient may complain of subjective shortness of breath. Bilateral blocks at the interscalene are contraindicated. The risk of pneumothorax is low when the needle is correctly placed at the C5 or C6 level because of the distance from the dome of the pleura. Blockade of the vagus, recurrent laryngeal, and cervical sympathetic nerves, as well as epidural and intrathecal injections, have been reported during interscalene block. Reports of catastrophic nerve damage resulting from cord injection or high-dose spinal underscore that **this block should not be performed in a heavily sedated or anesthetized patient.**

Block Technique. With the patient in the supine position, the head is turned away from the side to be blocked. The lateral border of the sternocleidomastoid muscle is palpated and marked; identification is facilitated by having the patient lift his or her head briefly. The interscalene groove may be palpated by rolling the fingers posterolaterally from the muscle border, over the belly of the anterior scalene muscle. A line is extended laterally from the cricoid cartilage to intersect the vertical line of the interscalene groove; this represents the level of the C6 transverse process. The external jugular vein often crosses at this level, but is not a reliable anatomic landmark.

A 22-gauge, 4-cm, short-bevel needle is inserted perpendicular to skin with a 45-degree caudad and slightly posterior angle (Fig. 125–1). The needle is advanced until a paresthesia is obtained or, if a nerve stimulator is being used, a motor response is observed in the forearm or hand. The brachial plexus is usually quite superficial in the interscalene area (1 to 2 cm). A "click" may be felt as the blunt needle penetrates the prevertebral fascia, giving another confirmation of accurate needle location. If the needle encounters bone within 2 cm of the skin surface, this is likely transverse process, and the needle should be gently "walked off" anteriorly. After a test dose is given, 20 to 50 mL of local anesthetic is injected incrementally with frequent aspiration. Caudad spread of the local anesthetic may be facilitated by maintaining digital pressure proximal to the injection site and placing the patient in a head-up position during or following blockade.

Supraclavicular Block

Because of the compact arrangement of the trunks of the brachial plexus at the level of the first rib, the supraclavicular approach is extremely efficient; relatively small volumes of local anesthetic result in rapid and profound neural blockade when

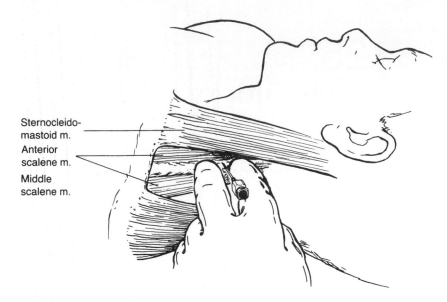

Sternocleido-
mastoid m.

Anterior
scalene m.

Middle
scalene m.

Figure 125–1. Interscalene block. The fingers palpate the interscalene groove, and the needle is inserted with a caudad and slightly posterior angle. (From Wedel DJ.[2])

injected accurately. The supraclavicular approach provides excellent surgical anesthesia for the elbow, forearm, and hand.

Side Effects and Complications. The major complication associated with supraclavicular blockade is pneumothorax, which usually presents in the postoperative period. Routine chest radiograph is not justified because of the delayed presentation. The incidence ranges from 0.5% to 6%, decreasing with the experience of the practitioner. Block of the phrenic (50% to 60%), recurrent laryngeal, and cervical sympathetic nerves are minor inconveniences requiring only reassurance. Nerve damage is uncommon and usually transient. Intravascular injection is largely preventable by careful technique, including the use of test doses, aspiration, and incremental injection.

Block Technique. The three trunks of the brachial plexus are compactly arranged cephaloposterior surrounding the subclavian artery at the level of the first rib, inferior to the clavicle at approximately its midpoint.

The patient is positioned in the supine position with the head turned away from the side to be blocked and the arm adducted and stretched as far as possible toward the ipsilateral knee. In the classic description, the midpoint of the clavicle is marked. The lateral border of the sternocleidomastoid muscle is identified (aided by the patient lifting the head), and the interscalene groove is palpated by rolling the fingers back from the muscle border over the anterior scalene muscle. A mark is then made 1.5 to 2.0 cm posterior to the clavicle at its midpoint within the interscalene groove. Palpation of the subclavian artery, if possible, provides further verification of the correct needle placement.

A 22-gauge, 4-cm, short-bevel needle is directed in a caudad, slightly medial, and posterior direction until a paresthesia or the first rib is encountered. This needle orientation lies in a plane parallel to a line joining the skin entry site and the patient's ear.

If the first rib is encountered before a paresthesia is elicited, then the needle can be walked anteriorly and posteriorly along the rib until a paresthesia or the subclavian artery is encountered (Fig. 125–2). If the artery is located, the needle should be redirected in a more posterolateral direction, a maneuver that usually results in elicitation of a paresthesia. A nerve stimulator can also be used to aid needle placement.

Axillary Block

The axillary approach to the brachial plexus is most commonly used because of its ease of perfor-

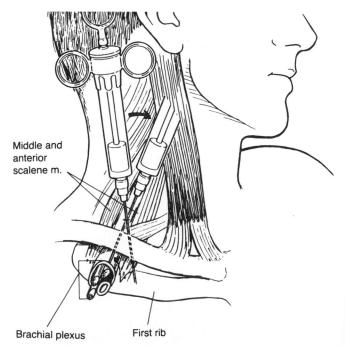

Middle and
anterior
scalene m.

Brachial plexus   First rib

Figure 125–2. Supraclavicular block. The needle is systematically walked anteriorly and posteriorly until the plexus is located. (From Wedel DJ.[2])

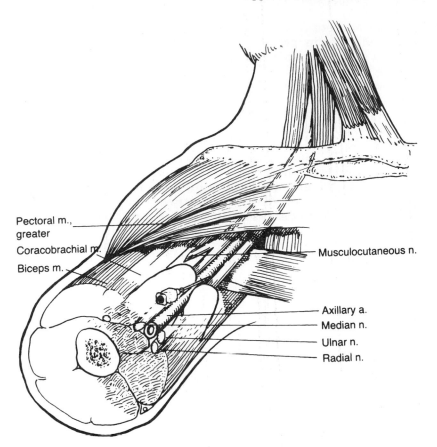

Figure 125–3. Axillary block. The arm is abducted at right angles to the body, and distal pressure is maintained during injection of the local anesthetic. (From Wedel DJ.[2])

Pectoral m., greater

Coracobrachial m.

Biceps m.

Musculocutaneous n.

Axillary a.
Median n.
Ulnar n.
Radial n.

mance, safety, and reliability, particularly for hand and forearm surgery. A variety of approaches to the axillary block have been described, including elicitation of paresthesias, transarterial injection, sheath blocks, and use of a nerve stimulator, and in experienced hands all seem to result in a reasonable success rate. Use of this technique is confined to patients who are able to abduct their arms sufficiently to allow access to the neurovascular bundle within the axilla. The musculocutaneous nerve may not always be blocked with this approach, but can be supplemented either at the level of the coracobrachialis muscle or as it courses superficially above the interepicondylar line at the elbow.

Side Effects and Complications. Because of the large volumes of local anesthetic often recommended for axillary blocks, the proximity of large blood vessels and the popularity of "immobile" needle techniques, local anesthetic toxicity from rapid uptake or intravascular injection may be a higher risk with this technique compared to other approaches to the brachial plexus. Frequent aspiration combined with incremental injection is an important feature of any method used in this block. Hematoma, sometimes with associated vascular compromise of the upper extremity, and infection are rare but reported complications. The assertion that paresthesia techniques are associated with a higher risk of neural complications has not been substantiated.

Block Technique. For all approaches to the ax-

illary block, the patient is positioned supine with the arm to be blocked abducted at right angles with the body and the elbow flexed to 90°. The axillary artery is palpated as close to the axillary crease as possible, and a line is drawn tracing its course distally. The artery is fixed against the humerus at the level of the axillary crease by the index and middle fingers of the nondominant hand. Placement of the needle proximal to the fingers along with maintenance of distal pressure encourages proximal spread of the local anesthetic solution, increasing the likelihood of blocking the musculocutaneous nerve (Fig. 125–3).

Paresthesia techniques involve elicitation of single or multiple paresthesias with a small gauge (22- to 25-g), 2-cm needle. A minimum volume of 10 ml local anesthetic is carefully injected at each paresthesia.

Nerve stimulator techniques can be used using a Teflon-coated (insulated) needle and commercially available nerve stimulators. This technique avoids sensory paresthesias, but requires additional equipment.

Sheath techniques are advocated by those experts who downplay the anatomical relevance of the multicompartmental nature of the axillary sheath. In this technique, a short-bevel needle is slowly advanced in proximity to the axillary artery until a "fascial click" is felt. At this point, the total volume of local anesthetic is injected after negative aspiration. This technique is associated with a slow and often incomplete onset of surgical anesthesia, but is quite effective in pediatric axillary blocks where patient cooperation may be absent and heavy sedation is often required.

Transarterial techniques have been described involving placement of a sharp needle through the axillary artery and injecting local anesthetic (40 to 50 mL) behind the artery, or in some descriptions dividing the total volume behind and superior to the artery. Obviously, great care must be taken to avoid intravascular injection with this technique.

Side Effects and Complications. As in other approaches to the brachial plexus, intravascular injection is a risk necessitating standard precautions as described earlier. Persistent paresthesias are usually self-limited and rarely result in permanent nerve damage.

Selected References

1. Urmey WF, Talts KH, Sharrock NE. One hundred percent incidence of hemidiaphragmatic paresis associated with interscalene brachial plexus anesthesia as diagnosed by ultrasonography. Anesth Analg 1991;72:498–503.
2. Wedel DJ. Nerve blocks. In Miller RD, ed. Anesthesia. 5th ed. New York: Churchill Livingstone, 2000:1520–1548.

Suggested References

Brown DL, Bridenbaugh PO. The upper extremity: Somatic blockade. In Cousins MJ, Bridenbaugh PO, eds. Neural Blockade in Clinical Anesthesia and Management of Pain. 3rd ed. Philadelphia: Lippincott-Raven, 1998:345–372.

Thompson GE, Rorie DK. Functional anatomy of the brachial plexus sheaths. Anesthesiology 1983;59:117–122.

126
Lower Extremity Blocks

Denise J. Wedel, M.D.

Blocks of the lower extremity have not achieved the popularity and widespread clinical application of upper extremity block techniques. One explanation for this difference lies in the well-accepted safety and efficacy of centroneuraxis blocks for lower extremity surgery. Furthermore, unlike the brachial plexus, the nerves supplying the lower extremity are not anatomically clustered where they can be easily blocked with a relatively superficial injection of local anesthetic. Because of the anatomic considerations, these blocks are technically more difficult and require more training and practice to acquire expertise. Finally, persistent block of any of the major nerves of the lower extremity makes the patient unable to ambulate, an unacceptable side effect in the outpatient population.

Nonetheless, there are advantages associated with nerve blocks of the lower extremity, and these techniques are gaining in popularity, due in part to the increased use of antithrombotic agents. Peripheral blockade is rarely associated with morbidity due to hematoma formation, even in anticoagulated patients. In addition, surgical anesthesia can be provided in one limb without complete sympathectomy, in contrast to centroneuraxis block. Peripheral nerve blocks of the lower extremity usually result in a prolonged duration of anesthesia, especially if long-acting agents are used, thus providing excellent postoperative pain relief for selected patients.

Femoral Nerve Block

Anatomy. The femoral nerve is formed within the psoas major muscle by the posterior divisions of L2–L4, emerges from the lateral border of that muscle, and descends in the groove between the psoas and iliacus muscles. It enters the thigh lateral to the femoral artery and divides into anterior and posterior branches distal to the inguinal ligament. The femoral nerve supplies the anterior compartment muscles of the thigh (quadriceps, sartorius) and skin of the anterior thigh from the inguinal ligament to the knee. Below the knee, it supplies sensation to the medial side of the leg extending to the big toe in the distribution of the saphenous nerve.

Clinical Applications. Because of its limited sensory distribution, the femoral nerve block is usually combined with other peripheral blocks in clinical practice. However, it can be used alone for muscle biopsies of the quadriceps muscle or other surgical procedures limited to the anterior thigh, and its use has been described for anesthetic management of knee arthroscopy and surgical repair of fractures of the mid-femoral shaft.

Side Effects and Complications. The proximity of the femoral artery to this nerve may increase the risk of hematoma and intravascular injection. However, anatomically the nerve and artery are located in a separate sheaths approximately 1 cm apart. In most patients with normal anatomy, the femoral artery can be easily palpated, allowing correct, safe needle positioning lateral to the pulsation. Blockade of the femoral nerve should probably be avoided in patients who have undergone femoral vascular grafts, in whom the distorted anatomy increases the risk of excessive bleeding or infection. Nerve damage from needle trauma or drug toxicity is an unlikely complication from this block.

Description of the Technique of Femoral Nerve Block. With the patient in the supine position, a line representing the inguinal ligament is drawn between the palpated anterior superior iliac crest and the pubic tubercle. A second line is drawn at right angles to the inguinal ligament, representing the femoral artery. A 22-gauge, 3- to 5-cm, short-beveled needle is advanced until a paresthesia is obtained (Fig. 126–1A). A nerve stimulator may also be used to correctly place the needle. Arterial pulsations transmitted to the hub of the needle from the femoral artery can often be observed when the needle is in position. Then, after negative aspiration, 10 to 20 mL of local anesthetic solution is injected incrementally through the needle, including 5 to 10 mL of solution injected fan-wise laterally to block branches of the femoral nerve, which can divide high at the level of the inguinal ligament.

Lateral Femoral Cutaneous Nerve Block

Anatomy. The lateral femoral cutaneous nerve arises from L2–L3 emerging at the lateral border of

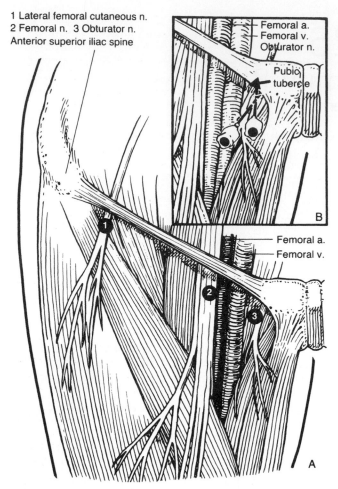

1 Lateral femoral cutaneous n.
2 Femoral n. 3 Obturator n.
Anterior superior iliac spine

Femoral a.
Femoral v.
Obturator n.

Pubic
tubercle

B

Femoral a.
Femoral v.

A

Figure 126–1. *A,* Anatomic landmarks for lateral femoral cutaneous, femoral, and obturator nerve blocks. *B,* Obturator nerve block. The needle is walked off the inferior pubic ramus in a medial and cephalad direction until it passes into the obturator canal. (From Wedel DJ.[1])

the psoas muscle inferior to the ilioinguinal nerve. It courses beneath the iliac fascia and enters the thigh deep in the inguinal ligament 1 to 2 cm medial to the anterior superior iliac spine. The nerve emerges from the fascia lata 7 to 10 cm caudad to the spine and divides into anterior and posterior branches. The anterior branches supply the skin of the anterolateral thigh to the knee, and the posterior branch supplies the skin of the lateral thigh from the hip to the midthigh.

Clinical Applications. This block is usually combined with other lower extremity blocks; however, it can provide adequate anesthesia for superficial procedures involving the skin of the anterolateral thigh such as skin graft harvests. It is an important part of lower extremity blockade when a thigh tourniquet is used.

Side Effects and Complications. Neuritis of this nerve secondary to needle trauma or drug toxicity is a potential but unlikely complication. Because there are no large blood vessels in the vicinity of this nerve, the likelihood of rapid uptake or intravascular injection is very small.

Description of the Technique of Lateral Femoral Cutaneous Nerve Block. The anterior superior iliac spine is palpated and a mark made at a point 2 cm medial and 2 cm caudad to this landmark. Using sterile technique, a 4-cm, 22-gauge, short-bevel needle is advanced through a skin wheal in an orientation perpendicular to the skin. As the needle is advanced, the fascia lata is encountered at a depth of 1 to 3 cm, with a sudden release indicating passage through this structure. Local anesthetic (10 to 20 mL) is injected above and below the fascia at several points as the needle is slowly moved fan-wise laterally and medially (see Fig. 125–1A).

The success rate of this block can be increased by depositing an additional 10 mL of solution just medial and posterior to the anterior superior iliac crest. The needle is advanced to the medial edge of the spine and then redirected to walk underneath the spine. The lateral femoral cutaneous nerve is a pure sensory nerve, so a nerve stimulator is not helpful in performing this block. Paresthesias may be elicited during needle placement; these confirm that the needle depth is correct.

Obturator Nerve Block

Anatomy. The obturator nerve is derived primarily from L3–L4, with variable minor contributions from L2. It lies deep in the obturator canal after descending from the medial psoas muscle border. It forms anterior and posterior branches as it leaves the obturator canal. The anterior branch supplies an articular branch to the hip, the anterior adductor muscles, and a variable cutaneous branch to the lower medial thigh. The posterior branch supplies the deep adductor muscles with a variable articular branch to the knee.

Clinical Applications. Usually the obturator nerve is blocked as part of regional anesthesia for knee surgery. Because it is primarily a motor nerve, it is rarely blocked on its own, although obturator nerve block can be useful in treating or diagnosing the extent of adductor spasm in patients with cerebral palsy and other muscle or neurologic diseases affecting the lower extremities before surgical intervention (adductor tenotomy).

Side Effects and Complications. Because of the deep location of the nerve in the obturator canal, this is a difficult block to learn and perform. An inadequate blockade of this nerve can mar an otherwise elegant regional anesthetic for knee surgery. The obturator canal contains vascular and neural structures, increasing the potential risk of intravascular injection or nerve damage.

Description of the Technique of Obturator Nerve Block. With the patient in the supine position, a mark is made 1 to 2 cm lateral and 1 to 2 cm caudad to the palpated pubic tubercle. Using sterile technique, a skin wheal is raised and a 22-

gauge, 8- to 10-cm, short-bevel needle is advanced slightly medially toward the pubic tubercle. Usually the inferior pubic ramus will be encountered at a depth of 2 to 4 cm. At that point the needle is walked medially and cephalad in small steps until it drops into the obturator canal. The obturator nerve is located 2 to 3 cm past the point of contact with the pubic ramus (Fig. 125–1A and 1B). After negative aspiration, 10 to 15 mL of local anesthetic solution is injected. A nerve stimulator is very useful for accurate location of this motor nerve; a twitch will be observed in the medial thigh adductor muscles as the needle approaches the obturator nerve.

Perivascular Technique ("3-in-1 Block")

The perivascular technique is based on the premise that injection of a large volume of local anesthetic within the femoral canal while holding distal pressure will result in proximal spread of the solution into the psoas compartment, resulting in a lumbar plexus block. The key anatomical assumption is that the fascial sheath surrounding the lumbar roots extends into the femoral canal and acts as an enclosed conduit for the spread of local anesthetic solutions.

Surface landmarks are described under femoral nerve block. Using sterile precautions, a skin wheal is made 1 cm lateral to the femoral artery and 2 cm distal to the inguinal ligament. A 22-gauge, 5-cm, short-bevel needle is advanced in the cephalad direction at a 30° to 45° angle to skin until a paresthesia is obtained. Alternatively, a nerve stimulator can be used to locate the femoral nerve. Once the needle is correctly located, firm pressure is applied just distal to the skin entry with the fingers of the other hand while the needle is held immobile. A total of 20 to 40 mL of local anesthetic is injected incrementally following negative aspiration. Reportedly reliable anesthesia of the femoral and lateral femoral cutaneous nerves is achieved with 20 mL of solution, whereas obturator nerve block requires volumes greater than 30 mL.

Sciatic Nerve

Anatomy. The sciatic nerve derives from L4–L5 and S1–S3. It is a large peripheral nerve with a width of 2 cm. It exits the pelvis with the posterior cutaneous nerve of the thigh, passes through the sacrosciatic foramen beneath the piriformis muscle, and courses between the greater trochanter of the femur and the ischial tuberosity. At the lower border of the gluteus maximus muscle, the sciatic nerve becomes superficial as it begins its descent down the posterior thigh toward the popliteal fossa. The sciatic nerve supplies sensation to the largest area of the lower extremity including the posterior thigh and everything below the knee, with the exception of a thin medial strip supplied by the saphenous nerve (terminal branch of the femoral nerve).

Clinical Applications. Because of its wide sensory distribution, the sciatic nerve block can be used alone for any surgery below the knee that does not require a thigh tourniquet. It can also be combined with other peripheral nerve blocks to provide anesthesia for surgical procedures involving the thigh and knee. This form of anesthesia avoids the sympathectomy associated with centroneuraxis blocks, and thus its use may be advantageous in cases where any shift in hemodynamics might be deleterious, such as patients with significant aortic stenosis.

Side Effects and Complications. Sciatic nerve block is technically difficult and can be quite painful. Adequate sedation is an important component if this procedure is to meet with patient and surgeon satisfaction; however, in the classic approach the patient is in a lateral position, which may complicate airway management during sedation. Hematoma formation and nerve damage are potential risks. Because of the large area of blockade with sciatic nerve block, vasodilation with venous pooling will occur in the affected extremity. Thus, although the risk is lower than with centroneuroaxis blocks, sciatic nerve block may be associated with hemodynamic changes in patients with decreased intravascular volume or low cardiac outputs.

Description of the Technique of Sciatic Nerve Block: Classic Approach of Labat (Posterior). The patient is positioned laterally, with the leg to be blocked fully flexed and rolled forward so that the heel of the upper (operative) leg rests on the knee of the dependent (nonoperative) leg, which is stretched out in a straight line with the torso (Fig. 126–2). A line is drawn between the palpated posterior superior iliac spine and the greater trochanter of the femur. This line is bisected with a perpendicular line extending approximately 5 cm caudad. Now a line is drawn between the

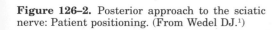

Figure 126–2. Posterior approach to the sciatic nerve: Patient positioning. (From Wedel DJ.[1])

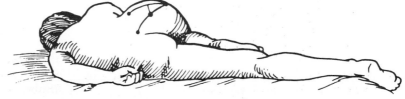

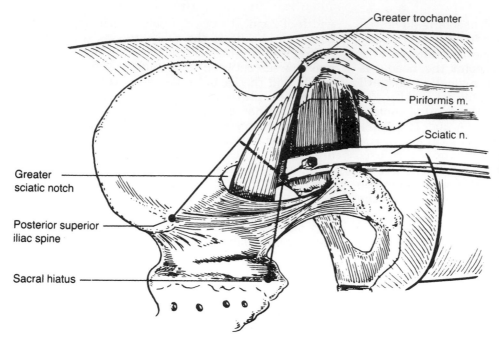

Figure 126–3. Anatomic landmarks for the posterior approach to sciatic nerve block. (From Wedel DJ.[1])

greater trochanter of the femur and the sacral hiatus, which will cross the perpendicular at a point 3 to 5 cm along the line. This represents the point of needle insertion. Using sterile technique, a 22-gauge, 10- to 12-cm, short-bevel needle is advanced perpendicular to the skin until a paresthesia is elicited or bone is encountered (Fig. 126–3). If bone is contacted, the needle is redirected to systematically

sweep in a lateral-medial direction until the nerve is located. A nerve stimulator is helpful in ascertaining the correct needle position. When the sciatic nerve is located, 25 to 30 mL of local anesthetic solution is injected.

Description of the Technique of Sciatic Nerve Block: Anterior Approach. This technique is useful for situations where the patient cannot be positioned for the classic posterior approach because of pain or lack of cooperation. The femoral nerve is blocked first, making this approach more comfortable for the patient.

The patient is placed in the supine position and a line drawn between the anterior superior iliac spine and the pubic tubercle, representing the inguinal ligament. This line is trisected, and a second parallel line is drawn from the point of the tuberosity of the greater trochanter of the hip. The intersection of this second line with the more medial of the perpendicular lines represents the point of needle entry (Fig. 126–4). Using sterile technique, a 22-gauge, 10- to 12-cm, short-bevel needle is advanced with a slight lateral angulation until the lesser trochanter of the hip is encountered. At this point, the needle is redirected slightly medially, walked off the femur, and advanced until a paresthesia is elicited, (approximately 5 cm past bone). A total of 20 to 25 mL of local anesthetic solution is injected incrementally after careful aspiration. A nerve stimulator is useful for locating the sciatic nerve in this technique.

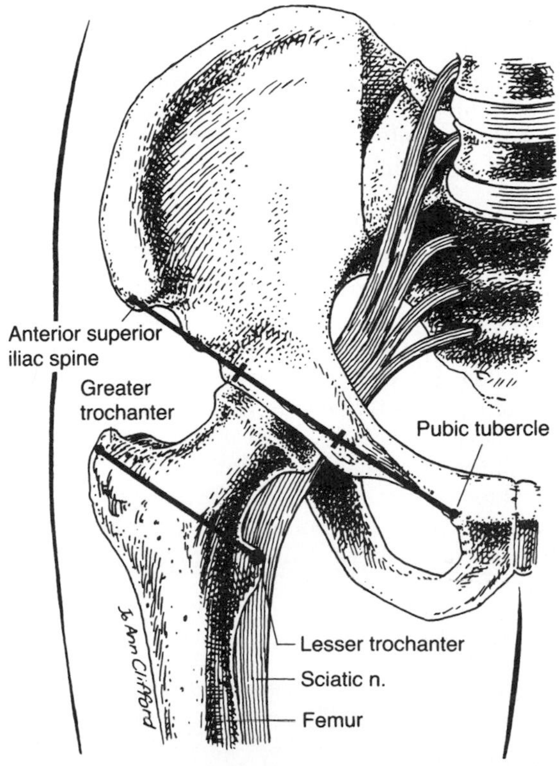

Psoas Compartment Block

Anatomy. The lumbar plexus lies in a fascial compartment between the psoas and the quadratus lumborum muscles at the level of L4-5.

Figure 126–4. Anatomic landmarks for the anterior approach to sciatic nerve block. (From Wedel DJ.[1])

Clinical Applications. All of the blocks discussed so far are peripheral nerve blocks. The psoas compartment block is a block of the lumbar plexus at the level of L4. This block was first described as a means of providing anesthesia to the hip flexors and the lower extremity through a single needle insertion. It has never been extremely popular because of the lack of definitive landmarks, the possibility of epidural spread, and the availability of other blocks. Recently, stimulating needles of the appropriate length have become more readily available, making this block technically easier than when first described. It may enjoy a renaissance of interest as practitioners search for a means of providing continuous postoperative pain relief away from the central neuraxis in patients receiving anticoagulation therapy.

Side Effects and Complications. The depth of needle insertion and location of the plexus increase the risk of epidural or spinal injection. Frequent aspiration and use of a test dose are important safeguards. In addition, nerve damage can occur.

Description of Technique. With the patient in the lateral position, knees tucked on the chest, the L4 spinous process is identified. A point 3 cm caudal and 5 cm lateral is marked. A 6-inch insulated epidural needle is inserted at the mark perpendicularly until the transverse process of L5 is encountered. The needle is then redirected cephalad until it passes the transverse process. A glass syringe can then be attached to the needle to identify a loss of resistance between the quadratus lumborum and the psoas. This usually is felt at a depth of 12 cm. Alternatively, a stimulating needle can be used, searching for quadriceps motion as the lumbar plexus is encountered. When the plexus has been identified, 20 to 25 mL of local anesthetic is injected to ensure adequate spread, or a catheter can be introduced for continuous infusion.

Selected References

1. Wedel DJ. Nerve blocks. In Miller RD, ed. Anesthesia. 5th ed. New York: Churchill Livingstone, 2000:1520–1548.
2. Bridenbaugh PO, Wedel DJ. The lower extremity: Somatic blockade. In Cousins MJ and Bridenbaugh PO, ed. Neural Blockade. 3rd ed. New York: Lippincott-Raven, 1998: 373–394.
3. Winnie AP, Ramamurthy S, Durrani Z. The inguinal paravascular technique of lumbar plexus anesthesia: The "3-in-1 block." Anesth Analg 1973;52:989–996.

127
Lower Extremity Block: Psoas Compartment Block

C. Jankowski, M.D.

The psoas compartment block (PCB) is a block of the lumbar plexus done through a posterior approach. It was first described in 1976. Initially, it did not achieve widespread use, because the loss-of-resistance technique first described was technically difficult and unreliable. The advent of uncomplicated nerve stimulator techniques has made PCBs easier to place and much more reliable. Further, PCB has been shown to be more effective at blocking the lateral femoral cutaneous and obturator nerves than anterior approaches to the lumbar plexus, such as Winnie's "3-in-1" block. This, along with recent enthusiasm for peripheral nerve blocks as primary and adjunct anesthetics and for postoperative analgesia, has renewed interest in PCBs.

Anatomy

The lumbar plexus arises from the ventral rami of L1–L4, with variable contributions from T12. It lies in a fascial compartment between the psoas and quadratus lumborum muscles (Fig. 127–1). The lumbar plexus gives rise to the femoral (L2-4), lateral femoral cutaneous (L2-3), obturator (L2-3), genitofemoral (L1-2), ilioinguinal (L1), and iliohypogastric (L1) nerves. It provides sensory innervation to the anterior thigh and to the medial portion of the lower leg via the saphenous nerve, a distal branch of the femoral nerve. It also provides sensory innervation to the bulk of the femur, ischium, and ilium.

Clinical Applications

The PCB has a variety of clinical applications. It can be used as the primary anesthetic for diagnostic knee arthroscopy and quadriceps muscle biopsy. However, it does not block the sciatic nerve, and

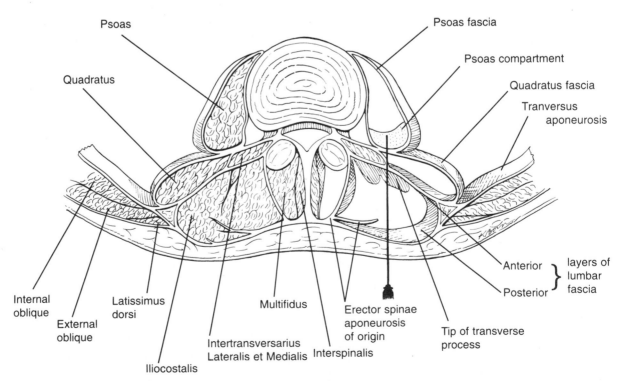

Figure 127–1. Cross-section at the level of L4-L5, illustrating the psoas compartment, within which lies the lumbar plexus. (From Ayers J, Enneking FK.[1])

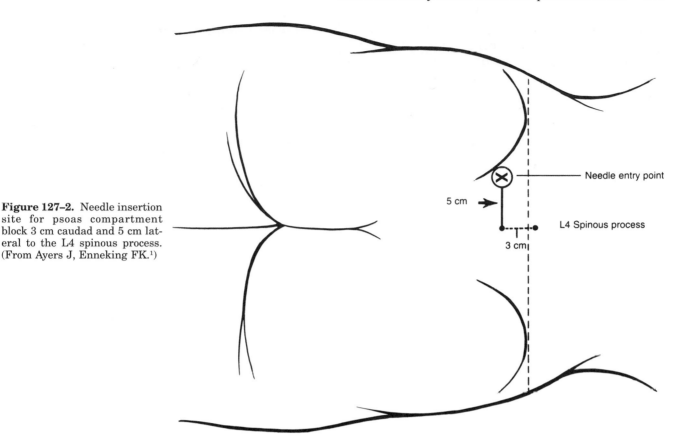

Figure 127–2. Needle insertion site for psoas compartment block 3 cm caudad and 5 cm lateral to the L4 spinous process. (From Ayers J, Enneking FK.[1])

will not provide sufficient anesthesia for most other lower extremity procedures. It can be used as a primary anesthetic for other lower extremity procedures when combined with a sciatic nerve block. This approach provides the advantages of a regional technique while avoiding the pitfalls of neuraxial blockade.

PCBs are useful for postoperative analgesia, especially in those for whom regional analgesia is indicated, but a neuraxial technique is not desirable. Both single-shot and continuous infusion techniques have been used. Specific procedures for which PCB have been used to provide postoperative analgesia include total knee arthroplasty, anterior cruciate ligament repair, total hip arthroplasty, and femoral procedures.

Finally, PCBs have been used for neurolytic procedures. Despite the large number of motor fibers in the lumbar plexus, motor block does not seem to be a significant problem with this approach.

Technique

A variety of techniques have been used for PCBs. The most reliable involve using a nerve stimulator. The patient is positioned laterally. The knees are drawn to the chest. The iliac crests are identified, and a line is drawn between them. This should be at the level of the L4 spinous process. The L4 spinous

process is identified. A mark is made 5 cm lateral and 3 cm caudad from the spinous process (Fig. 127–2). This is the site of needle insertion. An insulated needle is inserted perpendicular to the skin until the L5 transverse process is contacted. Using a current of 1 mA, the needle is "walked off" the transverse process in a slightly medial and cephalad manner until a quadriceps (femoral nerve) or adductor (obturator nerve) twitch is obtained or a lateral femoral cutaneous nerve paresthesia is elicited. Final needle depth is 8 to 11 cm. The needle location is refined so that a response is present with a current of ≤0.5 mA. Then 30 mL of local anesthetic solution is injected in 5-mL increments, with aspiration between each increment. Because the obturator nerve is the most medial, injection on an adductor twitch may increase the risk of epidural spread.

An alternate approach involves marking the intercristal line and a perpendicular line from the original line to the posterior superior iliac spine. The needle is inserted at the intersection of the lines, perpendicular to the skin in all planes. Twitches are elicited as described earlier.

Side Effects and Complications

As with most peripheral nerve blocks, hematoma, infection, persistent paresthesias, and local anesthetic toxicity are potential complications of PCB. Epidural spread of local anesthetic can occur, causing block of the contralateral leg. This typically occurs with local anesthetic volumes in excess of 30 mL or when the needle is placed too far medially. Subarachnoid injection of local anesthetic also can occur, bringing with it the possibility of total spinal.

Suggested References

1. Ayers J, Enneking FK. Continuous lower extremity techniques. Tech Reg Anesth 1999;3:47–57.
2. Farny J, Drolet P, Girard M. Anatomy of the posterior approach to the lumbar plexus. Can J Anaesth 1994;41:480–485.
3. Patt RB, Cousins MJ. Techniques for neurolytic neural blockade. In Cousin MJ, Bridenbaugh PO, eds. Neural Blockade in Clinical Anesthesia and Management of Pain. 3rd ed. Philadelphia: Lippincott-Raven, 1998;1007–1061.

128
Nerve Block at the Ankle

Douglas A. Dubbink, M.D.

Anesthesia distal to the ankle is accomplished by interrupting five major nerve trunks:

- Tibial nerve (posterior tibial nerve) (L4-5, S1-3).
- Sural nerve, consisting of a branch from the tibial nerve and one from the common peroneal nerve.
- Deep peroneal nerve (anterior tibial nerve) (L4-5, S1-2).
- Superficial peroneal nerve (L4-5, S1-2).
- Saphenous nerve, the sensory branch of the femoral nerve (L2-4).

The ankle block is a relatively easy block to learn if the anatomy is well understood. Ankle blocks can be effective for nearly any surgical procedure of the foot. Major complications are rare; however, prolonged paresthesias have been reported.

Technique

The **tibial nerve** supplies the sole and plantar portions of the toes up to the nails. It lies behind the posterior tibial artery anteromedial to the Achilles tendon and deep to the flexor retinaculum, which must be penetrated for a successful block (Fig. 128–1).

- A skin wheal is raised medial to the Achilles tendon at the level of the upper border of the medial malleolus.
- A 3- to 5-cm, 22- or 25-g needle is directed at right angles to the tibia. The needle tip is slowly advanced until a paresthesia is elicited (a nerve stimulator can be used) or bone is contacted. At this point, 5 to 7 mL of local anesthetic is injected near the posterior aspect of the tibia with an equal volume injected during withdrawal of the needle to the skin surface if a paresthesia is not elicited.

The **sural nerve** is a superficial nerve that provides cutaneous sensation to the lower posterolateral ankle, lateral foot, and fifth toe.

- This nerve is blocked by subcutaneous infiltration from the lateral malleolus to the Achilles tendon at the level of the upper border of the lateral malleolus.

- A total of 5 to 10 mL of local anesthetic should be sufficient.

The **deep peroneal**, **superficial peroneal**, and **saphenous** nerves can all be blocked using a single injection site.

The **deep peroneal** nerve courses midway between the malleoli before assuming its position between the anterior tibial tendon and the extensor hallucis longus tendon beneath the extensor retinaculum at the dorsum of the foot. It innervates the short extensors of the toes and provides skin sensation to the interdigital cleft between the great and second toes.

- While the patient dorsiflexes the foot, the tendons of the anterior tibial and extensor hallucis longus muscles can be readily identified at a level just

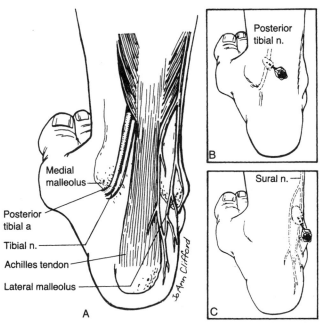

Figure 128–1. A, Anatomic landmarks for block of the posterior tibial and sural nerves at the ankle. B, Posterior tibial nerve: method of needle placement for block at the ankle. C, Sural nerve: method of needle placement for block at the ankle. (From Wedel DJ.[1])

319

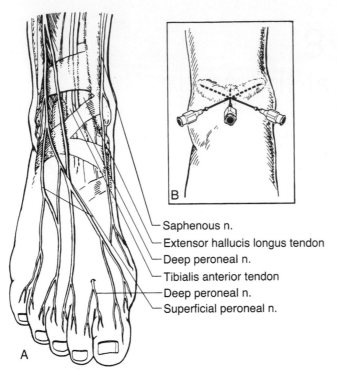

Saphenous n.
Extensor hallucis longus tendon
Deep peroneal n.
Tibialis anterior tendon
Deep peroneal n.
Superficial peroneal n.

Figure 128–2. *A,* Anatomic landmarks for block of the deep peroneal, superficial peroneal, and saphenous nerves at the ankle. *B,* Method of needle placement for block of the deep peroneal, superficial peroneal, and saphenous nerves through a single needle entry site. (From Wedel DJ.[1])

□ A 25-g, 3- to 5-cm needle is inserted perpendicular to skin, as depicted in Figure 128–2. A loss of resistance will often be felt during passage through the extensor retinaculum.

□ Between 3 and 5 mL of local anesthetic is usually adequate.

The **superficial peroneal nerve** supplies cutaneous sensation to the dorsum of the foot and toes (except between great and second toes).

□ The superficial peroneal nerve can be blocked by injecting local anesthetic subcutaneously laterally from the site of injection of the deep peroneal nerve toward the superior aspect of the lateral malleolus using 5 to 10 mL of solution.

The **saphenous nerve** runs anterior to the medial malleolus near the long saphenous vein to supply cutaneous innervation to the anteromedial side of the lower leg and medial foot midway to the toes.

□ The saphenous nerve is blocked with 3 to 5 mL of local anesthetic injected subcutaneously medially from the site of injection of the deep peroneal nerve toward the saphenous vein.

Selected Reference

1. Wedel DJ. Nerve blocks. In Miller RD, ed. Anesthesia. 5th ed. Philadelphia: Churchill Livingstone, 2000:1520–1548.

Suggested References

Adriani J. Labat's Regional Anesthesia: Techniques and Clinical Applications. 4th ed. St. Louis, Warren H Green, 1985.
McMinn RMH, Hutchings RT. Color Atlas of Human Anatomy. Chicago, Year Book Medical, 1992.

above a line connecting the malleoli. Often the pulsation of the anterior tibial (dorsalis pedis) artery will be felt. The nerve lies lateral to the artery and deep to the extensor retinaculum.

129
Retrobulbar Blocks

Michael P. Hosking, M.D.

Anatomy

The **ciliary ganglion**, a parasympathetic ganglion 1 to 2 mm in diameter, is located approximately 1 cm from the posterior boundary of the orbit between the lateral surface of the optic nerve and the ophthalmic artery. Parasympathetic fibers originating in the oculomotor nerve and postganglionic fibers supply the ciliary body and sphincter pupillae muscles. The **nasociliary nerve**, a branch of the ophthalmic nerve, supplies the sensory innervation of the cornea, iris, and ciliary body via the short ciliary nerves, 6 to 10 small filaments accompanying the ciliary arteries. Retrobulbar block primarily involves the ciliary ganglion, ciliary nerves, and cranial nerves II, III, and VI. Cranial nerve IV is not affected, because it lies outside the muscle cone (Figs. 129–1 and 129–2).[1,2]

Technique for Retrobulbar Block

In the adult, the distance to the ciliary ganglion from the skin is approximately 3.5 cm. Accordingly, a 25-gauge, 35-mm needle is typically used to minimize the risk of the needle passing beyond the ciliary ganglion and puncturing vessels in the retrobulbar apex.

- □ Palpate the inferolateral margin of the orbit and make a skin wheal.
- □ Ask the patient to look straight ahead. (Recently, ophthalmologists have cautioned against the conventional upward and inward positioning of the eye, because this places the routine needle path in close proximity to the optic nerve, and ophthalmic artery and vein.)
- □ Make the injection through the skin at the junction of the lateral and middle thirds of the inferior orbital rim.
- □ Advance slowly. The needle should penetrate only the retrobulbar fat and intermuscular septum. Resistance may indicate that the needle is in muscle, the optic nerve, or the wall of the eye; withdraw and redirect.
- □ Advance to 35 mm.

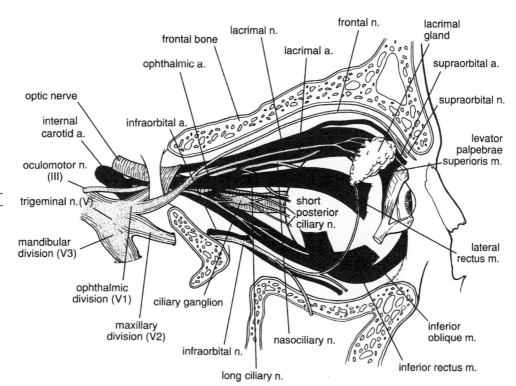

Figure 129–1. Orbital anatomy as seen from the lateral approach. (From Dutton JJ.[1])

lacrimal n.

frontal n.

lacrimal gland

frontal bone

ophthalmic a.

lacrimal a.

supraorbital a.

optic nerve

supraorbital n.

internal carotid a.

infraorbital a.

levator palpebrae superioris m.

oculomotor n. (III)

trigeminal n.(V)

short posterior ciliary n.

mandibular division (V3)

lateral rectus m.

ophthalmic division (V1)

ciliary ganglion

inferior oblique m.

maxillary division (V2)

nasociliary n.

infraorbital n.

inferior rectus m.

long ciliary n.

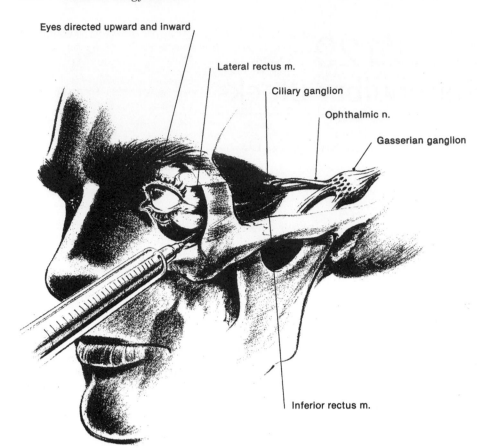

Eyes directed upward and inward

Lateral rectus m.

Ciliary ganglion

Ophthalmic n.

Gasserian ganglion

Inferior rectus m.

Figure 129–2. Retrobulbar block is performed by blocking the ciliary ganglion and nerves in the posterior muscle cone. Although the figure depicts a traditional upward, inward eye position, a straight-ahead gaze is now the usual preferred eye position to decrease the risk of injury to the optic nerve or ophthalmic artery or vein. (From Katz J.[2])

□ Aspirate. If negative, slowly inject 2 to 4 mL of local anesthetic solution over 20 to 30 seconds.

□ Ask the patient to close the eye and gently massage it intermittently for 3 to 4 minutes.

□ Observe the eye for proptosis or blood in lower fornix, which indicates retrobulbar hemorrhage.

□ Treat hemorrhage with firm pressure and massage. This complication may necessitate cancellation of surgery.

Local Anesthetic Agents

The most commonly used agents are a 1:1 mixture of 2% lidocaine with 0.5% or 0.75% bupivacaine. Some advise use of epinephrine or hyaluronidase.

Oculocardiac Reflex

Bradycardia, junctional rhythm, or asystole secondary to traction on the eye and ocular musculature is termed the oculocardiac reflex (OCR). Serious morbidity secondary to OCR has decreased because of increased knowledge and more aggressive treatment. Atropine or glycopyrrolate can be used for treatment or for prophylaxis. OCR can occur in an empty orbit from extraocular muscle stimulation. Hypoxia, hypercarbia, and light anes-

thesia potentiate this reflex. Retrobulbar block does not guarantee attenuation of this reflex; thus eye massage must be done carefully after the block is placed.

□ **Afferent pathway**: Ciliary ganglion to the ophthalmic division of the trigeminal nerve to the gasserian ganglion to the main trigeminal sensory nucleus fourth ventricle.

□ **Efferent pathway**: Vagus nerve.

Other complications are discussed in Chapter 223.

Peribulbar Anesthesia

Another technique that will produce orbital anesthesia has been described by Davis and Mandel.[3] This technique involves injections above and below the orbit, with local anesthetic deposited in and behind the orbicularis oculi muscle and beneath, above, and behind the globe. The potential for intraocular or intradural injection is decreased because the anesthetic is deposited outside the muscle cone. The risk of intraconal hemorrhage and direct optic nerve injury is also decreased. Davis and Mandel[3] reported no apparent complications in more than 1,600 cases using this technique.

Complications

Retrobulbar Hemorrhage. The **most common complication**, retrobulbar hemorrhage occurs secondary to puncture of the vessels within the retrobulbar space. It is characterized by simultaneous appearance of an excellent motor block of the globe, closing of the upper lid, proptosis, and a palpable increase in IOP. Many retrobulbar hemorrhages are minimal or even subclinical, and on rare occasions, surgery may be continued. But because of the significant risk of repeat hemorrhage with its devastating complications, surgery often must be postponed.

Oculocardiac Reflex. An oculocardiac reflex (see Chap. 223) manifested by bradycardia, dysrhythmias, and even periods of cardiac asystole may occur acutely with block placement or expanding retrobulbar hemorrhage. The latter may happen some hours after a retrobulbar hemorrhage as additional blood extravasates. The reflex is trigeminal-vagal via the ciliary branch of the ophthalmic division of the trigeminal nerve. If an arrhythmia develops, surgical manipulation should be stopped and intravenous atropine (0.007 mg/kg) given.

Central Retinal Artery Occlusion. Retrobulbar hemorrhage can result in central retinal artery occlusion that if not treated promptly and sufficiently may result in total loss of vision. This potentially blinding complication can also occur if the dura around the optic nerve is penetrated and local anesthetic is accidentally injected into the subarachnoid space.

Puncture of Posterior Globe. Perforation of the globe can occur during retrobulbar injection despite the use of a blunted needle in this procedure. The patient experiences immediate ocular pain and restlessness after perforation. Intraocular hemorrhage and retinal detachment may result from this complication.

Penetration of Optic Nerve. Optic atrophy and permanent loss of vision may occur even in the absence of retrobulbar hemorrhage. The postulated mechanisms include direct injury to the optic nerve, injection into the nerve sheath with compressive ischemia, and intramural sheath hemorrhage.

Inadvertent Brain Stem Anesthesia. Accidental access to the **cerebrospinal fluid** can occur during performance of retrobulbar block secondary to perforation of the meningeal sheaths surrounding the optic nerve. The patient may experience disorientation, amaurosis fugax, aphasia, hemiplegia, unconsciousness, convulsions, and respiratory or cardiac arrest. The incidence of central nervous system spread was 0.13% in one large series.

Direct **intravascular injection** via the optic nerve sheath or local anesthetic carried via the ophthalmic and internal carotid artery by retrograde flow to the thalamus and midbrain can also precipitate sudden obtundation, convulsions, and cardiopulmonary arrest. Prompt recognition and treatment necessitate careful patient monitoring.

Epinephrine Toxicity. In patients with hypertension, angina, or arrhythmias, the amount of exogenous epinephrine injected with local anesthetic should be reduced. A total injection of 0.05 mg (10 mL of 1:200,000) epinephrine does not contribute significantly to problems in these patients. In fact, the release of endogenous catecholamines secondary to anxiety of suboptimal analgesia may greatly exceed the relatively minute amount of exogenous catecholamine.

Other Complications. Other possible complications include

□ epinephrine toxicity.
□ immediate allergic reactions.

Contraindications

□ Age under 15 years.
□ Procedures lasting more than 90 minutes.
□ Uncontrolled cough, tremor, or convulsive disorder.
□ Disorientation or mental impairment.
□ Excessive anxiety or claustrophobia.
□ Language barrier or deafness.
□ Bleeding or coagulation disorders.
□ Perforated globe.
□ Inability to lie flat.

Selected References

1. Dutton JJ. Complications of orbital surgery. In Krupin T, Kolker AE, eds. Atlas of Complications in Ophthalmic Surgery. London: Wolfe, 1993:12.3.
2. Katz J. Atlas of Regional Anesthesia. East Norwalk, CT, Appleton-Century-Crofts, 1985.
3. Davis DB, Mandel MR. Posterior peribulbar anesthesia: An alternative to retrobulbar anesthesia. J Cataract Refract Surg 1986;12:182–184.

Suggested References

McGoldrick KE, Feitl ME, Krupin T. Neural blockade in ophthalmologic surgery. In Cousins MJ, Bridenbaugh PO, eds. Neural Blockade. Philadelphia: Lippincott-Raven, 1998:533–556.

Nicholl JMV, Acharya AP, Ahlen K, et al. Central nervous system complications after 6,000 retrobulbar blocks. Anesth Analg 1987;66:1298–1302.

Unsold R, Stanley JA, DeGroot J. The CT-topography of retrobulbar anesthesia: Anatomic-clinical correlation of complications and suggestions of a modified technique. Graefes Arch Clin Exp Ophthalmol 1981;217:125–136.

130
Regional Anesthesia and Pain Relief in Children

Robert J. Friedhoff, M.D.

Regional anesthesia in pediatric patients has been undergoing a revival since the early 1990s. This is advantageous especially for those undergoing outpatient surgery. Regional blocks can provide prolonged and predictable intraoperative anesthesia and postoperative analgesia. Regional techniques are usually performed along with general anesthesia in children. Performing the block after inducing anesthesia but before starting surgery will allow a reduction of general anesthetic agents once the block is established. The clinician needs to be familiar with the relevant anatomic, physiologic, and pharmacologic differences in children.

Anatomy

Target nerves are smaller, closer to other anatomic structures (e.g., vessels), and closer to the skin in children. The caudal extent of the dura and spinal cord extends approximately two interspaces lower in an infant compared with an adult, down to S3-4 and L3, respectively. By age 12 months, they are in the adult position. The epidural fat is more gelatinous and less fibrous in an infant, favoring the spread of local anesthetics and the passage of epidural catheters. This changes after 8 years of age.

Physiology

Clinically significant decreases in blood pressure secondary to sympathectomy from central neuraxis blockade are rare in children younger than 8 years.

Pharmacology

The potential for local anesthetic toxicity is increased in infants because of reduced binding proteins, resulting in increased free local anesthetic.

Maximum recommended doses for commonly used local anesthetics are:

- Lidocaine, 3 mg/kg
- Lidocaine with epinephrine 6 mg/kg.
- Bupivacaine, 2.6 mg/kg.
- Ropivacaine, 3.0 mg/kg.

Cooperation

For the high-risk premature infant, essentially all regional techniques with the exception of spinal anesthesia are performed under heavy sedation or anesthesia. A peripheral nerve stimulator can be useful.

Test Doses

Using epinephrine to detect unanticipated intravascular injection in patients under volatile anesthetics is unreliable and controversial. The local anesthetic should be injected slowly and with frequent aspiration.

Topical Blocks

EMLA cream is a combination of prilocaine and lidocaine. It is placed on the skin and covered with a Tegaderm dressing at least 1 hour before an invasive procedure (e.g., needle stick, circumcision, separation of prepubital adhesions). Iontophoresis of lidocaine takes approximately 10 minutes. A drawback to this technique is that the EMLA apparatus causes a tingling sensation that may be troublesome to the child.

Specific Techniques

Ilioinguinal/Iliohypogastric Nerve Block

Indication. Hernia repairs and orchidopexy.
Technique. Insert the needle one fingerbreadth

inferior and medial to the anterior superior iliac spine and fan the needle from lateral to medial. Wound edge infiltration or instillation of drug before closure (enough to fill the wound after dissection) can also be used.

Key. Identify the anterior superior iliac spine and place a 23-gauge needle 1 to 2 cm medial and inferior to it. Feel the "pop" through the fascia and fan the local anesthetic.

Drug. Bupivacaine 0.25% to 0.5%, 2 to 10 mL, depending on the size of the patient.

Penile Block

Indication. Circumcision, hypospadias repairs

Technique. Ring the base of the penis with a superficial wheal of local anesthetic or, while pulling the penis toward the feet, insert a needle at 90°, just below the symphysis pubis into the shaft. "Pop" through Buck's fascia and inject one-half of the drug at the 11 o'clock and one-half at 1 o'clock area of the top of the penis.

Key. Avoid epinephrine.

Drug. Bupivacaine 0.25% plain, 2 to 10 mL depending on the patient.

Femoral Nerve Block

Indication. Quadriceps muscle biopsy, femoral shaft fracture, knee surgery.

Technique. Remember NAVEL (nerve, artery, vein, empty space, ligament). The nerve is lateral to the artery. Draw a line from the anterior superior iliac spine to the pubic tubercle. This demarcates the inguinal ligament. Just below (0.5 to 1.0 cm) the inguinal ligament, place an insulated needle attached to a nerve stimulator lateral to the femoral artery pulsations. (The patient must not be paralyzed with a muscle relaxant.) Set the twitch monitor at 1 per second and stimulate at the lowest palpable setting until a twitch is noted in the patella.

Drug. Bupivacaine 0.25% to 0.5% or ropivacaine 0.2%, 5 to 20 mL depending on the patient's size.

Lateral Femoral Cutaneous Block

Indication. Often done in conjunction with a femoral nerve block.

Technique. Advance a needle 1 cm below and medial to the inguinal ligament and the anterior superior iliac spine. Deposit the drug after "popping" through the fascia lata.

Drug. Bupivacaine 0.5%, 0.1 to 0.2 mL/kg.

Axillary Block

Indication. Surgery on the arm or hand.

Technique. Use a nerve stimulator as in adults (in an unparalyzed patient). One can also palpate the axillary artery in the axilla, puncture the skin with a 20-gauge needle, then place a 22-gauge blunt needle through the puncture site, aiming toward the artery until you feel a "pop" through the fascia or "septa" of the axillary sheath. After negative aspiration, inject local anesthetic.

Drug. Bupivacaine 0.25% or ropivacaine 0.2% with epinephrine 1/200,000, 0.5 mL/kg up to 40 mL.

Single-Shot Caudal Block

Indication. Surgery below the diaphragm.

Technique. With the patient in the lateral decubitus position (left lateral for a right-handed clinician, right lateral for a left-handed clinician) with the knees flexed up into the abdomen, palpate and identify with a thumbnail the two sacral cornua above the gluteal fold. Using aseptic technique, place a 23-gauge needle at 45 degrees to the skin until a "pop" is felt through the sacrococcygeal ligament. Lower the needle parallel to the skin and advance 1 cm. After negative aspiration for blood and CSF, inject slowly while observing the ECG for T-wave changes. Injection of the local anesthetic should be easy. Any resistance indicates incorrect needle placement.

Drug. Bupivacaine 0.125% to 0.25% or ropivacaine 0.2% depending on the patient's age and incision location: penile surgery, 0.5 to 0.8 mL/kg; inguinal surgery, 1.0 mL/kg up to 20 mL. Other analgesics such as the α-adrenergic agonist clonidine (dose of 2 μg/kg) or preservative-free ketamine (dose of 0.5 mg/kg) can be added to the bupivacaine solution to prolong the duration of the block for an additional 3 to 12 hours. Adverse effects include sedation and minor hypotension.

Continuous Caudal Block

Indication. Prolonged pain relief and placement of catheter tip at level of incision.

Technique. Similar to single-shot. After identifying the caudal space under sterile technique, using either an 18-gauge angiocatheter or Crawford needle is advanced. The epidural catheter is then threaded through the needle 3 cm or to the level of the incision. Tegaderm dressing is applied. Note that maintaining a clean dressing in the sacral area and ensuring access to the site (i.e., no spica cast) are mandatory.

Drug. Dependent on catheter position and surgery.

Lumbar Epidural Block

Indications and Technique. Similar to adults. For patients weighing less than 30 kg, a 2-inch,

18-gauge Weiss or Crawford needle can be used. Contraindications are similar to those for adults.

Drug. Choices include lidocaine, bupivacaine, fentanyl, morphine (Duramorph), or hydromorphone, depending on the patient and the surgery.

Spinal Block

Indication. For former premature high-risk neonates undergoing lower abdominal surgery.

Technique. Try to place the anesthetic with the patient in the sitting position, upright with special attention given to the head, so as not to flex it and obstruct the airway. The depth of the subarachnoid space is about 0.7 cm in premature infants and 1.0 cm in full-term infants. It is best to avoid any sedation if possible, including ketamine to prevent postoperative apnea. Placing the blood pressure cuff on a lower extremity will avoid stimulating the restless infant.

Drug. Tetracaine 1 mg/kg plus dextrose (this block is done only in small neonates).

Suggested References

Cook B, Grubb DJ, Aldridge LA, et al. Comparison of the effects of adrenaline, clonidine and ketamine on the duration of caudal analgesia produced by bupivacaine in children. Br J Anaesth 1995;75:698–701.

Dalens BJ. Regional Anesthesia in Infants, Children and Adolescents. Baltimore, Williams & Wilkins, 1995.

Rice L. Regional Anesthesia in Pediatrics. ASA Refresher Course Lectures. Park Ridge, IL, American Society of Anesthesiologists, 1998.

Peutrell JM, Mather SJ. Regional Anaesthesia in Babies and Children. Oxford, UK, Oxford University Press, 1997.

131
Bronchopleural Fistula

Glenn E. Woodworth, M.D.

A bronchopleural fistula is a connection between the airways or lung parenchyma and the pleural space. If the fistula communicates with the surface of the chest, it is a bronchopleural cutaneous fistula. Causes include rupture or erosion of a lung abscess, bronchus, bulla, cyst, suture line, or parenchymal tissue into the pleural space. Chronic bronchopleural fistula formation has been reported to occur in 1% to 3% of patients after pulmonary resection. Persistent air leak, sepsis, empyema, purulent sputum, and respiratory distress characterize such fistulae. Predisposing factors include perioperative radiation therapy, residual neoplasm or infection at the resection site, and a long avascular bronchial stump.

Treatment is highly dependent on the etiology and nature of the fistula. In general, attempts are made to reduce the pleural space and seal the fistula. This is often accomplished by chest tube placement or pleurodesis. But if the fistula is large (e.g., disruption of a postpneumonectomy bronchial stump), surgical intervention will usually be necessary.

Anesthetic Considerations

The primary clinical concern when caring for patients undergoing surgical repair of bronchopleural fistulae relates to providing adequate alveolar gas exchange during positive-pressure ventilation. Other clinical concerns include preventing contamination (by a pulmonary abscess or empyema) of the healthy lung and avoiding tension pneumothorax. Tension pneumothorax is prevented or treated by chest tube placement. If empyema is present, drainage under local anesthesia should be considered before surgery. During anesthesia induction, spontaneous ventilation and discontinuation of chest tube suctioning will minimize loss of tidal volume during positive-pressure ventilation.

Small fistulas can be managed using a standard single-lumen endotracheal tube. However, patients with larger leaks or those with fistulas associated with pulmonary infection (e.g., abscess, empyema) will need one-lung ventilation using a double-lumen endotracheal tube or bronchial blocker.

Mechanical Ventilation

In patients with bronchopleural fistula, delivering adequate ventilation with conventional mechanical ventilators and single-lumen tubes may be difficult unless the fistula is small. Problems arise when a significant portion of the tidal volume is lost through the fistula into the pleural space or atmosphere. Besides reducing the effective alveolar ventilation, gas flow through the fistula also retards healing and closure. The following approaches to the management of positive-pressure ventilation attempt to reduce the gas flow across the fistula:

- Selective intubation of the contralateral lung. This method can be successful; however, underlying pulmonary disease may make oxygenation during one-lung ventilation difficult. Gas exchange may improve with the application of continuous positive airway pressure (CPAP) with 100% O_2 to the nonventilated lung.
- Valve systems. Several different types of chest tube valve systems have been designed. Flow across the fistula is reduced by increasing the pleural pressure during a positive-pressure breath, thereby decreasing the pressure gradient across the fistula. Usually, the inspiratory cycle of the ventilator triggers closure of the chest tube valve, which then opens during expiration.
- High-frequency ventilation. This method has been suggested as the nonsurgical treatment of choice for large fistulas. High-frequency ventilation reduces airway pressures and thus reduces the driving pressure across the fistula.
- Differential ventilation. This method is a modification of the selective intubation method. Instead of ventilating only one lung, each lung is managed with a different type of ventilation through a double-lumen tube with two synchronized ventilators. The nondiseased lung may be ventilated normally, whereas the affected lung is ventilated with a reduced tidal volume, exposed to CPAP, or ventilated with high-frequency ventilation.

Suggested References

Benumof JL. Anesthesia for Thoracic Surgery. Philadelphia, WB Saunders, 1987.
Benumof JL, Alfery DD. Anesthesia for thoracic surgery. In Miller RD, ed. Anesthesia. 5th ed. Philadelphia: Churchill Livingstone, 2000:1665–1752.

132
Pneumo-, Hemo-, and Chylothorax

Terese T. Horlocker, M.D.

Pneumothorax

Pneumothorax is an accumulation of air outside the lung but within the pleural cavity. The air occupies space needed for full lung inflation and cardiac filling. There is increased intrathoracic pressure and a reduction in vital capacity, minute ventilation, and venous return to the heart. Hypoxia results from increased shunt (continued perfusion of nonventilated lung). The decreased venous return may result in subsequent decrease in cardiac output.

Classification and Etiology. Pediatric pneumothorax may occur under several conditions.

□ Pneumothorax of the newborn occurs in 1% of vaginal deliveries, usually when delivery was difficult or complicated by meconium aspiration.
□ Neonates with respiratory distress syndrome, especially if mechanical ventilation and/or positive end-expiratory pressure are used, are also prone to pneumothorax.
□ Congenital diaphragmatic hernia results in a noncompliant underdeveloped lung ipsilateral to the defect in the diaphragm. The more compliant contralateral lung is prone to barotrauma and pneumothorax.

Spontaneous pneumothorax occurs without trauma.

□ Primary: No known pulmonary disease; occurs most often in tall, thin males, presumably from rupture of emphysematous blebs.
□ Secondary: Occurs in patients with underlying pulmonary disease and is associated with an increased mortality rate.

Traumatic pneumothorax occurs secondary to blunt or penetrating trauma to the chest wall (Tables 132–1 and 132–2). However, the most common cause is iatrogenic and is related to subclavian line placement.

□ Penetrating trauma (gunshot or knife wound) has virtually a 100% prevalence of pneumothorax.
□ Blunt trauma causes rupture of alveoli, with subsequent dissection of air into pleural space.
□ Iatrogenic pneumothorax can occur during line placement, cardiopulmonary resuscitation, regional blocks, mechanical ventilation, and surgical procedures.

Tension pneumothorax occurs when air enters the pleural cavity on inspiration but, because of the ball-valve mechanism, does not exit on expiration. This leads to progressive enlargement of the pleural space, which shifts the mediastinum and trachea away from the pneumothorax and decreases venous return. There is usually a rapid deterioration in vital signs and cyanosis that may progress to death.

Diagnosis. A pneumothorax is not likely to produce severe symptoms unless it is a tension pneumothorax, represents more than 40% of a single lung volume, or occurs in a patient with preexisting pulmonary disease. Patients complain of unilateral pleuritic chest pain or cough. Breath sounds may be diminished or absent. Intraoperatively, increased airway pressure, decreased pulmonary compliance, cyanosis, and hypotension may be seen. Radiographic examination is the best diagnostic tool, but it is difficult to estimate the percentage of pneumothorax from film. Blood gases show hypoxia and possibly hypercarbia (in cases of impending respiratory failure).

Treatment. Tension pneumothorax is a surgical emergency, and time should not be spent seeking radiologic evidence. If tension pneumothorax is sus-

Table 132–1. Prevalence of Thoracic Injuries in Closed Thoracic Trauma

Prevalence (%)	Injuries
>50	Fractured ribs
	Myocardial contusion
	Pulmonary contusion
10–50	Hemopneumothorax
	Flail segment
	Thoracic wall contusion
<10	Fractured thoracic spine
	Ruptured thoracic aorta
	Ruptured diaphragm
	Pulmonary laceration
	Fractured sternum
Occasional	Ruptured trachea or main bronchus
	Ruptured innominate artery
	Ruptured pulmonary artery or vein
	Hemopericardium
	Ruptured esophagus
	Disrupted aortic or tricuspid valve

From Marshall BE, Longnecker DE, Fairley HB.[1]

Table 132–2. Indications for Thoracotomy for Hemothorax

Persistent hypotension despite aggressive volume replacement
Bleeding greater than 300 mL/hr for 4 hours
Massive continuing hemorrhage greater than 2,000 mL
Left hemothorax in the presence of widened mediastinum

From Kaplan JA.[2]

pected, a large-bore needle should be placed in the second intercostal space in the midclavicular line, allowing air to drain freely.

Most patients with pneumothorax of more than 20% of the pleural volume require chest tube placement. Recurrence may necessitate tetracycline or surgical pleurodesis.

Nitrous oxide should be avoided until thoracotomy or chest tube placement has been completed. Solubility of N_2O compared with N_2 results in rapid diffusion of N_2O into the pleural space, which can double the size of the pneumothorax in 10 minutes.

Hemothorax

Hemothorax occurs in 70% of major chest injuries. The hemothorax volume is about 2000 mL, equivalent to almost one-half of total blood volume. To be radiographically visible, 500 mL of blood must accumulate. The bleeding may be from pulmonary parenchymal vessels (low perfusion pressure, easy to control) or from intercostal, subclavian, or other major vessels (high perfusion pressure, brisk and severe bleeding).

Etiology. Hemothorax can occur from any blunt or penetrating chest trauma, such as gunshot wounds, rib fractures, surgical procedure, line placement, or thoracentesis (see Table 132–1).

Diagnosis. Hypovolemia from blood loss is the most common problem. Examination reveals dullness to percussion, diminished breath sounds, and in severe cases, a deviated trachea. Upright chest radiographs are more sensitive in diagnosing hemothorax, because only 200 to 500 mL of fluid collection is needed, compared to 500 to 2000 mL for supine films. Thoracentesis is necessary to confirm the diagnosis. The hematocrit of the pleural fluid should be greater than 50% of systemic hematocrit.

Treatment. Chest tube placement is necessary for both diagnosis and treatment of hemothorax. Concurrent pneumothoraces are frequently present. Some 80% of patients presenting with hemothorax will need **only** chest tube placement, with no further surgical intervention. Bleeding from larger vessels or the heart necessitates thoracotomy (see Table 132–2).

Complications. Despite chest tube placement, retention of blood clots may occur, which may lead to fibrinous organization or empyema. Most residual hemothoraces are managed conservatively and completely resorb in 3 to 4 weeks.

A retained hemothorax should be decorticated if it causes lobar atelectasis, occupies more than one-third of a hemothorax, or is associated with a fever of 101°F.

Chylothorax

Chylothorax is accumulation of lymph fluid within the pleural cavity. At the T5 vertebra, the thoracic duct crosses over to the left side of the vertebral column and continues on to terminate at the junction of the subclavian and internal jugular veins. Anatomic variations are common, however, and the thoracic duct may enter on the right side. Fluid leakage from the thoracic duct may be as high as 1500 to 2500 mL per day.

Etiology. Chylothorax may result from blunt or penetrating trauma, especially cervical spine or thoracic dislocations, as well as surgical trauma during dissections near the descending thoracic aorta, ductus arteriosus, and cervical nodes. The thoracic duct can also be disrupted during central line placement. Patients with neoplasms, especially lymphoma, can develop chylothorax without trauma.

Diagnosis. The presentation resembles that of hemothorax: progressive respiratory distress with decreased breath sounds over the involved hemothorax. Thoracentesis yields straw-colored or white drainage containing fat globules (demonstrated on Sudan III stain) and chylomicrons (demonstrated by electrophoresis). The triglyceride level in pleural fluid may also be diagnostic.

Treatment. Chest tube placement with continued drainage usually results in spontaneous closure over several days. However, patients can become malnourished from loss of fat calories and lymphopenic from drainage of lymphocytes in chyle. Intravenous hyperalimentation with short-chain triglycerides will facilitate closure. Patients who are allowed to eat should be placed on a strict no-fat diet. For cases with large drainage amounts (more than 1500 mL/day), surgical ligation may be required.

Selected References

1. Marshall BE, Longnecker DE, Fairley HB. Anesthesia for Thoracic Procedures. Boston, Blackwell Scientific, 1988.
2. Kaplan JA. Thoracic Anesthesia. 2nd ed. New York, Churchill Livingstone, 1991.

Suggested References

Grenvik A. Textbook of Critical Care. 4th ed. Philadelphia, WB Saunders, 2000.

133
Double-Lumen Endotracheal Tubes

David J. Cook, M.D.

Double-lumen endotracheal tubes have been developed to enable functional separation of the lungs. This separation can prevent spillage or contamination from one lung to the other and control the distribution of ventilation. The most common indication for single-lung ventilation is to improve surgical exposure; this is a relative indication (Table 133–1).

While single-lung ventilation can also be achieved with single-lumen tubes or bronchial blockers, double-lumen tubes have the following advantages:

□ Relative ease of placement.
□ Rapid conversion from one-lung to two-lung ventilation.

□ Provision for suctioning from both lungs.
□ Application of continuous positive airway pressure to the nonventilated lung.

Lung separation can be lifesaving, but its initiation can produce sudden and dramatic impairment of oxygen exchange. Other disadvantages particular to double-lumen tubes are that they increase airway resistance and can make secretion clearance difficult.

Relative contraindications must also be considered when contemplating placement of these tubes (Table 133–2).

Tube Selection

Types of double-lumen tubes include Carlens, White, Bryce-Smith, and Robertshaw. All share common features. They have two lumina, one terminating in the trachea and the other in the right or left mainstem bronchus. They have two cuffs and are molded to conform to the oropharynx and mainstem bronchus. The Carlens is a left-sided tube with a carinal hook. The White is essentially a right-sided Carlens; the Bryce-Smith lacks a carinal hook and has a slotted cuff on its right-sided version to allow right upper lobe ventilation.

The modern Robertshaw design is clear plastic and disposable with left- and right-sided versions. It lacks a carinal hook and generally has a lower resistance to airflow than other designs. The tubes are available in sizes 41, 39, 37, 35, and 28 French (with an internal diameter of each lumen of approximately 6.5, 6.0, 5.5, 5.0, and 4.5 mm, respectively). Both cuffs are high-volume, low-pressure type with the bronchial cuff colored bright blue; this bronchial

Table 133–1. Indications for Separation of the Two Lungs (Double-Lumen Tube Intubation) or One-Lung Ventilation

Absolute

Isolation of one lung from the other to avoid spillage or contamination:
- Infection.
- Massive hemorrhage.

Control of the distribution of ventilation:
- Bronchopleural fistula.
- Bronchopleural cutaneous fistula.
- Surgical opening of a major conducting airway.
- Giant unilateral lung cyst or bulla.
- Tracheobronchial tree disruption.
- Life-threatening hypoxemia due to unilateral lung disease.

Unilateral bronchopulmonary lavage: Pulmonary alveolar proteinosis.

Relative

Surgical exposure (high priority):
- Thoracic aortic aneurysm.
- Pneumonectomy.
- Upper lobectomy.
- Mediastinal exposure.
- Thoracoscopy.

Surgical exposure (medium [lower] priority):
- Middle and lower lobectomies and subsegmental resections.
- Esophageal resection.
- Procedures on the thoracic spine.

Postcardiopulmonary bypass status after removal of totally occluding chronic unilateral pulmonary emboli.

Severe hypoxemia due to unilateral lung disease.

From Benumof JL.[1]

Table 133–2. Relative Contraindications to Use of Double-Lumen Tube

Presence of lesion along double-lumen tube pathway.
Difficult or impossible conventional direct vision intubation.
Critically ill patients with single-lumen tube in situ who cannot tolerate even a short period off mechanical ventilation.
Full stomach or high risk of aspiration.

Modified from Benumof JL.[1]

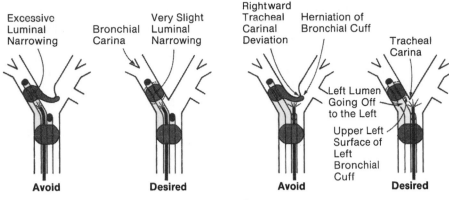

Figure 133–1. This schematic diagram depicts the complete fiberoptic bronchoscopy picture of left-sided double-lumen endotracheal tubes (both the desired view and the view to be avoided from both of the lumina). *A,* When the bronchoscope is passed down the left lumen of the left-sided tube, the endoscopist should see a very slight left luminal narrowing and a clear straight-ahead view of the bronchial carina off in the distance. Excessive left luminal narrowing should be avoided. *B,* When the bronchoscope is passed down the right lumen of the left-sided tube, the endoscopist should see a clear straight-ahead view of the tracheal carina and the upper surface of the blue left endobronchial cuff just below the tracheal carina. Excessive pressure in the endobronchial cuff, as manifested by tracheal carinal deviation to the right and herniation of the endobronchial cuff over the carina, should be avoided. (From Benumof JL.[1])

cuff is also slanted in the right-sided version to improve right upper lobe ventilation. Finally, this version has a radiopaque line at the end of both lumens to allow for radiographic detection of placement.

The left-sided double-lumen tube can be used for most thoracic procedures requiring one-lung ventilation regardless of the operative side. It should be used for right thoracotomies requiring right lung collapse and can also be used for left thoracotomies with left lung collapse. In left-sided surgery, the endobronchial portion of the left-sided tube can be withdrawn into the trachea at the time of left mainstem clamping and continue to be used for right lung ventilation through both lumens.

Conversely, use of the right-sided tube can be problematic. To ventilate the right upper lobe, the slot of the endobronchial portion of the right-sided tube must be closely opposed to the right upper lobe orifice. **Because the length of the right mainstem bronchus is shorter and more variable than the left mainstem, right-sided endobronchial intubation poses a significant risk for right upper lobe collapse and hypoventilation.**

The contraindications to left-sided placement are carinal or proximal left mainstem lesions that could be traumatized by a left-sided tube. Except for these

contraindications, a left-sided tube is preferred when possible.

Double-Lumen Tube Placement Technique

To place the double-lumen tube, perform the following steps:

- Review the history and examine the patient for conditions that may affect tube choice or require special intubation techniques.
- Check both cuffs (the bronchial cuff usually requires less than 3 mL of air); cuffs can be protected at intubation with a teeth guard.
- The MacIntosh blade is usually preferred, because it approximates the tube's curvature.
- Pass the tip of the Robertshaw–type tube through the larynx with the distal curvature concave anteriorly.
- Once the tip is through the larynx, remove the stylette and rotate the tube 90 degrees toward the appropriate side.

After intubation, the anesthesiologist must use an established routine to verify tube placement; this can comprise clinical signs, fiberoptic visualization, or chest radiography. Clinical signs alone may miss malpositioning 48% of the time. For this reason, fiberoptic bronchoscopy is routinely used to confirm proper positioning (Fig. 133–1).

Tube position **must** be reconfirmed after repositioning the patient. Head flexion may cause tube advancement, endobronchial placement of the tracheal lumen, or upper lobe obstruction. Head extension can cause bronchial decannulation. In addition,

Table 133–3. Complications of Double-Lumen Tubes

Malpositioning.
Tracheobronchial tree disruption.
Traumatic laryngitis.
Suturing of double-lumen tube to intrathoracic structure.

From Benumof JL.[1]

intraoperative surgical manipulation may displace the tube.

Complications of double-lumen tube placement are listed in Table 133–3. Most of these complications involve the use of older Carlens tubes and can be avoided by multiple checks on tube position, selection of appropriately sized tubes, attention to cuff inflation, extreme care in repositioning patients, and caution in patients with bronchial wall abnormalities.

Selected References

1. Benumof JL. Anesthesia for Thoracic Surgery. 2nd ed. Philadelphia, WB Saunders, 1995.

Suggested References

Benumof JL, Alfery DD. Anesthesia for Thoracic Surgery. In Miller RD, ed. Anesthesia. 5th ed. Philadelphia: Churchill Livingstone, 2000:1665–1752.

134
One-Lung Ventilation and Methods of Improving Oxygenation

Richard Belmont, D.O. □ Brian A. Hall, M.D.

One-lung anesthesia is performed using a double-lumen endotracheal tube or bronchial blocker. It is indicated when one lung can contaminate the other lung with either infected material or blood, or when the distribution of ventilation must be separated.

Mechanism of Hypoxia

The lateral decubitus position is often necessary for thoracic surgery. In this position, the dependent lung tends to be underventilated as it is compressed by the pressure of the abdominal contents and the weight of the mediastinum. The nondependent lung is relatively overventilated because its compliance is increased, particularly when the corresponding hemithorax is opened. Because of the mismatch, patients in this position may develop arterial hypoxemia.

During one-lung ventilation, there is an increased a-ADO$_2$ because of continued perfusion of the atelectatic lung, creating an increase in the transpulmonary shunt. However, CO$_2$ removal is usually not a problem, because CO$_2$ is 20 times more diffusible than O$_2$ in the lung.[1] In addition, the increased VD/VT ratio from one-lung ventilation facilitates CO$_2$ elimination.

Factors Affecting Oxygenation During One-Lung Ventilation

Many factors may affect oxygenation during one-lung ventilation:

□ Degree of active vasoconstriction in the hypoxic lung (hypoxic pulmonary vasoconstriction [HPV]). HPV is of greatest benefit when 30% to 70% of the lung is made hypoxic.
□ Vasodilating agents. Most systemic vasodilators inhibit regional HPV. Those that have been specifically studied include nitroglycerin, nitroprusside, dobutamine, calcium antagonists, and many β$_2$-receptor agonists.
□ Anesthetic drugs. Halothane has been demon-strated to inhibit this reflex in humans. Nitrous oxide has no reported effect.
□ Increased pulmonary vascular pressure. Pulmonary vascular smooth muscle is unable to constrict against increased vascular pressure; this occurs in, for example, mitral stenosis, volume overload, mitral insufficiency, and pulmonary embolism.
□ Vasoconstrictor drugs. Dopamine, epinephrine, phenylephrine, and other vasoconstrictors preferentially constrict normoxic lung vessels and defeat the HPV mechanism.
□ Hypocapnia. This has been thought to directly inhibit regional HPV. However, during one-lung ventilation, hypocapnia can be accomplished only through hyperventilation of the dependent lung, leading to increased airway pressure and resultant increased pulmonary vascular resistance in the ventilated lung. This directs blood flow into the hypoxic lung.

Surgical Manipulation

Although HPV is responsible for most blood flow redistribution away from the nonventilated lung, compression of the nondependent lung may further reduce nondependent lung blood flow. On the other hand, trauma may release vasodilator prostaglandins.

Ligation of the pulmonary artery for pneumonectomy improves oxygenation by removing perfusion to the unventilated lung.

Preoperative and Intraoperative Condition of the Dependent Lung

The pulmonary vascular resistance of the ventilated lung determines the lung's ability to accept redistributed blood flow from the dependent lung. Preoperative vascular disease may result in high vascular resistance and interfere with HPV. Clinical conditions that may increase dependent-lung HPV include low inspired oxygen tension and hypothermia.

Maintaining the lateral decubitus position for long periods may cause a transudate in the dependent lung, further reducing functional residual capacity and increasing airway closure.

Methods for Ventilating the Dependent Lung

Several methods are used to ventilate the dependent lung.

□ A FiO_2 of 1.0 protects against hypoxemia and has been associated with PaO_2 values between 150 and 250 mm Hg during one-lung ventilation. A high FiO_2 also promotes vasodilation in the dependent lung to accept blood flow redistribution from the hypoxic nondependent lung. However, high FiO_2 may lead to absorption atelectasis, oxygen toxicity, and bleomycin-induced injury. The risks and benefits of high FiO_2 should be assessed individually.

□ The dependent lung should initially be ventilated with a tidal volume of 10 to 12 mL/kg. Tidal volumes below 8 mL/kg may lead to decreased FRC and atelectasis in the dependent lung. Tidal volumes above 15 mL/kg may increase pulmonary vascular resistance and shunt blood to the nonventilated lung.

□ The respiratory rate should be adjusted to maintain $PaCO_2$ at approximately 40 mm Hg.[1] Hypocarbia has a vasodilatory effect in the lung and thus will inhibit HPV. In addition, hypocapnia will inhibit HPV in the nondependent lung and increase vascular resistance in the dependent lung.

□ CPAP to the nondependent lung is the most effective way to increase PaO_2 during one-lung ventilation. CPAP at 5 to 10 cm H_2O maintains patency of nondependent alveoli allowing gas exchange to occur and diverts blood away from the collapsed lung.

□ PEEP of 10 cm H_2O to the dependent lung increases FRC and improves gas exchange in the dependent lung. However, PEEP may compress small interalveolar vessels increasing pulmonary vascular resistance, which shunts blood to the nondependent lung and ultimately decreases PaO_2.

Miscellaneous Causes of Hypoxemia

Various other causes of hypoxemia in one-lung ventilation must be considered, including:

□ Mechanical failure of the oxygen supply.
□ Gross hypoventilation of the dependent lung.
□ Malfunction of dependent lung airway lumen; for example, blockage by secretions or malposition.
□ Resorption of residual oxygen from the clamped nonventilated lung.
□ Factors that decrease mixed venous oxygenation saturation, such as increased cardiac output or increased oxygen consumption (shivering, hypothermia, excessive sympathetic drive).

Selected References

1. Barash PG, Cullen BF, Stoelting RK, eds. Clinical Anesthesia. 3rd ed. Philadelphia, Lippincott-Raven, 1997.

Suggested References

Benumof J. Anesthesia for Thoracic Surgery. Philadelphia, WB Saunders, 1987.

Benumof JL, Alfery DD. Anesthesia for thoracic surgery. In Miller RD, ed. Anesthesia. 5th ed. New York: Churchill Livingstone, 2000:1665–1752.

Stoelting RK, Miller RD. Basics of Anesthesia. 3rd ed. New York, Churchill Livingstone, 1994.

135
High-Frequency Ventilation

Doris B. Ockert, M.D.

High-frequency ventilation (HFV) is the delivery of small tidal volumes (equal to or less than the anatomical dead space) at high rates. Four methods of HFV delivery have been developed:

- High-frequency positive-pressure ventilation (HFPPV).
- High-frequency jet ventilation (HFJV).
- High-frequency oscillatory ventilation (HFOV).
- High-frequency chest wall compression (HFCWC).

A general comparison of the major types of HFV is given in Table 135–1. HFV was developed to reduce the risk of barotrauma and cardiovascular compromise and to improve pulmonary gas exchange in ventilator-dependent patients.

Physiology

The mechanism of gas transport depends on convection, diffusion, and complex mechanisms different from normal gas transport and not well understood. Physiologic consequences include the following:

- Carbon dioxide elimination still occurs with tidal volumes as low as 50 to 75 mL. In general, an increase in tidal volume increases CO_2 elimination. Higher frequencies with fixed tidal volumes increase CO_2 elimination only up to a point (3 to 6 Hz, 180 to 360/min). A decrease in airway resistance increases the penetration of gas to the alveolar zone and increases CO_2 elimination.
- Oxygenation has not improved as initially hoped when compared with conventional ventilation. Mean and peak airway pressures are usually lower.
- The magnitude of the hemodynamic effect is re-

lated to the amount of positive pressure applied to the airway. At lower peak and mean airway pressures, the adverse effects should be less. Experimentally, this has not always been the case.
- The fluctuations in intracranial pressures are less, but the mean pressure is not decreased.

Clinical Applications

HPV has several clinical applications:

- Laryngeal and tracheal surgery. The aim is to minimize the intra-airway space occupied by the endotracheal tube and decrease ventilatory excursions. HFJV is used in operating rooms.
- Emergency airway management. After introduction of a small cannula through the cricothyroid membrane, a patient can be ventilated using HFJV.
- Bronchopleural fistula. Smaller volumes are thought to be lost through the fistula.
- Infant and adult respiratory distress syndrome. HFOV is regularly used in modern pediatric intensive care units, but its advantage over conventional ventilation in both infant and adult respiratory distress syndrome has not been shown.

Drawbacks

Problems with HFV include:

- Barotrauma.
- Difficulty in monitoring ventilation (tidal volume, FiO_2, $ETCO_2$, and airway pressures).
- Insufficient alarms.
- Possibility of aspiration with uncuffed tubes.
- Poor humidification of gases.
- No scavenging of anesthetic agents.
- High gas usage by the ventilator.

Table 135–1. General Comparison of the Major Types of HFV

	HFPPV	HFJV	HFOV	HFCWC
Frequency	1–2 Hz 60–110/min	2–6 Hz 110–400/min	2–15 Hz 400–2400/min	2–15 Hz 400–2400/min
Tidal volume	3–5 mL/kg	2–5 mL/kg*	*	*

*Actual value unknown because of entrainment.

Suggested References

Gillespie DJ. High-frequency ventilation. A new concept in mechanical ventilation. Mayo Clin Proc 1983;58:187–196.

Grundy E. High-frequency ventilation. Anesth Rev 1987;4:37.

Kallas HJ. Non-conventional respiratory support modalities applicable in the older child: High-frequency ventilation and liquid ventilation. Crit Care Clin 1998;14:655–683.

Sjostrand U. High-frequency positive-pressure ventilation. Clin Care Med 1980;8:345.

136
Preoperative Evaluation of the Patient with Cardiac Disease

Bradly J. Narr, M.D.

Heart disease has a high prevalence in most patient populations. Elective surgical procedures usually allow clinical evaluation of the patient with cardiac disease before the day of surgery. Significant abnormalities detected by history, physical examination, or in association with other risk factors may necessitate further testing. However, careful assessment by an anesthesiologist is by far the most important part of the process. Most cardiac testing should be done in the perioperative patient for the same reasons that it is done in the nonsurgical patient—that is, when it will affect the patient's treatment or outcomes.

Disorders with implications for anesthetic care include coronary artery disease, congestive heart failure (CHF), rhythm problems, and heart valve abnormalities. Clinical evaluation of the patient should allow detection of serious coronary syndromes, symptomatic congestive heart failure, severe valvular disease, and new or unstable rhythm problems. A consensus guideline has been written that integrates an individual's clinical presentation, known cardiovascular risk factors, and the invasiveness of the planned procedure with recommended testing algorithms.[1]

The clinical predictors of increased perioperative risk for myocardial infarction, congestive heart failure, and death are listed in Table 136–1. The major clinical predictors have the highest likelihood for risk modification by formalized testing and intervention. Modern treatment of unstable myocardial ischemia and myocardial infarction include anticoagulation and thrombolysis. In postoperative patients, thrombolysis is not an option, and full anticoagulation has risk; thus, it is important to intervene in unstable coronary syndromes before an elective surgical intervention.

An important clinical assessment parameter is functional capacity. Table 136–2 lists easily obtainable patient history information and correlates this with energy requirements estimated in metabolic equivalents (MET). Perioperative risk may be increased in patients unable to achieve a 4-MET activity level on a day-to-day basis. Obtaining this historical information may be impossible in patients with orthopedic problems or severe vascular disease, and further diagnostic testing should be undertaken if a high-risk surgical procedure is planned (Table 136–3).

A guideline, although not necessarily supported by randomized prospective studies, brings consistency and a logical progression to the complex topic of preoperative cardiovascular evaluation. The central concept is that clinical assessment findings integrated with the complexity of the planned procedure directs further testing. For example, a patient who has compensated CHF and angina and who

Table 136–1. Clinical Predictors of Increased Perioperative Cardiovascular Risk (Myocardial Infarction, Congestive Heart Failure, Death)

Major
Unstable coronary syndromes.
- Recent myocardial infarction* with evidence of important ischemic risk by clinical symptoms or noninvasive study.
- Unstable or severe† angina (Canadian Class III or IV).‡
Decompensated congestive heart failure.
Significant arrhythmias.
- High-grade atrioventricular block.
- Symptomatic ventricular arrhythmias in the presence of underlying heart disease.
- Supraventricular arrhythmias with uncontrolled ventricular rate.
Severe valvular disease.
Intermediate
Mild angina pectoris (Canadian Class I or II).
Prior myocardial infarction by history or pathologic Q waves.
Compensated or prior congestive heart failure.
Diabetes mellitus.
Minor
Advanced age.
Abnormal ECG (left ventricular hypertrophy, left bundle branch block, ST-T abnormalities).
Rhythm other than sinus (e.g., atrial fibrillation).
Low functional capacity (e.g., inability to climb one flight of stairs with a bag of groceries).
History of stroke.
Uncontrolled systemic hypertension.

*The American College of Cardiology National Database Library defines *recent MI* as greater than 7 days but less than or equal to 1 month (30 days).
†May include "stable" angina in patients who are unusually sedentary.
‡Campeau L. Grading of angina pectoris. Circulation 1976;54:522–523.
From J Am Coll Cardiol 1996;27:910–948. Reprinted with permission from the American College of Cardiology.

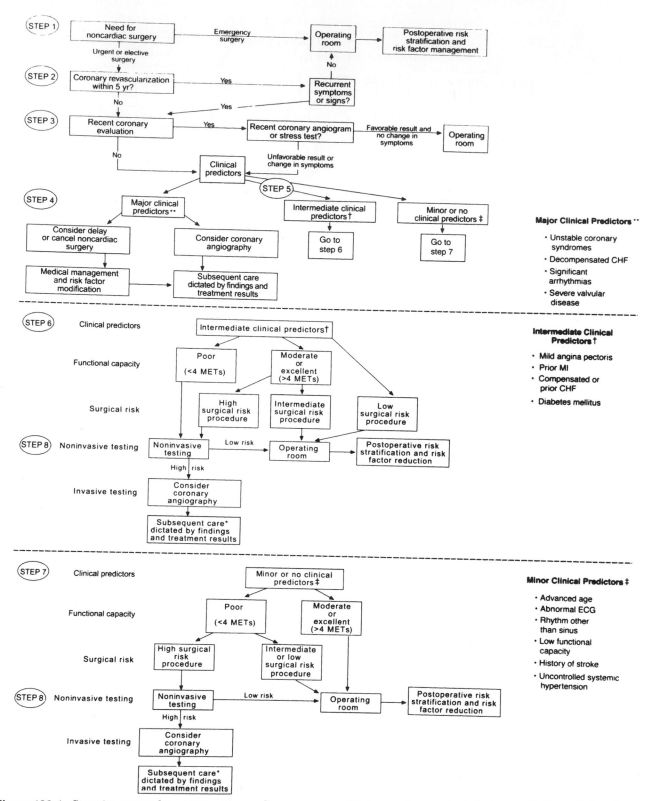

Figure 136–1. Stepwise approach to preoperative cardiac assessment. *Subsequent care may include cancellation or delay of surgery, coronary revascularization followed by noncardiac surgery, or intensified care. (From J Am Coll Cardiol 1996;27:910–948. Reprinted with permission from the American College of Cardiology.)

never exceeds 1 MET in activity level needs an anesthesiologist for his minor surgical procedure, not further testing.

Figure 136–1 details a stepwise approach to cardiac assessment. Several points bear emphasis.

Emergency surgery precludes preoperative evaluation and risk factor management may require intensive care or postoperative invasive cardiology interventions. Major clinical predictors for cardiac events generally demand intervention or further testing before elective surgery. A patient with moderate or excellent physical activity tolerance should proceed directly to the operating room for all but high-risk surgical procedures.

Summary

Careful clinical evaluation allows logical testing and intervention in patients with cardiac disease before surgery. Improved outcomes are not necessarily dependent on documenting the severity of disease in patients who are well compensated clinically when intermediate- and low-risk procedures are planned. The most important aspect of evaluation is that it be performed by a physician, preferably an anesthesiologist, who can complete a clinical

Table 136–2. Estimated Energy Requirements for Various Activities

| 1 MET | Can you take care of yourself? Eat, dress, or use the toilet? Walk indoors around the house? Walk a block or two on level ground at 2–3 mph or 3.2–4.8 km/h? Do light work around the house like dusting or washing dishes? | 4 METs | Climb a flight of stairs or walk up a hill? Walk on level ground at 4 mph or 6.4 km/h? Run a short distance? Do heavy work around the house like scrubbing floors or lifting or moving heavy furniture? Participate in moderate recreational activities like golf, bowling, dancing, doubles tennis, or throwing a baseball or football? |
| 4 METs | | >10 METs | Participate in strenuous sports like swimming, singles tennis, football, basketball, or skiing? |

MET indicates metabolic equivalent.
Adapted from the Duke Activity Status Index and American Heart Association Exercise Standards.
From J Am Coll Cardiol 1996;27:910–948. Reprinted with permission from the American College of Cardiology.

Table 136–3. Cardiac Risk* Stratification for Noncardiac Surgical Procedures

High	(Reported cardiac risk often >5%) • Emergent major operations, particularly in the elderly • Aortic and other major vascular • Peripheral vascular • Anticipated prolonged surgical procedures associated with large fluid shifts and/or blood loss
Intermediate	(Reported cardiac risk generally <5%) • Carotid endarterectomy • Head and neck • Intraperitoneal and intrathoracic • Orthopedic • Prostate
Low†	(Reported cardiac risk generally <1%) • Endoscopic procedures • Superficial procedure • Cataract • Breast

*Combined incidence of cardiac death and nonfatal myocardial infarction.
†Do not generally require further preoperative cardiac testing.
From J Am Coll Cardiol 1996;27:910–948. Reprinted with permission from the American College of Cardiology.

assessment and relate this to the invasiveness of the anticipated procedure.

Selected Reference

1. Guidelines for perioperative cardiovascular evaluation for noncardiac surgery. Report of the American College of Cardiology/American Heart Association Task Force on Practice Guidelines (Committee on Perioperative Cardiovascular Evaluation for Noncardiac Surgery). J Am Coll Cardiol 1996;27:910–948.

Suggested Reference

Roizen MF, Foss JF, Fischer SP. Preoperative evaluation. In Miller RD, ed. Anesthesia. 5th ed. Philadelphia: Churchill Livingstone, 2000:824–883.

137

Pacemakers

Mark F. Trankina, M.D.

Few areas in clinical medicine are more dependent on, and have been affected more, by advances in engineering technology than cardiac pacing. Approximately 150,000 permanent pacemakers are implanted each year in the United States. This places an ever-increasing burden on the anesthesiologist to properly manage this technology during the perioperative period, a period that still involves morbidity and mortality when associated with the presence of a pacemaker.

The key to perioperative management in patients with permanent pacemakers is to treat the underlying medical problems. Although the presence of a pacemaker indicates cardiac disease, the pacemaker should be considered an adjunct to successful anesthetic management and not a problem in itself.

Indications for permanent pacemakers include symptomatic bradyarrhythmias, asymptomatic Mobitz II or greater, sinus-node dysfunction, some types of supraventricular tachycardia (SVT) or ventricular tachycardia (VT), orthotopic heart transplantation, hypertrophic and dilated cardiomyopathy, and long QT syndrome.

Indications for the use of temporary pacemakers include following cardiac surgery, treatment of drug toxicity resulting in arrhythmias, certain arrhythmias complicating myocardial infarction, permanent generator failure, and cardiac arrest.

Pacemaker Codes

In a pacemaker code, the first letter refers to the chamber paced, the second letter refers to the chamber sensed, and the third letter refers to the response to the sensed event. The final two letters refer to programmability and antitachycardia (ICD) functions. In the first position, A refers to atrium, V refers to ventricle, and D implies that both the atrium and the ventricle are paced. For the second position, the same letters are used for chamber or chambers sensed. In addition, O indicates that no chamber is sensed. In the third position, I refers to inhibition; T, to triggering; D, to double (atrium triggered and ventricle inhibited); O, to none. A newer class of pacemakers, designated by R (rate-adaptive) in the fourth position (i.e., DDDR), are designed to deliver a more physiologic response by

changing rate in response to exercise. Table 137–1 summarizes common generator configurations.

Preoperative Evaluation

Pacemakers are common in the general population (1:460). Patients with permanent pacemakers typically have significant heart disease and should be evaluated in the usual fashion for medical problems. Approximately 50% of these patients have significant coronary artery disease, 20% are hypertensive, and 10% have insulin-dependent diabetes. Medications, acid base status, and electrolyte levels, as well as the pacemaker function itself, should be evaluated preoperatively.

The type of pacemaker generator (i.e., unipolar or bipolar, programmable) and indication for pacemaker placement should be elucidated. Knowledge of the preexisting arrhythmia is important to anticipate potential therapy should the generator fail during the anesthetic. Patients with complete heart block and severe bradycardia are more likely to be pacemaker dependent and thus potentially at higher risk should a malfunction occur. Patients with sick sinus syndrome and carotid sinus hypersensitivity are less likely to be pacemaker dependent. The patient should be questioned about the recurrence of symptoms similar to those experienced before placement of the pacemaker, such as dizziness or fainting.

To evaluate the pacemaker, the preoperative ECG and chest radiograph should be carefully reviewed. The pacemaker is usually checked electronically before and after surgery to verify its function. Each paced beat should correspond to a pulse beat. If the patient's intrinsic rate is faster than the programmed rate, then the pacemaker usually will be inhibited and thus difficult to evaluate. Interventions that increase vagal tone can be used to ascertain pacemaker function by slowing the patient's intrinsic rate and starting the pacemaker. The chest radiograph may help verify lead integrity and generator identification and reveal signs of heart failure.

Intraoperative Management

Most modern pacemakers can be programmed with an external device that emits either a coded

Table 137–1. Common Permanent Pacemaker Modes

Code	Indication	Function	Perioperative Management
VVI	Bradycardia without the need for preserved AV conduction.	Demand ventricular pacing.	Magnet use may be helpful and converts to asynchronous pacing usually at 72 beats/min.
VVIR	Bradycardia without the need for preserved AV conduction; chronotropic incompetence.	Allows a somewhat physiologic response to exercise.	Pacemaker may sense perioperative changes (e.g., temperature and respiratory rate) as related to exercise or unpredictable response to magnet placement; suggest postoperative interrogation.
DDD	Bradycardia when AV synchrony can be preserved.	Provides more physiologic response; maintains AV concordance.	Unpredictable response to magnet placement; suggest postoperative interrogation.
DDDR	Patients requiring physiologic response of heart rate (i.e., chronotropic incompetence).	Provides increased physiologic response to exercise; maintains AV concordance.	Pacemaker may sense perioperative changes (e.g., temperature and respiratory rate) as related to exercise or unpredictable response to magnet placement; suggest postoperative interrogation.

radiofrequency message or a pulsed magnetic field to the pacemaker. Currently, no universal programmer is available, and thus each generator requires a unique unit. Electrosurgical cautery (ESC), which emits radiofrequency energy, has the potential to cause transient or permanent changes in pacemaker function. The most common problem is inhibition of the pacemaker. As long as the electromagnetic interference (EMI), defined as an adverse change in the normal function of a device caused by electromagnetic energy, from the ESC is brief, it should be of little concern in most patients. But if the inhibition is continuous, many pacemakers will revert to a "noise mode" and pace asynchronously. This rarely leads to difficulty, however.

If ESC is to be used extensively, then consideration should be given to reprogramming the generator to an asynchronous mode preoperatively, to avoid intermittent inhibition. But conversion to an asynchronous mode does not prevent circuit damage from electrocautery. Magnets, which activate a reed switch in the generator, can also be used to convert many generators to an asynchronous mode. Routine use of magnets without knowledge of the expected pacemaker response is not advocated. ESC may rarely increase the rate of capture of the pacemaker and induce ventricular fibrillation.

Unfortunately, many programmable pacemakers are affected in an unpredictable fashion by EMI; thus, they should be evaluated on an individual basis. In 1987, Hayes found that 21% of patients exposed to electrocautery during various types of surgery had their pacemaker reprogram to the backup mode. The risk of reprogramming appears to be growing with increasing complexity of the newer generators, such as those that modulate rate.

Measures to decrease susceptibility to EMI in the operating theater include:

□ Using bipolar ESC rather than unipolar ESC whenever possible.
□ Keeping the ESC receiving plate as remote from the generator as possible.
□ Ensuring that the pacing generator/electrode axis is not in the line between the operative site and the receiving plate.

□ Using the lowest current and the shortest burst of ESC possible.
□ Shielding the generator from beams of therapeutic ionizing radiation, which can damage circuits.
□ Using nerve stimulators carefully, with lead placement away from the generator.

Diagnostic radiography does not interfere with pacemaker function. If ESC is to be used, a magnet should be available but not necessarily placed on the patient, unless the exact response of the pacemaker is known (see Table 137–1). Applying the magnet to a programmable generator (i.e., VVIR or DDD) in the presence of EMI increases the risk of reprogramming and is discouraged. If a programmable generator reprograms as a result of EMI, magnet placement can be done in an attempt to convert the generator to asynchronous mode (reed closure). Once a magnet is placed on a programmable generator, it should be left on the generator until a programming unit is available, because a new program can manifest itself after magnet removal.

Summary: Preoperative Preparation

□ Obtain complete information on the pacemaker from the manufacturer.
□ Program rate-adaptive off and/or predict implications in the OR.
□ Consider programming to be asynchronous.
□ Ensure that a pacemaker magnet is available.
□ Ensure that an alternate pacing modality is available (Table 137–2).
□ Ensure that intravenous chronotropes (e.g., isoproterenol, ephedrine) are available.
□ Discuss ESC precautions with the surgeon.
□ When practical, regional anesthesia should be chosen, to permit evaluation of adequacy of cerebral perfusion.
□ A cardiology consultation probably is not needed if the patient is asymptomatic and recent evaluations of the generator are satisfactory. Generator interrogation is always advisable, if feasible.

Table 137–2. Comparison of Temporary Pacing Techniques

Method	Time to Initiate	Chambers Paced	Advantages	Disadvantages	Uses
Transcutaneous	1–2 minutes	Right ventricle	Simple, rapid, safe.	Variable capture, patient discomfort.	Arrest, intraoperative, prophylactic.
Transesophageal	Minutes	Left atrium	Reliable atrial capture, safe, simple.	Unreliable ventricular capture, requires special generator.	Prophylactic atrial, intraoperative, overdrive SVT, atrial electrogram.
Transvenous semirigid	3–20 minutes	Atrium and/or ventricle	Most reliable, well tolerated.	Invasive, time-consuming, potential complications.	Arrest, prophylactic, maintenance.
Transvenous flow-directed	3–20 minutes	Right ventricle	Simple, does not require fluoroscopy.	Invasive, stability questions, less readily available.	Arrest, intraoperative, prophylactic, maintenance.
Pacing pulmonary artery catheter (PAC)	Minutes (if PAC is in place)	Atrium and/or ventricle	Reliable ventricular capture, well tolerated.	Requires specific PAC that must be placed first.	Arrest, intraoperative, prophylactic, maintenance.
Epicardial	<1 minute	Atrium and/or ventricle	Reliable short-term.	Postoperative only, early lead failure.	Arrest, prophylactic, maintenance.
Transthoracic	10–60 seconds	Ventricle	Rapid and simple.	Many potential complications.	Arrest only.

Any generator exposed to electrical intervention, such as ESC or cardioversion, should be subsequently evaluated for program integrity, circuit damage, and myocardial damage at the electrode site. The latter could lead to increased threshold requirements with subsequent loss of capture. These problems may manifest intraoperatively or may not become evident until far into the postoperative period.

Suggested References

Atlee JL. Management of patients with pacemakers or ICD devices. In Atlee JL, ed. Arrhythmias and Pacemakers: Practical Management for Anesthesia and Critical Care Medicine. Philadelphia: WB Saunders, 1996:293–329.

Bourke ME. The patient with a pacemaker or related device. Can J Anaesth 1996;43:R24–41.

Ducey JP, Fincher CW, Baysinger CL. Therapeutic suppression of a permanent ventricular pacemaker using a peripheral nerve stimulator. Anesthesiology 1991;75:533–536.

Mangar D, Atlas GM, Kane PB. Electrocautery-induced pacemaker malfunction during surgery. Can J Anaesth 1991;38:616–618.

Peters RW, Gold MR. Reversible prolonged pacemaker failure due to electrocautery. J Interv Card Electrophysiol 1998;2:343–344.

Rozner MA, Trankina MF. Intrathoracic Gadgets: Update on Pacemakers and Implantable Cardioverter Defibrillators. American Society of Anesthesiology Refresher Courses. Chicago: American Society of Anesthesiology, 2000:231.

138

Automatic Implantable Cardioverter-Defibrillator

Mark F. Trankina, M.D.

Overview

Approximately 300,000 Americans die each year from sudden cardiac arrest. Prophylactic antiarrhythmic drug therapy has not been as successful as was once hoped in controlling ventricular tachycardia and fibrillation. The automatic implantable cardioverter-defibrillator (AICD or ICD) has emerged as a practical and effective means of controlling lethal arrhythmias in patients whom medical therapy has failed. By the turn of the century, about 200,000 people had received defibrillators since federal approval for the devices was obtained in 1985. An estimated 100,000 recipients were still alive in 1999. Nine companies have produced 126 models of ICDs. These devices are costly, about $20,000 for the generator plus a comparable amount in hospital costs.

ICDs may be placed either transvenously or surgically via median sternotomy or thoracotomy. General anesthesia is required for surgical placement. Although transvenous placement is often done by cardiologists with intravenous sedation, consideration should be given to the stress associated with testing the unit. Many anesthesiologists prefer general anesthesia when providing anesthesia for transvenous placement, to allow better physiologic control of the patient throughout testing. After the unit is placed, it must be tested (ventricular fibrillation). This can lead to prolonged periods of asystole that can result in significant myocardial and cerebral ischemia. Enough time should be allowed between tests to ensure reperfusion and restoration of hemodynamic stability. It may be left to the anesthesiologist to monitor the duration and frequency of testing/ischemic periods. Vasoactive drugs are often used to stabilize these patients during and immediately after the testing period. High-dose narcotic therapy may be indicated to minimize cardiac depression. Minimum monitoring includes two-lead ECG and continuous arterial pressure monitoring.

The most commonly used generator (more than 80,000 placed), the Ventak, can deliver only a high-energy shock. More recently developed devices can deliver "tiered therapy" that under the correct conditions will attempt overdrive pacing first and then deliver a defibrillation shock if needed. Like a pacemaker, an ICD system consists of a generator and a set of leads. The shock is created by electronic circuitry in the generator that changes the battery voltage (typically 3 volts) to nearly 700 volts for a maximum energy discharge (roughly 30 joules). ICD function and lead placement are described by the North American Society of Pacing and Electrophysiology (NASPE) Generic Defibrillator Code (Table 138–1).

ICDs developed since 1993 have many programmable features, but essentially they measure each cardiac R-R interval and categorize the rate as normal, too fast (short R-R interval), or too slow (long R-R interval). When the device detects a sufficient number of short R-R intervals within a specified time period, it will begin an antitachycardia event. The internal computer will decide between overdrive pacing (less energy used, better tolerated by the patient, used for atrial flutter and ventricular tachycardia [VT]) or shock. If shock is chosen, then an internal capacitor is charged. Charging time depends on the desired output; a maximum shock can take 6 to 15 seconds.

Typically, ICDs deliver no more than 6 shocks per event, although some can deliver as many as 18. Within an event, each successive therapy must be at equal or greater energy than the previous attempt. Thus, once a shock is delivered, no further antitachycardia pacing can take place. Most devices can now be programmed to reconfirm VT or VF after charging, to prevent inappropriate shock therapy. Despite this reconfirmation, approximately 20% to 40% of shocks are for a rhythm other than VT or VF. Supraventricular tachycardia remains the most common etiology of inappropriate shock therapy.

Single- and dual-chamber pacemakers can function in the presence of an ICD as long as the electrodes are bipolar. An ICD with a built-in capability for antibradycardia pacing will begin pacing when the R-R interval is too long. Beginning about 1993, most ICDs incorporated backup VVI pacing to protect the patient from the common occurrence of postshock bradycardia. In July 1997, the FDA approved devices with sophisticated dual-chamber pacing modes and rate-responsive behavior for ICD

Table 138–1. NASPE Generic Defibrillator Code

Position I	Position II	Position III	Position IV*
Chamber(s) shocked	Antitachycardia pacing chamber(s)	Tachycardia detection	Antibradycardia pacing chamber(s)
O = None	O = None	E = Electrogram	O = None
A = Atrium	A = Atrium	H = Hemodynamic (not yet available)	A = Atrium
V = Ventricle	V = Ventricle		V = Ventricle
D = Dual (A + V)	D = Dual (A + V)		D = Dual (A + V)

*Position IV can be expanded into its complete NASPE pacemaker code to fully explain the device (e.g., VVE-DDDR).

patients who need permanent pacing (about 20% of ICD patients). If a patient with an ICD requires temporary pacing, bipolar leads, the lowest possible amplitude for capture, and the slowest rate associated with adequate hemodynamic status should be used. It is possible for a pacing spike followed by a QRS complex to be interpreted as VT, causing discharge of the unit. Inactivation of the ICD may be required during temporary pacing if interference occurs. Cardioverter units for atrial fibrillation are presently under investigation. The perioperative management of these devices is unknown, but most likely they will behave similar to ICDs.

External defibrillation can be used in a patient with an implanted ICD. However, the paddles should be oriented away from the implanted electrodes, if possible, and the lowest effective energy used. Gloves should be worn at all times when working with these patients, because the ICD can discharge at any time. Extra care should be taken to understand the psychological stress that these patients may feel; many of them have survived a cardiac arrest and do not expect to live long. The patient's perception may be that an anesthetic is exceptionally dangerous because of the ICD itself.

ICD Magnets

As in pacemakers, magnet behavior in many ICDs can be altered by programming. Most devices will suspend tachyarrhythmia detection (and thus therapy) when a magnet is appropriately placed to activate the reed switch. Antitachycardia therapy in some Guidant-CPI devices can be permanently disabled by magnet placement for 30 seconds. With the magnet mode enabled, Guidant-CPI devices emit tones synchronized to R waves, signifying adequate placement of the magnet and suspension of tachyarrhythmia detection (thus disabling therapy). If the device switches to a constant tone, then antitachycardia therapy has been programmed off. To reenable therapy, the magnet must be removed and then replaced until the constant tone reverts to tones synchronized to R waves. Subsequent removal of the magnet then returns the device to the enabled state. Any Guidant-CPI device that emits tones while a magnet is placed will be disabled during the magnet session. To ensure correct mag-

net placement on their devices, Medtronic plans to market a "smart magnet" that maintains communication with the device and reports on the device's status during the magnet session.

Again, interrogating the device and calling the manufacturer remain the most reliable ways to determine magnet response.

Preoperative Evaluation

All ICDs should have the antitachycardia therapy disabled before induction of anesthetic and commencement of the procedure. Devices with pacemaker capabilities should be handled as discussed in Chapter 137. As with pacing devices, monopolar electrosurgical cautery (ESC) has been reported to "confuse" an ICD into delivering inappropriate therapy. Also, many ICDs have no noise reversion behavior, so ESC-induced ventricular oversensing might cause nonpacing in a patient who depends on an ICD for pacing.

Intraoperative Management

No special monitoring or anesthetic technique is required for the patient with an ICD. However, ECG monitoring and the ability to deliver prompt external cardioversion or defibrillation must be present as the ICD is being disabled. Should external defibrillation become necessary, device manufacturers recommend using the lowest possible energy, placing the paddles perpendicular to the path of the implanted leads, and keeping the paddles away from the implanted generator, the same as with a standard pacemaker device. Postoperatively the ICD must be reinterrogated and reenabled.

In summary, patients receiving ICD therapy can present a challenge to the anesthesiologist, not because of the generator itself, but rather because of the underlying disease processes.

Suggested References

Atlee JL. Management of patients with pacemakers or ICD devices. In Atlee JL, ed. Arrhythmias and Pacemakers: Practical Management for Anesthesia and Critical Care Medicine. Philadelphia: WB Saunders, 1996:293–329.

Bourke ME. The patient with a pacemaker or related device. Can J Anaesth 1996;43:R24–41.

Cannom DS. A review of the implantable cardioverter defibrillator trials. Curr Opin Cardiol 1998;13:3–8.

Gross JN, Sackstein RD, Song SL, et al. The antitachycardia pacing ICD: Impact on patient selection and outcome. PACE Pacing Clin Electrophysiol 1993;16:165–169.

Rozner MA. Intrathoracic Gadgets: Pacemakers and Implantable Cardioverter-Defibrillators in the New Millenium. American Society of Anesthesiology Refresher Course Lectures. Chicago: American Society of Anesthesiology, 2000:231.

Saksena S, Madan N, Lewis C. Implanted cardioverter-defibrillators are preferable to drugs as primary therapy in sustained ventricular tachyarrhythmias. Prog Cardiovasc Dis 1996;38:445–454.

Vlay SC. Electromagnetic interference and ICD discharge related to chiropractic treatment. Pacing Clin Electrophysiol 1998;21:2001.

139
Detection and Treatment of Perioperative Acute Coronary Syndromes

Guy S. Reeder, M.D.

The acute coronary syndromes (ACS) constitute a spectrum of myocardial ischemia, including ST elevation myocardial infarction (MI), non-ST elevation MI, and unstable angina pectoris. (The old terms "Q-wave" and "non–Q-wave MI" have been replaced with "ST segment elevation" and "non–ST segment elevation MI.") Early in the course of presentation, it may be difficult to separate non-ST elevation MI from prolonged unstable angina, and thus these two conditions are initially managed in a similar fashion.

The pathogenesis of perioperative ACS is similar to that of spontaneously developing myocardial ischemia and MI. Plaque rupture or erosion leads to formation of partially or totally occlusive thrombus, most often at the site of preexisting angiographically modest coronary artery disease. Additional predisposing factors in the perioperative setting include increased oxygen demand due to catecholamine release from metabolic stress and a hypercoagulable state. Total coronary occlusion most often leads to ST segment elevation MI, whereas subtotal occlusion is most commonly associated with non–ST segment elevation coronary syndromes (although many other factors, including preexistent collaterals, level of oxygen demand, and coronary vasomotion, may alter this generalization).

Detection of ACS is enhanced by appropriate perioperative monitoring of high-risk patients (see Chaps. 85, 96, and 97). Intraoperative monitoring may include multilead electrocardiography (ECG), trend monitoring of pulmonary artery pressure and, in some cases, transesophageal echocardiography of regional and global left ventricular systolic function. The incidence rate of ACS peaks on the third postoperative day and declines thereafter. Although chest pain or pressure may be the major clinical presentation, more commonly the patient describes vague discomfort, dyspnea, or some other, less specific complaint. ST elevation or depression or elevated cardiac enzyme markers may be noted. Occasionally, pulmonary edema, new congestive heart failure, or ventricular arrhythmia may be the first manifestation.

A general approach to management of ACS is shown in Figure 139–1. Urgent cardiology consultation is warranted when ACS is suspected. Necessary adjustments in anesthetic and fluid management should be made to optimize oxygenation, blood volume, and hemoglobin while minimizing myocardial oxygen demand. Because the underlying problem in ACS is platelet-rich thrombus, pharmacotherapy includes antiplatelet and antithrombotic agents. These agents greatly increase the risk of bleeding in the intraoperative and perioperative settings, and thus must be used cautiously. In cases where the risk of postoperative hemorrhage is low, aspirin should be administered immediately, and intravenous heparin should be considered. Although low molecular weight heparin has been shown to be more effective than unfractionated heparin in treating ACS, its effects are more difficult to monitor and reverse quickly based on commonly available tests. Thus, unfractionated heparin is currently preferred. The potent intravenous glycoprotein IIb/IIIa platelet antagonists are generally contraindicated in the setting of ongoing or recent surgery, because of the high risk of hemorrhagic complications. Anti-ischemic therapy should include intravenous β blockade, preferably with a quickly reversible agent such as esmolol, as well as intravenous nitroglycerin.

The treatment approach then diverges based on ECG findings. Patients with ST segment elevation or new left bundle branch block will be considered separately from those with ST segment depression or nonspecific ECG changes (see Fig. 139–1).

Acute Myocardial Infarction

ST segment elevation is highly specific for acute MI. The differential diagnosis includes pericarditis and coronary spasm (transient ST segment elevation). Patients with persistent ST segment elevation or new left bundle branch block typically have total occlusion of an epicardial coronary artery and are

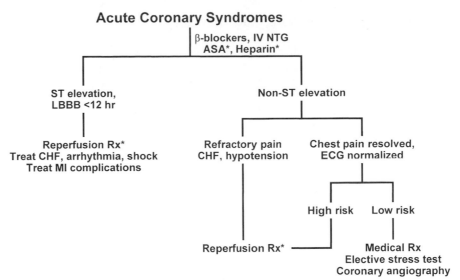

Figure 139–1. Therapy and decision making for patients with acute coronary syndromes. Reperfusion therapy includes angioplasty and/or thrombolysis. ASA, aspirin; LBBB, left bundle branch block; MI, myocardial infarction; NTG, nitroglycerine; CHF, congestive heart failure; Rx, therapy.

candidates for reperfusion therapy (thrombolysis or direct angioplasty), which is most beneficial if achieved early but is of some value up to 12 hours after event onset. Thrombolytic therapy is almost always contraindicated in the postoperative setting. However, if the patient's risk of bleeding will allow aspirin and intravenous heparin, then primary angioplasty, with or without stent implantation, is an excellent alternative to thrombolytic therapy if performed by an experienced physician in a timely manner. Most often this will be in the same center, but occasionally emergent patient transfer may be necessary.

Complications of MI include congestive failure, ventricular arrhythmias, and cardiogenic shock. These must be diligently monitored for and corrected with appropriate pharmacologic measures. Intra-aortic balloon pumping may be useful for hemodynamic support before patient transfer or with the development of delayed shock or heart failure. The use of angiotensin-converting enzyme inhibitors should be considered early for patients with ST elevation MI if systolic blood pressure is above 100 mm Hg, especially if left ventricular function is reduced or mitral regurgitation or left ventricular failure is present. Pharmacologic therapy may also include aspirin, β blockers, and appropriate lipid-lowering therapy, usually with a statin agent.

Non–ST Segment Elevation ACS

Non–ST segment elevation ACS most commonly results from incompletely occlusive coronary thrombus. Patients at high risk for subsequent mortality and morbidity include those with persistent ST segment depression, those with elevated cardiac serum markers such as troponin or CK-MB, and those manifesting hemodynamic instability, including hypotension, shock, congestive heart failure, pulmo-

nary edema, and frequent ventricular arrhythmia. High-risk patients, as well as those with refractory ischemic pain, should be considered for urgent reperfusion therapy similar to that used for ST segment elevation ACS. The same caveats regarding assessment of bleeding risk and use of potent platelet and thrombin inhibitors apply. For other patients who are hemodynamically stable and minimally symptomatic, urgent angiography is not necessary, as long as the patient remains stable on aspirin, heparin, β blockers, and nitrates. Bedside echocardiography to monitor wall motion and systolic function is appropriate. Further investigation can be delayed until later in the convalescence and usually includes stress imaging and/or angiography. Guidelines for the management of preoperative risk stratification, acute MI, and for the use of coronary angioplasty are available.

Special Situations

- Aspirin allergy: Clopidogrel, 75 mg daily, may be substituted.
- Heparin-induced thrombocytopenia: This typically does not occur during the first 5 days of therapy unless recent earlier exposure to heparin has occurred. Patients with this disorder will have an antibody to the heparin-platelet factor 4 complex. Substitute desirudin, a direct-acting antithrombin that is structurally and functionally unrelated to heparin.
- β blockers are contraindicated in second-degree or greater AV block and in patients with severe asthma but should not be withheld in diabetic patients.
- Calcium channel blockers are indicated for rate control of rapid atrial fibrillation, which may accompany or precipitate ACS in some individuals. However, there is no primary indication for these

agents in ACS otherwise, and they generally should be avoided.

□ For refractory ventricular tachycardia/ventricular fibrillation, the current drug of choice is intravenous amiodarone, 150 mg bolus and intravenous infusion.

□ Mechanical complications of MI: With anterior wall MI, pump failure is the most serious complication and is a strong indication for reperfusion therapy as well as for inotropic support and intra-aortic balloon pumping. With inferior wall MI, complications such as papillary muscle dysfunction or rupture, as well as hemodynamically significant right ventricular MI, are more common. Surface or transesophageal echocardiography allows rapid and accurate differentiation of these disorders.

□ Sudden hemodynamic collapse: Because preexisting symptoms of ACS may be vague in the postoperative patient, the differential diagnosis is wide and also includes pulmonary embolus, dissection, pneumothorax, cardiac tamponade, and sepsis.

Suggested References

Agency for Health Care Policy and Research, Unstable Angina Guideline Panel. Diagnosing and managing unstable angina. Am Fam Physician 1994;49:1459–1462, 1465–1468, 1473–1475.

Eagle KA, Brundage BH, Chaitman BR, et al. Guidelines for perioperative cardiovascular evaluation of noncardiac surgery. J Am Coll Cardiol 1996;27:910–948.

Reeder GS. Contemporary diagnosis and management of unstable angina. Mayo Clin Proc 2000;75:953–957.

Ryan TJ, Antman EM, Brooks NH, et al. ACC/AHA guidelines for the management of patients with acute myocardial infarction. J Am Coll Cardiol 1999;34:890–811.

Scanlon PJ, Faxon DP, Audet AM, et al. ACC/AHA Guidelines for coronary angiography: A report of the American College of Cardiology/American Heart Association Task Force on Practice Guidelines (Committee on Coronary Angiography). J Am Coll Cardiol 1999;33:1756–1824.

Verheugt FW. Acute coronary syndromes: Drug treatments. Lancet 1999;353(suppl II):20–23.

Warltier DC, Pagel PS, Kersten JR. Approaches to the prevention of perioperative myocardial ischemia. Anesthesiology 2000;92:253–259.

140
Anticoagulation and Reversal for Cardiopulmonary Bypass

Gregory A. Nuttall, M.D.

Mechanism of Action of Heparin

The surface of a non–heparin-coated cardiopulmonary bypass (CPB) circuit is extremely thrombogenic. Therefore, it is imperative that the patient be anticoagulated before and throughout CPB. Heparin is the anticoagulant of choice for cardiac surgery with CPB.

Standard heparin is composed of a heterogeneous group of polyanionic mucopolysaccharides. A unique pentasaccharide sequence of heparin has been identified that interacts with the serine protease antithrombin III (AT III).[1] The active center serines of procoagulants thrombin (IIa), factor Xa, factor XIa, factor XIIa, and factor IXa are inhibited by an arginine reactive center of the AT III molecule. Heparin binds to the lysine site on AT III, producing a conformational change at the arginine reactive center. Heparin binding converts AT III from a progressive slow inhibitor to a very rapid inhibitor. After AT III binds to its substrate, the heparin dissociates from the complex and is available to bind to another AT III molecule. The AT III remains covalently bonded to its substrate. Thrombin and factor Xa are the substances most sensitive to inactivation.

Heparin Monitoring

The heparin management protocol developed by Bull and colleagues[2] with activated clotting time (ACT) guidance has been the standard for CPB since 1975. This ACT-based system of heparin management with an initial loading dose of heparin (300 U/kg), followed by supplemental heparin to maintain the ACT at greater than 400 to 450 seconds, has been the standard heparin management system at many institutions.

The ACT is a sensitive but nonspecific assay. Its practicality is based on its ability to test whole blood in the operating room. Diatomaceous earth or another substance accelerates clotting until a rotating magnet is pulled away from the wall of the tube. The ACT is very sensitive to heparin, but values can also be abnormally prolonged in the setting of reduced factor XII activity, hypothermia, or platelet count below 50,000/mL or a fibrinogen level below 100 mg/dL. Heparin resistance, an abnormally short ACT value following a standard heparin dose, is most commonly caused by an acquired AT III deficiency. The most common cause for this is earlier chronic heparin therapy. AT III deficiency is treated with the administration of either AT III concentrate or several units of fresh frozen plasma.

The ACT provides a functional assay of heparin activity in whole blood, but it does not measure the exact blood concentration of heparin. Automated heparin assays based on the protamine titration test are also available. After termination of CPB, the ACT can be used to confirm the protamine antagonism of heparin therapy by return of the ACT to preheparinization values.

Protamine Reversal

After CPB, the anticoagulant effects of heparin must be reversed to prevent excessive bleeding. Protamine is the drug traditionally used for this purpose. A polycationic peptide derived from the sperm of fish, protamine antagonizes the anticoagulant effects of heparin by ionically binding to heparin and forming a complex that is cleared from the blood. Protamine is generally administered intravenously on a dosage schedule in which 1 to 1.3 mg of protamine is given to reverse 1 mg of heparin. More refined protamine dosing schedules have been developed based on the automated heparin assay devices described earlier. There are four types of adverse reactions to protamine.[3] The most common is a direct non–histamine-mediated systemic vasodilation with hypotension. This can be reduced or obviated by administering protamine slowly. Protamine can also induce anaphylactic, anaphylactoid, and severe pulmonary vasoconstriction reactions.

Selected References

1. Hirsh J. Heparin. N Engl J Med 1991;324:1565–1574.
2. Bull BS, Korpman RA, Huse WM, Briggs BD. Heparin therapy during extracorporeal circulation: 1. Problems inherent to existing heparin protocols. J Thorac Cardiovasc Surg 1975;69:674–684.
3. Horrow JC. Protamine: A review of its toxicity. Anesth Analg 1985;64:348–361.

141
Evaluation of the Coagulation System

Maria DeCastro, M.D.

Evaluation of the coagulation system facilitates preoperative assessment of coagulation, enables assessment of adequate anticoagulation after the administration of anticoagulant agents, and improves diagnostic accuracy in the setting of intraoperative coagulopathy. Although normal coagulation involves a complex interplay of vascular endothelium, platelets, and the soluble clotting factors, the classical divisions of the clotting cascade are useful in understanding the reactions measured by the various clotting tests (Fig. 141–1).[1]

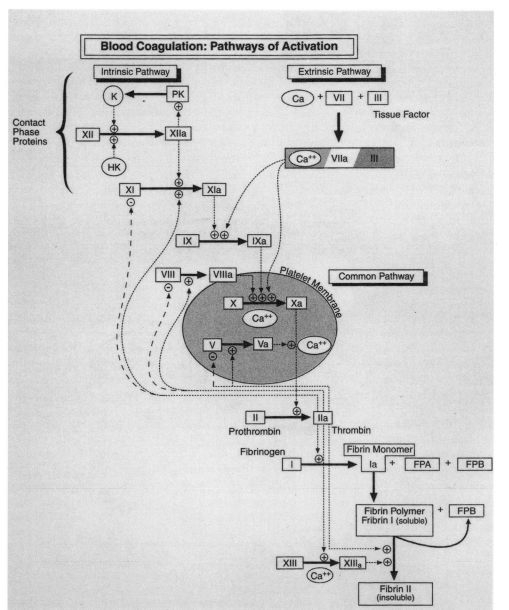

Figure 141–1. Activation of proteins leading to blood coagulation. A positive-feedback system (amplification) magnifies initial pathway reactions. A negative-feedback system (inhibition) serves as a countervailing force and limits coagulation. Dotted arrows and + signs indicate facilitation of the process; dashed arrows and − signs indicated inhibition of the process. The intrinsic pathway is initiated by the action of kallikrein (K) and high molecular weight kininogen (HK) and prekallikrein (PK) cofactors on Factor XII. Fibrinopeptide A (FPA) and fibrinopeptide B (FPB) are two peptides released when the fibrin monomer is formed. (From Carvalho ACA.[1])

Preoperative Assessment of Coagulation

Careful clinical history is the best preoperative screen for bleeding disorders. In the absence of clinical suspicion, routine preoperative clotting studies are not warranted. Table 141–1 summarizes some of the most common laboratory studies of coagulation in patients presenting for surgery.

Assessment of Anticoagulation

Activated Clotting Time. Because of its simplicity and speed, the activated clotting time (ACT) is the most commonly used test for monitoring adequacy of anticoagulation in the operating room. This test of whole blood clotting uses one of two activators (celite or kaolin) to stimulate contact activation of coagulation. The ACT thus measures the intrinsic and common pathways of coagulation. Clot formation either pulls away a small iron cylinder interrupting a magnetic field (Hemochron; International Technidyne, Edison, NJ) or slows the descent of a small plastic plunger (Hemotec; Medtronic, Parker, CO). Besides operator errors, prolonged ACT can be caused by hemodilution, hypothermia, thrombocytopenia, and platelet dysfunction. Importantly, the antifibrinolytic agent aprotinin acts as an inhibitor of contact activation and prolongs the reactions measured by the ACT. The presence of aprotinin affects celite-activated ACT measurements more than kaolin-activated measurements.[4]

Heparin Assays. Automated heparin–protamine titration devices are available that can measure blood heparin levels and calculate protamine reversal dosages intraoperatively. By correlating heparin levels with ACT, these devices can also calculate an individual heparin dose response.

Intraoperative Coagulation Monitoring

Thromboelastography. Thromboelastography (TEG) is a viscoelastic test of whole blood clotting that provides information about the clotting cascade, platelet function, and clot lysis. Figure 141–2 shows the variables measured by the TEG and common abnormalities. In liver transplantation[5] and cardiac surgery,[6] TEG use has been associated with reduced transfusion requirements.

Bedside Tests of Coagulation. Two bedside monitors of prothrombin time (PT) and activated partial thromboplastin time (APTT) are now available. Although earlier studies have demonstrated greater variability in bedside APTT results than in PT results, good agreement between these bedside monitors and simultaneously obtained laboratory results has recently been shown.[7]

Bedside Tests of Platelet Function. A convenient, reproducible bedside test of platelet function would be a useful addition in the diagnosis of platelet-associated coagulopathy. To date, no such test exists. Intraoperative bleeding time measurements are not practical to obtain or reliable under anesthesia, which alters skin blood flow. Although TEG (specifically, the maximum amplitude measurement) does provide information about platelets, it is not specific for platelet function and cannot distinguish between disorders of platelet number and disorders of platelet function. The HemoSTATUS device (Medtronic, Parker, CO) adds platelet-activating factor to a kaolin ACT. Shortening of the ACT measurement provides evidence of functioning

Table 141–1. Laboratory Studies of Coagulation

Coagulation Test	Measured Aspect	Utility
PT	Extrinsic pathway, common pathway	Prolonged in severe factor deficiency, severe hypofibrinogenemia.
		Indirect measure of liver function.
		Screening test for oral anticoagulants.
APTT	Intrinsic pathway, common pathway	Prolonged in severe factor deficiency, severe hypofibrinogenemia.
		Prolonged in hemophilias.
		Prolonged by heparin.
		Usually prolonged in von Willebrand's disease.
		Prolonged, not associated with bleeding, in deficiencies of XII, prekallikrein, HMWK, lupus anticoagulant.
Fibrinogen	Common pathway	Increased risk of hemorrhage if less than 100 mg/dL.
		May be useful preoperatively in the presence of thrombolytic therapy.
Bleeding time	Platelet function	Not useful in routine screening.
		Marked prolongation (greater than 2 times normal) associated with bleeding.
		Usually minor prolongation with aspirin.
		Prolonged in von Willebrand's disease, uremia, myeloproliferative diseases, congenital platelet defects.

Adapted from de Moerloose P[2] and Whalen J, Tuman KJ.[3]

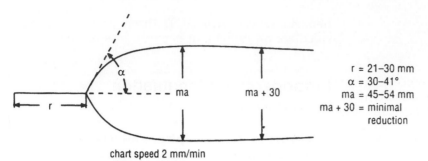

chart speed 2 mm/min

r = 21–30 mm
α = 30–41°
ma = 45–54 mm
ma + 30 = minimal
reduction

Variable	Measures		Abnormality	Example
r reaction time	thromboplastin generation via the intrinsic pathway	↑r	Factor deficiency Heparin Severe thrombocytopenia	Factor deficiency
α angle of divergence	rate of clot formation	↓α	Hypofibrinogenemia Thrombocytopenia Thrombocytopathy	Hypofibrinogenemia
ma maximum amplitude	maximum clot strength/elasticity	↓ma	Thrombocytopenia Thrombocytopathy Hypofibrinogenemia Factor XIII deficiency	Thrombocytopenia
ma + 30	clot retraction after 30 minutes	↓ma + 30	Fibrinolysis	Fibrinolysis

Figure 141–2. Typical TEG pattern and variables measured, normal values, and examples of some abnormal tracings.

platelets. Although some authors have correlated longer platelet-activated ACT measurements with blood loss in cardiac surgery,[8] others have not.[9]

Point-of-Care Testing

Refinement and miniaturization of technology have fostered the development of an auxiliary coagulation laboratory in the operating room. Because information from bedside (point-of-care) tests is obtained more quickly than in a standard hospital laboratory, these tests may lead to a more rational use of costly blood bank resources. Operator proficiency and quality control for bedside testing must be rigorously documented to ensure accurate results and to justify patient charges. Point-of-care testing is subject to regulation by a number of governing bodies, including the Joint Commission on Accreditation of Healthcare Organization, College of American Pathologists, State Health Departments, and local hospital departments of pathology.

Selected References

1. Carvalho ACA. Hemostasis and thrombosis. In Schiffman FJ, ed. Hematologic Pathophysiology. Philadelphia: Lippincott-Raven, 1998:161–243.
2. de Moerloose P. Laboratory evaluation of hemostasis before cardiac operations. Ann Thorac Surg 1996;62:1921–1925.
3. Whalen J, Tuman KJ. Monitoring hemostasis. Int Anesthesiol Clin 1996;34(3):195–213.
4. Wang JS, Lin CY, Hung WT, et al. In vitro effects of aprotinin on activated clotting times with different activators. J Thorac Cardiovasc Surg 1992;104:1135–1140.
5. Kang YG, Martin DJ, Marquez J, et al. Intraoperative changes in blood coagulation and thromboelastographic monitoring in liver transplantation. Anesth Analg 1985;64:888–896.
6. Shore-Lesserson L, Manspeizer HE, DePerio M, et al. Thromboelastographic-guided transfusion algorithm reduces transfusions in complex cardiac surgery. Anesth Analg 1999;88:312–319.
7. Boldt J, Walz G, Triem J, et al. Point-of-care (POC) measurement of coagulation after cardiac surgery. Intensive Care Med 1998;24:1187–1193.
8. Despotis GJ, Levine V, Filos KS, et al. Evaluation of a new point-of-care test that measures PAF-mediated acceleration of coagulation in cardiac surgical patients. Anesthesiology 1996;85:1311–1323.
9. Ereth MH, Nuttall GA, Santrach PJ, et al. The relation between the platelet-activated clotting test (HemoSTATUS) and blood loss after cardiopulmonary bypass. Anesthesiology 1998;88:962–969.

Suggested References

Despotis GJ, Gravlee G, Filos K, et al. Anticoagulation monitoring during cardiac surgery. Anesthesiology 1999;91:1122–1151.
Whitten CW, Greilich PE. Thromboelastography: Past, present, and future. Anesthesiology 2000;92:1223–1225.

142

Causes of Intraoperative Bradycardia

Karen S. Reed, M.D., Ph.D.

Bradycardia is one of several common arrhythmias that occur during anesthesia. It may be hemodynamically significant, particularly in patients with heart disease. Factors that cause sinus bradycardia under anesthesia can be classified into three categories: intrinsic, vagal responses, and direct effects (Table 142–1).

Intrinsic to the Patient

Hypoxemia causes both cardiovascular and respiratory depression, leading to bradycardia, hypotension, and decreased minute ventilation in a patient breathing spontaneously. Because of its critical nature, hypoxemia should be first on the list of possibilities in a patient with bradycardia.

Table 142–1. Causes of Intraoperative Bradycardia

Intrinsic
  Systemic
    Hypoxemia
    Hypercarbia
    Increased intracranial pressure
    Hypothermia
    Drugs
      Opiates
      β blockers
      Calcium channel blockers
      Potent inhalational agents
      Anticholinesterase inhibitors
      Succinylcholine
  Cardiac
    Sinus bradycardia
    Junctional rhythms
    Sick sinus syndrome
    Atrioventricular conduction defects
    Myocardial infarction
Vagal responses
  Reflex stimulation
    Oropharynx
    Extraocular muscles
    Peritoneum
    Bowel
    Right atrial distention
    Bladder distention
Direct effects
  Volatile anesthetics
  Narcotics
  Regional anesthetics
  High spinal or spinal shock

Sick sinus syndrome is characterized by severe sinus bradycardia with sinus pause or arrest with escape. The impulse from the sinus node is blocked before it depolarizes the atrium, which leads to sinoatrial (SA) block. A sinus pause results from repetitive SA block and can lead to atrial fibrillation. Sick sinus syndrome is seen in the elderly with coronary artery disease, and usually presents as syncope.

Increased intracranial pressure can, via medullary ischemia, cause the Cushing triad of systemic hypertension, sinus bradycardia, and respiratory irregularities. Nonanesthetic drugs such as β blockers or digoxin may be the cause of intraoperative bradycardia.

Hypothermia initially causes a transient increase in heart rate by sympathetic stimulation, especially in the presence of shivering. With temperature decreases below 34°C, the heart rate decreases proportionally. Bradycardia is thought to result from the direct effect of cold on the SA tissue. The bradycardia is not affected by atropine or vagotomy.

Bradycardia is commonly seen after myocardial infarction because of damage to the myocardium.

Vagal Responses

Stimulation of the oropharynx (by laryngoscopy, intubation, and extubation), extraocular muscles, bronchus, peritoneum, and rectum gives rise to autonomic reflexes that include bronchospasm, bradycardia or tachycardia, hypotension or hypertension, and cardiac arrhythmias. These effects are more common in lightly anesthetized, hypoxic, or hypercarbic patients. Preventive approaches include the use of atropine, topical anesthesia, intravenous local anesthetics, adrenergic-blocking agents, deep anesthesia, and vasodilating agents.

Acetylcholine-related drugs, such as succinylcholine and neostigmine, have also been shown to cause bradycardia. Bradycardia is seen in children after the first dose of succinylcholine. In 80% of adults, bradycardia is seen after the second dose of succinylcholine if given 5 minutes after the first dose. The bradycardia is thought to be related to the following: (1) the choline molecule from the breakdown of succinylcholine may sensitize the patient to subsequent succinylcholine; (2) succinylcholine may directly stimulate peripheral sensory receptors to produce reflex bradycardia; and (3) succinylcholine may stimulate the sympathetic and parasympathetic nervous systems. Other nondepolarizing muscle relaxants, such as vecuronium, may be associated with bradycardia because they lack vagolytic effects.

Direct Anesthetic Effect

Inhaled anesthetic gases, such as halothane, enflurane, and isoflurane, all depress the sinus node activity by altering the slope of phase IV depolarization. This appears to be related to an effect on calcium flux across the membrane.

Narcotics, such as fentanyl and morphine, have a direct action on the sinus node as well as central nervous system effects that cause bradycardia.

A mild decrease in heart rate may be seen in patients undergoing intravenous regional block on release of the tourniquet.

Fetal bradycardia can be seen after intravenous administration of local anesthetic in the mother even though no hypotension occurs in the mother. Paracervical injection of anesthetic is associated with a 20% to 30% incidence rate of fetal bradycardia. Local anesthetic toxicity causes a high mortality rate among newborns. Fetal bradycardia from local anesthetic is associated with apnea and convulsions at birth.

Suggested References

Doyle DJ, Mark PW. Reflex bradycardia during surgery. Can J Anaesth 1990;37:219.
Hillel Z, Thys DM. Electrocardiography. In Miller RD, ed. Anesthesia. 5th ed. Philadelphia: Churchill Livingstone, 2000: 1231–1254.
Kew MC, Lowe JP. The cardiovascular complications of intravenous regional anesthesia. Br J Surg 1971;58:179.
McGough ER. Cardiovascular system. In Gravenstein N, ed. Manual of Complications During Anesthesia. Philadelphia: JB Lippincott, 1991:181.

143
Aortic Stenosis

Martin L. DeRuyter, M.D.

Clinical Features

One-fourth of all patients with chronic valve disease have aortic stenosis (AS).[1] AS is generally subdivided into subvalvular, valvular, and supravalvular obstruction. Pure valvular stenosis is most common, representing 75% of patients with AS.

Traditionally, the cause of AS has been attributable to rheumatic heart disease, but as the incidence of rheumatic heart disease has decreased, other causes are becoming increasingly common. These include congenital stenosis, a bicuspid valve that later calcifies, and idiopathic degenerative calcification of aortic cusps (senile valve). Congenitally bicuspid valves occur in 1% to 2% of the population. Some 80% of adults with symptomatic valvular AS are male. Rheumatic AS is almost always associated with rheumatic involvement of the mitral valve. With AS, some degree of aortic insufficiency is likely. As the population ages, the prevalence of AS is likely to increase. A study of the elderly reported mild calcification in 40% and severe calcification in 13% of the patients studied. The prevalence of critical aortic valve stenosis was 2.9% in the over-age-75 group.[2]

Natural History

All patients are at increased risk of sudden death, yet the natural history of AS is more typical of a gradual onset of symptoms, mostly manifesting in the fifth to seventh decades. Although patients remain asymptomatic for many years, once the onset of symptoms occurs there is an acceleration toward death. Three cardinal symptoms are exertional dyspnea, angina, and syncope. Systolic hypertension is unusual, and a systolic pressure above 200 mm Hg generally excludes severe narrowing of the valve.

Untreated AS results in death, with CHF being the cause of death in one-half to two-thirds of these patients. Typical time frames from onset of symptoms till death are angina, 3 years; syncope, 3 years; dyspnea, 2 years; and congestive heart failure (CHF), 1.5 to 2 years. Sudden death is usually secondary to a cardiac arrhythmia.

Extent of Valvular Stenosis

The normal valve area is 2.5 to 3.5 cm^2; significant hemodynamic obstruction does not occur until the valve area is less than 1 cm^2. General classifications of AS by valve area are:

- Mild, greater than 1.2 cm^2.
- Moderate, 0.7 to 1.2 cm^2.
- Severe, 0.5 to 0.7 cm^2.
- Critical, less than 0.5 cm^2.

Critical AS is also defined as an outflow obstruction gradient exceeding 50 mm Hg. However, gradients are accurate at predicting severity of stenosis less than 50% of the time because they are flow-dependent.

Surgical Correction

Most patients undergo aortic valve replacement (AVR). The timing of surgery is based on symptoms and the degree of valve narrowing. Two major valve types are available, a bioprosthetic valve (tissue valve) and a mechanical valve. Choice of the type of valve a patient will receive relies mostly on weighing risks of anticoagulant-related bleeding, structural failure of the bioprosthetic valve, expected longevity of the patient and the likelihood of reoperation with its risk of death, and the patient's functional status. A review of an 11-year follow-up study of patients who were randomized to either a bioprosthetic valve or a mechanical valve noted no difference in survival rates between the two groups. Structural valve failure was observed in the bioprosthetic group, but this was offset by increased bleeding complications in the group who received mechanical valves.[3] In general, 10-year survival after AVR is approximately 67%.

Percutaneous transluminal valvuloplasty is mentioned for completeness. This may be an alternative to surgery in selected patients, but for all practical purposes indications are few.

Concomitant Diseases

Patients with AS often may have other, compounding medical problems. It is estimated that one half of the symptomatic patients also have anatomically significant coronary artery disease (CAD). Furthermore, the reported prevalence of significant CAD in asymptomatic patients ranges from 0% to 33%.[4] There is a less frequent association between gastrointestinal bleed and valvular heart disease.

Anesthetic Considerations for Aortic Valve Replacement

Many clinicians prefer a narcotic-based anesthetic. The principal advantages of narcotics are their lack of vasodilation and negative inotropy, which help promote hemodynamic stability. The negative features of inhalation agents have limited their role. Halothane depresses sinoatrial node automaticity, possibly causing a junctional rhythm and jeopardizing an optimal left ventricular end-diastolic volume that is dependent on a properly timed atrial contraction.[5] Isoflurane has undesirable effects on systemic vascular resistance (SVR) that may compromise coronary perfusion. Enflurane is a potent myocardial depressant.

In practice, most clinicians use a combination of a narcotic and either an inhalation agent or an intravenous hypnotic to produce optimal hemodynamics and allow for early extubation.

Monitoring usually includes arterial and pulmonary artery catheters, electrocardiograph with leads II (to assess presence of p-waves) and V_5 (to monitor for left ventricular ischemia).[6] Arrhythmias and hypotension should be treated aggressively. Anesthetic goals are summarized in Table 143–1.

Anesthesia for Noncardiac Surgery

Patients with AS who undergo noncardiac surgery are also at increased risk of perioperative myocardial infarction, CHF, and arrhythmias. An adequate history for symptoms and appropriate diagnostic testing should be done before elective surgery. Anesthetic goals for noncardiac surgery are similar to those for AVR, as summarized in Table 143–1. Given the potential for deleterious effects of a reduced SVR, spinal or epidural anesthesia is relatively contraindicated.

Table 143–1. Anesthetic Goals for Aortic Valve Replacement

Avoid hypotension.
Maintain sinus rhythm, avoiding both bradycardia and tachycardia.
Optimize intravascular volume to maintain venous return and left ventricular filling.
Avoid sudden increases or decreases in SVR.
Be aware of potential for myocardial ischemia and use appropriate monitoring.

Selected References

1. Braunwald E. Valvular heart disease. In Fauci AS, et al, eds. Harrison's Principles of Internal Medicine. 14th ed. New York: McGraw-Hill, 1998:1311.
2. Lindroos M, Kupari M, Heikkila J, et al. Prevalence of aortic valve abnormalities in the elderly: An echocardiographic study of a random population sample. J Am Coll Cardiol 1993;21:1220.
3. Hammermeister K, Sethi G, Henderson W, et al. A comparison of outcomes in men 11 years after heart-valve replacement with a mechanical valve or bioprosthesis. N Engl J Med 1993;328:1289.
4. Jackson JM, Thomas SJ. Valvular heart disease. In Kaplan JA, ed. Cardiac Anesthesia. 4th ed. Philadelphia: WB Saunders, 1999:727.
5. Stoelting RK, Dierdorf SF. Valvular heart disease. In Anesthesia and Co-Existing Disease. 3rd ed. New York: Churchill Livingstone, 1993:21–35.
6. Moore R, Martin D. Anesthetic management for the treatment of valvular heart disease. In Hennsley F Jr, Martin D, eds. The Practice of Cardiac Anesthesia. Boston: Little, Brown, 1990:351.

144
Heart Failure: Classification, Compensation, and Therapy

Karen S. Reed, M.D., Ph.D.

Heart failure is a condition in which the heart cannot provide sufficient cardiac output to satisfy the metabolic needs of tissues.

Causes of Heart Failure

Causes of heart failure include increased workload, disorders of the myocardium, and restriction to ventricular filling. Increased workload results from the following:

□ High output states: hyperthyroidism, anemia, systemic arteriovenous fistula, dermatologic disorders.
□ Valvular regurgitation or left-to-right shunts.
□ Increased impedance to ejection: systemic hypertension, pulmonary hypertension, pulmonary or aortic stenosis.

Disorders of the myocardium can result from cardiomyopathies and myocardial infarction. Restriction to ventricular filling may be linked to:

□ Pericardial constriction or effusion.
□ Mitral or tricuspid stenosis.
□ Increased ventricular stiffness: infiltrative myocardial disease, ventricular hypertrophy, hypertrophic cardiomyopathy.

New York Heart Association Functional Classification of Cardiac Patients

The New York Heart Association has developed a functional classification for cardiac patients:

□ Class I: No limitation. Greater than ordinary physical activity does not cause undue fatigue, palpitation, dyspnea, or angina. Prognosis good.
□ Class II: Slight limitation of physical activity. Comfortable at rest. Ordinary physical activity causes fatigue, palpitation, dyspnea, or angina. Prognosis good with therapy.
□ Class III: Marked limitation of physical activity. Less than ordinary activity will lead to symptoms. Comfortable at rest. Prognosis fair with therapy.
□ Class IV: Inability to carry on any physical activity without discomfort. Symptoms of heart failure or angina present at rest. Any physical activity increases discomfort. Prognosis guarded with therapy.

Compensation

Increased sympathetic activity mediated by elevated levels of plasma norepinephrine, angiotensin II, and endothelium leads to increased heart rate, increased contractility, and increased venoconstriction, which elevate venous return and preload. The enhanced sympathetic activity has an adverse effect because of increasing arteriolar constriction, thereby increasing afterload and oxygen requirements.

Cardiac hypertrophy will increase working muscle mass. Hypertrophy will have an adverse effect by increasing wall tension, decreasing coronary blood flow, and increasing oxygen requirements. Hypertrophic muscle also has abnormal systolic and diastolic properties.

The Frank-Starling mechanism has an adverse effect on pulmonary and systemic congestion. Left ventricular size also increases, leading to an increase in wall tension and oxygen requirements.

Renal salt and water retention, caused by elevated aldosterone and arginine vasopressin, increases venous return. Increased venous return has an adverse effect on pulmonary and systemic congestion. Elevated renin-angiotensin leads to increasing vasoconstriction and afterload. Elevated atrial natriuretic peptide leads to natriuresis, diuresis, and vasodilation. Increased peripheral oxygen extraction increases oxygen delivery and cardiac output.

Management

Heart failure is managed as follows:

□ Reduce cardiac workload by rest, treatment of exacerbating factors, vasodilators, and an intraaortic balloon pump if necessary.

357

□ Improve cardiac performance by correcting the underlying defect and rhythm abnormalities and by using positive inotropic agents. Therapeutic modalities include angiotensin-converting enzyme (ACE) inhibitors, nitrates, hydralazine, calcium channel blockers, diuretics, inotropes, and β blockers

□ Control excess salt and water by sodium restriction, diuretics, and mechanical fluid removal.

Suggested References

Kelly RA, Smith TW. Digoxin in heart failure: Implications of recent trials. J Am Coll Cardiol 1993;22:107A.

Lake CL. Chronic treatment of congestive heart failure. In Kaplan JA, ed. Cardiac Anesthesia. 4th ed. Philadelphia: WB Saunders, 1999:131.

Little WC, Applegate RJ. Congestive heart failure: Systolic and diastolic function. J Cardiothorac Vasc Anesth 1993;7:2.

Riegger GA. Lessons from recent randomized controlled trials for the management of congestive heart failure. Am J Cardiol 1993;71:38E.

Schwartz K, Chassagne C, Boheler KR. The molecular biology of heart failure. J Am Coll Cardiol 1993;22:30A.

Speakman MT, Kloner RA. Congestive heart failure. In Rakel RE, ed. Conn's Current Therapy. Philadelphia: WB Saunders, 1999:293.

Weintraub NL, Chaitman BR. Newer concepts in the medical management of patients with congestive heart failure. Clin Cardiol 1993;16:380.

145
Neonatal Cardiovascular Physiology

Robert J. Lunn, M.D.

To understand the normal and abnormal patterns of neonatal circulation, one needs to understand the normal fetal and transitional circulation. Abnormalities that develop in utero can dramatically affect subsequent cardiovascular development.

Fetal Circulation

The placenta is responsible for exchanging oxygen, nutrients, and metabolic wastes between fetal and maternal blood. Blood containing oxygen and nutrients is carried to the fetus via a single umbilical vein. The umbilical vein enters the liver and joins the inferior vena cava (IVC) via the ductus venosus, which allows 50% to 60% of umbilical venous blood to bypass the hepatic circulation. In the right atrium (RA), one-third of inferior caval blood is directed across the foramen ovale to the left atrium (LA). This occurs because of the geometric relationship between the IVC and the crista dividens at the anterior edge of the foramen ovale. This ensures that blood with the highest oxygen content perfuses the coronary and cerebral circulations. Blood returning from the superior vena cava (SVC) along with two-thirds of IVC blood enters the right ventricle (RV) and is ejected into the pulmonary artery (PA). The pulmonary vascular resistance (PVR) in the fetal lungs is very high because of the relatively hypoxic conditions and because the lungs are fluid filled and relatively collapsed. As a result of this high PVR, 90% of the blood that enters the PA is shunted across the ductus arteriosus (DA) into the descending aorta.

Left atrial blood, consisting mainly of blood directed across the foramen ovale, crosses the mitral valve and is pumped into the ascending aorta by the left ventricle (LV). Most of the blood that enters the ascending aorta from the LV perfuses the heart, brain, and upper extremities. Blood perfusing the lower body returns to the placenta via the paired umbilical arteries.

Several important points about the fetal circulation should be stressed. First, the fetal ventricles work in a parallel fashion, and thus fetal cardiac output is equal to the combined output of both ventricles. Second, the RV receives and pumps two-thirds of the fetal blood; as a result the RV at term has 25% more muscle mass than that of the LV. Finally, it is important to understand that the development of normal cardiac chambers and vessels requires that these structures receive normal blood flow. Abnormal restriction or augmentation of blood flow in utero will adversely affect development. For example, restriction of blood flow across the foramen ovale in utero results in a hypoplastic mitral valve, LV, and ascending aorta and is thought to be the central lesion in the hypoplastic left heart syndrome.

Transitional Circulation

The newborn infant must accomplish numerous cardiopulmonary changes to develop a normal adult type of circulatory system. Many of these changes occur in a gradual fashion over the first several days of life. The circulatory pattern that bridges the fetal type of circulation and the adult type of circulation is commonly referred to as the transitional circulation.

Several events occur in the first few minutes after an infant is born. With the first few breaths, lung water is removed and the lungs inflate, dramatically increasing the ambient oxygen content. Distention of the alveoli and increasing oxygen content result in a drop in the PVR. Separation from the placenta, which is a very low-resistance organ, results in an increase in systemic vascular resistance (SVR). The combined effects of decreasing PVR and increasing SVR result in increased pulmonary blood flow.

In the fetus and in the first few hours of life, the pressures in the PA and aorta are equal. In the fetus, about 90% of the blood that enters the PA is shunted across the DA into the aorta (right to left). Within hours after birth, this flow is reversed, and 30% to 50% of the left ventricular output is shunted into the PA. As a result, the pulmonary blood flow is higher during transition than in the fetus or the adult.

Physiologic closure of the DA begins 10 to 15 hours after birth and results from muscular constriction of the medial smooth muscle. It is important to remember that this closure is initially reversible. Common stresses that can cause the DA to open include hypoxemia, hypothermia, hypervolemia, sepsis, and acidemia. In addition, premature infants may have a persistent DA that results in very high pulmonary blood flow from left-to-right shunting and subsequent volume overload of the LV and congestive heart failure. In some forms of congenital heart disease, the DA supplies most of the pulmonary blood flow. Infants with these so-called ductal-dependent lesions develop extreme cyanosis and acidosis several hours after birth as the DA begins to close. Ductal patency can be maintained in these infants with an infusion of prostaglandin (PGE₁). Anatomic closure of the DA occurs by necrosis followed by fibrosis; this process normally takes several weeks.

The foramen ovale is a flap-like opening that allows RA blood to pass into the LA. After birth, the LA pressure increases above the RA pressure as a result of increased systemic pressure and an increase in blood coming from the lungs. This produces functional closure of the foramen ovale soon after birth. The foramen ovale remains a potential site of right-to-left shunting in all newborns and remains probe patent in many individuals into adulthood. The ductus venosus also closes 5 to 7 days after birth.

Neonatal Cardiovascular Physiology

Cardiac Output. At birth, the ventricles begin to work in series; thus the entire cardiac output passes through both ventricles. Because the newborn's myocardial fibers contain a large amount of noncontractile mass, the newborn's LV is relatively noncompliant. Although the Frank-Starling mechanism is intact, it is effective only over a normal preload. Large increases in preload result in volume overload and decreased cardiac output. Because of the noncompliant ventricles, newborns have a relatively fixed stroke volume, so the cardiac output is more dependent on heart rate than in adults. Likewise, newborns cannot tolerate large increases in afterload without compromising cardiac output.

Autonomic Control. The parasympathetic nervous system is fully functional at birth; the sympathetic system is not fully developed until 4 to 6 months of age. As a result, various noxious stimuli produce bradycardia in young infants. The baroreceptor reflex is intact in neonates, but its responsiveness may be reduced by volatile anesthetics. The chemoreceptor reflex differs in neonates compared with adults, in that the response to hypoxia is bradycardia rather than tachycardia.

Gross and Ultrastructural Development. Because of increasing demands on the LV and decreasing demands on the RV, the LV rapidly increases in size and mass after birth, and by 4 weeks of age the LV weighs more than the RV. This is reflected by the leftward shift of the QRS axis during infancy. The neonatal heart also retains a larger comple-

ment of anaerobic enzymes, which gives the newborn a greater tolerance for hypoxia.

Pulmonary Circulation. The pulmonary circulation undergoes major changes at birth and exhibits a greater sensitivity to physiologic manipulations during the newborn period. At birth, PA and aortic pressures are equal, but the PA pressure drops to 50% of aortic pressure after several days and continues to decline through the first month of life. Failure of the PVR to decline normally results in a condition known as persistent pulmonary hypertension of the neonate. The normal decrease in PVR also will not occur if the pulmonary bed is exposed to high pressure or flow, such as occurs in infants born with large ventricular septal defects or atrioventricular canal defects. In these situations, pulmonary hypertension is initially reversible, but irreversible pulmonary vascular obstructive disease will eventually develop. It is important to repair these defects in infancy to prevent fixed pulmonary hypertension.

Persistent pulmonary hypertension in the neonate (PPHN). Referred to in the past as persistent fetal circulation, leads to respiratory failure and death unless treated. It may be primary or secondary in causation. Secondary causes of PPHN include the following:

□ Meconium aspiration syndrome.
□ Hyaline membrane disease.
□ Neonatal sepsis with pneumonia.
□ Congenital diaphragmatic hernia.
□ Certain congenital heart defects.

The key pathologic process in this syndrome is increased pulmonary vascular resistance that prevents normal pulmonary blood flow and induces a right-to-left shunt through the persistent fetal channels (patent foramen ovale [PFO] and patent

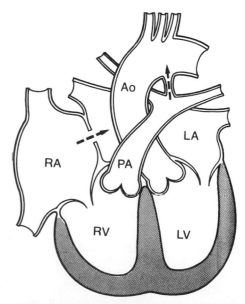

Figure 145–1. Diagram of right-to-left shunting (indicated by arrows) through the PFO and PDA, which results from PPHN. (From Graves ED, Redmond CR, Arensman RM.[1])

ductus arteriosus [PDA]) (Fig. 145–1). Therapeutic modalities for PPHN include the following:

□ Mechanical ventilation.
□ Tolazoline.
□ Prostaglandin E_2 and prostacyclin.
□ Isoproterenol.
□ Extracorporeal membrane oxygenation (ECMO).
□ Nitric oxide (endothelium-derived relaxing factor).

Selected Reference

1. Graves ED, Redmond CR, Arensman RM. Persistent pulmonary hypertension in the neonate. Chest 1988;93:638.

Suggested Readings

Benson LN, Freedom RM. The transitional circulation. In Freedom RM, Benson LN, Smallhorn JF, eds. Neonatal Heart Disease. London: Springer-Verlag, 1992:149.

Clarke WR. The transitional circulation: Physiology and anesthetic implications. J Clin Anesth 1990;2:192–211.

Hickey PR, Wessel DL, Reich DL. Anesthesia for treatment of congenital heart disease. In Kaplan JA, ed. Cardiac Anesthesia. 3rd ed. Philadelphia: WB Saunders, 1993:681.

Schiebar RA. Cardiovascular physiology of the fetus and newborn. In Cook DR, Marcy JH, eds. Neonatal Anesthesia. Pasadena, CA: Appleton Davies, 1988:1.

146
Congenital Heart Disease: Congestive Heart Failure

David J. Cook, M.D.

The anesthetic management of congenital congestive heart failure (CHF) requires a thorough understanding of neonatal physiology and the pathophysiologic effects of a great number and variety of congenital heart lesions.

Characteristics of the Neonatal Cardiovascular System

The Transitional Circulation. The right heart sees a low afterload as pulmonary vascular resistance (PRV) decreases with lung expansion. Furthermore, with the closure of the foramen ovale (FO), its volume load increases from only 66% to 100% of the cardiac output (CO).

The left heart at birth sees **large** increases in afterload and volume load as the ductus arteriosus (DA) and FO close. The ductus arteriosus functionally closes at 24 to 48 hours and becomes anatomically closed over several weeks. The FO functionally closes at 24 to 48 hours but will not become closed anatomically for months to years.

The pulmonary vasculature undergoes a large decrease in PVR in 24 to 48 hours that continues to decrease over years with pulmonary arterial tree remodeling. Note, however, that it is much more muscular than in adults. Therefore, it responds to stressors with dramatic increases in PVR.

The neonate undergoes a period of hemodynamic instability that usually resolves in days to weeks with the above changes, but in the presence of congenital defects, hemodynamic instability may persist and abnormal physiology may allow viability.

Functional Capacities of the Immature Heart. In the immature heart, there is ventricular equality; right ventricle (RV) and left ventricle (LV) thicknesses are equal at birth. By 4 weeks, the LV:RV mass ratio is 2:1, the adult ratio. Also, the immature heart is less compliant. Therefore, the Starling curves for the RV and LV are very similar in the neonate. Ventricular interaction is closely interrelated during the first few months of life, and CHF **rapidly** becomes biventricular.

The immature heart has a restricted ability to alter its stroke volume, making CO very rate dependent. It is therefore very susceptible to volume overload.

The immature ventricle is also less efficient at handling afterload; the Sterling plateau is reached at lower filling pressures.

In the normal neonate, the circulatory reserve is largely proportional to age until a mature cardiovascular physiology is established. Subtle changes are much more likely to result in failure than in adults.

Congenital Heart Defects

Congenital heart defects are classified clinically or anatomically. The defects may present primarily with cyanosis or primarily with congestive failure, the latter resulting from obstructive lesions or from shunts generating excessive pulmonary blood flow. Anatomically, defects can be classified as obstructions, shunts, or mixed (combining an obstructive and a shunt lesion). A description using both clinical and anatomic classifications can be used.

Obstructive lesions can be subvalvular, primary valvular, or supravalvular. The physiology of neonatal pure obstructive lesions is similar to that of adults, except that the obstruction may be more profound and is more likely to be right-sided than in the adult.

Shunt lesions vary with the hemodynamic state and can therefore be altered by anesthetic management. The orifice producing the shunt may be **restrictive** or **nonrestrictive.** If restrictive, the primary determinant of shunt fraction is the orifice radius and pressure gradient. If nonrestrictive, the shunt direction and magnitude depend on the relative resistances of the pulmonary and systemic vascular beds.

Anesthetic Management

To date, no pharmacologic agent can selectively alter the pulmonary and systemic vascular beds independently. Ventilatory maneuvers are much more useful.

Pure Obstructive Lesions. For pure obstructive lesions, the management strategies are similar to those in adults. The inotropic state can be modified with volatile agents or β blockers to help minimize outflow obstruction. The chronotropic state can be optimized to take advantage of the beneficial effects of atrial systole (via pacing or pharmacologic agents). Preload and afterload can be modified to alter gradients across obstructions.

Shunt Lesions. In shunt lesions, the PVR–systemic vascular resistance (SVR) ratios can be altered to improve ventricular workloads. No selective pulmonary vasodilator exists, but ventilatory manipulations can alter PVR independent of SVR (Table 146–1).

High doses of narcotics and deep levels of anesthesia can attenuate some pulmonary vascular responses.

Vasopressors, usually α agents, can be used to reduce right-to-left shunting and maintain coronary perfusion.

Vasodilators, especially prostaglandin E (PGE_1 and PGE_2), can maintain a patent ductus.

CHF may result from the interaction of the congenital lesion and an immature physiology. Inotropics and vasopressors can be used as in adults, but the results may be unpredictable.

Even if the particular anatomic defect is known, physiologic responses to anesthetic management can be unpredictable because of the following:

Table 146–1. Manipulations That Alter PVR

Increase PVR	Decrease PVR
Hypoxia	Oxygen
Hypercarbia	Hypocarbia
Acidosis	Alkalosis
Hyperinflation	Normal FRC
Atelectasis	Blocking sympathetic stimulation
Sympathetic stimulation	Low hematocrit level
High hematocrit level	
Surgical constriction	

From Hickey PR, Wessel DL, Reich DL.[1]

□ Transitional circulation.
□ Reduced functional capacities.
□ Anatomic defects.
□ Altered development due to chronic heart disease.
□ Previous surgical alteration.

Selected Reference

1. Hickey PR, Wessel DL, Reich DL. Anesthesia for treatment of congenital heart disease. In Kaplan JA, ed. Cardiac Anesthesia. 3rd ed. Philadelphia: WB Saunders, 1993:681.

Suggested References

Baum VC, Perloff JK. Anesthetic implications of adults with congenital heart disease. Anesth Analg 1993;76:1342.
Schwartz AJ, Campbell FW. Physiologic approach to congenital heart disease. In Lake CL, ed. Pediatric Cardiac Anesthesia. Norwalk, CT: Appleton & Lange, 1993:7.

147

Anesthesia for Patent Ductus Arteriosus and Other Neonatal Cardiovascular Problems

Robert J. Lunn, M.D.

Congenital heart disease can be classified in a number of different ways. The most useful method for the anesthesiologist involves a physiologic classification based on whether there is obstruction to flow or increased or decreased pulmonary blood flow. Some lesions, such as truncus arteriosus, can have either increased or decreased pulmonary blood flow depending on the particular anatomy and physiology of a given patient (Table 147–1).

Most patients with congenital cardiovascular disease present early in life. However, some patients (e.g., those with bicuspid aortic valves or mild coarctation of the aorta) may not be diagnosed until much later in life.

Table 147–1. Flow Characteristics of Various Congenital Cardiac Lesions

Increased pulmonary blood flow lesions
  Atrial septal defect
  Ventricular septal defect
  Patent ductus arteriosus
  Endocardial cushion defect (atrioventricular
    canal abnormality)
  Anomalous origin of coronary arteries
  Transposition of the great arteries*
  Anomalous pulmonary venous drainage*
  Truncus arteriosus*
  Single ventricle*
Decreased pulmonary blood flow lesions
  Tetralogy of Fallot
  Pulmonary atresia
  Tricuspid atresia
  Ebstein's anomaly
  Truncus arteriosus*
  Transposition of the great arteries*
  Single ventricle*
Obstructive lesions
  Aortic stenosis
  Pulmonary stenosis
  Coarctation of the aorta
  Asymmetric septal hypertrophy

*Systemic hypoxemia occurs as a result of the mixing of systemic and pulmonary venous returns. Classification as an increased or decreased pulmonary blood flow lesion depends upon the absence or presence within the anatomic variation of obstruction to pulmonary blood flow.
From Schwartz AJ, Campbell FW.[1]

Improvements in anesthesia, surgery, and the ability to safely place very small infants on cardiopulmonary bypass with deep hypothermic circulatory arrest have resulted in better long-term outcomes for patients with congenital heart disease. Because of these improved techniques, there is a trend to surgically correct congenital cardiac defects earlier in infancy. For example, in the recent past, patients with transposition of the great arteries were palliated in early infancy and then treated with some form of intra-atrial baffle repair later in childhood. But follow-up analysis of these patients revealed that over time, the right ventricle (which was the systemic ventricle) was unable to sustain this workload. The arterial switch procedure, which involves repositioning the great arteries on their respective ventricles early in the neonatal period, was developed with the hope of improving long-term outcome.

Even with the trend toward earlier corrective surgery, some patients with more complex lesions must be palliated early in infancy. For example, patients with pulmonary atresia frequently have pulmonary arteries that are too small to allow complete repair in infancy. These patients are treated with some form of surgical shunt, such as the modified Blalock-Taussig (BT) shunt. The surgical shunts accomplish two purposes. First, they improve pulmonary blood flow, which alleviates severe cyanosis. Second, the improved blood flow to the pulmonary arteries stimulates growth, which may allow complete correction at a later time.

Some forms of congenital heart disease are treated medically during the neonatal period and surgically corrected later in infancy. For example, large ventricular septal defects or atrioventricular canal defects can present in early infancy with signs of congestive heart failure and pulmonary congestion. These patients are managed initially with digitalis and diuretics. This allows the infant to grow, which makes the surgical correction technically easier. However, the pulmonary vascular bed will develop irreversible pulmonary artery obstructive disease if exposure to high blood pressure and flow is allowed to persist. For this reason, these lesions are corrected before 2 years of age, commonly around 6 to 12 months.

Correctable Cardiac Anomalies That Present in the Neonatal Period

Patent Ductus Arteriosus. Persistence of the ductus arteriosus is the most common cardiovascular anomaly that presents in the neonatal period. Causes of a patent ductus arteriosus are listed in Table 147–2. These infants are often premature; they frequently have other associated medical conditions, such as hyaline membrane disease, and present with congestive heart failure and pulmonary edema. Initial medical management involves digitalis, diuretics, and fluid restriction. With conservative management, often the ductus will close spontaneously. Indomethacin (0.1 to 0.3 mg/kg) can be given to stimulate closure of the ductus. This treatment can cause renal failure and platelet dysfunction. Surgical ligation of the ductus arteriosus through a left thoracotomy incision is done if conservative management fails.

These infants are frequently dehydrated when they present to the operating room, so they may tolerate volatile anesthetics poorly. Nitrous oxide, fentanyl, and ketamine in some combination are well tolerated in most of these infants. A fluid bolus of 5 to 10 mL/kg at the start of the case improves tolerance to anesthetics. Many of these patients will have indwelling umbilical or peripheral arterial catheters in place; these are useful monitors throughout the procedure. Noninvasive blood pressure monitoring, combined with pulse oximetry, is often adequate for these cases. Possible complications with anesthetic implications include damage to the phrenic nerve or recurrent laryngeal nerve.

Surgical Shunt Procedures. Patients who present early in infancy with severe cyanosis are frequently palliated with some type of surgical shunt procedure during the neonatal period. These are basically systemic to pulmonary artery connections that increase pulmonary blood flow, relieve cyanosis, and stimulate pulmonary artery growth.

Some of these infants receive pulmonary blood flow via the ductus arteriosus and become extremely cyanotic as the duct begins to close. Prostaglandin E_2 can be infused in these infants to maintain ductal patency until a more permanent surgical shunt is placed.

Table 147–2. Common Causes of Patent Ductus Arteriosus in Newborns

Prematurity	Acidosis
Neonatal sepsis	Hypoxemia
Pneumonia	

Table 147–3. Surgical Shunts

Blalock-Taussig shunt	Subclavian artery to pulmonary artery
Modified Blalock-Taussig shunt	Synthetic graft from subclavian to pulmonary artery
Potts' shunt	Descending aorta to left pulmonary artery
Waterston's shunt	Ascending aorta to right pulmonary artery
Central shunt	Aorta to main pulmonary artery
Glen's shunt	Superior vena cava to right pulmonary artery (nonconfluent pulmonary artery)
Bidirectional Glen's shunt	Superior vena cava to right pulmonary artery (confluent pulmonary artery)

The modified BT shunt is the most commonly used type of surgical shunt. The classic BT shunt involves anastomosis of either the right or left subclavian artery to the respective pulmonary artery. The modified BT shunt uses a synthetic graft between the subclavian and pulmonary artery and preserves patency of the subclavian artery. Other types of surgical shunts are listed in Table 147–3. These procedures are usually done through a thoracotomy incision, with the exception of central shunts, which are performed through a median sternotomy.

Obviously, blood pressure must be monitored on the opposite side of the shunt. These patients can become extremely cyanotic during the procedure. Minimizing pulmonary vascular resistance (Table 147–4) and maintaining acid-base balance is critical. After the shunt is opened, pulmonary blood flow is somewhat dependent on perfusion pressure across the shunt; thus maintaining an adequate blood pressure is critical in preventing hypoxemia and preventing the graft from becoming thrombosed.

Other Neonatal Lesions. Other complex forms of congenital heart disease present for surgical correction during the neonatal period. These include transposition of the great arteries, hypoplastic left heart syndrome, interrupted aortic arch, critical aortic stenosis, and occasionally severe coarctation

Table 147–4. Factors That Alter Pulmonary Vascular Resistance

Increase Pulmonary Vascular Resistance	Decrease Pulmonary Vascular Resistance
Hypoxia	Oxygen
Acidosis	Alkalosis
Hypercarbia	Hypocarbia
Hypothermia	Normothermia
Sympathetic stimulation	Decreases sympathetic stimulation
Atelectasis	Normal FRC
High airway pressures/ PEEP	Normal airway pressures

of the aorta. An understanding of the physiologic classification of these lesions, combined with an understanding of manipulations of systemic and pulmonary vascular resistance, will enable safe anesthetic management of these cases.

Selected Reference

1. Schwartz AJ, Campbell FW. Pathophysiological approach to congenital heart disease. In Lake CL, ed. Pediatric Cardiac Anesthesia. 3rd ed. Stamford, CT: Appleton & Lange, 1998:7.

Suggested References

Beynen FM, Tarhan S. Anesthesia for the surgical repair of congenital heart defects in children. In Tarhan S, ed. Cardiovascular Anesthesia and Postoperative Care. 2nd ed. Chicago: Year Book Medical, 1990:105.

Lake CL. Anesthesia for Patients with Congenital Heart Disease. In Kaplan JA, ed. Cardiac Anesthesia. 4th ed. Philadelphia: WB Saunders, 1999:785.

Rosen DA, Rosen KR. Anomalies of the aortic arch and valve. In Lake CL, ed. Pediatric Cardiac Anesthesia. 3rd ed. Stamford, CT: Appleton & Lange, 1998:431.

148
Cardiopulmonary Bypass

David J. Cook, M.D.

Cardiopulmonary bypass (CPB) replaces heart and lung function during cardiopulmonary arrest. The basic features of the circuit are a pump, an oxygenator, and venous return and arterial inflow lines. A heat exchanger and a blood reservoir are also essential elements.

CPB Circuit Structure

A right atrial cannula is the source for drainage of blood into the venous reservoir. Blood exits the reservoir, goes to a pump (roller or centrifugal), and is pumped through an oxygenator (typically hollow fiber), most of which have integrated heat exchangers. For hollow fiber oxygenators, PaO_2 is determined by the FIO_2 of the fresh gas flow passing countercurrent through the hollow fibers; $PaCO_2$ is determined by the total gas flow rate though the oxygenator. The pressurized, oxygenated blood then typically passes though an arterial line filter before entering the aortic cannula (usually placed in the proximal aorta).

Additional features of the CPB circuit include cardiotomy suction, temperature and oxygenation monitors, a cardioplegia delivery system, and a ventricular vent.

Control of Systemic Oxygenation During CPB

The factors that control systemic oxygenation during non-CPB conditions also control oxygenation during CPB. Oxygen requirements are most profoundly affected by body temperature, whereas oxygen delivery is determined by pump flow and hematocrit (Hct).

The Basic Relationships

- Arterial oxygen content (CaO_2) = 1.34 (Hgb) (sat%) + 0.003 (PaO_2).
- Arteriovenous oxygen content difference ($AVDO_2$) = CaO_2 − CvO_2.

- Systemic oxygen delivery (DO_2) = cardiac output or CPB pump flow × CaO_2.
- Systemic oxygen consumption (VO_2) = cardiac output × $AVDO_2$.
- The **temperature coefficient** (Q10) describes the ratio of metabolic rates at two temperatures separated by 10°C. Every 10°C decrease in body temperature decreases VO_2 by about 60% (Q10 is 2.0 to 2.2).

General Practice of CPB

- Nonpulsatile flow (2.0 to 2.5 L · min^{-1} · m^{-2}), based on the cardiac index under anesthesia in non-CPB conditions (also may be expressed as mL/kg/min).
- Mild to moderate hypothermia (28°C to 35°C).
- Moderate normovolemic hemodilution (Hct 20% to 30%).
- MAP (60 to 80 mm Hg). Even with moderate hypothermia, cerebral autoregulation begins to fail below a cerebral perfusion pressure of 50 to 55 mm Hg.

CPB Hemodynamics and Hemodilution. Under non-CPB conditions, moderate hemodilution decreases CaO_2 but may not decrease DO_2, because hemodilution is associated with increases in cardiac output. However, during CPB, pump flow is typically less than the cardiac output that would be seen with equivalent hemodilution under non-CPB conditions. This results in a decrease in whole body O_2 delivery during CPB, which is approximately equivalent to the degree of hemodilution. Additionally, in the absence of compensatory flow increases, MAP during CPB is typically reduced, because the lower blood viscosity associated with hemodilution reduces systemic vascular resistance (SVR).

Effect of Temperature Change on Systemic Oxygenation. Hypothermia to 27°C reduces systemic oxygen requirements approximately 60%. Because oxygen demand decreases so dramatically with hypothermia, adequate oxygenation can be maintained with reduced flows and/or greater degrees of hemodilution. However, during the early and late CPB, when patients approximate normothermia, the margin between systemic oxygen supply and demand is narrowed. A beneficial effect of hypothermia is that the associated increases in SVR may offset the reductions in SVR associated with hemodilution alone.

Effect of Anesthetic Depth. Anesthetic depth has less influence than hypothermia on Vo_2 during CPB. However, anesthetic depth is of greater relative importance at body temperatures above 32°C. Plasma levels of anesthetics decrease with the onset of CPB secondary to dilution from an increased circulatory volume. Therefore, IV infusion techniques or the use of inhalation agents during CPB helps ensure adequate anesthesia.

Monitoring the Adequacy of Perfusion During CPB

Systemic Oxygen Saturation (Svo_2). Svo_2 reflects venous oxygen content, the amount of oxygen left in the venous blood after systemic oxygen requirements are met. Although Svo_2 does not measure either Vo_2 or Do_2, it provides an index of the adequacy of their matching. As such, Svo_2 monitoring conveys extremely valuable information as to the interaction of systemic oxygen requirements, pump flow, arterial oxygen content, hematocrit level, and temperature. An Svo_2 above 65% generally indicates a satisfactory margin of safety for systemic oxygenation. A higher saturation is indicated during hypothermia given that hypothermia increases the oxygen affinity of Hgb.

□ In-line Hgb or Hct monitors are available and are usually coupled to the Svo_2 detector.
□ Temperature monitoring is performed in three areas: the venous line (reflecting the adequacy of whole body cooling or warming), the arterial inflow line, and the heat exchanger, where temperature should not exceed 38.5°C
□ Optional arterial in-flow line monitoring devices are available to monitor gases (Pao_2, pH, $Paco_2$, base deficit, and temperature).

Difficulties in Maintaining Systemic Oxygenation During CPB

During stable hypothermia, systemic oxygenation is easy to maintain, but the transitions to and from hypothermia can be a problem.

Initiation of CPB is associated with nearly instantaneous hemodilution and decreased SVR. In the absence of increased flow, hypotension commonly occurs until cooling is initiated, SVR is increased pharmacologically, or volume resuscitation occurs.

During rewarming from CPB, SVR and MAP will fall as vasodilation occurs and blood viscosity decreases. This occurs at a time when systemic oxygen demand may double (27°C to 37°C).

Cardioplegia

Cardioplegia with a high potassium solution results in depolarization and diastolic arrest. This induces electromechanical silence and reduces myocardial oxygen demand (MVo_2) by more than 80%. Cardioplegia is indicated when the aortic cross-clamp is in place, because there is no coronary blood flow at this time. Cardioplegia may consist of an oxygenated blood–high K^+ mixture (blood cardioplegia) or high K^+ solution alone (crystalloid cardioplegia). Cardioplegia is usually given intermittently into the aorta proximal to the cross clamp (antegrade), or directly into the coronary ostia. Retrograde cardioplegia via the coronary sinus is also used. Left ventricular hypertrophy and coronary artery disease make myocardial protection more difficult to achieve.

Suggested References

Cook DJ. Changing temperature management for cardiopulmonary bypass (review article). Anesth Analg 1999;88:1254–1271.

Cook DJ. Low-flow cardiopulmonary bypass is the preferred technique for patients undergoing open heart surgical procedures CON (editorial). J Cardiothorac Vasc Anesth 2001 (in press).

DiNardo JA. Anesthesia for Cardiac Surgery. Norwalk, CT, Appleton & Lange, 1998.

Gravlee GP, Davis RF, Kurusz M, et al. Cardiopulmonary Bypass, Principles and Practice. Baltimore, Lippincott Williams & Wilkins, 2000.

Kirklin JW, Barratt-Boyes BG. Hypothermia, Circulatory Arrest, and Cardiopulmonary Bypass in Cardiac Surgery. 2nd ed. New York: Churchill Livingstone, 1992:61–94.

Mangano CM, Hill L, Cartwright CR, et al. Cardiopulmonary bypass and the anesthesiologist. In Kaplan JA, ed. Cardiac Anesthesia. 4th ed. Philadelphia: WB Saunders, 1999:1061–1110.

Shanewise JS, Hug CC Jr. Anesthesia for adult cardiac surgery. In Miller RD, ed. Anesthesia. 5th ed. Philadelphia: Churchill Livingstone, 2000:1753.

149
Anesthesia for Coronary Artery Bypass Grafting Procedures

Roxann D. Barnes, M.D.

Management of a patient undergoing cardiopulmonary bypass (CPB) for coronary artery bypass grafting (CABG) requires preparation and vigilance.

Preoperative

Risk factors for coronary artery disease include smoking, hyperlipidemia, and genetic factors. Special attention should be given to associated cardiac disorders, such as regurgitant or stenotic valvular lesions, ventricular hypertrophy or dilation, arrhythmias, and congenital anomalies. The coronary angiogram gives detailed information about the anatomy and degree of stenosis, and the functional status of the heart (ejection fraction [EF]). Coexisting diseases such as atherosclerotic vascular disease, hypertension, pulmonary disease, renal disease, diabetes mellitus, and coagulation problems should be noted. Medications, especially β blockers, should be continued the morning of surgery.[1]

Monitors and Induction of Anesthesia

Standard monitors include a five-lead electrode system for ST segment analysis. Large-bore IVs are critical for rapid fluid resuscitation. An arterial line (radial, ulnar, brachial, or femoral) is placed, taking into account whether or not radial artery harvesting will be done.

Central venous access is necessary for assessing volume status and cardiac function and for fluid and vasoactive drug administration. A central venous catheter is sufficient for primary surgery in patients with a normal EF. A pulmonary artery catheter (PAC) can be used to measure pulmonary vascular resistance, filling pressures, and serial cardiac output/index (CO/CI) and to provide transvenous pacing. Core temperature monitoring (e.g., nasopharyngeal, tympanic) as well as more peripheral temperature monitoring (e.g., bladder, rectal, skin) are used to determine temperature gradients. Urine output is continuously monitored.

Any induction agent is suitable if used appropriately. Titration of induction drugs with concurrent monitoring of hemodynamics is key. Goals during induction include the following:

- Avoid increased myocardial oxygen consumption (tachycardia, increased wall tension from excessive preload or afterload, or increased contractility).
- Avoid decreased myocardial oxygen supply (from tachycardia diminishing diastolic perfusion time, diastolic hypotension, or hypoxemia).

Preparation for CPB

Baseline arterial blood gas (ABG), electrolytes, glucose, and activated clotting time (ACT) are measured. The on-CPB hemoglobin can be calculated to determine whether red blood cells are needed in the pump prime. Prophylactic antibiotics are administered. An antifibrinolytic may be used. A thermodilution CO/CI is obtained. The patient must be well anesthetized to prevent ischemia during periods of high stimulation, such as incision and sternotomy/sternal spreading. Mechanical ventilation is temporarily suspended during sternotomy to prevent injury to the lung and right side of the heart. Internal thoracic and/or radial artery dissection is a period of decreased stimulation, and hypotension may develop.

Heparin (300 units/kg) must be given centrally. There must be no confusion regarding heparin administration; proceeding with CPB without adequate heparinization can be fatal. Heparin is often included in the pump prime. After heparin administration, blood pressure is often pharmacologically lowered to 90 to 100 mm Hg to facilitate aortic cannula placement. The venous cannula is placed into the right atrium (single) or into the superior and inferior venae cavae (dual).

Initiation of CPB

The ACT is rechecked; it should exceed 350 seconds for safe initiation of CPB. The patient may need to be cooled down.[2] Continuation of mechanical ventilation is important during partial CPB (pulsatile arterial/PA waveforms from LV/RV ejection). Mechanical ventilation may be stopped when CPB is at full flow, typically 2.4 L/min/m^2.

Maintenance During CPB

Anesthetic dosage depends on whether or not the patient will be "fast-tracked." Fast-tracking emphasizes early extubation and shorter intensive care unit stays to minimize complications and cost. Fentanyl, 15 to 20 µg/kg, or sufentanil, 5 to 10 µg/kg, can be used in combination with inhalation or other intravenous agents. Relative contraindications for fast-tracking include low EF, congestive heart failure, pulmonary hypertension, pulmonary disease, reoperation, emergency cases, and use of an intraaortic balloon pump. A volatile agent delivered by a vaporizer connected directly to the oxygenator may be used during CPB. Muscle relaxation is necessary until sternal wiring.

During CPB, the ACT is maintained at greater than 450 seconds, with additional heparin given as needed. The ACT is rechecked every 30 to 60 minutes, more frequently if the patient remains warm, which speeds heparin elimination. An initial ABG on CPB is obtained and used to calibrate the in-line monitors. A mixed venous oxygen saturation exceeding 60% is desired to ensure adequate tissue perfusion. An MAP of 50 to 80 mm Hg is adequate; a precise target level is based on the patient's medical history.[3, 4] Methods of increasing MAP on CPB are limited, involving either increasing arterial flow or administering α-adrenergic agonists, such as phenylephrine.

The aortic cross-clamp is placed and cardioplegia solution is administered in the aortic root and retrograde through the coronary sinus, if necessary, for diastolic arrest. Repeat doses of cardioplegia solution may be required, depending on time or reappearance of electrical activity. Sinus rhythm often returns spontaneously during rewarming with cross-clamp removal; if it does not, antiarrhythmics and/or defibrillation (20 joules) may be necessary.

Separation from CPB and the Post-CPB Period

A useful checklist for separation from CPB is as follows:

□ Mechanical ventilation is resumed with 100% oxygen. Visual confirmation of full re-expansion of both lungs is essential.
□ Normothermia (core and venous return temperatures at least 36°C, with a gradient of <3°C between core and peripheral) should be established.

If it is not, redistribution of thermal energy ensues with postbypass hypothermia.
□ Adequate cardiac rate and rhythm are essential. Sinus rhythm is desirable with a slightly higher heart rate, because the myocardium is less compliant post-CPB. Pharmacologic methods and epicardial or transvenous (atrial, ventricular or AV sequential) pacing can be used.
□ Calcium is beneficial to treat hypocalcemia and hyperkalemia, increase systemic vascular resistance, and enhance contractility.

The perfusionist transfuses blood into the heart by slowly occluding the venous return. As the heart fills, the arterial flow is lowered on the pump while the anesthesiologist continuously watches the heart, to avoid overdistention. As acceptable pressure is generated, CBP is terminated. CO/CI is measured to determine the need for inotropes. CI exceeding 2.0 is sufficient for adequate organ perfusion. Transesophageal echocardiography may be performed to evaluate regional wall motion abnormalities and ventricular function and filling defects.

When the patient is stable off CPB, heparin is reversed with protamine (1.3 mg/100 units of heparin). Vents must be removed and suction to the CBP machine turned off before protamine is administered. Protamine is given slowly to minimize hypotension. Anaphylactic and complement-mediated reactions to protamine can be severe and result in catastrophic pulmonary hypertension. ABGs, electrolytes, and glucose are monitored. Intraoperatively salvaged blood can be washed, filtered, and given back to the patient. ACT, activated partial thromboplastin time, prothrombin time, platelet count, and thromboelastogram can guide further hemostatic interventions.

Selected References

1. Wallace A, Layug B, Tateo I, et al. Prophylactic atenolol reduces postoperative myocardial ischemia. Anesthesiology 1998;88:7–17.
2. Cook DJ. Changing temperature management for cardiopulmonary bypass. Anesth Analg 1999;88:1254–1271.
3. Hartman G. Pro: During cardiopulmonary bypass for elective coronary artery bypass grafting, perfusion pressure should routinely be greater than 70 mm Hg. J Cardiothorac Vasc Anesth 1998;12:358–360.
4. Cartwright CR, Mangano CM. Con: During cardiopulmonary bypass for elective coronary artery bypass grafting, perfusion pressure should *not* routinely be greater than 70 mm Hg. J Cardiothorac Vasc Anesth 1998;12:362–364.

Suggested Readings

Kaplan JA, Wynands JE. Anesthesia for myocardial revascularization. In Kaplan JA, ed. Cardiac Anesthesia. 4th ed. Philadelphia: WB Saunders, 1999:689.
Shanewise JS, Hug CC Jr. Anesthesia for adult cardiac surgery. In Miller RD, ed. Anesthesia. 5th ed. Philadelphia: Churchill Livingstone, 2000:1753–1804.

150

Off-Pump Coronary Artery Bypass and Minimally Invasive Direct Coronary Artery Bypass

Roxann D. Barnes, M.D.

Definitions and Indications

Cardiopulmonary bypass (CPB) can be avoided for coronary artery bypass grafting (CABG) by using either off-pump coronary artery bypass (OP-CAB) or minimally invasive direct coronary artery bypass (MIDCAB). OPCAB involves CABG of one or more vessels through a median sternotomy on the beating heart. MIDCAB consists of CABG done through a lateral anterior thoracotomy on the beating heart.

In both techniques, each diseased artery is identified and immobilized, often using a specialized stabilization device. The stenotic segments are bypassed without CPB or cardioplegia.

The initial indication for MIDCAB was to treat patients with single-vessel disease that was not amenable to PTCA.[1] The indications for OPCAB and MIDCAB include the desire or need to avoid cardioplegia and CPB.

Advantages and Disadvantages

The purported advantages of MIDCAB over a median sternotomy include decreased risk of sternal wound infection and reduced musculoskeletal injury.[1] However, MIDCAB may cause more trauma to costal cartilages (+/- rib segment removal), resulting in more pain.[2] A disadvantage of MIDCAB is that it allows only limited exposure, so fewer vessels can be grafted—often only the internal thoracic artery (ITA) to the left anterior descending (LAD). Other vessels must be treated with angioplasty. OPCAB allows grafting of multiple vessels.

OPCAB and MIDCAB can be used either as primary surgery or as reoperation. Both have become increasingly popular techniques for avoiding the adverse effects associated with cannulation and CPB, such as hypothermia, coagulation derangements, renal impairment, arrhythmias, manipulation and crossing-clamping of the ascending aorta (which increases the risk of aortic dissection/neurologic sequelae because of atherosclerotic disease), and prolonged postoperative ventilation. Purported advantages of MIDCAB and OPCAB over conventional CPB include decreased surgical time, shorter lengths of stay, and possibly decreased cost. A possible disadvantage of MIDCAB compared to CPB is the concern that the anastomoses may be less optimal because they are done under a less well-controlled approach than through a median sternotomy with cardioplegic arrest.[3]

Anesthetic Technique: Preparation and Monitoring

Large-bore IVs are needed for volume resuscitation. Cross-matched blood is made available, and intraoperative collection of shed autologous blood is used. A CPB circuit should be set up with a perfusionist on standby.

Patients are typically hemodynamically unstable, and thus extensive invasive monitoring is indicated. An arterial line is critical, with careful site selection mandatory if radial artery harvest is being done. A pulmonary artery catheter (PAC) is useful for assessing volume status and serial cardiac output (CO), and for providing transvenous pacing. Continuous thermodilution CO or oximetric PAC is especially useful. Multiple central ports allow concomitant instillation of various vasoactive drugs.

With MIDCAB, access to defibrillate and pace the heart is impaired, so external defibrillator and pacing pads are used.[4] Transesophageal echocardiography can assess global ventricular function, regional wall motion abnormalities, and volume status. Temperature monitoring is critical.

Anesthetic Technique: Induction and Maintenance

To avoid prolonged intubation, a "fast-track" anesthetic approach is used, limiting narcotics to 5 μg/kg sufentanil, 15 μg/kg fentanyl, or remifentanil infusion. Any anesthetic technique that facilitates early extubation and avoids ischemia is acceptable.

Some surgeons choose to use one-lung ventilation (OLV) for improved surgical exposure. For MIDCAB, OLV is useful if the ITA pedicle is harvested thoracoscopically. OLV is not necessary with OPCAB.

Antifibrinolytics are not indicated. There is some concern that their use might contribute to graft thrombosis.

Induced bradycardia facilitates surgical performance, especially with MIDCAB. Besides optimizing the surgical field, bradycardia reduces myocardial oxygen demand until the heart can be adequately revascularized. Bradycardia may be facilitated by anesthetic choice, which may include:

□ Narcotics such as fentanyl, sufentanil, and remifentanil.
□ Muscle relaxants that do not induce tachycardia.
□ β blockers such as esmolol as a bolus or infusion, or labetalol.
□ Calcium channel blockers.

Induced bradycardia is less critical with OPCAB since the advent of newer stabilization devices such as the CTS retractor, the Octopus, and the Cohn stabilizer (Fig. 150–1). These devices hold a segment of the diseased coronary artery immobile while the heart is beating so the anastomoses can be performed.

Surgery on the beating heart readily precipitates arrhythmias from ischemia, manipulation, and reperfusion. These arrhythmias must be treated aggressively. Lidocaine and magnesium are used routinely[6]; other antiarrhythmic agents must be readily available. Useful antiarrhythmic strategies include:

□ Ensuring that defibrillation paddles are prepared and ready.
□ Asking the surgeon to temporarily stop manipulation.

□ Keeping lidocaine and magnesium boluses and/or infusions ready at hand.
□ Preventing myocardial ischemia.
□ Correcting electrolyte and acid-base abnormalities.
□ Continuing antiarrhythmic medication.
□ Treating excessive bradycardia pharmacologically, or with epicardial or transvenous pacing.

Anesthetic Technique: Surgical Considerations

After anesthesia induction, saphenous vein and/or radial artery harvesting is accomplished. A median sternotomy (OPCAB) or anterior thoracotomy (MIDCAB) is used. One-half to two-thirds of a full heparinizing dose for CPB (150 to 200 units/kg) is given. The ITA is dissected. The ACT is checked every 30 minutes, and additional heparin doses of 3000 to 5000 units are given as necessary to maintain ACT above 300 seconds. Antiarrhythmic agents are given before vessel occlusion is done. Baseline CO, pulmonary artery pressures, and ST segment analyses are assessed before and after vessel occlusion to guide interventions.

To facilitate surgical exposure, the heart must be lifted and rotated. When the heart is repositioned, venous return is compromised, causing insufficient preload and a possibly precipitous drop in cardiac output. Fluid resuscitation, inotropic medications, and peripheral vasoconstrictors (e.g., phenylephrine) are used. Mean arterial pressures must be maintained at or above preoperative pressures to ensure adequate coronary perfusion.

Once the ITA is anastomosed to the LAD, improved hemodynamics are seen. If necessary, vein grafts or radial artery grafts are then grafted to other coronary arteries. For OPCAB proximal anastomoses, a side-biting C-clamp is placed on the aorta while the blood pressure is reduced temporar-

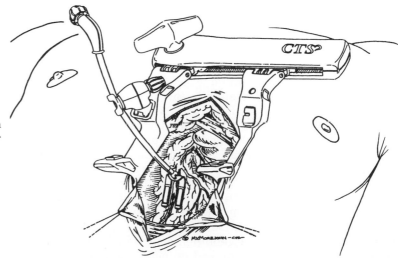

Figure 150–1. Example of an OPCAB stabilization device. (From Gayes JM.[5] Copyright Guidant Corporation, Indianapolis.)

ily. Nitroglycerin causes vasodilation of the coronary arteries, prevents vasospasm of the radial artery, and reduces wall stress during ischemic periods. Sodium nitroprusside can also be used for quick, titratable control of blood pressure.

If the patient's heart cannot tolerate the ischemia from vessel occlusion, options include stenting of the artery via an arteriotomy or emergent institution of CPB. Although the stented vessel provides blood flow to distal ischemic myocardium, there is a risk of intimal dissection.

Anesthetic Technique: Postoperative Considerations

The incision is closed after all anastomoses are completed. Heparin is not routinely reversed. The patient may be extubated.[2] Local anesthetic infiltration of the anterior thoracotomy wound reduces postoperative pain. Graft patency in the catheterization laboratory may be assessed postoperatively, so preparations must be made to transport the patient.

Selected References

1. Maslow AD, Park KW, Pawlowski J, et al. Minimally invasive direct coronary artery bass grafting: Changes in anesthetic management and surgical procedure. J Cardiothorac Vasc Anesth 1999;13:417–423.
2. Heres EK, Marquez J, Malkowski MJ, et al. Minimally invasive direct coronary artery bypass: Anesthetic, monitoring, and pain control considerations. J Cardiothorac Vasc Anesth 1998;12:385–389.
3. Bonchek L, Ullyot DJ. Minimally invasive coronary bypass: A dissenting opinion. Circulation 1998;98:495–497.
4. Maslow AD, Aronson S, Jacobsohn E, et al. Off-pump coronary artery bypass graft surgery. J Cardiothorac Vasc Anesth 1999;13:764–781.
5. Gayes JM. The minimally invasive cardiac surgery voyage. J Cardiothorac Vasc Anesth 1999;13:119–122.
6. Huss MG, Wasnick JD. Magnesium and off-pump coronary artery bypass. J Cardiothorac Vasc Anesth 1999;13:374–375.

151
Intra-Aortic Balloon Pump

David J. Cook, M.D.

The intra-aortic balloon pump (IABP) is a mechanical device used to provide temporary circulatory support during a period of acute cardiac failure.

Equipment

The adult IABP consists of a 8.5 to 12 Fr catheter whose distal 30 cm is covered with a polyurethane balloon (volume, 35 to 40 mL). The pediatric catheter is 5 to 7 Fr with a 5- to 12-mL balloon.

The catheter is inserted into the common femoral artery percutaneously by the Seldinger technique or by an open surgical procedure. It is then threaded proximally so that the balloon lies high in the descending thoracic aorta.

The catheter is controlled by a drive console that has a pneumatic pump capable of rapidly inflating and deflating the catheter balloon with helium. Balloon cycling is triggered either from the electrocardiogram R wave, inflating with diastole and deflating with onset of systole (Fig. 151–1), or from the aortic pressure waveform. It should be adjusted to inflate when the dicrotic notch occurs in the pressure cycle (Fig. 151–2). The balloon can be set to trigger with every beat, every other beat, etc.

Hemodynamic Effects

With balloon deflation at onset of systole, the peak aortic systolic pressure falls 10% to 15% (systolic unloading).

□ Balloon inflation can increase intra-aortic diastolic pressure by 70%.
□ Cardiac index increases 10% to 15%; pulmonary capillary wedge pressure falls by a similar amount.
□ Coronary blood flow increases as a result of increased diastolic pressure.

Initiation of balloon counterpulsation produces a reduction in myocardial oxygen demand and a shift of the Starling curve to the right. These effects appear to taper over 48 to 72 hours.

Indications

The IABP is used primarily for acute cardiac failure refractory to pharmacologic intervention. Most commonly it is used for low-output states after cardiopulmonary bypass, but it also has wide application in cardiogenic shock secondary to myocardial ischemia. The pump can also be placed preoperatively when the surgical stress is anticipated to exceed the functional capacity of a diseased heart. In recent years, the IABP has also found wider use as a bridge to cardiac transplantation.

Approximately 3% to 4% of patients undergoing cardiopulmonary bypass need IABP support. If the patient is not hypovolemic and the heart is in a rhythm suitable for IABP use, the criteria listed in Table 151–1 can be used to determine appropriate initiation of IABP support.

Weaning from IABP Support

Traditionally, patients have been weaned from IABP support by a gradual reduction in augmentation rate (1:1, then 1:2, then 1:3, etc.). Most hemodynamic changes occur while going from 1:1 to 1:2 augmentation.[3] To institute a more gradual reduc-

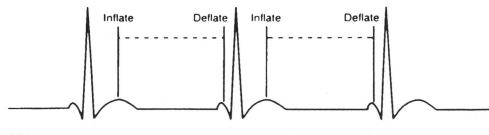

Figure 151–1. Inflation/deflation timing of an intra-aortic balloon correlated with the electrocardiogram. (From Gray JR, Faust RJ.[1])

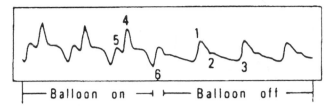

Figure 151-2. Arterial pressure tracing (balloon on 1:1 and balloon off). Note diastolic peak (4) balloon augmentation and systolic peak (1), dicrotic notch (2), diastolic low (3), diastolic peak (4), systolic peak (5), and end-diastolic dip (6). (From Gray JR, Faust RJ.[1])

Table 151-1. Criteria for Emergency Use of IABP After Cardiac Surgery

Relative
  Requirement for large doses of pressor agents.
  Malignant arrhythmia with evidence of intraoperative infarction not well controlled with drug therapy.
Definite
  Difficulty in weaning from cardiopulmonary bypass after 30 to 45 minutes (or three attempts) at flow rates above 500 mL/min.
  Hypotension (<60 mm Hg mean) and low cardiac index (<1.8 $L \cdot min^{-1} \cdot m^{-2}$) with high wedge pressure (> 25 mm Hg) despite pressor agents and afterload reduction.
  Continued postoperative use (if IABP was initiated before surgery).

Adapted from Bolooki H.[2]

tion in circulatory assist and to reduce the risk of thrombus formation around a static balloon, an alternate weaning approach is to maintain a 1:1 augmentation rate but gradually reduce balloon inflation, because the rate and degree of deflation are determined by changes in the intra-aortic diastolic pressure.[3] There is a paucity of literature on this subject.

Complications

Current literature reports a complication rate of 5% to 27%. Given placement of a large catheter in the common femoral artery, loss of distal pulses, bleeding, and infection occur as expected. The relative frequency of each of these complications varies widely between reports, and the literature is inconsistent as to the impact of chronic placement on complication rates. Nevertheless, it may be reasonable to expect an approximately 20% incidence of bleeding or vascular compromise in these patients. These complications may readily become life threatening.

Outcome

Two reports have evaluated immediate and long-term prognosis following IABP support with the aim of identifying reliable determinants of survival. Neither study was randomized to control. In a study by Hedenmark and colleagues,[4] the mean duration of inotropic support was 67 hours. Of 90 patients, 61% survived their hospitalization, and 51% had long-term survival at 23 months. The primary determinant of survival after placement of IABP was early recovery (within 24 hours) of cardiac function with maintenance of vital organ perfusion.

The study by Lund and colleagues[5] was restricted to post–cardiopulmonary bypass patients receiving IABP support. Of these 90 patients, 49% died while on IABP; the 30-day mortality rate was 61%, and

the 5-year survival rate was 22%. Independent predictors of 30-day mortality rate included the use of isoprenaline and norepinephrine, the number of direct current cardioversions, chronic left ventricular failure, and the functional severity of the patient's heart disease.

Theoretically, the predicted improvement in demand/supply ratio offered by IABP support can benefit patients with acute cardiac decompensation. Nevertheless, it remains to be determined to what extent IABP will improve survival and for whom this technology is best used.

Selected References

1. Gray JR, Faust RJ. Intra-aortic balloon counterpulsation and ventricular assist devices. In Tarhan S, ed. Cardiovascular Anesthesia and Postoperative Care. 2nd ed. Chicago: Year Book Medical, 1989:513.
2. Bolooki H. Application of Intra-aortic Balloon Pump. 2nd ed. Mount Kisco, NY, Futura, 1984.
3. Bolooki H. Current status of circulatory support with an intra-aortic balloon pump. Med Instrument 1986;20:266.
4. Hedenmark J, Ahn H, Nystrom S, et al. Intra-aortic balloon counterpulsation with special reference to determinants of survival. Scand J Thor Cardiovasc Surg 1989;23:57.
5. Lund O, Johansen G, Allermand H, et al. Intra-aortic balloon pumping in the treatment of low cardiac output following open heart surgery: Immediate results and long-term prognosis. J Thorac Cardiovasc Surg 1988;36:332.

Suggested References

Bates ER, Stomel RJ, Hochman JS, et al. The use of intra-aortic balloon counterpulsation as an adjunct to reperfusion therapy in cardiogenic shock. Int J Cardiol 1998;65:S37–42.
Curtis J, Boland M, Bliss D, et al. Intra-aortic balloon cardiac assist: Complication rates for the surgical and percutaneous insertion techniques. Am Surg 1988;54:142.
Melhorn U, Kroner A, de Vivie ER. 30 years of clinical intra-aortic balloon pumping facts and figures. J Thorac Cardiovasc Surg 1999;47:298–303.
Scheld HH. Mechanical support—risks and benefits. J Thorac Cardiovasc Surg 1997;45:1–5.

152
Increased Intracranial Pressure

C. Thomas Wass, M.D.

Intracranial pressure (ICP) is determined by the relationship of the volumes of the intracranial vault (formed by the skull) and the intracranial contents. The latter is composed of three volume compartments: brain parenchyma, cerebrospinal fluid, and blood. By definition, intracranial hypertension exists when ICP is sustained above 15 mm Hg.

Brain

The brain parenchyma is composed of cellular elements, intracellular and interstitial water. The average adult brain weighs 1350 to 1450 g and accounts for approximately 90% of the intracranial volume. This compartment may expand because of tumor growth or cerebral edema (vasogenic or cytotoxic).

Cerebrospinal Fluid

Cerebrospinal fluid (CSF) occupies approximately 5% of the intracranial volume (i.e., 75 mL, of which approximately 25 mL is within the ventricular system). The rate of CSF production is about 0.35 to 0.40 mL/min in the normal adult. Expansion of this compartment occurs with communicating or obstructive hydrocephalus.

Blood

Intracranial blood accounts for approximately 5% of the intracranial volume. The cerebral blood volume (CBV) is 3 to 7 mL/100 g brain weight. Elevation of the head decreases both CBV and ICP. Expansion of the blood compartment may result from cerebral hemorrhage or dilation of resistance and/or capacitance vessels. This compartment is most amenable to acute manipulation by the anesthesiologist (see following). With few exceptions (e.g., cerebral vasospasm, profound hypotension), increases in CBF usually result in parallel increases in CBV and ICP.

Intracranial Elastance

Historically, the intracranial pressure-volume relationship has been termed *compliance* in the medical literature. Compliance is defined as unit(s) of volume (e.g., intracranial volume) change per unit(s) of pressure (e.g., ICP) change (i.e., $\Delta V/\Delta P$). However, the pressure-volume curve (Fig. 152–1)[1] presented in our textbooks actually depicts the reciprocal of compliance, or *elastance*.

Elastance is defined as $\Delta P/\Delta V$. In normal patients, small volume increases in any one of the three intracranial compartments result in little or no change in ICP. The compensatory mechanisms that initially protect against an elevation in ICP are (a) translocation of intracranial CSF through the foramen magnum to the subarachnoid space surrounding the spinal cord, (b) increased CSF absorption through the arachnoid granulations, and (c) translocation of blood out of the intracranial vault. Once these mechanisms are exhausted, an abrupt increase in ICP occurs in association with small increases in intracranial volume (see Fig. 152–1). That is, intracranial compliance is de-

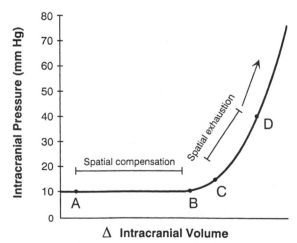

Figure 152–1. Idealized intracranial pressure-volume curve. Points A and B represent spatial compensation with expanding intracranial volume. The elastance of the intracranial compartment is low. At point C, spatial exhaustion occurs as compensatory mechanisms fail. Between points C and D, the elastance is increased and small changes in volume result in large changes in ICP. (From Sulek CA.[1])

creased or, more correctly, ***intracranial elastance is increased***.

Anesthetic Considerations

The goals of managing a patient with intracranial hypertension include preventing cerebral ischemia and preventing brain herniation (Fig. 152–2).[1,2]

Respiratory. $PaCO_2$ is the single most potent physiologic determinant of CBF and CBV. Between $PaCO_2$ values of 20 to 80 mm Hg, CBF increases by 1 mL · 100 g brain weight^{-1} · min^{-1} and CBV increases by 0.05 mL · 100 g brain weight^{-1} for each 1 mm Hg increase in $PaCO_2$ (see Fig. 25–1). Decreasing $PaCO_2$ to 25 to 28 mm Hg should provide near-maximal reductions in ICP, lasting up to 24 to 36 hours, without adversely affecting acid-base/electrolyte status or decreasing cerebral oxygen delivery (i.e., resulting from a leftward shift in the oxyhemoglobin dissociation curve). Hypoxia (PaO_2 below 50 mm Hg) will increase CBF and ICP (see Fig. 25–1). Positive end-expiratory pressure (PEEP) may decrease venous effluent from the cranium and aggravate intracranial hypertension.

Coughing against a closed glottis (i.e., Valsalva's maneuver) will increase ICP. Intravenous lidocaine, esmolol, and narcotic may be used to attenuate the ICP response to direct laryngoscopy, tracheal intubation, and coughing.

Cardiovascular. Mean arterial pressure (MAP) is a determinant of cerebral perfusion pressure (i.e., CPP = MAP − ICP). The blood-brain barrier and autoregulation may be disrupted at the site of cerebral pathology from ischemic, traumatic, hemor-

rhagic, or osmolar insults. In these regions, it is correct to assume that regional CBF is passively dependent on CPP. Before the dura is opened, it is prudent to treat all hypertensive episodes by deepening the level of anesthesia and/or administering antihypertensive drugs that lack the ability to dilate cerebral vessels and thus elevate ICP (e.g., esmolol, labetalol, metoprolol).

Intravenous fluid administration should not be spared at the expense of hemodynamic stability. Osmolar, not oncotic, pressure is the primary determinant of fluid shifts within the brain.[3] Therefore, maintaining intravascular isovolemia with a near iso-osmolar solution (normal saline, lactated Ringer's) is safe and beneficial to end-organ preservation. Hypo-osmolar glucose-containing fluids (D5%W) have the ability to (a) aggravate cerebral edema, (b) increase ICP, and (c) induce hyperglycemia, which exacerbates ischemic neurologic injury.

Electrocardiographic abnormalities that occur with subarachnoid hemorrhage may not be as benign as once thought. For example, abnormal thallium scintigraphy, regional wall motion abnormalities, and elevated creatine kinase-MB isoenzymes have been noted in approximately 30%, 30%, and 50%, respectively, of patients with acute subarachnoid hemorrhage.[4]

Renal. Both osmotic and loop diuretics are effective in reducing the parenchymal fluid compartment and decrease CSF formation (V_f). Mannitol administration in patients with intracranial hypertension is not associated with a transient increase in ICP.[5]

Metabolic. Cerebral metabolism decreases approximately 6% per 1°C of temperature reduction. Mild hypothermia (i.e., temperature reductions of 1 to 6°C) has been reported to improve neurologic outcome following focal or global brain ischemia in laboratory studies.[6] Conversely, fever worsens postischemic neurologic outcome.[6] Proposed mechanisms for temperature modulation of postischemic neurologic outcome include alterations in cerebral metabolism, blood-brain barrier stability, membrane depolarization, ion homeostasis (e.g., calcium), neurotransmitter release (e.g., glutamate or aspartate), enzyme function (e.g., phospholipase, xanthine oxidase, or nitric oxide synthase), and free radical production or scavenging. Large clinical trials are currently being conducted to evaluate the affect of mild hypothermia on neurologic outcome in humans.

Musculoskeletal. A nondepolarizing muscle relaxant without histamine-releasing properties (e.g., vecuronium, cisatracurium) is ideal for facilitating tracheal intubation and maintaining muscle paralysis. In the pathologic brain, pancuronium and gallamine can induce systemic and intracranial hypertension. Succinylcholine also has the ability to increase ICP, possibly by increasing muscle afferent activity. This response may be prevented by deep anesthesia or pretreatment with metocurine.

Specific Anesthetics. In general, all volatile anesthetics are vasodilators that, with normocap-

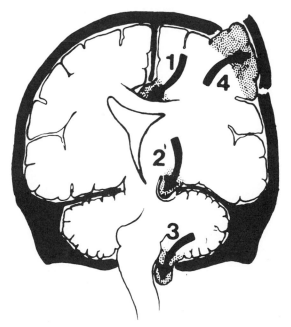

Figure 152–2. Schematic representation of different types of brain herniation: (1) cingulate gyrus, (2) temporal lobe (uncal), (3) cerebellar, and (4) transcalvarial (postoperative or traumatic). (From Fishman RA.[2])

nia, will increase CBF, CBV, and ICP. The order of vasodilator potency is approximately halothane $>>$ enflurane $>$ isoflurane $=$ sevoflurane $=$ desflurane. This effect can be overcome by hyperventilation. For halothane, hyperventilation must begin before administration to overcome the drug-induced increased CBF. In contrast, cerebral vasodilation is overcome by hyperventilating patients before, during or after initiating inhaled isoflurane, sevoflurane, and desflurane. Hyperventilation during the use of deep enflurane has been associated with seizures.

All intravenous anesthetics except ketamine cause some degree of reduction in cerebral metabolism, CBF, and ICP (provided that ventilation is not depressed). Todd and colleagues[7] were unable to demonstrate a significantly different outcome (incidence of new neurologic deficits, total hospital stay, or hospital cost) in neurosurgical patients anesthetized with either propofol/fentanyl, isoflurane/nitrous oxide, or fentanyl/nitrous oxide.

Postoperative. Rapid and smooth emergence enables the neurosurgeon to evaluate the patient's neurologic status before discharge from the operative suite.

Selected References

1. Sulek CA. Intracranial pressure. In Cucchiara RF, Black S, Michenfelder JD, eds. Clinical Neuroanesthesia. 2nd ed. Philadelphia: Churchill Livingstone, 1998:73–123.
2. Fishman RA. Brain edema. N Engl J Med 1973;293:706–711.
3. Kaieda R, Todd MM, Cook LN, et al. Acute effects of changing plasma osmolality and colloid oncotic pressure on the formation of brain edema after cryogenic injury. Neurosurgery 1989;24:671–678.
4. Szabo MD, Crosby G, Hurford WE, et al. Myocardial perfusion following acute subarachnoid hemorrhage in patients with an abnormal electrocardiogram. Anesth Analg 1993;76:253–258.
5. Ravussin P, Abou-Madi M, Archer D, et al. Changes in CSF pressure after mannitol in patients with and without elevated CSF pressure. J Neurosurg 1988;69:869–876.
6. Wass CT, Lanier WL. Hypothermia-associated protection from ischemic brain injury: Implications for patient management. Int Anesthesiol Clin 1996;34:95–111.
7. Todd MM, Warner DS, Sokoll MD, et al. A prospective, comparative trial of three anesthetics for elective supratentorial craniotomy. Anesthesiology 1993;78:1005–1020.

Suggested References

Drummond JC, Patel PM. Cerebral physiology and the effects of anesthetics and techniques. In Miller RD, ed. Anesthesia. 5th ed. Philadelphia: Churchill Livingstone, 2000:695–734.
Drummond JC, Patel PM. Neurosurgical anesthesia. In Miller RD, ed. Anesthesia. 5th ed. Philadelphia: Churchill Livingstone, 2000:1895–1933.

153
Anesthesia for Hypophysectomy

Mary B. Weber, M.D.

Hypophysectomy is the excision or destruction of the pituitary gland, also called the hypophysis. Lesions of the pituitary gland requiring or resulting from this procedure can be hyper- or hypofunctioning. They can cause a variety of anatomic and physiologic abnormalities that affect anesthetic management.

Review of Pituitary Function

Anterior Pituitary. The function of the anterior pituitary (adenohypophysis) is controlled by the hypothalamus via the hypophyseal portal system, which transports releasing factors to the anterior pituitary. The adenohypophysis secretes the following:

- Growth hormone.
- Thyroid-stimulating hormone.
- Adrenocorticotropic hormone (ACTH).
- Luteinizing hormone.
- Follicle-stimulating hormone.
- Prolactin.
- Melanocyte-stimulating hormone.

Hyposecretion. Hyposecretion usually reflects panhypopituitarism from various causes, including compression of the gland by a tumor, necrosis after postpartum hemorrhagic shock, head injury, radiation therapy, and surgical or chemical hypophysectomy. Treatment is accomplished with specific hormone replacement.

Hypersecretion. A basophilic adenoma of the anterior pituitary gland may produce excessive ACTH, resulting in hyperadrenocorticism, or Cushing's disease. An adenoma secreting excess growth hormone results in gigantism if the epiphyses have not yet closed or in acromegaly after puberty. Excessive secretion of thyroid-stimulating hormone may cause hyperthyroidism. The most frequent hormonal abnormality associated with an anterior pituitary tumor is excess prolactin resulting in galactorrhea and amenorrhea.

Posterior Pituitary. Antidiuretic hormone (ADH, vasopressin) and oxytocin are the hormones synthesized in the hypothalamus and stored and released by the posterior pituitary. Disorders involving the posterior pituitary include diabetes insipidus caused by a deficiency of ADH and inappropriate ADH secretion.

Anesthetic Considerations

Patients scheduled to undergo hypophysectomy may present with pressure effects from tumor growth, resulting in headaches, palsies of cranial nerve III, IV, or VI; or, most often, visual disturbances from optic nerve damage. They also may present with altered endocrine function. These patients must be evaluated, especially in regard to physiologic and anatomic changes from endocrine dysfunction. Any abnormalities should be corrected preoperatively, because further impairment may occur after surgical manipulation.

Cushing's Disease

Patients with Cushing's disease need special attention. The patient with hyperadrenocorticism may suffer from hyperglycemia, hypertension, hypokalemia, increased intravascular volume, and skeletal muscle weakness. Increased intraoperative blood loss is common.

Acromegaly

The acromegalic suffers from a general overgrowth of skeletal, soft, and connective tissues, resulting in coarse facial features and enlarged hands and feet. Altered airway anatomy includes overgrowth of soft tissues of the upper airway, including enlargement of the tongue and epiglottis, overgrowth of the mandible with increased distance from lips to vocal cords, glottic and subglottic narrowing, enlarged vocal cords, nasal turbinate enlargement, and possible paralysis of recurrent laryngeal nerves. This may predispose to sleep apnea and impaired face mask fit and difficult intubation during anesthesia induction. If difficult airway management is anticipated, it is prudent to perform an awake fiberoptic intubation. A smaller internal-diameter endotracheal tube should be used, and mechanical trauma to the upper airway should be minimized to prevent postintubation edema and airway obstruction. Rarely, a tracheostomy is required.

These patients are also susceptible to hyperglycemia, hypertension, congestive heart failure, enlarged lung volumes, increased mismatch of ventilation and perfusion, peripheral neuropathy, skeletal muscle weakness, osteoarthritis, osteoporosis, and inadequate ulnar blood flow. One must consider the possibility of this inadequate collateral circulation when placing a radial arterial line. A peripheral nerve stimulator should be used to guide administration of nondepolarizing muscle relaxants.

Surgical Considerations

The transsphenoidal or bifrontal craniotomy approach may be used to gain access to the pituitary gland. Advantages of the transsphenoidal approach include elimination of frontal lobe retraction, microsurgical removal of small adenomas with sparing of normal tissue, reduced blood loss, and shorter hospital stay. Special anesthetic considerations include oral endotracheal intubation, oropharyngeal packing to prevent bleeding into the esophagus, and surgical use of epinephrine, cocaine, and lidocaine injected submucosally to reduce bleeding. A malleable spinal needle or a catheter may be placed in the lumbar subarachnoid space for the draining of cerebrospinal fluid or the injection of air to facilitate surgical exposure. Injected air flows up to the head and delineates the brain stem from the pituitary on fluoroscopy.

The cavernous sinus forms the lateral border of the sella turcica and includes the internal carotid artery, venous structures, and cranial nerves III, IV, V, and VI. Complications from operative manipulation therefore include carotid arterial spasm or hemorrhage, venous hemorrhage or venous air embolism (especially with head-up tilt), and cranial nerve damage. With tight surgical packing of the sella turcica, any bleeding in the field may result in backward pressure on the brain stem. Sudden new postoperative visual defects or changes in mental status require immediate reexploration to relieve possible hematomas impinging on the optic nerve or brain stem.

Other complications include altered endocrine function, including the development of diabetes insipidus. If diabetes insipidus occurs, fluid status must be assessed frequently and fluid replacement should cover urinary losses, maintenance fluids, and electrolyte imbalance. Exogenous vasopressin (desmopressin) may be administered intravenously or intranasally after nasal packing is removed.

Suggested References

Black S, Cucchiara RF. Tumor surgery. In Cucchiara RF, Black S, Michenfelder JD, eds. Clinical Neuroanesthesia. 2nd ed. New York: Churchill Livingstone 1998:343–365.

Messick JM, Cucchiara RF, Faust RJ. Airway management in patients with acromegaly. Anesthesiology 1982;56:157.

Messick JM, Faust RJ, Cucchiara RF. Anesthesia for transsphenoidal microsurgery. In Laws ER Jr, Randall RV, Kern EB, et al, eds. Management of Pituitary Adenomas and Related Lesions with Emphasis on Transsphenoidal Microsurgery. New York: Appleton-Century-Crofts, 1982:253–261.

Roizen MF. Anesthetic implications of concurrent diseases. In Miller RD, ed. Anesthesia. 5th ed. Philadelphia: Churchill Livingstone, 2000:903–1015.

Stoelting RK, Dierdorf SF. Anesthesia and Co-Existing Diseases. 3rd ed. New York, Churchill Livingstone, 1993.

154
Carotid Endarterectomy

Wolf H. Stapelfeldt, M.D.

Carotid endarterectomy is offered to patients at risk for cerebral ischemia caused by thromboembolic and/or obstructive atherosclerotic lesions in the area of the carotid bifurcation. There is also a significantly increased risk of myocardial ischemia with a threefold increase in perioperative morbidity and mortality in patients with a history of angina or prior myocardial infarction. Myocardial ischemia represents the predominant cause of perioperative mortality (1% to 2%) associated with this procedure. During carotid clamping, adequate cerebral blood flow may be dependent on collateral circulation and thus dependent on sufficient **cerebral perfusion pressure.** The imperative to protect the myocardium by controlling systemic blood pressure puts the anesthesiologist in a challenging situation.

Physiologic Effects

Carotid endarterectomy causes physiologic changes related to temporary total blood flow obstruction through the carotid artery. Surgical technique requires temporary total occlusion of the carotid artery, thereby rendering the ipsilateral hemisphere dependent solely on collateral blood flow from the vertebral arteries and the contralateral carotid artery through the circle of Willis. If high to normal cerebral perfusion pressure is maintained, collateral blood flow is usually sufficient. Frequently, however, adequate collateral blood flow cannot be achieved during intraoperative carotid occlusion, and a temporary shunt must be used. Because of an inherent increased risk of thromboembolic complications (an incidence rate of about 0.7%), shunts are not used routinely in carotid endarterectomy. A number of techniques have been developed to determine the need for shunt insertion. Each has its own theoretical or practical advantages and limitations in view of the ultimate goal of avoiding persistent changes in neurologic function and performance.

Techniques for Brain Monitoring

Neurologic Status. Neurologic status can be monitored in the awake patient under local anesthesia. This is effective in detecting ischemic episodes. In some institutions, less postoperative hypertension has been noted in patients who had an endarterectomy done under field block. However, awake patients may panic and become combative if they become aphasic or hemiplegic intraoperatively, leading to loss of control of the surgical field. Awake patients may also be more susceptible to anxiety-related sympathetic responses, thus posing a potentially increased risk for myocardial ischemia. Neurologic status assessment is an important diagnostic tool immediately following the conclusion of general anesthesia. Not all surgeons can routinely finish a carotid endarterectomy quickly enough to make field block anesthesia practical.

Carotid Stump Pressure. A carotid stump pressure (the pressure in the distal stump of the occluded carotid) is used by some to predict collateral flow distal to the occluded carotid artery. However, this does not indicate per se that adequate regional flow is adequate through potentially compromised zones. Pressure and flow do not necessarily correlate. Stump pressures of 60 mm Hg or above do not necessarily ensure adequate regional perfusion.[1] Conversely, in some patients regional perfusion may be adequate at stump pressures considerably below 60 mm Hg.

EEG or SSEP. Changes in **EEG or somatosensory evoked potential (SSEP)** signals are sensitive parameters for ischemia, because electrophysiologic activity accounts for about 60% of normal cerebral energy expenditure. For the same reason, changes in electrical activity are not necessarily specific for ischemia that is severe enough to threaten cellular integrity. Moreover, they are affected by changes in physiologic parameters, such as temperature, $Paco_2$, and the depth of anesthesia. EEG and SSEP signals are reflective of only parts of the brain, the cortical rim (EEG) or specific sensory central nervous system pathways (SSEP), and thus may not detect regional ischemic events in other parts of the brain. EEG changes occur in about 20% of patients during carotid occlusion and are considered indicative of potentially serious ischemia. This is supported by data demonstrating a strong correlation of EEG changes persisting for more than 10 minutes with postoperative neurologic deficit. Thus EEG changes are considered an indication for immediate shunt placement. The predictive value of EEG monitoring is decreased in the presence of preexisting neurologic deficits and/or EEG changes.

The 16-lead EEG is considered the gold standard for monitoring cerebral function in anesthetized patients. It responds in seconds and can detect regional ischemia, but requires continuous observation by a technician. Alternatively, processed EEGs have been developed that use fewer leads and are more easily interpreted.

Regional Cerebral Blood Flow. Regional cerebral blood flow can be calculated by measuring the washout of radioisotopes from the distribution of the middle cerebral artery. These studies allow the determination of the **critical regional cerebral blood flow, the flow rate below which 50% of patients show EEG signs of ischemia.** This is dependent on the anesthetic used, measuring about 20 $mL \cdot kg^{-1} \cdot min^{-1}$ in the presence of halothane versus 10 $mL \cdot kg^{-1} \cdot min^{-1}$ in the presence of isoflurane (at normocarbia).[2]

Dissection of the Carotid Bifurcation

The surgical dissection of the carotid bifurcation may be associated with direct and indirect hemodynamic effects. Although postoperative neurologic deficit is attributed predominantly to thromboembolic complications (65% to 95%), regional cerebral hyperperfusion—likely on the basis of impaired autoregulation—was also recognized as a possible mechanism of postoperative neurologic deficit.[3] Postoperative hypertension was identified as a major risk factor for neurologic deficit as well as myocardial ischemia. This may possibly be related to postoperatively impaired carotid baroreceptor function. Denervation of the carotid sinus per se was found to cause sympathomimetic electrocardiographic changes. On the other hand, dissection of the bifurcation may improve previously impaired baroreceptor function if carotid sinus afferent fibers are left intact, possibly causing postoperative hypotension. Finally, carotid body function may be impaired, particularly following bilateral carotid endarterectomy, thus abolishing cardiorespiratory responses to hypoxemia and rendering respiratory regulation totally dependent on changes in Pa_{CO_2}.

Selected References

1. McKay RD, Sundt TM, Michenfelder JD, et al. Internal carotid artery stump pressure and cerebral blood flow during carotid endarterectomy: Modification by halothane, enflurane, and Innovar. Anesthesiology 1976;45:390.
2. Michenfelder JD, Sundt TM, Fode N, et al. Isoflurane when compared to enflurane or halothane decreases the frequency of cerebral ischemia during carotid endarterectomy. Anesthesiology 1987;67:336.
3. Sundt TM, Sharbrough FW, Piepgras DG, et al. Correlation of cerebral blood flow and electroencephalographic changes during carotid endarterectomy. Mayo Clin Proc 1981;56:533.

Suggested References

Angell-James JE, Lumley JSP. Changes in the mechanical properties of the carotid sinus region and carotid sinus nerve activity in patients undergoing carotid endarterectomy. J Physiol (Lond) 1975;244:80.

Mahla ME, Trankina MF. Extracranial vascular disease. In Cucchiara RF, Black S, Michenfelder JD, eds. Clinical Neuroanesthesia. 2nd ed. Churchill Livingstone, New York, 1998:319–341.

Messick JM Jr, Casement B, Sharbrough FW, et al. Correlation of regional cerebral blood flow (rCBF) with EEG changes during isoflurane anesthesia for carotid endarterectomy: Critical rCBF. Anesthesiology 1987;66:344–349.

155
Cerebral Aneurysm Surgery

Paul E. Stensrud, M.D.

At autopsy, 4% to 6% of individuals are found to have cerebral aneurysms, but only an estimated 20% of these aneurysms rupture and produce subarachnoid hemorrhage (SAH).[1] SAH (most frequently due to cerebral aneurysm rupture) is heralded by sudden onset of severe headache, neurologic deficit, or alteration in consciousness.

The Hunt-Hess modification of the Botterell classification is used to clinically grade the severity of SAH (Table 155–1).[2] Grades I and II are characterized by increasing headache, grades III and IV are characterized by increasing neurologic deficits and alteration in consciousness, and grade V is characterized by deep coma. Grades III to V are associated with significantly worse outcome.

Likelihood of rupture of a cerebral aneurysm is affected by:

- Aneurysm size.
- Strength of the aneurysm wall.
- Previous rupture.
- Transmural pressure gradient.

The peak age range for SAH is 55 to 60 years, but SAH is also seen during pregnancy. Cerebral aneurysms that rupture during pregnancy most commonly do so between the 30th and 40th weeks of gestation or in the postpartum period and only rarely rupture at the time of delivery. This is in contrast to arteriovenous malformations, which commonly bleed at delivery.[1] Cerebral aneurysms may also manifest by compressing adjacent structures such as cranial nerves or portions of the brain stem, without frank rupture and SAH.[3]

Two major sources of morbidity and mortality associated with SAH are rebleeding and cerebral vasospasm. **Rebleeding** is noted in **29%** of patients, most often during the first 48 hours following the initial SAH[4] (although 11% of rebleeds occur more than 1 year after initial aneurysm rupture[3]). The mortality rate in patients who rebleed is 42%.[1] Factors determining the probability of rebleeding are the same as those predisposing to the initial rupture. In addition, rebleeding may occur intraoperatively if surgical access is difficult.

Cerebral vasospasm is angiographically detectable in **70% to 90%** of patients after SAH, whereas 50% of patients with detectable vasospasm have neurologic symptoms. Vasospasm is more likely with advancing clinical grade.[4] The peak incidence occurs 5 to 12 days after the initial SAH. Diagnosis is based on cerebral angiography or, alternatively, transcranial Doppler studies. Mortality of cerebral vasospasm has declined from 40% in the 1960s to 8% today.[4] The mechanism of cerebral vasospasm is poorly understood but is felt to be multifactorial. Promising vasospastic agents under investigation include hemoglobin and endothelin. Treatment of vasospasm includes induced hypertensive, hypervolemic hemodilution (triple H therapy), and administration of nimodipine. Nimodipine is a calcium-channel blocker that appears to have little hemodynamic effect during anesthesia. Nimodipine has little effect on the cerebral angiogram but does appear to reduce the symptoms and mortality due to vasospasm. In addition, some have advocated removal of subarachnoid blood during operation or even local application of thrombolytic agents such as recombinant tissue plasminogen activator (rTPA) or urokinase to remove a putative vasospastic agent from the subarachnoid space.[3, 4]

Preoperative Care

Following initial resuscitation, the diagnosis is established by computed tomography (CT) scanning, followed by cerebral angiography.[4] Thorough preoperative assessment concentrates on history of previous SAH, current neurologic status, and concurrent medical conditions. **Electrocardiographic (ECG) changes** are common with SAH and include ST segment changes, T wave inversion, and prolonged QT interval with U waves. These ECG

Table 155–1. Hunt-Hess Classification of Clinical Grade

Grade	Description
Unruptured	
I	Mild headache or nuchal rigidity
II	Moderate to severe headache, nuchal rigidity, ± cranial nerve palsy
III	Drowsiness, confusion, or mild focal deficit
IV	Stupor, hemiparesis, early decerebrate rigidity, vegetative disturbances
V	Deep coma, decerebrate rigidity, moribund

changes render the diagnosis of myocardial ischemia difficult, and patients with a history of coronary artery disease may require serial ECGs and cardiac enzyme studies, along with echocardiography. Many patients are prophylactically fluid-loaded to reduce the impact of vasospasm and may require central venous or pulmonary arterial pressure monitoring to optimize fluid status or to rule out myocardial ischemia. Analgesia must be provided and extreme hypertension avoided.

Induction

Of the four previously noted factors that affect the probability of aneurysm rupture, the only one under the control of the anesthesiologist is the **transmural pressure gradient** (blood pressure − intracranial pressure). A smooth induction is critical to avoid large increases in the transmural pressure gradient and aneurysm rupture or rebleeding. Preoperative sedation is continued as appropriate. Usual monitors (ECG, pulse oximeter, and blood pressure cuff) are supplemented by awake arterial line placement under local anesthesia. Thiopental induction plus use of a nondepolarizing neuromuscular relaxant is a reasonable approach. Ventilation is controlled and normocarbia is maintained. Before intubation, lidocaine and/or a β-blocker such as esmolol may be given intravenously to blunt the cardiovascular response to intubation.

Maintenance

Anesthesia may be maintained with any technique (narcotics, volatile agents, barbiturates), keeping in mind that it is desirable to awaken the patient promptly postoperatively in order to assess neurologic status. To aid surgical dissection, mild hyperventilation to a $PaCO_2$ of 32 mm Hg, cerebrospinal fluid drainage via a spinal catheter, or barbiturate or mannitol administration may improve surgical exposure. These measures are delayed until the dura is opened, to avoid a sudden increase in the transmural pressure gradient. Induced hypotension may be used to reduce the risk of aneurysm rupture and to facilitate aneurysm clipping, although its use may present increased risk in patients with vasospastic ischemia. Increased surgical use of temporary vascular clips has obviated the need for induced hypotension with most neurosurgeons. Indeed, induced hypertension is used in some patients to improve collateral blood flow.

Emergence

Rapid emergence is desirable to allow neurologic assessment so that prompt reexploration or further diagnostic procedures (CT, angiography) may be undertaken if neurologic deficits are discovered. Hypertension during emergence is undesirable and may be prevented by cautious administration of labetalol, esmolol, hydralazine, or sodium nitroprusside.[3]

Selected References

1. Smith RR, Miller JD. Pathophysiology and clinical evaluation of subarachnoid hemorrhage. In Youmans JR, ed. Neurosurgical Surgery. 3rd ed. Philadelphia: WB Saunders, 1990:1644.
2. Hunt WE, Hess RM. Surgical risk as related to time of intervention in the repair of intracranial aneurysms. J Neurosurg 1968;28:14.
3. Black S, Sulek CA, Day AL. Cerebral aneurysm and arteriovenous malformation. In Cucchiara RF, Black S, Michenfelder JD, eds. Clinical Neuroanesthesia. 2nd ed. New York: Churchill Livingstone, 1998:265–318.
4. Kassell NF, Shaffrey ME, Shaffrey CI. Cerebral vasospasm following aneurysmal subarachnoid hemorrhage. In Apuzzo MLJ, ed. Brain Surgery: Complication Avoidance and Management. New York: Churchill Livingstone, 1993:847.

156
Cerebral Protection

Robert E. Grady, M.D.

Cerebral ischemia results when the metabolic demands of cerebral tissue exceed substrate (primarily oxygen) delivery. Ischemia can be categorized as either **global**, with interruption of blood flow to the entire brain as occurs in cardiac arrest, or **focal**, with interruption of blood flow to a defined region of the brain, such as produced by embolic cerebral artery occlusion. **Cerebral protection** is an attempt to prolong the ischemic tolerance of neuronal tissues and to reduce or abolish neuronal injury.

Traditional Concepts

The traditional concept of cerebral metabolism is illustrated in Figure 156–1. Cerebral metabolism may be divided into a **functional** component and a **cellular integrity** component. The functional component comprises 60% of the neuronal oxygen use. This component is responsible for generating action potentials and may be assessed by evaluating the electroencephalogram (EEG). The remaining 40% of oxygen is used for protein synthesis and other activities geared toward maintaining cellular integrity.

Anesthetics and hypothermia are both capable of reducing the functional component of cerebral metabolism. However, only hypothermia decreases the integrity component of cerebral metabolism. Certain anesthetics (e.g., barbiturates, etomidate, propofol, and isoflurane) and hypothermia are capable of depressing EEG activity, and thus are thought to provide brain protection. The magnitude of cerebral protection is not necessarily proportional to the extent of EEG suppression (see below). Because anesthetics affect only the functional component, they should produce at most a 60% reduction in oxygen use. In contrast, hypothermia reduces both the functional and integrity components of cerebral metabolism.

Contemporary Concepts and Experimental Evidence

Brain protection in its most basic form depends on **limiting the duration of ischemia** while **optimizing cerebral oxygen delivery**. Research has also demonstrated that neurologic outcome is worse if hyperglycemia is present during the time of cerebral ischemia. Accordingly, **avoiding hyperglycemia** is thought to be "cerebral-protective."

As demonstrated in animal studies, barbiturates are considered the gold standard of brain-protective anesthetics during focal brain ischemia. That is, barbiturates administered before **focal ischemia** have been credited with improving neurologic out-

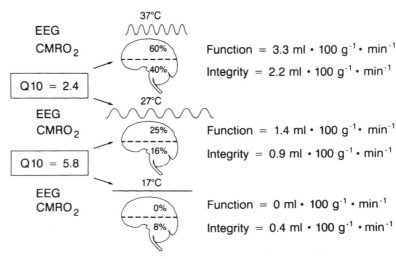

Figure 156–1. Theoretical interaction of temperature, brain function, CMRO₂, and calculated Q10 values. Q10 is defined as the ratio of metabolic rates at two temperatures separated by 10°C. In reducing temperature from 37° to 27°C, function is maintained, and both of the energy-consuming processes (i.e., function and integrity) are presumed to be affected equally with a reduction of CMRO₂ of slightly more than 50%, thus generating a Q10 value of about 2.4. With a further 10°C reduction in temperature to 17°C, function is abolished, resulting in a step decrease in CMRO₂ such that the calculated Q10 value is 5.0 or greater. At this point, the total oxygen consumed by the brain is reduced to less than 8% of the normothermic value of oxygen. (From Michenfelder JD.[1])

come. However, only one nonreproduced human study supports this supposition.[2] No cerebral-protective benefits have derived from barbiturates given either before or during a period of **global ischemia**. Furthermore, barbiturates administered after an ischemic event do not improve neurologic outcome. Close attention must be given to systemic hemodynamics when administering barbiturates; they may decrease cardiac contractility and produce hypotension, thereby compromising cerebral oxygen delivery.

The mechanism of barbiturate-mediated cerebral protection is thought to be related to both metabolic depression and a favorable redistribution of cerebral blood flow to ischemic areas (i.e., the Robin Hood effect). However, a 1996 report suggested that the extent of cerebral protection from barbiturates does not correlate with the degree of EEG suppression.[3] For example, barbiturate doses that maximally suppress the EEG (i.e., produce a flat or isoelectric EEG) may have equivalent cerebral-protective effects as smaller doses.[3] Therefore, factors other than metabolic suppression, such as membrane stabilization, free radical scavenging, and altered ion homeostasis, may account for all or part of the cerebral-protective effects of barbiturates observed in animal research.

Hypothermia has exhibited beneficial cerebral-protective effects through reductions in both the functional and the cellular integrity components of cerebral metabolism. Deep hypothermic circulatory arrest (DHCA) is a classic example of the use of hypothermia for cerebral protection. Using DHCA at temperatures of 15 to 18°?C, intact cerebral function may be regained after up to 60 minutes of complete global ischemia. Recent evidence points to a potential benefit from smaller, 1 to 2°C reductions in temperature.[4] Mild or profound hypothermia provides brain protection during both focal and global ischemia.[4] The mechanism of action partially involves decreased functional and integrity components of cerebral metabolism. Other proposed mechanisms include decreased levels of excitatory amino acids or free radicals, maintenance of ion homeostasis, and increased blood-brain barrier stability. An extreme reduction in body temperature requires cardiopulmonary bypass for temperature control and circulatory support. Regardless of the magnitude of hypothermia, one must be prepared to deal with potential complications, such as reduced drug metabolism, coagulation disorders, and cardiac rhythm disturbances.

Selected References

1. Michenfelder JD. The awake brain. In Michenfelder JD, ed. Anesthesia and the Brain. New York: Churchill Livingstone, 1988:14.
2. Nussmeier NA, Arlund C, Slogoff S. Neuropsychiatric complications after cardiopulmonary bypass: Cerebral protection by a barbiturate. Anesthesiology 1986;64:165–170.
3. Warner DS, Takaoka S, Wu B, et al. Electroencephalographic burst suppression is not required to elicit maximal neuroprotection from pentobarbital in a rat model of focal ischemia. Anesthesiology 1996;84:1475–1484.
4. Wass CT, Lanier WL. Hypothermia-associated protection from ischemic brain injury: Implications for patient management. Int Anesthesiol Clin 1996; 34:95–111.

Suggested Reference

Polis TZ, Lanier WL. An evaluation of cerebral protection by anesthetics with a special reference to metabolic depression. In Heyer EJ, Young WL, eds. Anesthesiology Clinics of North America: Anesthesia for the Patient With Neurologic Disease. Philadelphia: WB Saunders, 1997:691–717.

157

Anesthesia for the Sitting Position

Robert M. Craft, M.D.

The sitting position may be used for posterior approaches to the cervical spinal column and for surgery involving the posterior cranial fossa (see Chap. 78). Alternative positions for these procedures include park bench, prone, and supine with the head turned to the side. A properly positioned patient for a "sitting" case is actually in a modified recumbent position (Fig. 157–1).[1] Patients requiring cervical spine surgery should be carefully evaluated preoperatively, because decreased cervical range of motion, instability, or position-related neurologic symptoms may necessitate awake intubation. Patients with posterior fossa tumors should be approached with the knowledge that brain stem structures may be adversely affected by compression and obstructive hydrocephalus may result in elevated intracranial pressure. Relative contraindications to the sitting position are listed in Table 157–1.[2]

Potential Advantages of the Sitting Position

- Less blood loss.[3]
- Improved surgical exposure with less tissue retraction.
- Better access to the endotracheal tube, extremities, and chest.
- Reduced facial swelling.

Potential Complications of the Sitting Position

Venous Air Embolism (VAE) and Paradoxical Air Embolism. These complications are discussed in Chapter 158. A large study revealed that although the incidence of VAE was greater in sitting patients than in horizontal patients (45% vs. 12%), there was no difference in morbidity or mortality rate.[3]

Tension Pneumocephalus. Although there is a high frequency of pneumocephalus in the sitting position, symptomatic pneumocephalus is uncommon. Cerebrospinal fluid (CSF) is more likely to drain through the wound in sitting patients with cortical atrophy, allowing the entrapment of air (in-verted Coke bottle phenomenon). The effect of nitrous oxide on the frequency and severity of pneumocephalus is controversial.[4]

Circulatory Instability. Hypotension may ensue secondary to decreased venous return. This can be minimized by preoperative hydration, compression stockings, slow positional change, and maintenance of hips and knees in flexed position. A large retrospective comparison failed to show a difference in the incidence of hypotension between sitting and horizontal patients.[3]

Jugular Venous Obstruction. This may be avoided by limiting head flexion to allow two fingerbreadths between mandible and sternum.

Postoperative Central Apnea. Potential causes include a brain stem hematoma and surgical damage to the respiratory centers. Rigorous prevention and treatment of postoperative hypertension are indicated to help prevent hematoma formation.

Cranial Nerve Dysfunction. Cranial nerves V, VII, IX, X, XI, and XII may be involved (see Fig. 78–2).[5] Postoperative airway protection may be impaired by dysfunction of IX, X, or XII.

Quadriplegia. Reported cases are thought to have been caused by mechanical compression of the spinal cord or by ischemia resulting from stretching

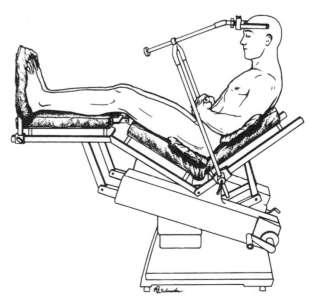

Figure 157–1. Standard sitting position. (From Milde LN.[1])

Table 157–1. Relative Contraindications to the Sitting Position

Ventriculoatrial shunt in place and open
Cerebral ischemia upright awake
Left atrial pressure (PCWP) < right atrial pressure
Platypnea-orthodeoxia*
Preoperative demonstration of patent foramen ovale or right-to-left shunt
?Cardiac instability ⎫ Chest compression and resuscitation not
                      ⎬ really better in prone or lateral
?Age extremes   ⎭ position

*Platypnea-orthodeoxia is a condition in which there is a right-to-left shunting of the blood at the atrial level only with assumption of the upright position.

From Black S, Cucchiara RF.[2]

of the spinal cord blood vessels. Preventive measures include preoperative examination of the cervical range of motion and radiographic determination of cervical canal dimensions, as well as prompt intraoperative treatment of hypotension.

Peripheral Nerve Injury. This may be prevented by careful positioning and padding of pressure points.

Monitoring

Frequently utilized monitoring for the sitting position includes electrocardiography (ECG), pulse oximetry, direct arterial monitoring (zeroed at the base of the skull), capnography and/or mass spectrometry, right atrial catheter, precordial Doppler, and transesophageal echocardiography. Electrophysiologic monitoring, such as brain stem auditory evoked response (BAER), somatosensory evoked potential (SSEP), and electromyography (EMG), is becoming more common. The following physiologic parameters may be monitored:

□ The **cardiopulmonary system** may be assessed with ECG, pulse oximetry, and arterial and central venous pressures.
□ The **brain stem** may be evaluated for signs of surgical trespass via the ECG, with potential warning signs including tachycardia, bradycardia, and ectopic beats. BAER or SSEP may also provide evidence of surgical transgression.

□ Evidence of **cranial nerve** stimulation may be revealed through examination of the ECG, arterial line, EMG, and BAER. Manipulation of cranial nerve V results in hypertension and bradycardia, whereas manipulation of cranial nerve X results in hypotension and bradycardia. Mechanical stimulation of cranial nerves V, VII, and XI may be revealed via EMG monitoring of the corresponding muscle groups, and insult to cranial nerve VIII will be evident on examination of BAER.
□ **Venous air embolism (VAE)** (see Chap. 158).

Choice of Anesthetics

Anesthetic concerns that may influence the choice of anesthetic agents include maintenance of cardiovascular stability, the risk of air embolism, possible increased intracranial pressure, and the desire to evaluate an awake patient immediately postoperatively. To these ends, no particular technique has proved superior. Many clinicians favor isoflurane, nitrous oxide, and low-dose fentanyl with muscle relaxation provided by nondepolarizing neuromuscular blocking agents (or high-dose isoflurane without relaxant in cases where EMG monitoring is used). The use of volatile anesthetics and nitrous oxide allows for easily controlled anesthetic depth, stable hemodynamic parameters, and rapid emergence, but their use must also be tempered by the knowledge of their effects on intracranial pressure and VAE (see Chap. 158).

Selected References

1. Milde LN. The head-elevated positions. In Martin JT, Warner MA, eds. Positioning in Anesthesia and Surgery. 3rd ed. Philadelphia: WB Saunders, 1997:71–93.
2. Black S, Cucchiara RF. Tumor surgery. In Cucchiara RF, Michenfelder JD, eds. Clinical Neuroanesthesia. 2nd ed. New York: Churchill Livingstone, 1998:343–365.
3. Black S, Ockert DB, Oliver WC, et al. Outcome following posterior fossa craniectomy in patients in the sitting or horizontal position. Anesthesiology 1988;69:49–56.
4. Artru AA. Breathing nitrous oxide during closure of the dura and cranium is not indicated. Anesthesiology 1987;66:719.
5. Duke DA, Lynch JJ, Harner SG, et al. Venous air embolism in sitting and supine patients undergoing vestibular schwannoma resection. Neurosurgery 1998;42:1282–1287.

158
Physiology and Treatment of Venous Air Embolism

Susan Black, M.D.

Etiology

Venous air embolism (VAE) can occur whenever a noncollapsible vein is opened and a pressure gradient exists favoring air entrainment rather than bleeding. This classically occurs when the operative site is above the level of the heart. It may also occur when noncollapsible veins are opened in an operative field into which gas has been insufflated under pressure.

Prevalence

VAE has been reported in most neurosurgical procedures, with the highest prevalence (50%) during posterior fossa craniotomy in the sitting position (Table 158–1).[1] VAE has been reported in many other surgical procedures that involve positioning the operative site above the level of the heart or using gas for insufflation or to cool some surgical instruments (gas may be inadvertently injected into a cavity or a joint or directly into vascular structures).[2]

Pathophysiology

The consequences of the VAE depend on the rate of air entry. Rarely, massive VAE may create an "air lock" in the right ventricle (RV), resulting in RV outflow obstruction, RV failure, and cardiovascular collapse. More commonly, VAE is a slow entrainment of air into the venous system, right heart, and the pulmonary vasculature, leading to increasing pulmonary vascular resistance (PVR) via two mechanisms. Mechanical obstruction of small arteries and arterioles and release of endogenous vasoactive agents cause pulmonary vasoconstriction, leading to increasing PVR, increasing RV afterload, increased pulmonary artery pressure (PAP), and ultimately increased central venous pressure (CVP) as the RV begins to fail. As VAE continues, hypotension develops as cardiac output falls. Adult respiratory distress syndrome may develop after large VAE episodes.

Paradoxical air embolism (PAE) or arterial air embolism may also develop. Air may pass from the right to the left side of the heart through either an intracardiac defect or the pulmonary vasculature. Once PAE occurs, more serious complications may develop from obstruction of coronary and cerebral arteries.

Diagnosis

The most sensitive monitors for VAE are transesophageal echocardiography (TEE) and Doppler

Table 158–1. Procedures with Risk for Venous Air Embolism

Procedure	Incidence of VAE
Neurosurgical Procedures	
Sitting posterior fossa craniotomy	45–55%
Posterior fossa craniotomy "horizontal" position	10–15%
Sitting cervical laminectomy	5–15%
Transsphenoidal pituitary resection	12%
Craniosynostosis	85%
Lumbar spine procedures	Case reports
OB/GYN	
Cesarean section	11–44%
Hysteroscopy, laser endometrial ablation	Case reports
Orthopedic	
Total hip replacement	67%
Intramedullary femur nailing, irrigation pelvic fractures, removal bone cyst, arthroscopy	Case reports
General Surgery	
Laparoscopy, laser tumor resection, liquid nitrogen instillation, insertion peritoneovenous shunt, hepatic resection, GI endoscopy, venovenous bypass during liver transplant	Case reports
Plastic Surgery	
Removal tissue expander	Case reports
Trauma	
Head and neck trauma, penetrating lung trauma	Case reports
Dental Procedures	
Dental implant	Case reports
Urologic Procedures	
Transurethral & open prostatectomy	Case reports
Intensive Care Patients	
Mechanical ventilation, central line placement and removal	Case reports

From Black S.[2]

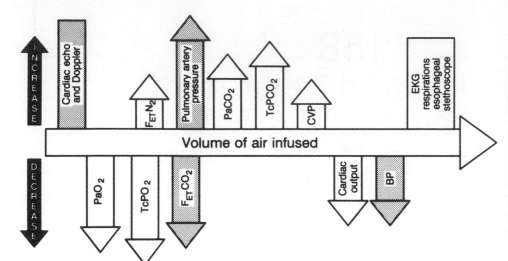

Figure 158–1. Changes in detection parameters for VAE with increasing volumes of air. Data are aggregated from human and animal studies. PaO$_2$, partial pressure of oxygen; TcPO$_2$, transcutaneous partial pressure of oxygen; FetCO$_2$, fraction of end-tidal carbon dioxide; PaCO$_2$, partial pressure of carbon dioxide; TcPCO$_2$, transcutaneous partial pressure of carbon dioxide; FetN$_2$, fraction of end-tidal nitrogen; CVP, central venous pressure; BP, blood pressure; ECG, electrocardiogram.

echocardiography, followed by expired nitrogen (ETN2), end-tidal carbon dioxide (ETCO2), PAP, CVP, right atrial (RA) catheter, and (least sensitive) the esophageal stethoscope (Fig. 158–1).[3]

The precordial Doppler is advocated as the basic monitor because it is reasonably priced, relatively easy to use, noninvasive, and very sensitive. TEE is a very sensitive monitor for VAE that detects localized air in the cardiac chambers. The multiorifice RA catheter can be used to confirm Doppler diagnosis of VAE, and rarely for life-saving aspiration of significant volumes of air during massive VAE. Proper placement of the right atrial catheter in the high right atrium by ECG control can increase its effectiveness by placing it where the air tends to collect during sitting neurosurgical procedures (Fig. 158–2).[4]

Treatment of VAE

The goals of treatment are to support the cardiovascular system to stop the influx of air at the surgical site. Flooding the field with saline should submerge the area of air entry. The application of jugular venous pressure for about 15 seconds will frequently raise the venous pressure in the wound sufficiently that the vessel will back-bleed and can be identified.

Because nitrous oxide (N$_2$O) has low solubility, it will diffuse into the VAE, increasing the size (see Chap. 44). Therefore, it should be discontinued. Vasopressors and volume infusion will increase preload, increase cardiac output, and aid in moving the VAE through the heart and peripheral pulmonary circulation. Aspiration of air from the RA catheter should be attempted. Use of PEEP to increase CVP and cerebral venous pressure to decrease VAE has been suggested, but most studies have demonstrated that it is ineffective. Also, with release of PEEP, increased right-sided heart pressures may increase the risk of PAE. In cases of VAE-related cardiovascular compromise, the classic recommendation has been to place the patient in Durant's position (left lateral decubitus position) to relieve RV outflow obstruction. Recent studies have not proved the efficacy of this manuever.[5]

Initial treatment of PAE is aimed at stopping further air entry. If myocardial ischemia develops, positive inotropic agents, usually epinephrine, are recommended to support the hemodynamics and increase contractility of the ventricles, causing breakup of the emboli. If symptomatic cerebral ischemia occurs, hyperbaric oxygen therapy should be considered as soon as the patient can be transported into a hyperbaric chamber.

Anesthetic Considerations

Certain conditions increase the risk of either significant VAE- or PAE-related morbidity should VAE develop (see Chap. 157). In the presence of these risk factors, efforts should be focused on decreasing the likelihood of VAE.

The use of N$_2$O in procedures that carry a risk for VAE is controversial. Animal and human data

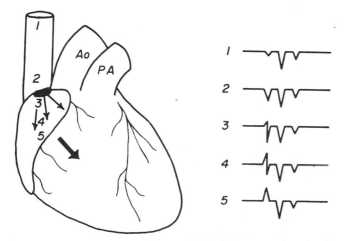

Figure 158–2. The intracardiac ECG from each position. With a single-orifice catheter, tracing 4 indicates the mid-right atrium. Because the ECG tracing originates from the middle orifice of a multiorifice catheter, and the desired position of the middle orifice is the high right atrium, tracing 2 should be sought. (From Cucchiara RF, Messick J, Gronert GA, et al.[4])

suggest that if N_2O is discontinued when VAE is diagnosed with precordial Doppler, the incidence and severity of VAE are not increased.[1]

Selected References

1. Losasso TJ, Muzzo DA, Dietz NM, et al. Fifty percent nitrous oxide does not increase the risk of venous air embolism in the sitting position. Anesthesiology 1992;77:21–30.
2. Black S. Venous air embolism. In Prough DS, Zornow MH, eds. Problems in Anesthesia. Vol. 9, No. 1. Philadelphia: Lippincott-Raven, 1997:113–124.
3. Cucchiara RF, Black S, Steinkeler JA. Anesthesia for intracranial procedures. In Barash PG, Cullen BF, Stoelting RF, eds. Clinical Anesthesia. Philadelphia: Lippincott-Raven, 1989:849–876.
4. Cucchiara RF, Messick JM, Gronert GA, et al. Time required and success rate of percutaneous right atrial catheterization: Description of a technique. Can Anaesth Soc J 1980;27:572–573.
5. Melhorn U, Burke EJ, Butler BD, et al. Body position does not affect the hemodynamic response to venous air embolism in dogs. Anesthesiology 1994;79:734–739.

159

Management of Acute Spinal Cord Injury

Scott A. Gammel, M.D.

Pathophysiology

Respiratory. Respiratory pathophysiology involves multiple factors. A lesion at T7 or higher is the critical level for significant alteration in respiratory function. With high thoracic or cervical cord lesions, vital capacity, expiratory reserve volume, and forced expiratory volume in 1 second are decreased.

Diaphragmatic paralysis is level dependent. A cord lesion at C4 or higher results in a paralyzed diaphragm with gross impairment of ventilation. A C5 lesion results in partial paralysis with significantly reduced ventilation, and a C6 lesion leaves the diaphragm intact so the patient can breathe.

Because 60% of tidal volume is attributed to rib cage expansion, **intercostal paralysis** will result in decreased cough. Paradoxical breathing also results when the diaphragm is intact while intercostal and accessory muscles are paralyzed.

Because of a spreading hematoma, ischemia, or edema, a **cord lesion** may extend to involve cervical segments important in maintaining ventilation. **Sleep apnea** (Ondine's curse) is secondary to an initial lesion or extension of a lesion involving anterolateral portions of the C2-4 cord.

Pulmonary embolism, even if small, may be significant given that there may already be decreased alveolar ventilation and reserve. Pulmonary edema often results from overtransfusion of fluid. It may also be neurogenic in origin alone or related to other associated injuries.

Gastrointestinal. Abdominal distention infringes on ventilatory reserve, a result of gastric paralysis and paralytic ileus. Several factors contribute to an increased risk of **aspiration**: increased secretions secondary to paralyzed sympathetic nervous system, gastric dilation, and ineffective cough.

Cardiovascular. Cardiovascular pathophysiology can be quite dramatic. Immediately postinjury, there is often a massive **sympathetic discharge** with subsequent hypertension and tachycardia. Following this, **parasympathetic reflexes** can result in sinus pauses, sick sinus syndrome, shifting sinus pacemaker, nodal escape beats, atrial fibrillation, multiform premature ventricular contractions, ventricular tachycardia, and ST-T changes.

Spinal shock (loss of vascular tone and vasopressor reflex, flaccid paralysis below level of injury, paralytic ileus, visceral and somatic sensory loss) occurs immediately after injury and lasts a few hours to 3 to 6 weeks. Loss of the sympathetic nervous system from T1-L2 leads to vasodilation, blood pooling, orthostatic hypotension, and potential bradycardia. A transection above T1 may result in a blood pressure of 40 mm Hg.

Because of the loss of sympathetic tone and paralyzed cardiac acceleration nerves (T1-4), **bradycardia** may result. This may be a clue to differentiating spinal shock from hemorrhagic shock, where tachycardia is expected.

Metabolic. Electrolyte and acid-base abnormalities must also be considered. **Hyperkalemia** after succinylcholine administration, significant enough to cause ventricular fibrillation, results from development of extrajunctional cholinergic receptor sites and supersensitive muscle membrane that acts like an endplate. Large amounts of potassium are released when a depolarizing muscle relaxant is given. The hyperkalemic response is not related to the succinylcholine dose, nor is it completely blocked by pretreatment with a nondepolarizing relaxant. It is related to the amount of muscle involved (whether flaccid or spastic paralysis) and generally occurs not in the acutely injured patient, but within the first week to 6 months of injury.

Hypercalcemia, resulting from mobilization of calcium related to reduced muscle activity, starts 10 days postinjury and peaks 10 weeks postinjury.

Respiratory acidosis may occur secondary to alveolar hypoventilation. **Metabolic alkalosis**, caused by vomiting and/or gastric suctioning, may also lead to **hypokalemia,** which can be potentiated by spillage of potassium into the dilated gut.

Thermoregulation is lost because sympathetic nerves normally relay to the hypothalamic regulatory center. Patients tend to be poikilothermic. Transection above C7 abolishes sweating, and resulting hyperthermia may increase oxygen demand and threaten an already decreased respiratory reserve.

Anesthetic Management

Preoperative. Because respiratory compromise is the leading cause of morbidity and mortality in the acute spinal cord–injured patient, preoperative respiratory management will determine the patient's postoperative pulmonary course.

□ **Chest physiotherapy** and postural drainage are associated with less atelectasis and a decreased need for mechanical ventilation and tracheostomy.
□ Deep venous **thrombosis prophylaxis** is also recommended preoperatively.
□ Preoperative administration of **oxygen** may minimize ischemic changes in the acutely injured cord.
□ Preoperative assessment of **arterial blood gases** and **ventilatory function** is recommended.
□ Placement of a **nasogastric tube** to suction the stomach before induction may be useful.

Airway Management. Airway management can be critical. Preparation for a **difficult intubation** should be anticipated, particularly if there is, or may be, associated facial or airway trauma. The patient is usually in cervical traction; maintaining the head in fixed neutral position with cervical cord lesions is imperative. **Awake fiberoptic intubation** is most commonly used for airway management. Awake nasotracheal intubation may be preferred in this situation, but it is contraindicated in the presence of a basilar skull fracture. An emergency tracheostomy might also be anticipated.

Cardiovascular. Cardiovascular management will depend on the level of cord lesion and other trauma associated with significant hemorrhage. In general, patients with cord lesions high enough to paralyze the sympathetic nervous system will be at risk for hypotension and resulting spinal cord ischemia, but also prone to pulmonary edema related to overzealous fluid replacement and inadequate cardiac compensation. Management is controversial.

In cervical cord injury, a pulmonary artery catheter is often recommended to balance fluid therapy and the cardiovascular effects of anesthetics. A preoperative fluid challenge in patients with cervical cord lesions or high thoracic cord lesions is recommended.

Spinal cord perfusion pressure must be maintained. Monitoring sensory- and motor-evoked potentials during stabilization and instrumentation of the vertebral column may be indicated.

Methylprednisolone, a 30 mg/kg bolus followed by 5.4 mg/kg/hr for 24 to 48 hours starting within 8 hours of injury, **improves neurologic outcome**.

Other considerations include maintaining normothermia and being prepared for electrolyte and pH abnormalities.

□ It is controversial whether succinylcholine is safe at time of injury or up to 2 hours later if needed for rapid sequence induction. Increased intubating doses of a nondepolarizing relaxant, such as vecuronium or rocuronium, may be preferable. If hyperkalemia occurs, it should be treated with glucose, insulin, bicarbonate, and calcium.
□ Serum calcium level should be measured preoperatively, and appropriate antiarrhythmic drugs should be available.
□ Monitoring should include direct arterial monitoring, urine output measurement, and possibly a pulmonary artery catheter.

In summary, the goals in the anesthetic management of the patient with acute spinal cord injury are to avoid exacerbating the cord injury by maintaining cord perfusion and avoiding cord ischemia. Steroid therapy should be started within 8 hours of injury, if possible. Respiratory insufficiency, cardiovascular instability, spinal shock, electrolyte/pH imbalance, and hypo- or hyperthermia should be treated as appropriate. Associated multiple trauma must also be anticipated.

Suggested References

Atkinson JLD, Faust RJ. Central nervous system trauma. In Cucchiara RF, Black S, Michenfelder JD, eds. Clinical Neuroanesthesia. 2nd ed. New York: Churchill Livingstone, 1998:539–556.

Bracken M, Shepard MJ, Holford TR, et al. Administration of methylprednisolone for 24–48 hours or tirilazad mesylate for 48 hours in the treatment of acute spinal cord injury. JAMA 1997;277:1597–1604.

Cottrell JE, Turndorf H. Anesthesia and Neurosurgery. St. Louis, CV Mosby, 1986.

Drummond JC, Patel PM. Neurosurgical anesthesia. In Miller RD, ed. Anesthesia. 5th ed. New York: Churchill Livingstone, 2000:1895–1933.

Quimby CW Jr, Williams RN, Greiferstein FE. Anesthetic problems of the acute quadriplegic patient. Anesth Analg 1973;52:3.

Stoelting RK, Dierdorf SF. Anesthesia and Co-Existing Disease. 3rd ed. New York, Churchill Livingstone, 1993.

160
Autonomic Hyperreflexia

Michael L. Bishop, M.D.

Autonomic hyperreflexia (AH) is a syndrome characterized by acute generalized sympathetic hyperreactivity in response to triggering stimuli. It occurs primarily in patients with spinal cord injury at or above T4-7. Its prevalence among the spinal cord injury population ranges from 66% to 85% of individuals and has been reported in a milder form among normal individuals, especially in response to urinary bladder distention. The triggering stimulus can be nearly any endogenous or exogenous stimulus occurring below the level of the cord lesion. It may occur in response to stimuli occurring during routine daily life but is especially common during operative procedures performed on patients with spinal cord injury. The reflex most commonly occurs intraoperatively but has also been reported postoperatively following recovery from both spinal and general anesthesia. Distention of a hollow viscus, such as the rectum or urinary bladder, is the most common precipitant, but the reflex may occur from spasm or distention of other viscera or from tactile or thermal stimulation of the skin. The magnitude of the response is generally proportional to the magnitude of the stimulus and is greater with increasing distance between the level of the cord lesion and the level of the dorsal root entry zone of the sensory stimulus. The syndrome usually appears from 6 months to 2 years from the time of injury.

Signs and Symptoms

Patients may experience sweating, flushing, nasal obstruction, severe headache, difficulty breathing, nausea, shivering, gooseflesh, visual field defects, and blurring of vision. Clinical observations may include severe acute hypertension, bradycardia, arrhythmias, profuse sweating, vasodilation above the level of the cord lesion, pallor, vasoconstriction below the level of the cord lesion, changes in skin and rectal temperature, visceral contraction, muscle spasm, ischemic electrocardiographic changes, and changes in the level of consciousness, convulsions, and cessation of respiration.

Cord lesions at or above T5 generally result in the full-blown syndrome; lesions at or below T10 generally result in minimal, if any, blood pressure response and no sweating; and lesions between T5 and T10 result in mild blood pressure elevation with either no sweating or sweating beginning at the level of the precordium and diminishing progressively to ankle level.

Morbidity and mortality rates occur from retinal, subarachnoid, and cerebral hemorrhages; strokes; symptoms of basilar artery insufficiency; and hypertensive encephalopathy.

Pathophysiology of the Reflex

Afferent pathways originating in the mucosa and muscle of the hollow organs ascend in the spinothalamic tracts and dorsal columns, respectively. Afferent pathways also originate in the cutaneous sensory endings and ascend via both spinothalamic tract and dorsal columns. Reflex motor outflow occurs via sympathetic neurons in the lateral horns of the spinal cord targeting blood vessels and viscera. Somatic efferent nerves may also be involved.

In normal patients, the reflex is inhibited by outflow from higher centers. In a patient with high spinal cord injury, this inhibitory outflow fails to reach the effector organs innervated by roots below the level of the cord lesion. The sudden rise in blood pressure is detected by the aortic arch, carotid sinus, and cerebral vessel pressure receptors with subsequent outflow via the intact cranial nerve X effector pathway, resulting in bradycardia. Stimulation of afferent pathways from these receptors to the vasomotor center in the medulla causes vasodilation of vessels above the level of the cord lesion, in contrast to the intense vasoconstriction occurring in response to the massive sympathetic outflow below the level of the cord lesion. In a patient with spinal cord injury, the remaining intact effector response is not sufficient to correct the severe reflex hypertension elicited by the reflex sympathetic outflow.

Prevention and Treatment

One potential approach to prevention when performing instrumentation of the urinary bladder is the application of topical anesthesia to the bladder mucosa. Unfortunately, this technique is unreliable, because it does not affect the proprioceptors in the underlying muscular layer.

Spinal anesthesia has repeatedly been cited as a reliable technique for prevention of AH when operative procedures are performed in the lower abdomen, pelvis, and lower extremities. However, Johnson and Thomason[1] suggested potential problems with spinal anesthesia in patients with spinal cord injury. In contrast, Schonwald et al[2] reported only infrequent technical difficulty in administration of spinal anesthesia in their series of 106 patients. In addition, Lambert et al[3] found no evidence of intraoperative hypotension in their series of 46 patients with spinal cord injury undergoing spinal anesthesia.

Stirt et al[4] reported adequate control of AH using a bupivacaine epidural anesthetic technique in a pregnant patient during childbirth. However, most investigators consider this technique unreliable, especially for urologic procedures, because there may be incomplete anesthesia of the sacral roots with epidural anesthesia.

General anesthesia also appears to be reliable in the prevention of AH, provided that good anesthetic depth is achieved. Inhalation techniques are effective; the occurrence of AH with nitrous/narcotic techniques has been reported.

Epidural meperidine has been reported to be effective in preventing AH in an obstetric patient.[5] Abouleish et al reported that fentanyl is ineffective in controlling AH in pregnant females with C4-5 quadriplegia.[6]

α-Adrenergic blocking drugs are not effective in treating AH, indicating that these drugs are more effective in blocking the effect of circulating sympathomimetics than in blocking sympathetic myoneural transmission. Sodium nitroprusside has been cited as effective in the treatment of the hypertension associated with AH.

The reflex may be terminated by removal of the inciting stimulus. This may be the best option in certain circumstances.

Selected References

1. Johnson B, Thomason R. Autonomic hyperreflexia: A review. Military Med 1975;140:345.
2. Schonwald G, Fish KJ, Perkash I. Cardiovascular complications during anesthesia in chronic spinal cord injured patients. Anesthesiology 1981;55:550–558.
3. Lambert DH, Deane RS, Mazuzan JE. Anesthesia and the control of blood pressure in patients with spinal cord injury. Anesth Analg 1982;61:344–348.
4. Stirt JA, Marco A, Conklin KA. Obstetric anesthesia for a quadriplegic patient with autonomic hyperreflexia. Anesthesiology 1979;51:560–562.
5. Baraka A. Epidural meperidine for control of autonomic hyperreflexia in a paraplegic parturient. Anesthesiology 1985;62:688–690.
6. Abouleish EI, Hanley ES, Palmer SM. Can epidural fentanyl control autonomic hyperreflexia in a quadriplegic parturient? Anesth Analg 1989;68:523–526.

Suggested References

Amzallag M. Autonomic hyperreflexia. Int Anesthesiol Clin 1993;31:87.

Broecker BH, Hranowsky N, Hackler RH. Low spinal anesthesia for the prevention of autonomic dysreflexia in the spinal cord injury patient. J Urol 1979;122:366.

Fraser A, Edmonds-Seal J. Spinal cord injuries. Anaesthesia 1982;37:1084.

161
Prematurity: Anesthetic Risks

Wayne H. Wallender, D.O. □ Randall P. Flick, M.D.

Approximately 6% of infants are born prematurely. Anesthetic morbidity increases directly with the degree of prematurity. Infants are considered premature if they are born before 38 weeks of gestation or weigh less than 2500 g at birth.

Intrauterine asphyxia is common in preterm fetuses and is often the cause of early labor and premature delivery. Preterm fetuses are more prone to asphyxia because of their reduced oxygen-carrying capacity. These infants rarely present for surgery unless severely ill, and most will have multiorgan pathology (Table 161–1). The underlying medical conditions are usually life-threatening respiratory, cardiovascular, or bowel crises. Premature infants have a higher perioperative complication rate following even minor surgery (Table 161–2).

Table 161–1. Organ System Pathology in Intensive-Care-Nursery Graduates

Airway
Subglottic stenosis
Tracheomalacia
Lungs
Chronic lung disease
Reactive pulmonary vasculature
Bullae
Pneumonia
Heart
Cardiomyopathy
Persistent PDA
Central nervous system
Delayed development
Seizures
Hydrocephalus
Gastrointestinal tract
Disordered swallowing/sucking
Gastroesophageal reflux
Bowel obstruction
Liver
Hepatic failure
Hyperalimentation hepatitis
Kidneys
Chronic renal failure
Renal tubular acidosis
Eyes
ROP
Other
Malnutrition

From Finholt DA.[1]

Anesthetic Considerations In Premature Infants

Impaired Temperature Regulation. Reasons for impaired temperature regulation in premature infants include:

□ Increased surface-to-volume ratio, resulting in heat loss.
□ Lack of fat insulation.
□ Fewer brown fat cells (cells stimulated by norepinephrine to increase heat production) than in full-term infants.
□ Thin skin, resulting in heat and water loss.

The clinical consequences of hypothermia are varied and may include hypoglycemia, apnea, bradycardia, and/or metabolic acidosis.

Respiratory Distress Syndrome (Hyaline Membrane Disease). Many premature infants have respiratory distress syndrome (RDS).

□ RDS is rare after 34 weeks of gestation in otherwise normal neonates.
□ RDS occurs three times more often in those born by cesarean section than in those born vaginally.
□ Other prenatal risk factors include maternal diabetes and perinatal asphyxia.
□ RDS is responsible for 50% to 75% of deaths occurring in preterm neonates.
□ RDS is caused by a deficiency in surfactant (functions to maintain alveolar stability) resulting in alveolar collapse, right-to-left shunting, hypoxemia, and metabolic acidosis.
□ Inadequate amounts of surfactant (produced by type II pneumocytes) are produced before 26 weeks of gestation.
□ Pneumothorax should be considered if oxygenation deteriorates abruptly.
□ Immediate treatment with artificial surfactant has reduced mortality associated with RDS.

Bronchopulmonary Dysplasia (BPD). This is defined as a continued oxygen requirement at 28 days of life in an neonate with a history of RDS.

□ This is a chronic disorder usually occurring in infants with a history of RDS (mechanism not known); the more severe the RDS, the greater the degree of BPD.

Table 161-2. Perioperative Complications in 33 Preterm Infants Following Minor Surgery

Complications	No. of Patients
Apnea	6
Atelectasis	2
Aspiration pneumonia	2
Extubation stridor	1
Excessive secretions*	1
Coughing and cyanosis	1

*Requiring suction to clear airway.
From Steward DJ.[2]

□ Risk factors associated with BPD include increased FIO_2, positive-pressure ventilation, infection, patent ductus arteriosus (PDA), and fluid overload in the first 5 to 6 days of life.
□ BPD is characterized by increased airway resistance, decreased pulmonary compliance, ventilation/perfusion mismatch, decreased Po_2, tachypnea, increased oxygen consumption, and increased pulmonary infections.
□ Pulmonary hypertension and cor pulmonale can result from severe BPD.

Apnea. Spells of apnea will be occur in many premature infants.

□ Defined as cessation of breathing that lasts for 15 to 20 seconds or produces cyanosis and bradycardia.
□ All premature infants have some degree of periodic breathing.
□ The more premature the infant, the greater the likelihood of developing apnea spells.
□ Risk of apnea spells is increased postoperatively, especially in preterm infants less than 44 weeks postconception age (risk is reduced after 44 to 60 weeks postconception age). In-hospital respiratory monitoring is recommended for at least 12 hours after surgical procedures.

Patent Ductus Arteriosus. PDA may result in congestive heart failure and respiratory distress.

□ PDA results in a left-to-right shunt, left ventricular hypertrophy, and increased pulmonary blood flow, and can lead to congestive heart failure, which manifests as respiratory failure.
□ The first line of treatment is usually an attempt to close the PDA medically with indomethacin before surgical ligation.

Infection. Infection is a threat to premature infants.

□ Because premature infants have reduced cellular and tissue immunity, pneumonia, sepsis, and meningitis are common.
□ Sepsis can develop in the absence of a positive blood culture, elevated white blood cell count, or fever.
□ First signs of infection may be apnea, bradycardia, or acidosis.

Necrotizing Enterocolitis. Primarily a disease of small preterm infants, this disorder has a multifactorial etiology with the common feature of hypoperfusion of the gastrointestinal tract, resulting in ischemia.

□ Small preterm infants (less than 32 weeks of gestation and 1500 g) are at greatest risk.
□ Initial signs are abdominal distention and bloody feces; shock may develop from multiple bowel perforations.
□ Patients are often hypovolemic and require fluid resuscitation before anesthesia is induced. Rapid fluid administration to preterm neonates may cause intracranial hemorrhage or reopening of ductus arteriosus.
□ Necrotizing enterocolitis is often associated with disseminated intravascular coagulopathy and thrombocytopenia.
□ Nitrous oxide should be avoided and preoperative blood pressure maintained.

Retinopathy of Prematurity. Premature infants are susceptible to retinopathy of prematurity (ROP).

□ ROP is inversely related to birth weight; the risk is highest in infants weighing less than 1000 g.
□ Although the role of oxygen as a risk factor is controversial, it remains prudent to minimize oxygen exposure in premature infants less than 44 weeks old. There is little convincing evidence that brief exposure of 100% oxygen is a risk factor for the development of ROP in infants of any age. Nonetheless, it is recommended that Po_2 be maintained between 60 and 80 mm Hg whenever possible to reduce the risk of ROP in susceptible infants.

Intracranial Hemorrhage. There are four types of intracranial hemorrhage in premature neonates:

□ Subdural.
□ Primary subarachnoid.
□ Periventricular-intraventricular (most common).
□ Intracerebral.

The incidence of periventricular-intraventricular hemorrhage is 40% to 45% in neonates under 35 weeks of gestational age. (Newborn immaturity is the single most important risk factor.) Intracranial hemorrhage is unusual after 10 days of life, with the vast majority of bleeds occurring in the first 3 days.

Mechanisms involved with intracranial hemorrhage include the following:

□ Impaired autoregulation of cerebral blood flow (CBF) occurs in stressed neonates. Elevated blood pressure increases CBF, which may result in hemorrhage.
□ Arterial hypoxemia and hypercapnia that occur during asphyxia can precipitate hemorrhage.
□ Effects of anesthesia on CBF in neonates are not known, but it is prudent to avoid hypoxemia and

hypercapnia and to avoid cerebral hyperperfusion by maintaining blood pressure in the normal range.

▫ Hyperosmolarity is a contributing factor; avoid hyperosmolar fluids (e.g., dilute bicarbonate and give slowly).

Selected References

1. Finholt DA. The anesthetic management of the premature nursery graduate. In Berry FA, ed. Anesthetic Management of Difficult and Routine Pediatric Patients. New York: Churchill Livingstone, 1986:315.
2. Steward DJ. Preterm infants are more prone to complications following minor surgery than are term infants. Anesthesiology 1982;56:304.

Suggested References

Gregory FA, ed. Pediatric Anesthesia. 2nd ed. New York, Churchill Livingstone, 1989.
Stoelting RR, Dierdorf SF. Anesthesia and Co-Existing Disease. 3rd ed. New York, Churchill Livingstone, 1993.

162
The Infant Airway Versus the Adult Airway

Pamela Jensen-Bundy, M.D.

Successful intubation of the infant larynx and trachea requires complete knowledge of the anatomy of these structures, as they differ from those of the adult in many respects. Major anatomic differences of the infant airway and their anesthetic significance are discussed here.

Position

The infantile larynx is more cephalad than the adult larynx. At birth, the rima glottidis is opposite the interspace of the third and fourth cervical vertebrae (C3 and C4), with the lower border of the cricoid cartilage opposite the lower border of C4. At age 13, the adult position is achieved. At that time, the lower cricoid cartilage is opposite the top of C7, and the rima glottidis is opposite the C4-5 interspace. Clinically, these differences cause the larynx to be more anterior in infants than in the typical adult.

Epiglottis

The infantile epiglottis is longer and stiffer than that of the adult. It tends to be U- or V- shaped, where the adult epiglottis is flatter and more flexible. The hyoid bone in the infant is attached to the thyroid cartilage, causing the base of the tongue to depress the epiglottis, leading to increased protrusion into the pharyngeal cavity. With age, the hyoid and thyroid cartilage separate, and the epiglottis becomes more erect. The angle of the epiglottis with the anterior pharyngeal wall changes from 45 degrees to become much closer to the base of the tongue in the adult (Fig. 162–1).[1]

Tongue

The infant tongue is relatively larger and more bulky than the adult tongue.

Laryngeal Exposure

To visualize the larynx in an infant or child, the laryngoscope blade may have to be passed perpendicularly with the head in the neutral position. Lifting an infant's upper back and shoulder area is helpful in obtaining proper neck extension. The epiglottis should be visualized to avoid folding it down over the larynx with the tip of the blade. Gentleness in manipulation of the laryngeal tissues is important; the use of excessive force is unnecessary and leads to bleeding and airway injury.

Vocal Cords

The vocal cords are composed of the vocal ligament anteriorly and the cartilaginous vocal process of the arytenoid posteriorly. With age, the increase in vocal cord length is because of an increase in the ligamentous portion, which increases from 50% to 80% of the entire length. As the cartilaginous portion is angled down the trachea and inward, the infantile cords are concave, whereas concavity is minimal in the adult. Forward movement of the

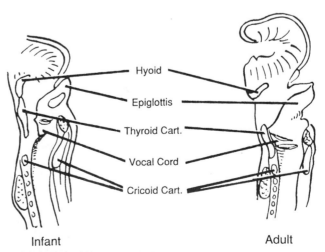

Figure 162–1. The infant larynx and the adult larynx in sagittal section. (From Eckenhoff J.[1])

399

Table 162–1. Endotracheal Tube Sizes (Internal Diameter)

Age	ID
Premature (<2.5 kg)	2.5
Term neonate	3.0
2–8 months	3.5
8–12 months	4.0
18–24 months	4.5
Older than 24 months	Age (yr)/4 + 4

thyroid cartilage with growth also straightens the cords. The concavity of the cords in the infant may impede passage of a curved endotracheal tube. Pushing the tube slightly posteriorly with the blade will aid advancement. With vigorous laryngoscopic lifting, occasionally the trachea is angled forward so much that tube advancement is prevented, even when the tip of the endotracheal tube may be beyond the cords. Slight relaxation of the blade allows the tube to be advanced successfully.

Cricoid Ring

The narrowest point of the infant larynx is at the level of the cricoid cartilage, whereas the rima glottidis is the narrowest point of the adult upper respiratory tract. A tube that cannot be advanced through the cricoid ring should be replaced with a smaller endotracheal tube or the anesthetic should be completed without a tube. A tube size that permits a slight leak when positive pressure is applied will usually be preferred. If too large a tube is left in place, laryngeal edema can result in airway compromise, stridor, and croup after extubation.

Table 162–2. Laryngeal Mask

Size	Weight (kg)
1	<6.5
2	6.5–20
2½	20–30
3	30–50
4	adult

Table 162–3. Endotracheal Tube Position

1-2-3/7-8-9 rule
(1-kg infant: 7 cm at lip)
ID × 3 gives the approximate position at the lip.
Add 2 to 3 cm for a nasotracheal ET tube.

Selection of Endotracheal Tube Size

Various formulas for determining endotracheal tube size in infants and children are available. Formulas for small infants are different than those for larger children. One recommendation is given in Table 162–1. Small endotracheal tubes with cuffs make selection of endotracheal tube size less critical. Tubes one size smaller and larger should be immediately available during intubation. Table 162–2 gives sizes for estimation of pediatric laryngeal mask airways.

Confirmation of Tube Placement

One technique to ensure proper endotracheal tube positioning is suprasternal notch palpation during intubation. The index or fifth fingertip of the palpator is placed in the suprasternal notch. As the tube and stylet are introduced, the trachea is compressed slightly. As the tube passes the fingertip, the intubator is told to stop. The head is turned to one side, drawing the tube slightly cephalad to be palpated again. The tube is then taped in place. This technique reliably places the tip of the endotracheal tube at the midpoint of the trachea with good safety margins, decreasing the chance of endobronchial intubation or extubation.[2] Table 162–3 gives another means of estimating the correct position to secure a pediatric endotracheal tube between the carina and the glottis.

Selected References

1. Eckenhoff J. Some anatomic considerations of the infant larynx influencing endotracheal anesthesia. Anesthesiology 1951;12:401.
2. Bednarek F, Kuhns L. Endotracheal tube placement in infants determined by suprasternal palpation: A new technique. Pediatrics 1975;56:224.

163
Congenital Pediatric Airway Problems

Wayne H. Wallender, D.O.

The pediatric upper airway is more easily compromised than that of adults. Anatomically, pediatric airways are narrower, resulting in greater resistance to air flow, and the tongue is relatively larger within the mouth. Other congenital abnormalities associated with airway problems (e.g., Hurler's syndrome, Treacher Collins syndrome, Pierre Robin syndrome, Goldenhar's syndrome, cleft lip or palate) can further complicate airway management.

As a general approach, these patients can be divided into those who will be difficult to intubate but can be ventilated by mask and those who are difficult or impossible to ventilate by mask. The latter group poses a more difficult anesthetic challenge and may require emergency tracheostomy. If a child can be ventilated by mask, then a number of options, including fiberoptic intubation, blind nasal intubation, or the use of a retrograde transtracheal wire, can be attempted until the trachea is successfully intubated.

Patients intubated at one stage in life may become more difficult to intubate years or even months later as growth affects their facial development. Those caring for these patients should be prepared with a variety of equipment and alternate plans for airway management.

Hurler's Syndrome (Mucopolysaccharidosis Type 1H)

Hurler's syndrome is associated with severe mental retardation, gargoyle facies, deafness, stiff joints, dwarfism, pectus excavatum, kyphoscoliosis, abnormal tracheobronchial cartilage, hepatosplenomegaly, and severe valvular and early coronary artery disease. Upper airway obstruction and difficult intubation are common because of infiltration of lymphoid tissue, enlarged tongue and small mouth, and profuse, thick secretions.

Pierre Robin Syndrome

Children with Pierre Robin syndrome may have cleft palate, micrognathia, glossoptosis (posterior displacement of the tongue), and congenital heart disease (CHD). Affected infants can present with significant airway problems almost immediately after birth. Intubation may be very difficult and should initially be attempted awake. Tracheostomy should be considered early. Airway obstruction may be relieved by positioning the patient prone, pulling the tongue forward, or using a nasopharyngeal airway. A suture may be placed to maintain the tongue position.

Treacher Collins Syndrome

This syndrome is the most common of the mandibulofacial synostoses. Clinical features include micrognathia, aplastic zygomatic arches, microstomia (small mouth), choanal atresia, and CHD. Usually these children present with less severe airway and intubation difficulties than are seen with Pierre Robin deformities.

Goldenhar's Syndrome

Patients with Goldenhar's syndrome are characterized by unilateral facial hypoplasia associated with mandibular hypoplasia (60%), CHD (20%), and eye, ear, and vertebral abnormalities on the affected side. Difficulty of tracheal intubation is highly variable in these patients.

Crouzon's Syndrome

This form of congenital craniofacial synostosis combines a wide, towering skull with proptosis, maxillary hypoplasia, and a beaked nose. Premature closure of cranial sutures does not begin until after birth; thus, cranial shape can vary. Life span and intelligence are usually normal. A high-arched palate and malocclusion can occur. Maxillary hypoplasia can make mask ventilation difficult, but intubation is usually not a challenge. Two cases of serious postoperative airway problems have been reported.

401

Table 163–1. Congenital Anomalies Associated with Cleft Lip with or Without Cleft Palate

Frequent	Occasional
Fetal hydantoin syndrome	Cri du chat syndrome
Fetal trimethadione syndrome	Facioauriculovertebral
Mohr's syndrome	anomalad
Orofaciodigital syndrome	Larsen's syndrome
Robert's syndrome	Meckel-Graber syndrome
Trisomy-18 syndrome	Oculodentodigital syndrome
	Trisomy-18 syndrome
	Waardenburg's syndrome

From Davis PJ, Hall S, Deshpande JK, et al.[1]

Cleft Lip and Palate

Considered together, cleft lip and palate represent a very common congenital anomaly and are associated with more than 150 syndromes. The incidence of cleft lip (with or without cleft palate) is 1:1000 births; that of cleft palate alone is approximately 1:2500 births. These patients may have other associated anomalies (Table 163–1). Middle ear infections are quite common in this population. Infants with this problem have difficulty swallowing and are at risk for pulmonary aspiration. Preoperatively, this risk can be decreased by feeding affected infants in the upright position with specially designed nipples.

Anesthetic management depends on the degree of airway abnormality and can be relatively straightforward in uncomplicated cases. Large defects of the palate are usually not associated with airway obstruction, unless the defect is so extensive that the tongue prolapses into the nasopharynx. However, large defects can cause difficulty with intubation if the laryngoscope blade wedges into the cleft or the oral endotracheal tube migrates into the cleft, resulting in extubation. Postoperative airway problems are also common after a palatoplasty. Surgical edema in children with small oral cavities can result in airway obstruction requiring reintubation.

Anesthetic Management

Regardless of the congenital anomaly presenting as a difficult airway, problems should be anticipated and managed expectantly. In most cases, preservation of spontaneous ventilation is strongly recommended in these patients. Suggestions for management include the following:

□ H_2 blockers may be considered preoperatively in infants at risk for aspiration.
□ Several intubation approaches should be considered (e.g., awake, blind nasal, fiberoptic), but alternative methods must be immediately available, including facilities for emergency bronchoscopy, cricothyrotomy, or tracheostomy.
□ Prepare a variety of laryngoscopy blades, endotracheal tubes, and stylets.
□ Preoxygenation is recommended.
□ Avoid giving intravenous sedatives, narcotics, or muscle relaxants.
□ Induction with sevoflurane or halothane/oxygen via spontaneous ventilation is preferred if awake intubation is not possible. Intravenous (IV) access should be established either before or as soon as possible after induction. Administer atropine before laryngoscopy.
□ Maintain spontaneous ventilation.
□ Perform laryngoscopy under deep anesthesia.
□ The administration of lidocaine, 1 mg/kg IV, before intubation may decrease the risk of laryngeal spasm.
□ Fiberoptic intubation is becoming more desirable in pediatric patients as smaller bronchoscopes become available. Currently, pediatric bronchoscopes are available that will fit through a 3.0-mm endotracheal tube, although they do not have suction ports.

Because children are very prone to laryngospasm at the time of extubation, all equipment for ventilation and reintubation must be available before extubation is attempted. Usually these children should not be extubated until awake. Mild laryngospasm can be treated with positive-pressure ventilation with oxygen by mask. Severe laryngospasm usually responds to a small dose of succinylcholine (0.3 mg/kg).

Selected References

1. Davis PJ, Hall S, Deshpande JK, et al. Anesthesia for general, urologic, and plastic surgery. In Motoyama EK, Davis PJ, eds. Smith's Anesthesia for Infants and Children. 6th ed. St. Louis: Mosby, 1996:571–604.

Suggested References

Gregory GA, ed. Pediatric Anesthesia. 2nd ed. New York, Churchill Livingstone, 1989.
Steward DJ. Manual of Pediatric Anesthesia. 3rd ed. New York, Churchill Livingstone, 1990.
Ward CF. Pediatric head and neck syndromes. In Katz J, Steward DJ, eds. Anesthesia and Uncommon Pediatric Diseases. 2nd ed. Philadelphia: WB Saunders, 1993:319–363.

164
Effects of High Maternal Oxygen Concentrations on the Fetus

Jerald O. Van Beck, M.D.

Increasing maternal oxygenation will increase oxygen tension (PO_2) in the fetal umbilical artery and umbilical vein (UV). Because of limited flow exchange, an increase in maternal arterial PO_2 does not produce an increase of equal magnitude in the fetus. Figures 164–1 and 164–2 demonstrate this. Even with a maternal inspired oxygen concentration (FIO_2) of 100%, fetal PO_2 in the UV will be less than 50 mm Hg. It has been shown in an animal model that by increasing the maternal FIO_2 from 0.21 to 1.0, the PO_2 in the UV increases by only 10 mm Hg at 1 atmosphere pressure.[1]

Hyperbaric oxygen delivery to the mother will significantly increase fetal PO_2, although to a lesser extent. It has been shown that hyperbaric oxygen delivery to a pregnant ewe to achieve an arterial PO_2 of 1300 mm Hg will raise UV PO_2 to nearly 600 mm Hg. No fall in uteroplacental or umbilical blood flow occurs.[1]

Toxicity

No fetal abnormalities have been found in human or animal models with administration of up to 100% oxygen at 1 atmosphere pressure. Hyperbaric oxygen delivery has been shown to be teratogenic in animal models. In hamsters, 100% oxygen at 2 atmospheres for 3 hours or 3 atmospheres for 2 hours resulted in a number of congenital anomalies including spina bifida, exencephaly, and limb defects. Hyperbaric oxygen administration to rabbits late in pregnancy resulted in retrolental fibroplasia, retinal detachment, microphthalmia, and stillbirth.

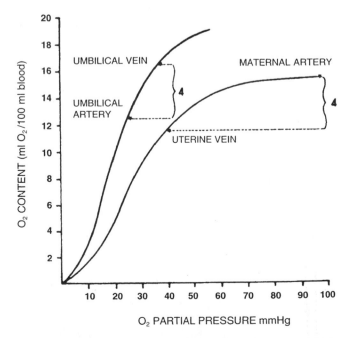

Figure 164–1. Oxygen contents and tensions, and arteriovenous oxygen concentration differences (brackets), on the fetal and maternal sides of the placenta. These are probable values in the undisturbed human, although use has been made of data from many sources, including experimental animals. (From Parer JT.[2])

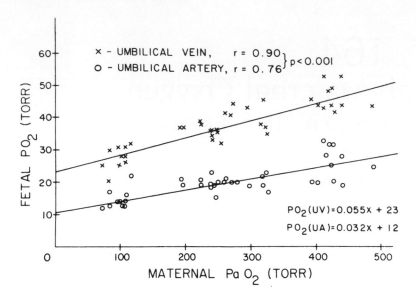

Figure 164–2. Relationship between maternal and fetal PaO₂. (From Ramanathan S, Gandhi S, Arismendy J, et al.[3])

Selected References

1. Pritchard JA, MacDonald PC, Gant NF. Williams Obstetrics. 18th ed. Norwalk, CT, Appleton-Century-Crofts, 1989.
2. Parer JT. Uteroplacental circulation and respiratory gas exchange. In Shnider S, Levinson G, eds. Anesthesia for Obstetrics. 2nd ed. Baltimore: Williams & Wilkins, 1987:14.
3. Ramanathan S, Gandhi S, Arismendy J, et al. Oxygen transfer from mother to fetus during cesarean section under epidural anesthesia. Anesth Analg 1982;61:576.

Suggested References

Levinson G, Shnider S. Anesthesia for surgery during pregnancy. In Shnider S, Levinson G, eds. Anesthesia for Obstetrics. 3rd ed. Baltimore: Williams & Wilkins, 1993:259.
Ramanathan S. Obstetric Anesthesia. Philadelphia, Lea & Febiger, 1988.

165
Fluid Management in Infants

Roger E. Hofer, M.D.

A major challenge during maintenance of anesthesia is the preservation of normal fluid and electrolyte balance. This is especially critical in children because of the smaller volumes involved. Normal daily water consumption in the infant is 10% to 15% of body weight, contrasted to only 2% to 4% in adults. Anesthesia affects the normal turnover of body water and electrolytes.

Fluid Replacement

Maintenance. Holliday and Segar[1] estimated infant maintenance fluids based on energy requirements: 1- to 10-kg infants need about 100 cal·kg^{-1}·24 h^{-1}; each kilogram over 10 and up to 20 requires an additional 50 cal·kg^{-1}·24 h^{-1}; after 20 kg, each additional kilogram requires 20 cal·kg^{-1}·24 h^{-1}. Approximately 1 mL of water is needed for each calorie expended (Table 165–1).

Estimated Fluid Requirements. Estimated fluid requirements (EFR) can also be calculated as follows:
- Weight less than 10 kg, 4 mL·kg^{-1}·h^{-1}.
- 10 to 20 kg, add 2 mL·kg·h^{-1}.
- More than 20 kg, add an additional 1 mL·kg^{-1}·h^{-1}.

Electrolyte Requirements

Preoperative dehydration can be classified as follows: mild, 50 mL/kg (5% body weight loss); moderate, 100 mL/kg (10% body weight loss); severe, 150 mL/kg (15% body weight loss). The fluid deficit in a patient receiving nothing by mouth (NPO) can be calculated by multiplying the number of hours that the patient is NPO by the maintenance fluid requirement. A child develops a deficit being NPO from fluids for only 4 to 6 hours; infants, for 2 to 4 hours. Replacing one-half of the deficit in the first hour and one-fourth in the second and third hours in addition to maintenance requirements has been suggested. Replacement for third-space losses is described in Table 165–2. In the neonate, insensible water loss is increased by crying, sweating, hyperventilation, bilirubin lights, and radiant heaters. Fever increases water loss by 12% per degree centigrade. Insensible loss is decreased by 30% to 35% when the infant is maintained in a high-humidity atmosphere or ventilated with humidified gases. Adequacy of fluid therapy is monitored by clinical signs (heart rate, blood pressure, urine output).

- The sodium deficit (in mEq) can be calculated as normal sodium − measured sodium × 0.6 × weight (kg).
- For metabolic acidosis, give one-half of the HCO$_3^-$ calculated requirement and then reassess the acid-base status: calculated HCO$_3^-$ (mEq) = base deficit × weight (kg) × 0.3 (0.4 for infants).
- Potassium replacement is initiated only after adequate urinary output has been established. Replace at a maximum of 3 mEq·kg^{-1}·24 h^{-1} at a rate not to exceed 0.5 mEq·kg^{-1}·h^{-1}. Ideally, urine output should be maintained at 0.5 to 1.0 mL·kg^{-1}·h^{-1}.

Blood Replacement

Intraoperative blood replacement must be aimed at maintaining an adequate oxygen-carrying capac-

Table 165–1. Maintenance Fluid Requirements

Body Weight (kg)	Daily Water Requirements
0–10	100 mL·kg^{-1}· 24 h^{-1}
11–20	1000 mL + 50 mL·kg^{-1}·24 h^{-1} for each kg over 10
>20	1500 mL + 20 mL·kg^{-1}·24 h^{-1} for each kg over 20

From Lockhart CH.[2]

Table 165–2. Guidelines for Third-Space Fluid Replacement

Probability of Fluid Translocation	Example	Additional Fluid Replacement (mg·kg^{-1}·h^{-1})
Little or none	Craniotomy	0
Mild	Inguinal hernia	2
Moderate	Thoracotomy	4
Severe	Bowel obstruction	6

From Lockhart CH.[2]

Table 165–3. Normal Infant Hemoglobin Values

Age	Value (g/dL)
Birth	13.5–22.0
1–7 days	13.5–22.0
8–14 days	12.5–21.0
15–30 days	10.0–20.0
2–5 months	10.0–14.0
6–11 months	10.5–13.5
1–2 years	10.5–13.5
2 years	11.0–14.0

Table 165–4. Calculation of Acceptable Blood Loss for a 2-Year-Old Child Weighing 10 Kg

Estimated blood volume	80 mL/kg × 10 kg = 800 mL
Normal red blood cell mass	800 mL × 45% = 360 mL
Red cell mass at 30% Hct	800 mL × 30% = 240 mL
Acceptable red blood cell loss	120 mL
Maximum acceptable range of whole blood loss	120 × 2.2 = 266 mL
	120 × 3 = 360 mL

From Lockhart CH.[2]

ity. Oxygen delivery = cardiac output × hemoglobin × oxygen saturation. Normal hemoglobin values for pediatric patients are given in Table 165–3.

Preoperatively, estimate blood volume and note starting hemoglobin. Estimated blood volume (EBV) ranges from 90 mL/kg in neonates to 65 mL/kg in teenagers.

The decision to transfuse depends on (1) preoperative hemoglobin level, (2) estimated surgical loss, and (3) the patient's cardiovascular response. An acceptable blood loss can be calculated as follows:

Estimated red cell mass (ERCM)
= EBV × Hct/100.

ERCM for 30% Hct = EBV × 30/100.

Acceptable red cell loss (ARCL)
= ERCM − ERCM$_{Hct\ 30\%}$.

Maximum acceptable whole blood loss can be calculated as shown in Table 165–4.

Cardiovascular status is the most reliable indicator of blood volume, because blood volume cannot be directly measured intraoperatively and blood loss estimates are often inaccurate.

Red Cell Products

The hemoglobin content of stored whole blood is 12 g/dL, that of packed red blood cells is 24 g/dL, and that of buffy coat–poor washed red blood cells is 28 g/dL. Approximately 4 mL of packed red blood cells per kilogram of body weight is required to increase the hemoglobin level by 1 mg/dL.

Fluid and Blood Replacement

For fluid and blood replacement:

□ Always use blood warmers with children. HCO_3 and calcium are rarely needed.

□ Generally, anything less than one-third acceptable blood loss (ABL) is replaced with 3 to 4 mL of crystalloid per mL of blood loss.

□ Between one-third ABL and ABL, replace either with 3 to 4 mL of crystalloid per mL of blood loss or with 5% albumin, mL for mL of blood loss.

□ Above ABL, replace the **total** blood loss with red blood cells along with sufficient colloid or crystalloid to supply volume equal to whole blood.

Glucose Management

Much controversy exists over the need for supplemental glucose in infants and children. Some recommend the use of glucose-containing fluids for all children under anesthesia, whereas others suggest that only infants and younger children need glucose supplementation intraoperatively. A third option is to measure glucose during surgery and supplement only when needed. Any of these options are acceptable as long as care is taken to prevent hyperglycemia and hypoglycemia. The simplest means of preventing either is to use a solution of 2.5% dextrose in lactated Ringer's solution run at a maintenance rate. This solution should be used in all infants and young children, as well as those at risk for hypoglycemia (metabolic or liver disease). Premature infants and neonates, however, may require a solution containing 5% dextrose, as their glucose consumption may be as high as 8 mg/kg/min.

Selected References

1. Holliday MA, Segar WE. Maintenance need for water in parenteral fluid therapy. Pediatrics 1957;19:823.
2. Lockhart CH. Maintenance of general anesthesia. In Gregory G, ed. Pediatric Anesthesia. New York: Churchill Livingstone, 1989:561.

Suggested References

Steward DJ. Manual of Pediatric Anesthesia. 3rd ed. New York, Churchill Livingstone, 1990.

166
Meconium Aspiration

Scott A. Lockwood, M.D.

Meconium aspiration pneumonitis is the leading cause of respiratory death in the full-term newborn. Meconium staining is present in 12% to 13% of all live births, and 36% of postdate pregnancies have meconium-stained amniotic fluid. Of infants born through meconium-stained fluid, 55% to 60% have meconium in their tracheas. If left untreated, 35% to 50% of these infants develop meconium aspiration syndrome. Meconium-stained infants have a mortality rate of 3.3%, compared with 1.7% for non–meconium-stained live births. The mortality rate for infants with meconium aspiration syndrome is 6 per 10,000 live births.

History

The immediate tracheal suctioning of infants born through meconium was first suggested in 1960. Infants who failed to receive immediate suctioning had a 24% increase in mortality rate. Tracheal suctioning resulted in a lower 1-minute Apgar score but did not lead to prolonged respiratory depression. Recently, the value of routine intratracheal suctioning has been questioned.

Conditions Associated with Meconium Staining

The following conditions are associated with the presence of meconium-stained amniotic fluid:

□ Uteroplacental insufficiency, as indicated by late decelerations.
□ Post-term pregnancies (average length of 10 days after due date).
□ Maternal hypertension.
□ Placenta previa.
□ Maternal pulmonary disease.
□ Placental abruptions.
□ Cord prolapse and cord compression.

Mechanisms

Four proposed mechanisms explain the presence of meconium-stained amniotic fluid:

□ Hypoxia results in shunting of circulation away from the gut to preserve vital organs. This exacerbates intestinal ischemia and causes hyperperistalsis and rectal sphincter relaxation with resultant passage of meconium. Increased vagal tone is involved in the mechanism.
□ Temporary compensated fetal distress results in peripheral ischemia without cardiac or cerebral depression; this may explain why many of these infants do not have low Apgar scores.
□ Umbilical cord compression causes a vagal response in a mature fetus associated with increased gastrointestinal motility and anal sphincter relaxation.
□ Passage of meconium may represent a normal physiologic function in a mature fetus (42 weeks and older).

Pathophysiology

Meconium is the sterile breakdown product of swallowed amniotic fluid, gastrointestinal cells, and intestinal secretions. With normal fetal breathing, the fetus inhales about 1 mL of fluid. With gasping, the infant can inhale up to 60 mL of amniotic fluid and debris. Mechanical airway obstruction by particles of meconium plays the most important role in the pathophysiology of meconium aspiration syndrome. Meconium in large amounts is capable of completely obstructing the trachea, resulting in rapid death. Smaller amounts move quickly to the lung periphery, resulting in obstruction of the distal airways. With complete obstruction, atelectasis of distal alveoli occurs, causing right-to-left intrapulmonary shunting, partially explaining the hypoxemia that is seen in these infants. Partial airway obstruction produces a ball-valve effect, allowing air to move around the obstruction during inspiration but not expiration. This trapped air can increase in volume and is responsible for the high incidence of pneumothorax in meconium aspiration syndrome. Sixty percent of patients have normal chest radiographs. However, characteristic radiologic findings include infiltrates, hyperexpansion, and extra-alveolar air. Episodes of in utero hypoxemia that increase the likelihood of meconium passage also increase the newborn's risk of developing persistent fetal circulation (PFC)/persistent pulmonary hypertension (PPH) after birth. Though the airway obstruction/air leak problems may be life-threatening, PPH usually poses the greatest risk.

Treatment

Respiratory failure from meconium aspiration can be prevented in more than 99% of cases by removing the meconium from the airways at birth.

□ Current recommendations include the early suction of fetal mouth and pharynx before the delivery of the shoulders. Intubation and tracheal suction are reserved only for those infants who are depressed or exposed to thick particulate matter on emergence. When there is evidence of hypoxia or bradycardia, the infant should be oxygenated. Heart rate should be monitored while the airway is suctioned. After the airway has been cleared and the infant is spontaneously breathing, oralgastric aspiration should be performed.

□ After initial resuscitation, the infant's respiratory status should be closely observed. The infant may require humidified oxygen, chest physiotherapy, postural drainage, and observation for hypoxemia, acidosis, and persistent pulmonary hypertension.

If mechanical ventilation is necessary to treat hypoxemia or hypercarbia, it is best to use a short inspiratory time, perhaps 0.15 to 0.2 second maximum, to avoid air trapping from partial obstruction from the meconium. Positive end-expiratory pressure may be beneficial for expansion of collapsed airways. Infants with persistent hypoxemia may respond to muscle relaxation with a rise in PaO_2 resulting from an increase in chest wall compliance and decreased struggling. Surfactant is effective therapy if started within 6 hours of birth, but corticosteroids and tracheobronchial lavage are not recommended. Extracorporeal membrane oxygenation and inhaled nitric oxide have also been used successfully.

Despite all of the treatment modalities that have been proposed and tested over the years, the best treatment continues to be the prevention of meconium aspiration by aggressive airway suctioning at birth.

Suggested References

Datta S, Ostheimer GW. Common Problems in Obstetric Anesthesia. Chicago, Year Book Medical Publishers, 1987.

Findlay RD, Taeusch HW, Walther FJ. Surfactant replacement for meconium aspiration syndrome. Pediatrics 1996;97:48–52.

Katz VL, Bowes WA. Meconium aspiration syndrome. Reflections on a "murky" subject. Am J Obstet Gynecol 1992;166:171–183.

Perg TCC, Gutcher GR, VanFrosten JP. A selective aggressive approach to the neonate exposed to meconium-stained amniotic fluid. Am J Obstet Gynecol 1996;175:296–303.

Shnider SM, Levinson G. Anesthesia for Obstetrics. 3rd ed. Baltimore, Williams & Wilkins, 1993.

Zuckerman R, Aucott S. Neonatal assessment and resuscitation. In Chesnut D, ed. Obstetric Anesthesia Principles and Practice. 2nd ed. St. Louis: Mosby, 1999:135–162.

167
Congenital Diaphragmatic Hernia

Wayne H. Wallender, D.O.

Congenital diaphragmatic hernia (CDH) most commonly presents shortly after birth as a true surgical emergency with respiratory distress and cyanosis. The primary problem in CDH is hypoplasia of the lung parenchyma and pulmonary vasculature. CDH is often associated with other congenital problems that may affect anesthetic management (Table 167–1).

Incidence and Classification

The estimate of the incidence of CDH varies from 1 in 600 to 1 in 18,000 births (average of 1 in 5,000 births). Classification is based on location of the defect, with the most common and significant being the posterior lateral aspect of the diaphragm, through the foramen of Bochdalek (80%). Left-sided hernias occur five times more often than right-sided ones. Hernias through the esophageal hiatus are generally small with no compromise of pulmonary function and do not usually present in the neonatal period. Other sites are shown in Figure 167–1. Incomplete muscularization of the diaphragm (eventration) may occur, resulting in the development of a hernia sac. Many cases are asymptomatic, but severe cases may present identically to CDH.

Embryology

In the fetus, the pleuroperitoneal cavity begins as a single compartment. The development and closure of the diaphragm are usually complete by the 9th fetal week, with return of the gut to the peritoneal cavity in the 10th week. Gut return from the yolk stalk occurring early or diaphragmatic formation occurring late produces the potential for a diaphragmatic hernia.

Anatomic defects of the lung occur because bronchial development can be impeded by the herniated abdominal contents.

Clinical Presentation

Suspicion of CDH can begin in utero, because about 30% of cases are associated with polyhydramnios. Severe CDH is usually discovered by ultrasound prenatally, immediately after birth, or within the first 6 hours of life. The infant presents with cyanosis and respiratory distress. Physical findings include shifted cardiac sounds, scaphoid abdomen, and diminished breath sounds on the affected side. The primary cause of death is progressive hypoxemia and acidosis. Radiographs are usually confirmatory. The immediate therapy is endotracheal intubation along with placement of a nasogastric tube to decompress the gut. Significant degrees of postsurgical hypoxemia and acidosis may result in persistent fetal circulation (PFC), with right-to-left shunting of desaturated blood. Progressive deterioration and death can result from the subsequent high pulmonary pressures. Ligation of patent ductus arteriosus in infants with severe PFC is controversial, because acute right ventricular failure and death can occur.

Anesthetic Management

Most infants are urgently intubated in the delivery room. If the infant is not intubated, the endotracheal tube can be placed while the infant is awake or after breathing halothane/oxygen spontaneously. Positive-pressure ventilation with bag and mask should be avoided, because it may cause further distention of the gut. Standard monitors along with arterial and central venous pressure catheters are recommended. Because heat loss is rapid, the operating room should be warmed and a source of radiant heat provided.

Selection of anesthetic depends on the infant's

Table 167–1. Associated Congenital Problems

Polyhydramnios: 30% (without gastrointestinal anomalies)
Central nervous system anomalies: 28% (spina bifida, hydrocephalus, encephalopathy)
Gastrointestinal anomalies: 20% (intestinal atresia, malrotation)
Genitourinary abnormalities: 15% (hypospadias)
Congenital heart disease: 13% to 23% (atrial septal defect, ventricular septal defect, tetralogy of Fallot, coarctation)

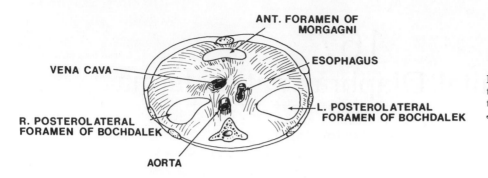

Figure 167–1. Potential sites of herniation of abdominal contents with congenital diaphragmatic hernia. (From Morray JP, Krane EJ.[1])

condition. The usual technique is oxygen/narcotic/relaxant. Nitrous oxide is contraindicated. Any sudden deterioration in heart rate, blood pressure, PaO_2, or lung compliance suggests a contralateral pneumothorax, which should be promptly treated by inserting a chest tube. Preoperative prophylactic contralateral chest tube insertion is recommended by some.

Two factors that affect pulmonary vascular resistance (PVR) are PO_2 and PCO_2. PaO_2 should be maintained in the 90- to 100-mm Hg range. The lungs should be hyperventilated to achieve a $PaCO_2$ of 25 to 30 mm Hg (to decrease PVR). The infant's abdomen may be primarily closed, or a staged closure may be performed with a Silastic pouch. After surgery, the infant should be transferred to an intensive care unit, intubated, and paralyzed in a warmed isolette. Attempts to reexpand the contralateral lung may lead to a pneumothorax from hypoplasia and atelectasis.

Postoperative Care

The postoperative care of infants with CDH is critical. Proposed therapeutic interventions include muscle relaxation and hyperventilation, tolazoline (an α-blocker used to improve pulmonary hypertension), and extracorporeal membrane oxygenation (ECMO) which is addressed in the next section. Infants with relatively normal lungs usually do well, but those with varying degrees of pulmonary hypoplasia have difficulty maintaining adequate oxygenation because of PFC. Postoperative intermittent positive-pressure ventilation will usually be necessary. Bilateral chest tubes are also frequently needed. Gastric suction should be continued.

Extracorporeal Membrane Oxygenation

Geggel et al[2] suggested criteria to identify infants who do not respond to pharmacological and ventilatory therapy, a group who might benefit from a period of extracorporeal membrane oxygenation (ECMO) to provide time for pulmonary growth and remodeling. Selection criteria for ECMO include hemodynamic instability, persistent acidosis, and severe barotrauma, as well as patients with severe pulmonary hypertension unresponsive to pharmacologic intervention.

ECMO is associated with significant risks. Contraindications include the following:

□ Gestational age less than 35 weeks.
□ Weight less than 2000 g.
□ Preexisting intracranial hemorrhage.
□ Congenital or neurological anomalies incompatible with good outcome.
□ More than 1 week of aggressive ventilatory therapy.
□ Congenital heart disease.

ECMO is discontinued if irreversible brain damage or lethal organ failure occurs, or when lung function improves. The overall survival rate of infants with CDH treated with ECMO is reported to be between 50% and 87%.[3]

Overall mortality rate in CDH remains high (20% to 80%, average 50%). The survivors lead fairly normal lives, despite some residual hypoplastic lung disease. Long-term sequelae include bronchopulmonary dysplasia, pulmonary hypoperfusion, and decreased FEV_1 and ventilatory capacity with normal functional residual capacity on pulmonary function testing.

Selected References

1. Morray JP, Krane EJ. Anesthesia for thoracic surgery. In Gregory GA, ed. Pediatric Anesthesia. 2nd ed. New York: Churchill Livingstone, 1989:893.
2. Geggel RL, Murphy JD, Langleben D, et al. Congenital diaphragmatic hernia: Arterial structural changes and persistent pulmonary hypertension after surgery. J Pediatr 1985; 107:457.
3. Heiss K, Manning P, Oldham KT, et al. Reversal of mortality for congenital diaphragmatic hernia with ECMO. Ann Surg 1989;209:225.

Suggested References

Berry FA. Basic considerations. In Berry FA, ed. Anesthetic Management of Difficult and Routine Pediatric Patients. New York: Churchill Livingstone, 1986:57.
Brands W, Kachel W, Wirth H, et al. Indication for using extracorporeal membrane oxygenation in congenital diaphragmatic hernias and pulmonary hypoplasia. Eur J Pediatr Surg 1992;2:81.

168
Other Neonatal Emergencies: Tracheoesophageal Fistula, Omphalocele

Robert J. Friedhoff, M.D.

Tracheoesophageal Fistula

Tracheoesophageal fistula (TEF) results from failure of the division of endoderm of the trachea and esophagus. TEF occurs in several forms (Fig. 168–1). Type C, esophageal atresia with a distal TEF, is the most common (90%) type. Maternal polyhydramnios may indicate the presence of the lesion before birth. Diagnosis is suspected at birth from excessive drooling, cyanotic episodes, coughing relieved by suctioning, and the inability to pass a soft catheter into the stomach. This can be confirmed by radiography showing a curled catheter in the upper esophageal pouch with an air bubble in the stomach. Contrast medium is unnecessary and contraindicated, because it may be aspirated. Associated conditions include prematurity (20% to 25%), congenital heart disease (20% to 25%), and other midline defects.

Preoperative Management. Preoperative assessment is directed at detecting associated congenital lesions and assessing the pulmonary status.

◻ Nurse the infant in the semi-upright position and apply continuous suction to the upper esophageal pouch to prevent further aspiration.

◻ Provide respiratory support with humidified oxygen.
◻ Obtain routine newborn preoperative laboratory tests (i.e., hemoglobin, electrolytes, glucose, calcium, arterial blood gases).
◻ Perform echocardiography to detect cardiac anomalies, including a right aortic arch (5% of neonates).

Pulmonary complications of TEF will not resolve until the fistula is ligated. Often a preliminary gastrostomy may be performed under local anesthesia.

Intraoperative Management

◻ Induction techniques include inhalation, rapid sequence, and awake intubation.
◻ Avoid nitrous oxide, which will contribute to gastric distention.
◻ Avoid intubating the fistula. Insert the endotracheal tube with the Murphy eye facing anteriorly while placing the endotracheal tube in the right mainstem and listen for unilateral breath sounds; then pull back until you hear bilateral breath sounds. Some clinicians may prefer to cut the

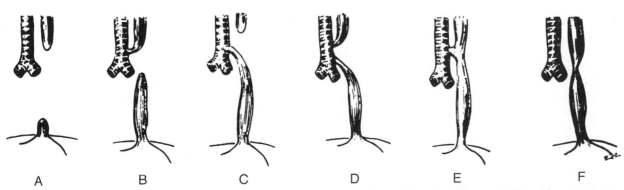

Figure 168–1. Types of congenital abnormalities of the esophagus. *A*, Esophageal atresia with no esophageal communication with the trachea; *B*, esophageal atresia with the upper segment communicating with the trachea; *C*, esophageal atresia with the lower segment communicating with the back of the trachea (representing more than 90% of all esophageal malformations); *D*, esophageal atresia with both segments communicating with the trachea; *E*, esophagus with no disruption of its continuity but with a tracheoesophageal fistula; *F*, esophageal stenosis. (From Gross RE.[1])

distal end of the endotracheal tube, eliminating the Murphy eye. Use of a cuffed endotracheal tube to both ventilate and occlude the fistula has been reported.

□ Place a Fogarty catheter to identify and occlude the fistula using a pediatric bronchoscope.
□ Attempt spontaneous ventilation to avoid gastric distention until the fistula has been ligated, then controlled ventilation.
□ Place a precordial stethoscope under the dependent lung.
□ Maintain routine intraoperative monitoring and an arterial catheter.
□ Regional anesthesia can be added as an adjuvant.

Postoperative Care

□ Optimize respiratory status in the intensive care unit with endotracheal intubation and mechanical ventilation.
□ Avoid damage to the esophageal anastomosis by **marking a suction** catheter, not to extend past the anastomosis for nasopharyngeal suctioning.

Postoperative Complications

□ Tracheal compression secondary to tracheomalacia may occur.
□ Swallowing is abnormal; 68% have gastroesophageal reflux leading to possible aspiration. Esophageal stricture is common.
□ A tracheal diverticulum may persist, causing problems with subsequent intubations.

Omphalocele

Anesthetic management is essentially the same for omphalocele and gastroschisis, but knowledge of the associated anomalies will influence anesthetic decisions. Omphalocele and gastroschisis are congenital defects of the anterior abdominal wall permitting external herniation of abdominal viscera. Gastroschisis is **not** midline (usually occurs on the right), has a normally situated umbilical cord (**not** covered with a hernia sac), and is **rarely** associated with other congenital anomalies, but does have an increased incidence of **prematurity.** Omphalocele has a 75% prevalence of other congenital defects, including cardiac anomalies (ventricular septal defects most common), trisomy 21, and Beckwith-Wiedemann syndrome (omphalocele, organomegaly, macroglossia, and hypoglycemia). **Epigastric** omphaloceles are associated with cardiac and lung anomalies. **Hypogastric** omphaloceles are associated with exstrophy of the bladder and other genitourinary anomalies.

Preoperative Care

□ The exposed viscera must be covered with a sterile plastic bag or film to limit evaporative **heat loss** from exposed bowel.
□ Deficits of fluid and electrolytes (often excessive) should be replaced aggressively.
□ Hypoglycemia should be corrected slowly with a **glucose infusion** (6 to 8 mg·kg^{-1}·min^{-1}). Severe rebound hypoglycemia may occur after bolus doses of glucose.
□ Decompress the stomach using a nasogastric tube.

Intraoperative Management

□ General endotracheal anesthesia with controlled ventilation is required for adequate ventilation. Combined volatile/narcotic techniques are most commonly used. N_2O should be avoided.
□ Routine monitors, arterial catheter, and +/- CVP are used.
□ Preoxygenation followed by **awake or rapid sequence** intubation is preferred.
□ Elevated intra-abdominal pressures, high ventilatory pressures, and inferior vena cava (IVC) compression can cause circulatory stasis in the lower limbs.

Postoperative Management

□ Problems seen intraoperatively with ventilation, elevated intra-abdominal pressure causing compression of the IVC and impaired visceral blood flow, prolonged ileus, and decreased hepatic clearance of drugs can continue postoperatively.
□ Urine output should be monitored closely.

Selected References

1. Gross RE. The Surgery of Infancy and Childhood. Philadelphia, WB Saunders, 1953.

Suggested Readings

Bray RJ. Congenital diaphragmatic hernia. Anaesthesia 1979;34:467.
Bray RJ, Lamb WH. Tracheal stenosis or agenesis in association with tracheo-oesophageal fistula and oesophageal atresia. Anaesthesia 1988;43:654.
Greeley WJ, Miller RD, eds. Atlas of Anesthesia. Vol VII. Philadelphia, Churchill Livingstone, 1999.
Greenberg L, Fisher A, Katz A. Novel use of neonatal cuffed tracheal tube to occlude tracheo-oesophageal fistula. Paediatr Anaesth 1999;9:339–341.
Katz J, Steward DJ, eds. Anesthesia and Uncommon Pediatric Diseases. 2nd ed. Philadelphia, WB Saunders, 1993.
Levin DL. Congenital diaphragmatic hernia: A persistent problem. J Pediatr 1987;111:390.
Motoyama EK, Davis PJ. Smith's Anesthesia for Infants and Children. 5th ed. St. Louis, Mosby, 1990.

169
Pediatric Neuromuscular Disorders

Terrence L. Trentman, M.D.

Cerebral Palsy

Although genetic abnormalities, perinatal anoxia, infection, and trauma have been proposed as etiologic factors in cerebral palsy, no clear single cause has been identified. Cerebral palsy has a prevalence of 2:1000 population. Patients will have a variety of presentations, from near normal functional status to complete incapacitation. The disorder is nonprogressive. Clinical manifestations include disorders of posture such as spasticity of lower or upper extremity muscle groups, mental retardation, behavioral abnormalities, and abnormal speech or vision. Gastroesophageal reflux is a common problem. These children typically take antiseizure drugs and may use dantrolene for muscle spasticity.

Patients with cerebral palsy often present for elective surgical procedures to correct various deformities. Some of these are listed in Table 169–1. Anesthetic concerns include the possibility of aspiration of gastric contents on induction of anesthesia, intraoperative hypothermia, and slow emergence. Succinylcholine does not cause hyperkalemia in these patients, and a rapid-sequence induction may be indicated. Temperature should be monitored and an effort made to keep the patient warm. Cerebral abnormalities may lead to slow awakening; the patient should remain intubated until fully awake and airway reflexes have returned. Pulmonary infections can complicate the postoperative course.

Hydrocephalus

Hydrocephalus is caused by abnormal circulation or absorption of cerebrospinal fluid (CSF). A choroid plexus papilloma can cause hydrocephalus via excess production of CSF, but this would be an unusual cause. Normal CSF volume is about 1 mL/pound in an adult and about 50 mL in an infant. The choroid plexus in the lateral ventricles produces CSF, which then flows via the foramina of Monroe to the third ventricle. CSF enters the fourth ventricle through the aqueduct of Sylvius, and the cisterna magna is entered through the foramina of Luschka and Magendie. The arachnoid villi absorb CSF; nonobstructive hydrocephalus occurs when there is inadequate absorption or excessive production of CSF. Obstructive or noncommunicating hydrocephalus results from blockage anywhere along the path of CSF flow. This can result from congenital structural abnormalities, infection, tumor, or trauma. There are three primary congenital causes of obstructive hydrocephalus:

- **Arnold-Chiari malformation**, in which a hindbrain anomaly leads to fourth ventricle elongation and displacement of brain stem and cerebellum inferiorly.
- **Dandy-Walker malformation**, where abnormal development of the fourth ventricle leads to outlet occlusion and cystic expansion of the ventricle.
- **Aqueduct of Sylvius stenosis**, in which there is narrowing between the third and fourth ventricles.

Enlarged head, irritability, vomiting, poor feeding, and "setting sun" sign (eyes deviated downward) are common signs of hydrocephalus and elevated intracranial pressure.

Treatment of hydrocephalus depends on the cause of the problem. Patients may present for excision of obstructive lesions or placement of ventriculoperitoneal or ventriculoatrial shunts. Ventriculospinal, ventriculocholecystostomy, and ventriculoureterostomy shunts are rarely used. Ventriculoatrial shunts may be placed with electrocardiographic or transesophageal echocardiographic guidance. Shunt revision is a common procedure, because the shunts are subject to displacement or obstruction as the child grows. The one-way valves in the shunts occasionally malfunction. Increased intracranial pressure may accompany the hydrocephalus; avoidance of succinylcholine, if possible, is advantageous in these situations. Use of potent

Table 169–1. Common Procedures for Children with Cerebral Palsy

Achilles tendon lengthening
Derotational osteotomy of the femur
Hip adductor release
Iliopsoas release
Dental restorations
Antireflux procedures
Stereotactic operations

inhalation agents, nitrous oxide, and narcotics is acceptable. Arrhythmias or hypotension may occur after shunt placement decreases intracranial pressure. Elevating the patient's head to encourage CSF drainage and minimizing pressure on the subcutaneous shunt are important considerations.

Myelomeningocele

Children with neural tube defects will present for a variety of surgical procedures, such as shunts for hydrocephalus, orthopedic operations on the lower extremities, and corrective or diversionary urinary tract procedures. Spina bifida is a defect of the midline vertebral arch, neural tube, and skin. If a sac containing meninges bulges through the defect, a meningocele is present; if the sac contains neural elements, it is called a myelomeningocele. Below the defect, nerve roots are abnormal, and bowel, bladder, and neuromuscular dysfunction results. Myelomeningocele is often associated with hydrocephalus and Arnold-Chiari malformation. Newborns with myelomeningocele require prompt closure of the defect to prevent infection. Induction of anesthesia can be accomplished with the patient in the lateral position, or supine if the sac is protected by a support that avoids pressure on it (i.e., doughnut pad). Consideration should be given to awake tracheal intubation if general anesthesia is required. Succinylcholine does not cause hyperkalemia in children with myelomeningocele; however, surgical needs (nerve stimulation) may preclude the use of longer-acting muscle relaxants. These patients are prone to aspiration secondary to gastroesophageal reflux and vocal cord motility abnormalities, and are at increased risk for postoperative hypoventilation. Chronic exposure to latex catheters has been proposed as the cause of the latex allergy seen in these children, and a careful history plus radioallergosorbent testing is indicated preoperatively.

Duchenne's Muscular Dystrophy

Duchenne's muscular dystrophy (DMD) is present in about 1 in 3500 male births. It is more severe than Becker muscular dystrophy, although both disorders result from abnormalities of the dystrophin protein in muscle membranes. DMD has an X-linked recessive genetic inheritance; there are few reports of females with the disorder. In DMD patients, muscle is gradually replaced with fat and connective tissue, although body habitus may be normal. Muscle weakness may not be noted until the child is several years old; hence the FDA's guideline that succinylcholine not be used in children except in airway emergencies.

It was once believed that patients with DMD were at increased risk for malignant hyperthermia (MH). Although patients with MH and DMD may present with similar clinical pictures (hyperkalemia, elevated creatine kinase, and cardiac arrest) after exposure to triggering agents, it is likely that the underlying mechanisms are different. Obviously, it is prudent to avoid triggering agents (succinylcholine and potent inhalation agents) in patients with DMD. Other anesthetic considerations include respiratory weakness, prolonged response to nondepolarizing muscle relaxants, cardiomyopathies, and cardiac arrhythmias. Most DMD patients die by age 25.

Suggested References

Behrman RE, ed. Nelson Textbook of Pediatrics. 15th ed. Philadelphia, WB Saunders, 1996.

Dierdorf SF, McNiece WL, Rao CC, et al. Failure of succinylcholine to alter plasma potassium in children with myelomeningocele. Anesthesiology 1986;64:272–273.

Karan SM, Colonna-Romano P, Rosenberg H. Evaluation of the patient with neuromuscular disease. In Longnecker DE, Tinker JH, Morgan GE, eds. Principles and Practice of Anesthesiology. 2nd ed. Philadelphia: CV Mosby, 1998.

McLeod ME, Creighton RE. Central nervous system diseases. In Katz J, Steward DJ, eds. Anesthesia and Uncommon Pediatric Diseases. 2nd ed. Philadelphia: WB Saunders, 1993:74–99.

Stoelting RK, Dierdorf SF. Anesthesia and Co-Existing Disease. 3rd ed. New York: Churchill Livingstone, 1993:599–604.

170
Pyloric Stenosis

Robert J. Friedhoff, M.D.

Pyloric stenosis is one of the most common gastrointestinal abnormalities occurring during the first 6 months of life. The incidence is 1 in 500 live births in the white population and 1 in 2000 in blacks.[1] Incidence is two to four times higher in males than in females. It is especially common in first-born males of parents who had pyloric stenosis.[2]

Pyloric stenosis usually presents at age 3 to 5 weeks in the preterm or term infant. The etiology is unknown. Proposed mechanisms include an imbalance in the autonomic nervous system, humoral imbalances, infection, or edema with muscular hypertrophy.[2, 3] Pyloric stenosis was first described in 1888 by Hirschsprung, although he could offer no effective treatment. Ramstedt described the optimal surgical therapy in 1912. Since then, improvements in fluid therapy and anesthetic technique have decreased morbidity from 25% down to 0.1% to 0.01%.[4]

Presentation

Pyloric stenosis is caused by thickening of the circular muscular fibers in the lesser curvature of the stomach and pylorus that result in obstruction of the pyloric lumen. There is both hypertrophy and an increased number of fibers. The typical presentation is characterized by persistent, bile-free vomiting. The infant is dehydrated and lethargic. The skin is cool to touch, capillary refill usually exceeds 15 seconds, and the eyes are sunken. The infant may present at less than its birth weight.[4] Vomiting can be projectile (2 to 3 feet), occurring after every feeding, causing loss of hydrogen, chloride, sodium, and potassium ions from the stomach. The vomitus does not contain any of the alkaline secretions of the small intestine, because the obstruction is proximal (at the gastric outlet). Bicarbonate remains in the plasma instead of being secreted by the pancreas.

Initially, the kidneys secrete bicarbonate and potassium from the distal tubules and collecting ducts, producing an alkaline urine to maintain a normal systemic pH. This results in hypokalemic, hypochloremic metabolic alkalosis. Eventually acidic urine is produced because of the preferential conservation of sodium from aldosterone secretion caused by volume depletion from continued vomiting. Maximal chloride ion conservation in the kidney results in a urinary chloride level below 20 mEq/L.

On physical examination, an olive-sized mass may be palpated in the mid-epigastrium. This, along with history, is diagnostic in 99% of cases. Noninvasive diagnostic tests include ultrasound, which can confirm the diagnosis. The "string sign" on barium swallow shows elongation and narrowing of the pyloric canal. Elevated levels of unconjugated bilirubin are seen in 20% of patients.[1, 2, 4]

Pyloric stenosis is a **medical emergency,** not a surgical emergency. Assessment of the degree of dehydration is made by noting the infant's weight loss and measuring bicarbonate and chloride levels. Treatment is instituted with intravenous normal saline with 5% dextrose. Addition of 40 mmol/L of potassium can be done after urine output is established. The solution is administered at a rate of 3 L/m³/day. Therapy is aimed at repletion of intravascular volume and correction of electrolyte and acid base abnormalities.[1, 2, 4] Urine chloride concentration greater than 20 mEq/L implies that the volume status has been corrected. The plasma chloride concentration should then be greater than 105 mEq/L.[4]

Management of Anesthesia

Anesthetic considerations for pyloric stenosis include usual neonatal anesthetic concerns; fluid, electrolyte, and glucose balance; anesthesia for a patient with a full stomach; and consideration of postoperative complications. Patients with pyloric stenosis are at increased risk for pulmonary aspiration of gastric contents.[5] After administration of intravenous atropine (20 µg/kg), the stomach should be emptied as completely as possible by passing a large-bore (14 F multiorifice) orogastric tube two to three times immediately before the induction of anesthesia.

After the application of routine monitors, the induction of anesthesia is variable. It can be accomplished either through a rapid sequence or modified rapid sequence intravenous induction using cricoid pressure, an awake oral endotracheal intubation, or even as an inhalation induction, although this method is rare today.[2]

After the induction of general anesthesia, a nasogastric tube should be inserted and left in place during the operative procedure. This will allow testing of the integrity of the pyloric wall after pyloromyotomy by the surgeon.[1] Anesthesia is maintained with volatile agents with or without nitrous oxide. Skeletal muscle relaxation is usually not needed after induction. Narcotic analgesia is seldom necessary in this age group with increased respiratory sensitivity. Rectal acetaminophen can be given in the postanesthesia recovery room. Caudal anesthesia is effective for intraoperative analgesia and muscle relaxation and for postoperative pain management.

Postoperatively, the infant may be lethargic. Respiratory depression and apnea may occur and are related to cerebrospinal fluid pH and hyperventilation. For these reasons, the infant should be fully awake and able to sustain a regular respiratory pattern before extubation. Hypoglycemia may occur 2 or 3 hours after surgical correction.[3] This is probably caused by cessation of intravenous glucose infusions and the depletion of glycogen stores from the liver. Small, frequent feedings are usually begun 4 to 6 hours postoperatively. An uneventful recovery should result in discharge from the hospital in 12 to 36 hours.

Selected References

1. Spear RM, Deshpande JK, Davis PJ. Anesthesia for general, urologic, and plastic surgery. In Motoyama EK, Davis PJ, eds. Smith's Anesthesia for Infants and Children, 6th ed. St. Louis, Mosby, 1996.
2. Bissonnette B, Sullivan P. Continuing medical education: Pyloric stenosis. Can J Anaesth 1991;38:668.
3. Stoelting RK, Dierdorf SF. Diseases common to pediatric patients. In Stoelting RK, Dierdorf SF (eds): Anesthesia and Co-Existing Disease. 3rd ed. New York: Churchill Livingstone, 1993:579.
4. Yemen TA. Gastrointestinal diseases. In Berry FA, Steward DJ, eds. Pediatrics for the Anesthesiologist. New York: Churchill Livingstone, 1993:101.
5. Cook-Sather SD, Tulloch HV, Liacouras CA, et al. Gastric fluid volume in infants for pyloromyotomy. Can J Anaesth 1997;44:278–283.

171
VATER Association and Trisomy-21

Paul E. Stensrud, M.D.

VATER Association

The acronym VATER is used to describe a non-random constellation of congenital defects that are not related closely enough to compose a discrete syndrome. VATER association comprises[1]:

- **V**ertebral defects.
- **A**nal malformation.
- **T**racheo-**e**sophageal fistula (TEF) with esophageal atresia.
- **R**adial and **r**enal dysplasia.

Components of the VATER association may manifest as isolated abnormalities, but these are more likely to be associated with one or more of the other components of the association. Following the early reports of the VATER association, additional defects, mainly cardiac (most commonly ventricular septal defect [VSD]), have been noted to occur in these patients. Associated abnormalities have led some to term the association VACTER or VACTERL, although VATER remains the most accepted acronym.[2, 3]

Certain congenital syndromes, including Klippel-Feil syndrome, Sprengel deformity, and Goldenhar syndrome, have been associated with components of the VATER association.[4] The VATER association is not inherited in a Mendelian fashion, and there is no well-defined number or type of anomalies necessary to classify a patient as having the VATER association. It is not clear why the anomalies making up the VATER association and the related syndromes are associated, but the multiple sites suggest an early global insult during early embryogenesis.[4]

The vertebral defects seen in the VATER association include hemivertebrae (most commonly), absent pedicles, fused vertebrae, and sacral dysgenesis. Imperforate anus is the most common anal malformation and may include rectovaginal or rectourethral fistulae. TEF occurs commonly, most frequently as esophageal atresia with distal TEF. Limb abnormalities include radial dysplasia, absent digits (usually the thumb), and duplication of the thumb. Renal dysgenesis is most commonly reported to involve unilateral renal agenesis, but multiple other renal abnormalities have been reported. Many other defects have been reported, including rib abnormalities and kyphoscoliosis associated with the vertebral anomalies, lower limb anomalies, genital anomalies (including cryptorchidism, hypospadias, and ambiguous genitalia), choanal atresia, duodenal atresia, deformed ears, and inguinal hernias.[2-4] Neurological problems are related only to the other abnormalities noted. Death is most commonly due to cardiac arrest and is most closely associated with the degree of cardiac abnormality.[3] Patients surviving the surgical repair of multiple anomalies involved are reported to do very well.

Anesthetic considerations in patients with VATER association are mainly determined by the multiple abnormalities that may be present. A complete and intensive workup is necessary in any patient who manifests any component(s) of this association, with special attention given to cardiac and renal function.[4] Early surgical intervention most commonly involves amelioration followed by correction of the tracheoesophageal and anal anomalies. The most common approach reported has been gastrostomy under local anesthesia followed by thoracotomy and repair of TEF, and diverting colostomy followed by pull-through procedure for repair of anal atresia.[2] Such a staged approach allows stabilization of the infant's cardiorespiratory status before the delayed major operations for repair of the defects involved.

Anesthetic considerations are the same as for any infant with TEF or anal atresia. Subsequent surgical procedures involve repair of other associated anomalies, mainly the radial, vertebral, and urogenital defects. **Gastroesophageal reflux** is common following repair of TEF, and subsequent anesthetic planning should reflect this. The anesthesiologist should continue to suspect associated **cardiac and renal abnormalities** and should be aware that these patients frequently require **antibiotic prophylaxis for endocarditis**.[2, 4]

Trisomy-21 (Down Syndrome)

Trisomy-21 (duplication of chromosome 21, commonly known as Down syndrome) is the most common chromosomal abnormality (1:700 to 1,100 live births). The risk of trisomy-21 increases with increasing maternal age, approaching 1:40 in mothers over age 45.[5] Patients with trisomy-21 exhibit characteristic oblique palpebral fissures and flat facies, single palmar crease, and dysplastic middle phalanx of the fifth digit. Trisomy-21 is associated with mental retardation (IQ below 65). Patients with this syndrome tend to be content and affectionate and function at a low normal social level, but they can be obstinate regarding changes in routine, which may affect the course of anesthetic induction.

Many features of the **airway** are abnormal in trisomy-21 patients. These patients are known to have a narrow nasopharynx and large tonsils and adenoids. As the child approaches maturity, the tongue becomes progressively larger because of papillary hypertrophy. A small cross-sectional area of the subglottic region is reported. The characteristic mouth-open, tongue-protruding appearance of these patients is an adaptation to the limited size of the upper airway. Nonetheless, intubation is usually not difficult.[5]

Cervical spinal malformations have been reported in association with trisomy-21, with 10% demonstrating cervical spinal stenosis and 31% demonstrating **atlantoaxial subluxation**, although only 1% to 2% of these patients will become symptomatic.[6] Lateral cervical spine radiographs in flexion and extension may be useful to rule out atlantoaxial instability. Such radiographs should be performed on all trisomy-21 patients with cervical range of motion or gait abnormalities.

Congenital heart disease has been reported in approximately 40% of trisomy-21 patients (Table 171–1). About 50% of the congenital cardiac anomalies are **endocardial cushion defects**, with **ventricular septal defects (VSD)** occurring in about 25%. Other reported anomalies include tetralogy of Fallot, secundum atrial septal defect (ASD), and patent ductus arteriosus (PDA).[5] A high rate of postoperative morbidity and mortality in trisomy-21 patients following cardiac surgery has been attributed to an increased incidence of respiratory complications because of the upper airway abnormalities and abnormal development of alveoli and the pulmonary vasculature, which predispose to the development of **pulmonary hypertension**.[7]

Other findings associated with trisomy-21 include obesity (which may make intravenous access difficult), laxity of the skin and joints, duodenal atresia, cataract and strabismus, otitis media and hearing loss, hypothyroidism, and hematologic malignancy.[5,6]

Anesthetic management in trisomy-21 is dictated by the patient's mental status and associated abnormalities, especially congenital cardiac anomalies and atlantoaxial instability. Atropine premedication, previously thought inadvisable in trisomy-

Table 171–1. Anesthetic Concerns in Trisomy-21

General
    Poor intravenous access
    Mental retardation
    Obesity
Airway
    Large tonsils and adenoids
    Large tongue
    Small subglottic area
Spine
    Cervical spinal stenosis
    Atlantoaxial subluxation
Cardiac
    VSD
    Other endocardial cushion defects
    ASD
    Tetralogy of Fallot
    PDA
    Pulmonary hypertension

21 patients, is now considered safe.[8] Response to preoperative sedation is variable because of varying degrees of mental deficiency. Induction may be accomplished using either inhalation or intravenous techniques, although difficulty obtaining intravenous access may be anticipated. The MAC of inhalation anesthetics is not reported to vary in these patients, and maintenance of anesthesia may be achieved with either inhalation or intravenous agents. Care must be taken in choosing an appropriately sized endotracheal tube, with awareness of the possibility of subglottic narrowing. Intubation should be performed with care taken to not hyperextend the cervical spine. Due caution should be exercised on extubation, and possible upper airway obstruction and postextubation stridor anticipated.[5–7]

Selected References

1. Quan L, Smith DW. The VATER association. J Pediatr 1973;82:104–107.
2. Weber TR, Smith W, Grosfeld JL. Surgical experience in infants with the VATER association. J Pediatr Surg 1980;6:849–854.
3. Weaver DD, Mapstone CL, Yu P. The VATER association. Analysis of 46 patients. Am J Dis Children 1986;140:225–229.
4. Beals RK, Rolfe B. VATER association. A unifying concept of multiple anomalies. J Bone Joint Surg 1989;71:948–950.
5. Stoelting RK, Dierdorf SF. Anesthesia and Co-Existing Disease. 3rd ed. New York, Churchill Livingstone, 1993:602–603.
6. Harris M. Neurologic and neuromuscular diseases. In Berry FA, Steward DJ, eds. Pediatrics for the Anesthesiologist. New York: Churchill Livingstone, 1993:215.
7. Morray JP, MacGillvray R, Duker G. Increased perioperative risk following repair of congenital heart disease in Down's syndrome. Anesthesiology 1986;65:221–224.
8. Wark HJ, Overton JH, Marian P. The safety of atropine premedication in children with Down's syndrome. Anaesthesia 1983;38:871–874.

172
Croup Versus Epiglottitis

Stephen T. Gott, M.D.

Respiratory distress is one of the most common presenting complaints in pediatric emergency departments. Both acute epiglottitis (supraglottic inflammation) and croup, or laryngotracheobronchitis (subglottic inflammation), present with evidence of airway obstruction. In 80% of all pediatric patients with acquired stridor, infection is the etiology. Of these, 90% are due to laryngotracheobronchitis and a minority are cases of epiglottitis. Other causes of respiratory distress, such as a foreign body, subglottic stenosis, tracheitis, and retropharyngeal abscess, also must be considered in the differential diagnosis.

Because of the possibility of rapid clinical progression to complete obstruction, acute epiglottitis requires early intervention. To provide the appropriate therapeutic interventions, one must be able to differentiate between acute epiglottitis and laryngotracheobronchitis. Table 172–1 compares these two causes of severe stridor.

Management

Croup (Laryngotracheobronchitis). Treatment of croup varies according to the severity. In mild cases, conservative measures such as humidification of air, fever control, and hydration are usually effective. In other cases, racemic epinephrine inhalations delivered by intermittent positive-pressure breathing or a simple nebulizer mask produce improvement. Add 0.2 to 0.5 mL of 2.25% racemic epinephrine to 3.0 to 5.0 mL of distilled water. Administer the solution through the vaporizer attachment via a patient-triggered ventilator at 15 to 20 cm H_2O pressure and a high inspiratory flow rate. Add at least 40% oxygen to the inspired gases. Administer the treatment for 15 to 20 minutes. If no improvement is seen, reconsider the diagnosis. Some patients require more than a single treatment, however. Rarely (less than 3%) is intubation or tracheostomy needed if dyspnea persists after treatment. Antiviral agents such as amantadine have been proven to be beneficial against influenza A. Antibiotics are needed only if a secondary bacterial infection develops. Steroid therapy is controversial because study findings are not uniform.

Acute Epiglottitis. The child with acute epiglottitis must be disturbed as little as possible. Transport the child to the operating room in the

Table 172–1. Acute Epiglottitis Versus Croup

	Acute Epiglottitis	Croup
Age	3–7 years	6 months–5 years
Family history	No	Yes
Prodrome	Usually none ± sore throat	Usually URI
Onset	Abrupt (6–24 hours)	Gradual (days)
Clinical course	Rapid, may progress to cardiorespiratory arrest	Usually self-limited
Signs and symptoms		
Fever	38–40°C	38–40°C
Hoarseness	No	Yes
Dysphagia	Yes	No
Dyspnea	Severe	No
Inspiratory stridor	Yes	Yes
Appearance	Toxic, anxious, sitting upright, leaning forward, mouth open, exaggerated sniffing position	Nontoxic
Oral cavity	Pharyngitis with excessive salivation	Minimal pharyngitis
Epiglottis	Cherry red, edematous	Normal
Radiograph		
Neck	Enlarged epiglottis	Narrow epiglottis
Anteroposterior	Tracheal narrowing	Subglottic narrowing (Steeple's sign)
Laboratory		
White blood cell count	Marked elevation with left shift	Variable
Bacteriology	*Haemophilus influenza*, type B isolated from throat and blood cultures	Viral etiology, parainfluenza usually

sitting position with airway equipment for possible ventilatory support. Do not attempt to visualize the pharynx because acute obstruction may ensue. The operating room should be set up for direct laryngoscopy, emergency bronchoscopy, and possible tracheostomy. Monitoring should include blood pressure, electrocardiography, precordial stethoscope, and pulse oximetry. Induce anesthesia with oxygen and an inhalation anesthetic with the child in the sitting position. Because of the unpredictable variation in the amount of edema, and the potential anatomical distortion and difficulty with ventilation, muscle relaxants and barbiturates should be avoided.

When anesthesia is induced, lie the child down gently. Assisted ventilation may be needed. Establish an intravenous line and administer intravenous atropine (0.02 mg/kg) to attenuate reflex bradycardia and lidocaine (1 mg/kg) to minimize the risk of coughing and laryngospasm. Avoid racemic epinephrine, which may precipitate complete airway obstruction. Perform laryngoscopy and intubate with an oral endotracheal tube (0.5 to 1.0 mm smaller than predicted for age). Once the child is anesthetized and well oxygenated, the oral endotracheal tube can be replaced with a nasotracheal tube (again, 0.5 to 1.0 mm smaller than predicted for age). Obtain a chest radiograph to confirm tube placement and to identify any infiltrate or atelectasis. Because of the potential resistance to ampicillin, a cephalosporin, such as cefotaxime (200 $\mu g \cdot kg^{-1} \cdot day^{-1}$), is initiated after blood and epiglottic cultures have been obtained. Steroids have not been shown to be beneficial. Postoperatively, monitoring in an intensive care unit is essential. Intravenous sedation and restraints help prevent accidental extubation. Inspired gases should be humidified and the nasotracheal tube regularly suctioned. Extubation should be done after the pyrexia has resolved (usually within 12 to 36 hours) and an air leak has developed around the endotracheal tube.

Suggested References

Fleisher GR, Ludwig S, eds. Textbook of Pediatric Emergency Medicine. 4th ed. Philadelphia, Lippincott Williams & Wilkins, 2000.

Gregory GA, ed. Pediatric Anesthesia. 3rd ed. New York, Churchill Livingstone, 1994.

Steward DJ. Manual of Pediatric Anesthesia. 4th ed. New York, Churchill Livingstone, 1995.

173
Neuromuscular Blockers in Neonates

Wayne H. Wallender, D.O.

The neuromuscular system is incompletely developed at birth and matures throughout the first year of life. During the first months of life, the infant diaphragm and intercostal muscles both show a progressive increase in the percentage of slow muscle fibers, which support prolonged repetitive efforts. The neonatal diaphragm is paralyzed simultaneously with peripheral muscles, in contrast to the resistance to diaphragmatic relaxation seen in adults. Infants have a greater extracellular fluid and blood volume in proportion to skeletal muscle weight than older children or adults, resulting in increased drug requirements for some agents. The reduced glomerular filtration rate in neonates is responsible for slower elimination of agents excreted by the kidneys, such as curare.[1] The neonatal myoneural junction is more sensitive to neuromuscular blockade and has less neuromuscular reserve when exposed to tetanic stimulation.[2, 3]

Specific Agents and Unique Characteristics in Neonates

Succinylcholine is the only depolarizing muscle relaxant commonly used today but is problematic in children. Neonates have a decreased sensitivity to its effects (50% less response than an adult to an equivalent dose). There is evidence that this resistance to succinylcholine persists even when the larger relative volume of distribution in the infant is taken into consideration, suggesting that the acetylcholine receptors are immature at birth. Succinylcholine is hydrolyzed rapidly in plasma (90%) by pseudocholinesterase. Even though term neonates have only about 50% of the plasma pseudocholinesterase of an adult, no prolongation of effect is seen. Neonates have adult levels of plasma pseudocholinesterase by 2 weeks of age. The duration of muscle paralysis from succinylcholine is shorter in neonates, probably because of dilutional factors and more rapid redistribution away from effector sites resulting from the high cardiac output. Neonates develop tachyphylaxis after about 3 mg/kg of succinylcholine.

It is uncommon for neonatal muscles to fasciculate after being given succinylcholine 1 to 2 mg/kg intravenously. An increase in plasma myoglobin occurs in 60% of prepubescent children. Elevated plasma creatine phosphokinase (CK), an indicator of muscle injury, occurs in 75% of patients and is not age related. An increase in serum potassium of about 0.5 mEq/L occurs after intravenous succinylcholine and is not prevented by pretreatment.

Masseter spasm can occur after succinylcholine administration. There is a 1% incidence with halothane induction followed by intravenous succinylcholine. Controversy exists as to the actual incidence of malignant hyperthermia (MH) associated with masseter spasm. Approximately 50% of such patients have positive halothane-caffeine contracture testing on muscle biopsy.

Bradycardia can occur with an intravenous bolus of succinylcholine. This is vagally mediated and can be prevented by pretreatment with atropine or glycopyrrolate. The incidence of bradycardia increases with repeated doses and is higher with halothane than with isoflurane.

Curare has been reported to have a more rapid onset of paralysis in neonates and a longer recovery time than in adults.[4] This sensitivity is observed even when the increased volume of distribution in infants is taken into consideration. Conflicting data support the observation that responses to nondepolarizing muscle relaxants are unpredictable in the neonate. Administration of these drugs should be closely monitored and the dose carefully titrated to achieve the level of muscle relaxation desired.

Pancuronium is 5 to 10 times more potent than curare and has a similar onset of action and recovery time. Children of all ages are reported to be more resistant to pancuronium than adults. Recovery may be prolonged in sick premature infants because of renal disease or increased volume of distribution from anasarca. There is also an increased incidence of intracranial hemorrhage in premature infants who are given pancuronium and who are **not anesthetized**, possibly because of a combination of increased blood pressure and increased levels of circulating catecholamines.

The recovery time for **metocurine** does not vary with age. The doses for relaxation are increased about 2.5-fold in acutely burned children (as are doses of curare and pancuronium).

Atracurium is an intermediate agent that is

metabolized by nonspecific esters and spontaneously decomposes by Hofmann degradation. The ED_{50} of atracurium varies with age and is lowest in neonates (i.e., neonates are most sensitive to its effects). Effects are further influenced by age and temperature. Neonates under 48 hours old require less atracurium to induce nearly complete paralysis than those who are 48 hours old (300 µg/kg versus 500 µg/kg). Recovery also takes longer in neonates under 48 hours old, and neonates with body temperatures below 36°C have a longer duration of paralysis.

Vecuronium induces paralysis more rapidly in infants than in adults, has a longer duration of block in neonates (probably because of the larger volume of distribution), and recovery time is longer.

Mivacurium is a short-acting agent metabolized by plasma cholinesterase. Preliminary data are similar in children and adults. In infants, the time required to produce complete blockade is similar to that of succinylcholine, although coughing and diaphragmatic movements may be more common with intubation. In can cause histamine release in large doses. Clearance in infants is more rapid than in children, presumably because of a larger volume of distribution.

Rocuronium is a nondepolarizing steroidal drug similar to vecuronium but with one-tenth the potency. The onset is more rapid than that of vecuronium. Time to recovery is twice as long in infants than in children age 1 to 5 years.

Reversal of Neuromuscular Blockers

In the past, pediatric patients were believed to need more neostigmine than adults to reverse neuromuscular blockade.[5] However, it has been demonstrated that neostigmine dose requirements are actually lower in pediatric patients.[6] The dose-response relationship for edrophonium does not differ between pediatric and adult patients, although the elimination half-life is shorter in neonates, resulting in more rapid clearance. A larger dose of edrophonium is usually recommended for children (1 mg/kg) compared with adults (0.5 mg/kg). To minimize cardiovascular changes, atropine 0.01 mg/kg should be given 30 seconds before edrophonium.

Table 173–1. Factors Prolonging Neuromuscular Blockade

Deficient pseudocholinesterase
Abnormal variant of pseudocholinesterase
Anticholinesterase-containing drugs
Phase II block
Hepatic dysfunction
Hypermagnesium
Hypothermia
Respiratory acidosis
Hypokalemia
Antibiotics
    Aminoglycosides
    Tetracyclines
    Lincomycins
    Polymyxins
Other drugs, including inhalation agents, local anesthetics, lithium, dantrolene, and certain chemotherapeutic agents, can have profound effects on muscle relaxation.

After adequate dosages of reversal agents, failure of reversal or the recurrence of blockade indicates the presence of other factors that can prolong neuromuscular blockade (Table 173–1).

Selected References

1. Fisher DM, O'Keeffe C, Stanski DR, et al. Pharmacokinetics and pharmacodynamics of d-tubocurarine in infants, children and adults. Anesthesiology 1982;55:203.
2. Kroenigsberger MR, Patten B, Lovelace RE. Studies of neuromuscular function in the newborn. I. A comparison of myoneural function in the full-term and the premature infant. Neuropaedtriatrie 1973;4:351.
3. Caumrine RS, Yodlowski EH. Assessment of neuromuscular function in infants. Anesthesiology 1981;54:29.
4. Gregory GA. Pharmacology. In Gregory GA, ed. Pediatric Anesthesia. 3rd ed. New York: Churchill Livingstone, 1994:13.
5. Cook DR. Muscle relaxants in infants and children. Anesth Analg 1981;60:335.
6. Fisher DM, Cronnelly R, Miller RD, et al. Neuromuscular pharmacology of neostigmine in infants and children. Anesthesiology 1983;59:220.

Suggested References

Cook DR, Davis PJ, Lerman J. Pharmacology of Pediatric Anesthesia. In Motoyama EK, Davis PJ, eds. Smith's Anesthesia for Infants and Children. 6th ed. St. Louis: CV Mosby, 1996:159.
Meretoja OA. Neuromuscular blocking agents in paediatric patients: Influence of age on the response. Anaesth Intensive Care 1990;18:440.

174
Pediatric Breathing Circuits

Karen S. Reed, M.D., Ph.D.

Circuits Without Valves

Ayre introduced the T-piece (Fig. 174–1) into clinical practice in 1937. The T-piece was used initially for spontaneous ventilation during anesthesia for infants. The anesthetic gases enter the tube at an inlet set at a right angle to the tube. Alveolar gas from expiration is flushed through the reservoir tube by the fresh gas flow. On inspiration, the patient inspires fresh and expired gas from the inlet and reservoir tube. Although a fresh gas flow of only 1.5 to 2 times the minute volume is required to prevent rebreathing or dilution of inspired gases, minimal airway resistance and improved humidification were advantages of this system.

Circuits with Overflow Valves

Mapleson added overflow valves and a reservoir bag to the T-piece. This modification allowed for better controlled ventilation. The Mapleson A, B, C, D, and E circuits differ in the position of the inflow of fresh gas, overflow valve, and the reservoir bag (see Fig. 91–1). The Mapleson A and D circuits remain in use; the Mapleson D circuit is the one used frequently in pediatrics.

Mapleson D Circuit. Fresh gas enters the Mapleson D circuit (Fig. 174–2) at the patient end, and the overflow valve is near the reservoir bag. In controlled ventilation, the overflow valve is partially closed and opens only at end inspiration with the generation of higher pressures. With exhalation, the deadspace gas, alveolar gas, and fresh gas enter the

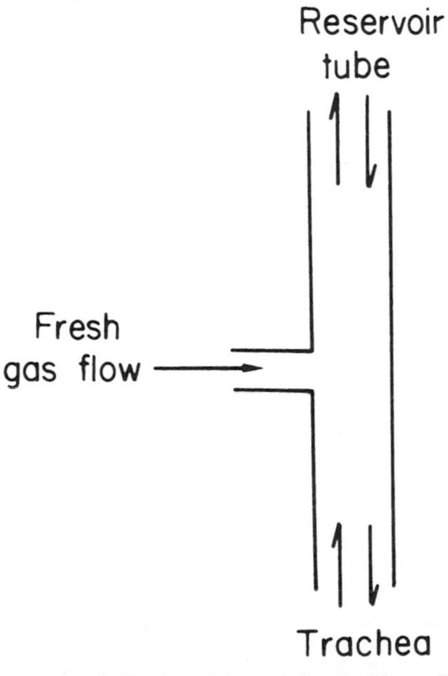

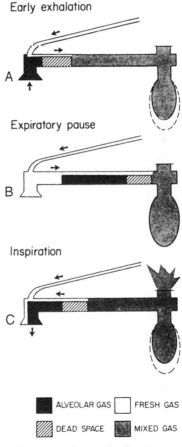

Figure 174–2. Mapleson D circuit. During controlled ventilation, the overflow valve is partially closed. *A,* During exhalation, deadspace, alveolar, and all fresh gas enter the corrugated tube. *B,* During the expiratory pause, fresh gas continues to enter the circuit, moving the mixed contents of the corrugated tube toward the reservoir bag. *C,* On inspiration, the patient receives the contents of the corrugated tube as well as all fresh gas. (From Fisher DM.[1])

Figure 174–1. Ayre's T piece (the original). (From Fisher DM.[1])

423

corrugated limb near the patient. The fresh gas continues to flow, moving the mixed gases into the reservoir bag. With inspiration, the patient inspires a mixture of fresh gas, alveolar gas, and deadspace gas. With increased pressure, the overflow valve opens and the contents exit the reservoir bag. In spontaneous ventilation, the overflow valve remains open and the mixture of gas exits when the airway pressure is maximal at the end of exhalation. With the Mapleson D circuit, many factors influence the gas mixture delivered to the patient. Changes in the respiratory rate may increase, decrease, or have no effect on the $PaCO_2$, depending on the amount of rebreathing. The fresh gas flow determines the gas mixture in the corrugated tube. As fresh gas flow increases, the alveolar gas is flushed away from the patient and the inspired gas is mostly fresh gas. Tidal volume may have an effect on the CO_2 exchange, depending on the fresh gas flow. If the fresh gas flow is high, increasing the tidal volume will decrease the $PaCO_2$. **Because of rebreathing, all of these systems require relatively high fresh gas flows to prevent hypercarbia** (Table 174–1). In general, with infants, a fresh gas flow that is three times the minute ventilation can be used. For older children and adults, use of a circle system will allow the use of lower fresh gas flows.

Bain Circuit. Bain and Spoerel introduced the Bain circuit (Fig. 174–3) into anesthesia in 1972. The Bain circuit places the fresh gas flow coaxial to the expiratory limb. The fresh gas still enters the circuit at the patient end, and the alveolar gas is exhausted through the expiratory limb to the overflow valve. The Bain circuit functions identically to the Mapleson D circuit. The advantages of the Bain circuit over the Mapleson D include (1) less equipment to interfere with the surgical field; (2) less likelihood of kinking the endotracheal tube or extubating the patient because the system is light-weight; and (3) the ability to mount the Bain circuit on the anesthesia machine, allowing for expired

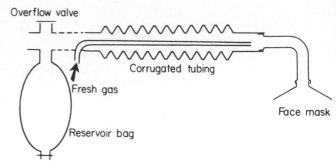

Figure 174–3. Bain circuit. This is a modification of the Mapleson D in which the fresh gas hose is coaxial with the corrugated tube. Because fresh gas enters the circuit at the patient end and the overflow valve is located near the reservoir, the Bain circuit functions identically to the Mapleson D. (From Fisher DM.[1])

gases to be scavenged. Gas flows and minute ventilation requirements are similar to those for the Mapleson D circuit.

Circuits with Inspiratory, Expiratory, and Overflow Valves

All pediatric circle systems (Fig. 174–4) have the basic components of the adult circle. Modifications of the adult circle are seen with the Bloomquist pediatric circle absorber, which can be placed on either the inspiratory or the expiratory limb. The Ohio infant circle absorber has the fresh gas inlet downstream from the inspiratory valve, so that the fresh gas flow flushes the deadspace of the mask. All circles have smaller inspiratory and expiratory tubing, reservoirs, canisters, and Y-connectors. The resistance in the pediatric circle systems is low, less than 0.3 cm H_2O at a flow rate of 10 L/min.

Devices have been designed to reduce the deadspace of the circle system, although technically, **the deadspace includes only the Y-piece and connectors between it and the patient**. Divided airway adapters separate the inspiratory and expiratory gases, thereby reducing the deadspace of the

Table 174–1. Two Sets of Recommendations for Fresh Gas Flow and Minute Ventilation to Produce Normocapnia During Controlled Ventilation with the Mapleson D Circuit

Recommendations by Bain JA and Spoerel WE[2]

Weight (kg)	Fresh Gas Flow	Tidal Volume (mL/kg)	Respiratory Rate (breaths/min)
<10	2000	10	12–14
10–50	3500	10	12–14
>50	70 mL·kg^{-1}·min^{-1}	10	12–14

Recommendations by Rose DK and Froese AB

Weight (kg)	Fresh Gas Flow		Minute Ventilation
10–30	1,000 mL/min + 100 mL·kg^{-1}·min^{-1}		2 × fresh gas flow
>30	2,000 mL/min + 50 mL·kg^{-1}·min^{-1}		2 × fresh gas flow

From Fisher DM.[1]

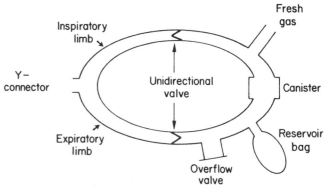

Figure 174–4. Components of the circle system and their usual arrangement. (From Fisher DM.[1])

connector. Circulators have been developed to decrease the deadspace under the mask. Use of these devices is not widespread.

Selected References

1. Fisher DM. Anesthesia equipment for pediatrics. In Gregory GA, ed. Pediatric Anesthesia. 3rd ed. New York: Churchill Livingstone, 1994;197–225.
2. Bain JA, Spoerel WE. Flow requirements for a modified Mapleson D system during controlled ventilation. Can Anaesth Soc J 1973;20:629.
3. Rose DK, Froese AB. The regulation of $PaCO_2$ during controlled ventilation of children with T-piece. Can Anaesth Soc J 1976;26:104.

Suggested References

Andrews JJ. Inhaled anesthetic delivery systems. In Miller RD, ed. Anesthesia. 5th ed. Philadelphia: Churchill Livingstone, 2000:174–206.

175
Maternal Physiologic Changes in Pregnancy

Gurinder Vasdev, M.D. □ Peter A. Southorn, M.D., F.R.C. Anes.

Physiologic changes in pregnancy begin within a few weeks of implantation and persist for 3 to 4 weeks after delivery.

Respiratory System

Difficulty in securing the airway is the most common cause of anesthesia-related mortality in the United States. Changes in maternal physiology contributing to this problem include:

□ Increased upper airway edema, necessitating a smaller endotracheal tube.
□ Increased vascularity of the upper airway and nasal congestion.
□ Decreased chest wall compliance, leading to early desaturation.
□ Decreased functional residual capacity (20%) and increased oxygen demand (60%), resulting in rapid desaturation during apneic episodes.
□ High risk for aspiration (see the section on Gastrointestinal System).

Physiologic compensatory mechanisms to improve fetal oxygenation include:

□ Rightward shifting of the maternal oxyhemoglobin dissociation curve (P_{50} = 30 mm Hg).
□ Increased (by 50%) minute ventilation. Progesterone is responsible for increasing the sensitivity of the central respiratory center to carbon dioxide. This causes respiratory alkalosis; however, neutral pH is maintained by increased renal excretion of bicarbonate.

Cardiovascular System

A myriad of cardiovascular changes occur during pregnancy. For example, maternal cardiac output increases 40%, to meet metabolic demands of both the mother and fetus. Gravid cardiovascular changes include:

□ Increased aldosterone production, causing increased plasma volume (45%) and dilutional anemia and improved rheology.
□ Increased stroke volume (30%) and heart rate (10%). Heart rate elevation occurs in response to increased oxygen demand. Progesterone decreases pulmonary and systemic vascular resistance, yet central venous pressure (CVP) and pulmonary capillary wedge pressure (PCWP) remain unchanged.
□ Uterine compression of the internal vena cava (IVC) and aorta, causing supine hypotension. A 15-degree lateral tilt can resolve this problem.
□ IVC compression and fluid retention, producing ankle edema and varicose veins and enlarging portal-systemic shunts.
□ ECG changes (e.g., left axis deviation, T-wave inversion in Lead III) occurring with cardiac enlargement and rotation of the heart cephalad and leftward.
□ Hyperdynamic flow murmurs.

These cardiovascular changes return to nongravid status within 8 weeks after delivery.

Gastrointestinal System

Pregnant patients are more prone to gastroesophageal (GE) reflux and aspiration because:

□ Gastric pH is decreased, resulting from production of gastrin by the placenta beginning after 15 weeks gestation.
□ Gastric emptying is delayed because of hormonal changes and mechanical obstruction by the gravid uterus. As a result, intragastric pressure is increased.
□ Lower esophageal sphincter (LES) competency is compromised when the gravid uterus causes the GE junction to shift cephalad and posterior. Additionally, LES tone is altered by high progesterone and estrogen levels.

Emergency C-section (2% of U.S. deliveries) further increases the risk of aspiration.

After 18 to 20 weeks gestation, women are at risk of aspiration pneumonia and suitable precautions should be taken. Patients with larger intrauterine size (e.g., multiple gestations or polyhydramnios) are at risk earlier in pregnancy.

Renal Function

Elevated intra-abdominal pressure and changes in bladder size and shape lead to mechanical obstruction and ureteric reflux. This increases the incidence of ascending urinary tract infection. Glomerular filtration is increased by 50% above nonpregnant values and is responsible for a 40% reduction in blood urea nitrogen and creatinine during normal pregnancy. Glucosuria and proteinuria (up to 300 mg/d) are fairly common.

Hepatic Function

Minor changes in hepatic transaminases (e.g., AST, LDH) may occur. Dilution of plasma proteins causes a decrease in the albumin:globulin ratio. Accordingly, the free fraction of albumin-bound medications is increased. Plasma cholinesterase levels are decreased (by dilution) without significant prolongation of succinylcholine-induced muscle block.

Hematologic System

There is activation of platelets, with an increased platelet turnover and shorter half-life. Factors VII, VIII, X, XII, and fibrinogen are increased. The fibrinolytic system is depressed by a relative reduction of antithrombin III. This results in a hypercoagulable state and renders pregnant patients more susceptible to thromboembolic disease.

Neurologic System

Local anesthetic requirements for neuraxial blockade are decreased during pregnancy secondary to reduced epidural space volume (epidural vein engorgement), decreased spinal cerebrospinal fluid (CSF) volume, increased CSF pH, and enhanced neural sensitivity to local anesthetics. The minimum alveolar concentration (MAC) of volatile anesthetics also is reduced 40% because of hormonal changes of pregnancy.

Uterine Physiology

Uterine blood flow and placental perfusion are affected by:

▫ Systemic vascular resistance.
▫ Aortocaval compression.
▫ Uterine contraction.

Placental blood supply is determined by spiral intervillous arteries, which are maximally dilated. They are supplied by arcuate and radial arteries, the ovarian, and uterine arteries. Myometrial tension decreases the caliber of spiral arteries reducing placental perfusion. Spiral arteries are maximally dilated and sensitive to α-adrenergic agonists (e.g., phenylephrine). Vasoconstriction can cause dramatic changes in placental blood supply. The surface area and integrity of the placenta are affected by maternal and placental disorders.

Prolonged uterine contraction (hypertonia) can cause fetal asphyxia. Treatment options include fluids, bed rest, oxygen, and tocolytics (e.g., nitroglycerine and albuterol). After delivery, uterine contraction is potentiated with massage, oxytocin, methylergonovine maleate, and carboprost tromethamine. Approximately 500 mL of blood are added to the maternal circulation with uterine contraction.

Fetal Oxygenation

Fetal oxygenation is dependent on placental blood supply, surface area integrity, and fetal cardiac output.

▫ Fetal cardiac output is rate-dependent.
▫ Mechanical compression of the umbilical cord decreases fetal oxygen delivery.
▫ Maternal-fetal oxygen transfer is facilitated by a leftward shifting of the fetal oxyhemoglobin curve.

Suggested References

Cheek TG, Gutsche BB. Maternal physiologic alterations during pregnancy. In Shnider SM, Levinson G, eds. Anesthesia for Obstetrics. 3rd ed. Baltimore: Williams & Wilkins, 1993:3–17.

Conklin KA, Backus AM. Physiologic changes of pregnancy. In Chestnut DH, ed. Obstetric Anesthesia: Principles and Practice. 2nd ed. St. Louis: CV Mosby, 1999:17–42.

Steer P, Flint C. ABCs of labour care: Physiology and management of normal labour. BMJ 1999;318:793–796.

176
Nonobstetric Surgery During Pregnancy

Elizabeth Noël Lumpkin, M.D.

Most women who undergo nonobstetric surgery during pregnancy are relatively healthy and experience uneventful operative and postoperative outcomes. It is estimated that up to 2% of pregnant women will have nonobstetric surgery during their pregnancy, which translates into approximately 75,000 cases per year in the U.S. This situation is unique, as the anesthesiologist cares not for one patient, but rather for two patients simultaneously. Anesthetic delivery needs to provide appropriate levels of anesthesia and analgesia while paying attention to the effects on the fetus.

Maternal Physiology

Pregnancy affects every organ in the mother, but those that require attention from an anesthetic standpoint include:

☐ **Respiratory:** decreased functional residual capacity, increased oxygen consumption, increased airway friability, higher incidence of difficult intubation.
☐ **Cardiovascular:** increased cardiac output, increased plasma volume, physiologic anemia of pregnancy, hypercoagulability.
☐ **Gastrointestinal:** decreased lower esophageal sphincter tone, increased gastric residual volumes.
☐ **Central nervous system:** decreased minimum alveolar concentration (MAC) for inhalation and local anesthetics.

Teratogens

Known teratogens are listed in Table 176–1. Traditionally, there have been concerns regarding the use of nitrous oxide and benzodiazepines. Nitrous oxide had been shown to decrease uterine blood flow in animal studies. This has not been demonstrated in humans. The cleft lip anomalies associated with benzodiazepines have only anecdotal evidence to support such a relationship.

Drugs that have a long history of safety in pregnancy include thiopental, morphine, meperidine, local anesthetics, muscle relaxants, and inhalation agents.

Uterine Blood Flow

Adequate uteroplacental perfusion is maintained by ensuring left uterine displacement and avoiding maternal hypotension. Other factors that can influence uterine blood flow include increased uterine activity, severe hyperventilation, and vasoconstrictors, such as endogenous or exogenous epinephrine. Special care must be taken when administering epidural and spinal anesthesia or when inducing general anesthesia.

Anesthetic Management

Preoperative

Preoperative goals include assessing the timing of surgery. If the procedure can be delayed until the second trimester, then the risks of teratogenicity of the first trimester, as well as the risk of preterm labor in the third trimester, can be reduced (Table 176–2).

If surgery cannot be delayed, then aspiration prophylaxis with a nonparticulate antacid, metoclopramide, or a histamine-2 blocker or a combination

Table 176–1. Known Teratogens

ACE inhibitors	Lithium
Alcohol	Mercury
Androgens	Phenytoin
Antithyroid drugs	Radiation (>0.5 Gy)
Carbamazepine	Streptomycin/kanamycin
Chemotherapy agents	Tetracycline
Cocaine	Thalidomide
Coumadin	Trimethadione
Diethylstilbestrol	Valproic acid
Lead	Vitamin A derivatives

Adapted from Hawkins JL.[1]

Table 176–2. Anesthetic Management for the
Parturient <20 Weeks Gestation

Postpone surgery if possible until the second trimester.
Ensure preoperative assessment by an obstetrician.
Provide aspiration prophylaxis.
Use regional anesthesia when possible.
Document fetal heart tone before and after the procedure.

Adapted from Hawkins JL.[1]

thereof should be used. The obstetrician should be consulted regarding the tocolytic administration and peripartum fetal monitoring (Table 176–3). Premedication with sedatives should be avoided. The use of magnesium as a tocolytic can potentiate the effects of muscle relaxants.

Intraoperative

No one technique has proved superior over any other. As long as maternal oxygenation is maintained and hypotension is avoided, most techniques can be effective. Routine monitoring, including blood pressure, oxygenation, ventilation, and temperature, should be done. If possible, instituting fetal monitoring after 20 weeks helps assess the intrauterine environment.

During general anesthesia, preoxygenation and rapid sequence induction with cricoid pressure are recommended. The anesthesiologist should be aware that the pregnant airway has a tendency to be more friable and edematous, hindering routine direct laryngoscopy. Maintenance of general anesthesia can include inhalation agents and nitrous oxide. Keeping inhalation agents below 2.0 MAC to prevent reduced cardiac output is advisable. Volatile agents are potent tocolytics that can help prevent preterm labor associated with surgical manipulation. The use of nitrous oxide is still somewhat controversial, although it has been suggested that 50% nitrous oxide should be safe in all but very long cases. Laparoscopic procedures are relatively contraindicated.

Regional anesthesia can allow a reduction in drug exposure, which can help reduce concerns

Table 176–3. Anesthetic Management for the
Parturient >20 Weeks Gestation

Consider prophylactic tocolytic agents with obstetrician.
Aspiration prophylaxis.
After 24 weeks, use left uterine displacement pre-, intra-, and
postoperatively.
Fetal monitoring when possible to assess intrauterine
environment.
Monitor uterine contractions postoperatively.

Adapted from Hawkins JL.[1]

about teratogenicity in the first trimester. Hypotension can be prevented with adequate preload and treatment with ephedrine as needed. As a general guideline, the usual dose of local anesthetic should be reduced by about one-third. Another added benefit of regional anesthesia is the ability to provide postoperative pain control without increasing maternal and fetal depression.

Postoperative

Fetal heart rate monitoring should continue in accordance with American College of Obstetricians and Gynecologists (ACOG) guidelines. The risk of preterm labor is still present in the immediate postoperative period. Contractions should also be monitored in any patient beyond 20 weeks gestation. Prophylaxis against deep venous thrombosis should be considered. Early mobilization is particularly important in the pregnant patient, who is at increased risk for thrombotic events. It should also be remembered that any systemic pain medications given could reduce fetal heart rate variability. Antiemetics should be used with caution, because many carry special risks during pregnancy. Ondansetron and metoclopramide are relatively safe.

Summary

Nonobstetric surgery can and does occur during pregnancy. Trauma, ovarian cysts, appendectomy, cholecystectomy, and cervical cerclages are most common. In addition, major operations such as aneurysm clipping, cardiopulmonary bypass, and liver transplants have been successfully performed on pregnant patients. Maternal disease is primarily responsible for the morbidity and mortality seen postoperatively and in utero. Nevertheless, the anesthesiologist should focus on prevention of hypoxemia, hypotension, and aortocaval compression to optimize the perioperative environment.

Selected References

1. Hawkins JL. Anesthesia for the obstetric patient for nonobstetric surgery. Anesth Analg 1997;84:S60–S65.

Suggested References

Cohen SE. Nonobstetric surgery during pregnancy. In Chestnut DH, ed. Obstetric Anesthesia: Principles and Practice. 2nd ed. St. Louis: CV Mosby 1999:273–289.
Duncan PG, Pope WD, Cohen MM, et al. Fetal risk of anesthesia and surgery during pregnancy. Anesthesiology 1986;64:790–794.
Rosen MA. Management of anesthesia for the pregnant surgical patient. Anesthesiology 1999;91:1159–1163.
Vincent RD. Anesthesia for the Pregnant Patient. Clin Ob and Gyn 1994;37:256–273.

177

Anesthesia for the Patient with Preeclampsia

Joseph J. Sandor, M.D.

Preeclampsia is a syndrome occurring after week 20 of gestation characterized by hypertension, proteinuria, and generalized edema. Preeclampsia is considered to be severe based on the criteria listed in Table 177–1. Preeclampsia becomes eclampsia if a grand mal seizure occurs. Preeclampsia/eclampsia abates within 48 hours after delivery of the entire placenta.

Etiology/Pathophysiology

The cause of preeclampsia remains unknown, although immunologic and genetic factors may play a role. Decreases in uterine blood flow and vasoconstriction of the spiral arteries of the myometrium are associated with the disorder. In addition to vasoconstriction, endothelial cell damage contributes to platelet activation and an imbalance of two circulating prostaglandins, prostacyclin and thromboxane.

Manifestations

Preeclampsia is a multisystem disease:

- **Central nervous system (CNS):** Headache, vertigo, cortical blindness, hyperreflexia, cerebral edema, cerebral hemorrhage, hyperirritability, and seizures.
- **Cardiovascular:** Hypovolemia, hemoconcentration, hypoproteinemia, elevated systemic vascular resistance, left ventricular hypertrophy, pulmonary edema, myocardial dysfunction, and increased sensitivity to catecholamines, sympathomimetics, and oxytocics.
- **Respiratory:** Interstitial edema, $\dot{V}/\dot{Q}$ mismatching, airway edema, and gastric aspiration.
- **Renal:** Decreased renal blood flow, decreased glomerular filtration rate, proteinuria, elevated creatinine and blood urea nitrogen, and hyperuricemia.
- **Hepatic:** Decreased hepatic blood flow, decreased plasma cholinesterase levels, periportal hepatic necrosis, subcapsular hemorrhage, and abnormal liver function tests.
- **Hematologic:** Prolonged bleeding time (25% of patients), platelet dysfunction, thrombocytopenia, and disseminated intravascular coagulation (20% of patients). The **HELLP syndrome** comprises *h*emolysis, *e*levated *l*iver enzymes, and *l*ow *p*latelets.
- **Placenta:** Uteroplacental insufficiency, placental abruption, chronic fetal hypoxia, fetal malnutrition, intrauterine growth retardation, premature labor, and premature birth.

Treatment

The definitive treatment for preeclampsia is delivery of the fetus and the placenta. Goals of the anesthesiologist include treatment of hypertension, volume replacement, and control of CNS irritability.

Intravenous fluid administration should be guided by **urine output** (greater than 1 ml·kg^{-1}·h^{-1}) and **central venous pressure** (4 to 6 cm H_2O). In patients manifesting cardiopulmonary dysfunction, a pulmonary artery catheter is the preferred method of hemodynamic monitoring. Intra-arterial cannulation allows continual blood pressure monitoring and provides easy access for blood sampling (e.g., clotting parameters, arterial blood gases, electrolytes, and Mg^{2+} levels). Loop diuretics are used to treat pulmonary edema, and mannitol may be given to treat cerebral edema. Magnesium sulfate has both anticonvulsant and antihyperten-

Table 177–1. Criteria for Classification as Severe Preeclampsia

Systolic blood pressure > 160 torr, diastolic blood pressure
 >110 torr or mean blood pressure > 120 torr
Proteinuria > 5 g/24 hr
Oliguria < 500 mL/24 hr
Headache, visual disturbances, epigastric pain, pulmonary
 edema, or cyanosis
HELLP syndrome (hemolysis, elevated liver enzymes,
 thrombocytopenia)

Adapted from Glosten B.[1]

Table 177–2. Effects of Increasing Plasma Magnesium Levels

Observed Condition	mEq/L
Normal plasma level	1.5–2.0
Therapeutic range	4.0–6.0
ECG changes (prolonged P-Q interval, widened QRS complex)	5.0–10
Loss of deep tendon reflexes	10
Sinoatrial and atrioventricular block	15
Respiratory paralysis	15
Cardiac arrest	25

From Glosten B.[1]

sive properties. It reduces CNS irritability and irritability of the neuromuscular junction, and has direct vasodilating action on the smooth muscles of arterioles and uterus. In excess of therapeutic range, $MgSO_4$ may cause skeletal muscle weakness, respiratory depression, and cardiac arrest. $CaCl_2$ counteracts the adverse effects of $MgSO_4$. Neuromuscular blockade is potentiated by $MgSO_4$, as is the sedative effect of opioids. Other useful antihypertensive agents include labetalol, hydralazine, nitroglycerin, methyldopa, clonidine, prazosin, nifedipine, and trimethaphan. Use of sodium nitroprusside (SNP) is discouraged by some authors because the fetus is susceptible to cyanide toxicity resulting from continuous SNP infusion. Table 177–2 summarizes the effects of increasing plasma magnesium levels.

Anesthetic Management

Vaginal delivery may be performed if the fetus is not distressed. Lumbar epidural analgesia provides pain relief and a method to control blood pressure during labor. Before catheter placement, it should be ascertained that the parturient has no coagulopathy and that adequate volume replacement (1 to 2 L) has been achieved. With regional anesthesia there is less pushing (less blood pressure elevation), less need for opioid analgesics, and an improvement in placental and renal blood flow. Because these patients demonstrate increased sensitivity to catecholamines, epinephrine is usually not added to the local anesthetic solution. Saddle block may be performed if the fetus is carefully monitored.

Cesarean section is indicated for delivery of a distressed fetus. If an epidural catheter has been previously placed (or if the cesarean section is elective), it may be used to provide surgical anesthesia, assuming appropriate intravascular volume restoration (1.5 to 2 L). Although previously considered controversial, spinal anesthesia has proven to be a safe technique for cesarean section for severely preeclamptic patients.

General anesthesia is an acceptable way to manage preeclamptic patients, but there are associated risks of pulmonary aspiration, airway compromise from edema, and acute blood pressure elevations during laryngoscopy. The brief but severe elevations in systemic and pulmonary pressures seen during laryngoscopy and intubation in preeclamptic parturients can lead to a significant risk of cerebral hemorrhage and pulmonary edema. A rapid-sequence induction technique is used. Sodium thiopental (4 mg/kg) plus succinylcholine (1.5 mg/kg) are given intravenously. Earlier IV treatment with intravenous hydralazine, lidocaine, sodium nitroprusside, nitroglycerine, and/or esmolol will attenuate the hypertensive response to laryngoscopy.

Because of the occasional severe degree of **oropharyngeal edema**, a smaller than usual size cuffed endotracheal tube is used to intubate the trachea. Anesthesia is then maintained with volatile agents, N_2O/O_2, and neuromuscular blockade as needed, guided by a peripheral nerve stimulator. Oxytocics may cause exaggerated blood pressure elevation, and ergot preparations should not be used. **Coagulopathies** are managed with transfusions of platelets, fresh frozen plasma, and cryoprecipitate as needed. After completion of surgery, the patient may be extubated once fully awake.

Selected References

1. Glosten B. Anesthesia for obstetrics. In Miller RD, ed. Anesthesia. 5th ed. Philadelphia: Churchill Livingstone, 2000:2024–2068.

Suggested References

Douglas MJ. Coagulation abnormalities and obstetric anaesthesia. Can J Anaesth 1991;38:17.

Friedman SA. Preeclampsia: A review of the role of prostaglandins. Obstet Gyncol 1988;71:122.

Hood DD, Curry R. Spinal versus epidural anesthesia for cesarean section in severely preeclamptic patients: A retrospective survey. Anesthesiology 1999;90:1276–1282.

Lim KH, Friedman SA. Hypertension in pregnancy. Curr Opin Obstet Gynecol 1993;5:40.

Morison DH. Anaesthesia and pre-eclampsia. Can J Anaesth 1987;34:415.

Stoelting RK, Dierdorf SF. Anesthesia and Co-Existing Disease. 3rd ed. Churchill Livingstone, New York, 1993.

178
Maternal Diabetes: Neonatal Effects

Jerald O. Van Beck, M.D.

Diabetes is a common, serious medical problem affecting pregnant women. The successful control of diabetes mellitus with insulin has led to the survival of increasing numbers of diabetic women who bear children. Diabetic mothers have an increased incidence of complications, including preeclampsia/eclampsia, polyhydramnios, intrauterine infections, intrauterine fetal distress, and dystocia. The fetal morbidity rate is greater than 10 times that of children of nondiabetic mothers for all gestational ages but especially after 32 weeks. Similarly, the neonatal mortality rate is greater than five times that of nondiabetic mothers and is higher in all gestational ages and in every birth weight for gestational age. Diabetic ketoacidosis remains a major cause of perinatal morbidity and mortality rates. The incidence of mortality and morbidity is related to the severity of diabetes and the quality of its management. Tables 178–1, 178–2, and 178–3 give a classification of maternal diabetes and data on risk.

Neonatal Morbidity Associated with Diabetes Mellitus

No single physiologic or biochemical event completely explains the diverse clinical manifestations associated with diabetes. The probable pathologic sequence is as follows: Maternal hyperglycemia causes fetal hyperglycemia and fetal hyperinsulinemia; these result in increased hepatic glucose up-

Table 178–1. A Summary of White's Classification of Diabetic Pregnant Women

Class	Characteristics	Implications
Gestational diabetes	Glucose intolerance diagnosed during pregnancy	Diagnosis before 30 weeks gestation is important to prevent macrosomia; treatment with diabetic pregnancy diet of adequate calories to prevent maternal weight loss; goal is fasting plasma glucose < 105 mg/dL, 2-hr postprandial plasma glucose < 120 mg/dL; if insulin is necessary, manage as in classes B, C, D.
A	Chemical diabetes diagnosed before pregnancy; managed by diet alone; onset at any age	Management similar as for gestational diabetes.
B	Insulin treatment necessary before pregnancy; onset $\geq$ age 20 yr; duration < 10 yr.	Some endogenous insulin secretion may persist; insulin resistance at the cellular level in obese women; fetal and neonatal risks equivalent to class C and D, as in management.
C	Onset age 10–20 yr, or duration 10–20 yr.	Insulin-deficient diabetes of juvenile onset.
D	Onset < age 10 yr, or duration > 20 yr or chronic hypertension (not preeclampsia) or benign retinopathy (tiny hemorrhages)	Fetal macrosomia or intrauterine growth retardation possible; so-called retinal microaneurysms may progress during pregnancy, then regress after delivery.
F	Diabetic nephropathy with proteinuria	Anemia and hypertension common; proteinuria increase in third trimester, declines after pregnancy; fetal intrauterine growth retardation common; perinatal survival about 85% under optimal conditions; bed rest necessary (class T [postrenal transplant] outlook is good).
R	Malignant proliferative retinopathy	Neovascularization; risk of vitreous hemorrhage or retinal detachment; laser photocoagulation is useful; abortion usually not necessary; route of delivery is controversial.
H	Coronary artery disease	Grave maternal risk.

From Datta S.[1]

Table 178–2. Neonatal Morbidity and Mortality in Diabetes

Disorder	Percentage
Deaths	3.2
Hypoglycemia < 40 mg%	12.0
Hypocalcemia < 7 mg%	26.0
Hypomagnesemia < 1.2 mg%	4.0
Polycythemia	11.0
Hyperbilirubinemia	16.0
Respiratory distress syndrome	3.0

Total number of infants is 217 (100%).
Adapted from Lemons JA, Vargas P, Delaney JJ.[2]

Table 178–4. Teratogenic Abnormalities in Infants

Location	Disorder
CNS	Anencephaly, meningomyelocele, spina bifida
Cardiac	Transposition of vessels, ventricular septal defect, situs inversus
Renal	Agenesis
Pulmonary	Hypoplastic lungs
Gastrointestinal	Anal and rectal atresia, small colon

Adapted from Cousins L.[4]

take and glycogen synthesis, accelerated lipogenesis, increased skeletal growth and augmented protein synthesis. As a result, infants tend to have a characteristic appearance, being large and plump with plethoric faces and enlarged viscera. Neonatal complications associated with maternal diabetes mellitus are outlined in Table 178–2.

Metabolic Derangements. Chronic fetal hyperinsulinemia at delivery results in neonatal hypoglycemia (below 30 mg/dL) in 50% to 75% of infants of diabetic mothers and 25% of infants of mothers with gestational diabetes. Only a minority of these neonates are symptomatic. Other problems include hyperglycemia, hypocalcemia, hypomagnesemia, and hyperbilirubinemia.

Macrosomia. Morbidity occurs due to mechanical birth injury and asphyxia as a consequence of fetal macrosomia, with disproportion between size of the infant and the maternal pelvis. As a result, the need for cesarean delivery with its attendant risks is increased. All viscera except the brain can be affected by the macrosomic process.

Respiratory Distress Syndrome. Fetal hyperinsulinemia is implicated in delaying surfactant production. Although respiratory distress can occur despite normal indices of fetal lung maturity (such

as lecithin-sphingomyelin ratio) in amniotic fluid, these determinations are helpful in assessing fetal lung maturity. The etiology of disturbed lung function is unknown, but rigorous control of maternal glucose concentration minimizes pulmonary complications.

Cardiovascular Problems. Cardiomegaly is seen in 30% of these neonates, with heart failure occurring in 5% to 10%. Asymmetric septal hypertrophy can also occur. Other complications include polycythemia and renal vein thrombosis.

Congenital Anomalies. The incidence of birth defects is up to three times that in the general population. Almost any organ system may be involved, but cardiac and skeletal systems are most commonly affected.[5] Studies have shown a correlation between these anomalies and poor maternal glucose control during the first trimester of pregnancy (Table 178–4).

Selected References

1. Datta S. Anesthesia for the pregnant diabetic patient. In Shnider SM, Levinson G, eds. Anesthesia for Obstetrics. 3rd ed. Baltimore: Williams & Wilkins, 1993:539–550.
2. Lemons JA, Vargas P, Delaney JJ. Infant of the diabetic mother: Review of 225 cases. Obstet Gynecol 1981;57:187.
3. Hill DE. Fetal endocrine pancreas. Clin Obstet Gynecol 1980;23:837.
4. Cousins L. Congenital anomalies among infants of diabetic mothers. Etiology, prevention, and prenatal diagnosis. Am J Obstet Gynecol 1983;147:333.
5. Reece EA, Homko CJ. Why do diabetic women deliver malformed infants? Clin Obstet Gynecol 2000;43:32–35.

Table 178–3. Current Perinatal Mortality in Diabetes Mellitus

White's Classification	Mortality/1000 Live Births
A	16
B	48
C	79
D	100
F-R	186

From Hill DE.[3]

Suggested References

D'Alessio JG, Ramanathan J, Allen G. Diabetes mellitus in pregnancy. In Norris MC, ed. Obstetric Anesthesia. 2nd ed. Philadelphia: Lippincott Williams & Wilkins, 1999:103–134.
Stoelting RK, Dierdorf SF. Anesthesia and Co-Existing Disease. 3rd ed. Philadelphia, Churchill Livingstone, 1993.

179

The Pregnant Patient with Cardiac Disease

John K. Erie, M.D.

The prevalence of heart disease during pregnancy is as high as 4%. It is the leading nonobstetric cause of maternal mortality. Maternal mortality ranges from 0.4% among patients assigned New York Heart Association functional classification I or II to 6.8% among patients in classes III and IV. Cardiac complications and death occur most commonly in the third trimester, during labor and delivery, and in the immediate postpartum period.[1, 2]

In 1960, rheumatic heart disease was responsible for the vast majority of heart disease in pregnant patients. Rheumatic heart disease still accounts for the majority of cardiac disease in pregnant patients, but congenital heart disease accounts for an increased proportion, because advanced medical and surgical care has allowed women with these conditions to reach child-bearing age.

Cardiovascular Changes During Pregnancy

The normal cardiovascular changes that occur during pregnancy are listed in Table 179–1. Note that blood pressure does not normally change from the nonpregnant state because the increase in cardiac output is counterbalanced by the decrease in systemic vascular resistance (SVR).

Mitral Stenosis

Mitral stenosis is the sole or predominant valvular lesion in most parturients with rheumatic heart disease. With mitral stenosis, there is impedance to filling of the left ventricle during diastole due to the diminished mitral valve area. Because of this stenotic valve, left ventricular filling is very dependent on atrial contraction. In addition, the left atrium must generate increased pressure to drive blood across the stenotic valve. This increase in left atrial pressure is eventually transmitted into the pulmonary vasculature, producing pulmonary edema and pulmonary hypertension.

Cardiovascular changes in pregnancy that can adversely affect a patient with mitral stenosis include:

□ The inability of the heart with mitral stenosis to generate the increased cardiac output needed by the pregnant patient.
□ The increase in blood volume further increases left atrial pressure and may lead to atrial fibrillation or pulmonary edema.

Anesthetic considerations in the pregnant patient with mitral stenosis include the following:

□ Avoid sinus tachycardia, because this allows less time for ventricular filling during diastole.
□ Avoid atrial fibrillation, because the loss of atrial contraction can produce episodes of failure. Cardioversion should be considered if drug therapy fails to decrease ventricular rate.
□ Avoid increases in blood volume, because this may precipitate pulmonary edema.

Mitral Insufficiency

Mitral insufficiency is the second most common valve defect in pregnant patients. It is usually toler-

Table 179–1. Normal Cardiovascular Changes During Pregnancy

Variable	Direction of Change	Average Change
Blood volume	↑	+35%
Plasma volume	↑	+45%
Red blood cell volume	↑	+20%
Cardiac output	↑	+40%
Stroke volume	↑	+30%
Heart rate	↑	+15%
Femoral (uterine?) venous pressure	↑	+15 torr
Total peripheral resistance	↓	−15%
Mean arterial blood pressure	↓	−15 torr
Systolic blood pressure	↓	−0–15 torr
Diastolic blood pressure	↓	−10–20 torr
Central venous pressure	↔	No change

From Cheek TG, Gutsche BB.[3]

ated reasonably well in pregnant patients. Important anesthetic considerations include the following:

□ Avoid increases in systemic vascular resistance.
□ Avoid decreases in contractility.
□ Avoid bradycardia.
□ Maintain sinus rhythm.
□ Consider afterload reduction.

Aortic Insufficiency

Pure aortic insufficiency is similar to mitral insufficiency. It is seldom a problem in parturients. Important anesthetic considerations include the following:

□ Avoid increases in systemic vascular resistance.
□ Avoid bradycardia.
□ Avoid decreases in contractility.
□ Consider afterload reduction.

Aortic Stenosis

Aortic stenosis is a relatively rare lesion in parturients as it is most prevalent in older age groups. Important anesthetic considerations include the following:

□ Avoid decreases in systemic vascular resistance.
□ Avoid bradycardia.
□ Avoid hypovolemia.

Congenital Heart Disease

Congenital heart disease can be categorized as follows:

□ Left-to-right shunt (ventricular septal defects, atrial septal defects, patent ductus arteriosus).
□ Right-to-left shunt (tetralogy of Fallot, Eisenmenger's syndrome).
□ Congenital valvular and vascular lesions (coarctation of the aorta, pulmonary stenosis, aortic stenosis).

Left-to-Right Shunt

The most common lesions producing left-to-right shunting in the pregnant patient include:

□ Ventricular septal defect.
□ Atrial septal defect.
□ Patent ductus arteriosus.

Although each of the foregoing conditions produces left-to-right shunting in different anatomic locations, the cardiovascular changes that occur with pregnancy affect all three in a similar manner.

□ The decrease in SVR is helpful, because it decreases the magnitude of left-to-right shunting.
□ The increase in blood volume can precipitate failure, because in each of these conditions the patient is in a state of compensatory hypervolemia.

The main anesthetic considerations in managing patients with a left-to-right shunt include the following:

□ Avoid excessive fluid administration, overtransfusion, and Trendelenburg position.
□ Avoid increases in SVR.

Right-to-Left Shunt

The most common congenital lesion in this category is tetralogy of Fallot characterized by right ventricular hypertrophy, right ventricular outflow obstruction, ventricular septal defect, and overriding aorta.

The cardiovascular changes associated with pregnancy affect patients with tetralogy of Fallot in the following manner:

□ The decrease in SVR enhances the magnitude of right-to-left shunt.
□ The increase in blood volume is beneficial since adequate right ventricular preload is necessary to eject blood past the outflow obstruction and increase pulmonary blood flow.

Anesthetic considerations include the following:

□ Avoid decreases in SVR, which can lead to episodes of cyanosis. Cyanotic episodes can be treated with phenylephrine.
□ Maintain adequate blood volume and venous return.
□ Avoid myocardial depressants, because any decrease in right ventricular contractility can diminish the amount of blood injected into the pulmonary circulation.

Selected References

1. Santos AC, Pederson H, Finster F. Obstetric anesthesia. In Barash PG, Cullen BF, Stoelting RK, eds. Clinical Anesthesia. 3rd ed. Philadelphia: Lippincott Williams & Wilkins, 1997:1075–1076.
2. Mangano DT. Anesthesia for the pregnant cardiac patient. In Schnider SM, Levinson G, eds. Anesthesia for Obstetrics. 3rd ed. Baltimore: Lippincott Williams & Wilkins, 1993:485.
3. Cheek TG, Gutsche BB. Maternal physiologic alterations during pregnancy. In Shnider SM, Levinson G, eds. Anesthesia for Obstetrics. 3rd ed. Baltimore: Lippincott Williams & Wilkins, 1993:3.

Suggested References

Glosten B. Anesthesia for obstetrics. In Miller RD, ed. Anesthesia. 5th ed. New York: Churchill Livingstone, 2000: 2024–2068.

180
Drugs Affecting the Uterus: Tocolytics and Oxytocics

K.A. Kelly McQueen, M.D.

The management of uterine contractibility during the peripartum period may provide special challenges for the anesthesiologist caring for the parturient. Preterm labor necessitates tocolytic therapy (Table 180–1), which may affect the parturient presenting for nonobstetric surgery or for cesarean section (C/S) if the fetus demonstrates distress. Oxytocics (oxytocin, Pitocin, methylergonovine maleate, prostaglandin F_2) are used to initiate and augment labor, to correct uterine atony and postpartum bleeding in the postpartum period, and to induce abortion.

Tocolytic Agents

Tocolytic agents inhibit uterine contractibility and thus may be used to treat preterm labor or undesired spontaneous term labor, such as occurs with breech presentation and previous C/S scar of unknown type.

The **β2-receptor agonists** terbutaline and ritodrine are commonly used to treat preterm labor. Ritodrine is the only drug specifically approved by the FDA for tocolysis. These agents interact with β-2 receptors on the uterine myometrial cells, activating adenyl cyclase, which catalyzes the conversion of ATP to cAMP. The increase in cAMP decreases intracellular calcium and inhibits myosin light-chain kinase. The combination of these effects decreases the interaction between actin and myosin and produces uterine relaxation. These agents may be administered intravenously, subcutaneously, or orally. Generally, these agents have little effect on the administration of either regional or general anesthesia; however, the side effects of large doses of these drugs may be of concern to the anesthesia provider. Such side effects include hypotension,

tachycardia, arrhythmias, myocardial ischemia, and pulmonary edema. Fetal tachycardia commonly occurs because of the rapid placental transfer of β-adrenergic agents.

Magnesium ($MgSO_4$) is often used to treat preterm labor, because it has fewer cardiovascular side effects than the β2-receptor agonists. But although $MgSO_4$ is known to decrease uterine activity, there is little evidence that it is effective as a tocolytic agent. $MgSO_4$ is often used to treat blood pressure and to lower the seizure threshold in patients with pregnancy-induced hypertension (PIH). The side effects of $MgSO_4$ include hypotension, maternal obtundation, muscle weakness, and prolonged effects of muscle relaxants administered during general anesthesia. $MgSO_4$ causes muscle relaxation by affecting the uptake and binding of cellular calcium. $MgSO_4$ also decreases the release of acetylcholine and alters the sensitivity of the neuromuscular junctions to acetylcholine. These effects alter the neuromuscular junction in skeletal muscle, producing prolonged muscle relaxation in the parturient needing general anesthesia. The loading intravenous dose of $MgSO_4$ is 4 g over 15 minutes, followed by a continuous intravenous infusion of 1 to 4 g/hr.

Prostaglandin synthase inhibitors and the calcium channel blocker **nifedipine** have been shown to effectively relax the uterus. **Indomethacin**, a prostaglandin synthase inhibitor, is commonly used for long-term tocolysis in high-risk parturients with preterm labor. Indomethacin inhibits cyclooxygenase and thereby prevents the synthesis of the prostaglandins that play an important role in the stimulus of uterine contractions. The maternal side effects of indomethacin are minimal, most commonly nausea and heartburn. But fetal concerns with long-term administration of indomethacin include premature closure of the ductus arteriosus and oligohydramnios resulting from decreased fetal urine excretion. Despite these fetal effects, indomethacin is commonly used either alone or with another agent for refractory preterm labor. Indomethacin can be given orally or rectally, with an initial dose of 50 mg followed by 25 mg every 4 to 6 hours.

Table 180–1. Tocolytic Pharmacologic Agents

Beta-adrenergic agonists (terbutaline)
Magnesium sulfate
Prostaglandin synthase inhibitors (indomethacin)
Calcium channel blockers (nifedipine)

Nifedipine acts by blocking cell membrane channels that are selective for calcium and by preventing the release of calcium, resulting in relaxation of smooth muscle. The side effects of nifedipine include hypotension, vasodilation, myocardial depression, and conduction defects. Like $MgSO_4$, nifedipine may prolong muscle relaxation. Nifedipine is not commonly used for tocolysis in the United States.

Oxytocics

These drugs stimulate the smooth muscle of the uterus, thereby producing or augmenting uterine contractions. **Oxytocin** is a posterior pituitary hormone that stimulates uterine smooth muscle. The synthetic derivative Pitocin is used to limit the antidiuretic and cardiovascular side effects of vasopressin that may contaminate oxytocin in vivo because of its proximity of production. Pitocin is generally given as an intravenous bolus and/or continuous infusion titrated to effect of stimulating and monitoring uterine contractions during labor and in the postoperative period. Pitocin generally affects the uterus by causing slow generalized contractions with periods of relaxation between contractions. The side effects of Pitocin include hypotension, especially when given as a bolus, and secondary tachycardia. The effects usually occur immediately and are transient. Transient ECG changes, including T-wave flattening and inversion and a prolonged Q-T interval, may occur. When given in large doses or over extended periods, antidiuretics may produce water intoxication and hyponatremia.

Methylergonovine maleate (Methergine), 0.2 mg given intramuscularly, a purified ergot alkaloid, is used to augment uterine contractions if Pitocin does not produce the desired effect. Methergine is exclusively used in the postpartum period because it produces tonic contractions faster, which significantly limit blood flow. Methergine's major side effects include nausea, vomiting, and significant hypertension due to direct peripheral vasoconstriction. For this reason, intravenous administration of Methergine is controversial, and the drug must be carefully administered to parturients with essential hypertension or PIH.

Severe uterine atony and postpartum hemorrhage may necessitate the use of **prostaglandin $F_{2\text{-alpha}}$ ($PGF_{2\alpha}$)**, although the drug can cause bronchospasm. The 15-methyl analog of $PGF_{2\alpha}$ acts similarly to $PGF_{2\alpha}$ produced by the pregnant uterus but promotes stronger, sustained uterine contractions, limiting blood flow to the uterus. 15-Methyl prostaglandin $F_{2\alpha}$ (250 μg) is administered intramuscularly or intramyometrially only after Pitocin and Methergine have been used because of the associated nausea, vomiting, and diarrhea.

Suggested References

Benedetti TJ. Maternal complications of parenteral β-sympathomimetic therapy for premature labor. Am J Obstet Gynecol 1983;145:1–6.

Caritis SN. Treatment of preterm labour: A review of the therapeutic options. Drugs 1983;26:243–261.

Mayer DC, Spielman FJ. Antepartum and postpartum hemorrhage. In Chestnut DH, ed. Obstetric Anesthesia: Principles and Practice. 2nd ed. St. Louis: CV Mosby, 1999:725–748.

Muir HA, McGrath JM, Chestnut DH. Preterm labor and delivery. In Chestnut DH, ed. Obstetric Anesthesia: Principles and Practice. 2nd ed. St. Louis: CV Mosby, 1999:665–693.

Niebyl JR, Witter FR. Neonatal outcome after indomethacin treatment for preterm labor. Am J Obstet Gynecol 1986;155:747–749.

181
Analgesia for Labor

K.A. Kelly McQueen, M.D.

Pain relief during labor provides maternal comfort and, perhaps more importantly, prevents the maternal and fetal sequence of maternal sympathetic activation. The drugs used for labor analgesia must be potent enough to provide relief of severe pain, and they must be used in doses that will not significantly affect the fetus.

Labor Pain

The first stage of labor begins with the onset of regular painful contractions and ends at complete dilation of the cervix. Pain in the first stage of labor is visceral and is caused by dilation of the cervix and lower uterine segment as well as the uterine contractions themselves (Fig. 181–1). These visceral afferent impulses are carried along the sympathetic nerves, where they connect with the somatic mixed spinal nerves through the rami communicants at T10, T11, T12, and L1. Referred pain can present over the cutaneous distribution of these dermatomes in the lumbar and sacral areas.

The second stage of labor begins with complete cervical dilation and ends with delivery of the baby. Pain in the second stage of labor is somatic, as stretching and tearing of the pelvic ligaments and muscles occurs. This pain is conducted along the pudendal nerves at S2, S3, and S4. In addition, uterine pain impulses continue as in the first stage of labor. Also, pain impulses during distension of the vagina and perineum just before delivery are conducted along the genitofemoral (L1, L2), ilio-inguinal (L1), and posterior cutaneous nerves of the thighs (S2, S3), although they have a small role in labor pain. Regional techniques producing analgesia/anesthesia during labor are summarized in Figure 181–2.

Epidural analgesia provides excellent relief of labor pain while preserving maternal motor function and fetal circulation. There are many drugs, used alone or in combination, that can effectively obliterate labor pain (Table 181–1). Fentanyl used alone provides good pain relief in early labor and allows maternal ambulation ("walking epidural"). Local anesthesia, used alone or in combination with fentanyl, provides excellent pain relief throughout labor but necessitates maternal confinement because of the risk of motor weakness and hypotension. The introduction of ropivacaine into practice has increased safety due to the decreased risk of hemodynamic collapse with intravascular injection. Bupivacaine is also commonly used in many labor and delivery departments. Lidocaine is frequently added for epidural "top up," increasing the density of nerve block during a period of intense pain, such as the second stage of labor or episiotomy repair. In many birthing centers after the epidural catheter is placed and boluses are given incrementally, a con-

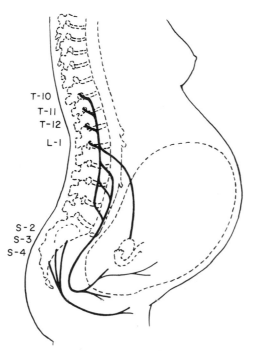

Figure 181–1. Parturition pain pathways. Afferent pain impulses from the cervix and uterus are carried by nerves that accompany sympathetic fibers and enter the neuraxis at the T10, T11, T12, and L1 spinal levels. Pain pathways from the perineum travel to S2, S3, and S4 via the pudendal nerve. (From Bonica JJ, Chadwick HS.[1])

Table 181–1. Drugs for Epidural Analgesia

Ropivacaine (0.1%–0.2%)
Bupivacaine (0.08%–0.125%)
Fentanyl (2 μg/mL in either of the above)

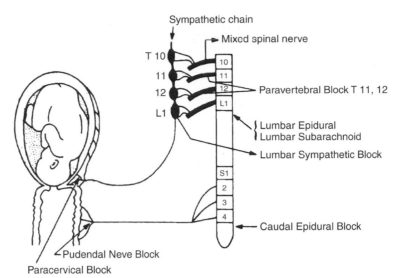

Figure 181–2. Summary of blocks available for producing analgesia during labor. (From Ramanthan S.[2])

tinuous infusion is initiated to maintain the desired level.

An epidural for labor is usually placed in a vertebral interspace between L2 and L5. Alternatively, a caudal block may be performed. A caudal block primarily affects the sacral segments and produces excellent analgesia in the second stage of labor. It can be extended to the lumbar and thoracic segments by increasing volume. Advantages of caudal anesthesia are few in the parturient, and sacral edema often distorts the caudal space in pregnancy, making this technique difficult and infrequently used.

Single-Shot Spinal

Multiparity and the rapid progression of labor often make the time required for epidural placement and incremental dosing of anesthetic impractical. In this setting, a patient who desires pain relief can be rapidly treated with a single intrathecal dose of narcotic or narcotic combined with local anesthetic (Table 181–2). Pain relief occurs within several contractions and predictably lasts 1.5 hours. The disadvantages of a single-shot spinal include increased risk of postdural puncture headache (PDPH) (Chap. 115) and the potential for labor outlasting pain relief.

Combined Spinal/Epidural

The need for rapid pain control combined with an unpredictable length of labor, as is the case in the young primipara, makes the option for a combined technique desirable. Spinal and epidural analgesia can be combined to provide rapid and continuous pain relief. A double-stick or needle-through-needle technique can be used (Fig. 181–3). Using either method, a dose of intrathecal narcotic or local and narcotic is given, followed by insertion of an epidural catheter. Because of concern for intrathecal catheter placement, two options for continued analgesia exist. One option is to test the epidural catheter at the limit of the intrathecal dose, thereafter bolusing the epidural and starting a continuous infusion. The second option is to start a continuous infusion in the untested catheter following the intrathecal injection. Both techniques have been effectively used, and as long as the mother and fetus are adequately monitored, a clear distinction in safety is not apparent. The advantage of this technique is rapid onset and the option of

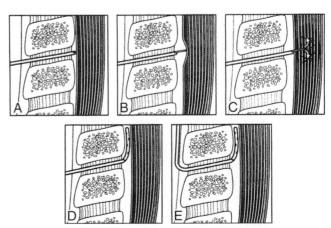

Figure 181–3. The combined spinal-epidural technique. Typically, an epidural needle is inserted in the epidural space (A) and a spinal needle is inserted through it (B). Because of the presence of air in the epidural space, the pencil-point spinal needle may deform the dura considerably before puncturing it (C). After injection through the spinal needle, it is withdrawn, and an epidural catheter is inserted (D), and the epidural needle is withdrawn (E). (From Eisenach JC.[3])

Table 181–2. Drugs for Subarachnoid Analgesia

Fentanyl (20 μg)
Sufentanyl (10 μg)
Either of the above diluted to 1 mL with preservative-free
  saline (bupivacaine [2.5 mg] and fentanyl [20 μg])

continuous analgesia with an indwelling catheter. The disadvantage is a small increased risk of PDPH.

Other Regional Blockade

Several options exist for blockade of specific nerve plexus. These include paravertebral, lumbar sympathetic, paracervical, and pudendal blocks. Risk versus benefit profiles for these blocks during labor discourage their mainstream use when other options are available.

Systemic Medication

Narcotics are the most effective of the systemic medications. No narcotic can produce analgesia without some respiratory depression, which is the most significant side effect, and none can produce complete analgesia without the risk of severe hypoventilation and obtundation. Therefore, systemic narcotics are used in labor to reduce pain, not completely eliminate it, when regional analgesia cannot be used. All systemic analgesics cross the placenta and have the potential to cause neonatal respiratory depression. Other side effects common to systemic narcotics are orthostatic hypotension, nausea and vomiting, decreased gastric motility, and the possibility of decreased uterine activity in the early stages of labor.

When regional anesthesia is not possible and narcotic analgesia may be required, labor pain can be successfully attenuated with fentanyl patient-controlled analgesia (PCA). Fentanyl can be dosed to decrease labor pain and the associated sympathetic stimulation (50 to 200 µg/hr) and is redistributed rapidly through the mother and the fetus. However, neonatal depression may occur as the neonate is more sensitive to narcotics than the mother.

Selected References

1. Bonica JJ, Chadwick HS. Labour pain. In Wall PD, Melzack R, eds. Textbook of Pain. 2nd ed. New York: Churchill Livingstone, 1989:482.
2. Ramanthan S. Obstetric Anesthesia. Philadelphia, Lea & Febiger, 1988.
3. Eisenach JC. Combined spinal-epidural analgesia in obstetrics. Anesthesiology 1999;91:299–302.

Suggested References

Belin Y, Leibowitz AB, Bernstein HH, et al. Controversies of labor epidural analgesia. Anesth Analg 1999;89:969–978.
Belin Y, Galea M, Zahn J, et al. Epidural ropivacaine for the initiation of labor epidural analgesia: A dose finding study. Anesth Analg 1999;88:1340–1345.
Chestnut D. Obstetric Anesthesia: Principles and Practice. 2nd ed. St. Louis, Mosby, 1999.

182
Fetal Monitoring

Stephen T. Gott, M.D.

The fetus can be evaluated in utero by several tests. These tests can aid in the diagnosis of placental dysfunction, assess fetal maturity, detect congenital anomalies, and assess fetal well-being.

Maternal Urinary and Plasma Estrogens. The placenta is the primary site of production of estrogens in the pregnant patient. A downward trend or sudden drop in estriol (E_3) can indicate placental dysfunction.

Human Placental Lactogen. There is a direct relationship between human placental lactogen (HPL) levels and placental and fetal weight. Low HPL levels may be associated with intrauterine growth retardation, hypertensive disorders of pregnancy, and postmaturity.

Ultrasonography. Ultrasonography is a reliable, noninvasive, sensitive method of determining fetal age, growth, and weight as well as placental location and presence of anomalies.

Amniotic Fluid Analysis. Fetal lung maturity may be assessed by measuring the ratio of the major phospholipids lecithin (L) and sphingomyelin (S). An L/S ratio exceeding 2.0 indicates the fetus is at low risk for developing respiratory distress syndrome. Chromosomal anomalies can be diagnosed from fetal cells acquired from amniotic fluid. α-Fetoprotein, which is primarily synthesized in the fetal liver, is detected in maternal plasma and amniotic fluid. In early gestation, elevated levels suggest a central nervous system anomaly such as spina bifida, hydrocephaly, or anencephaly. During late pregnancy, elevated levels may indicate congenital nephrosis or esophageal atresia.

Nonstress Test. A scoring system using a scale of 0 to 2 evaluates baseline fetal heart rate, accelerations, decelerations, baseline variability, and fetal movements during a 30-minute period. Uterine contractions are not required. A score of 9 to 12 indicates fetal well-being. A score below 9 indicates the need for an oxytocin challenge test, as described below.

Stress Test. Uterine contractions can compromise placental blood flow. If there is inadequate placental/fetal respiratory reserve, the heart rate will change. An oxytocin challenge test is positive if persistent, late fetal heart rate decelerations occur repeatedly with uterine contractions.

Fetal Blood Sampling During Labor. Fetal capillary blood pH is normally 7.25 to 7.45. A pH below 7.2 indicates fetal acidosis.

Fetal Heart Rate. The fetal heart rate monitor is a two-channel recorder that measures fetal heart rate and uterine activity. Monitoring may be direct (fetal ECG obtained from an electrode attached to the presenting part and intrauterine pressure measured by a saline-filled catheter inserted transcervically) or indirect (data obtained from transducers secured to the mother's abdomen). Variables to consider include baseline heart rate, beat-to-beat variability, periodic patterns, and uterine activity.

Fetal Heart Rate Patterns

The characteristics of fetal heart rate patterns are divided into baseline and periodic features (Fig. 182–1).

Figure 182–1. Normal fetal heart rate pattern and rate (upper trace) and uterine contractions (lower trace). No periodic changes. Paper speed, 3 cm/min.

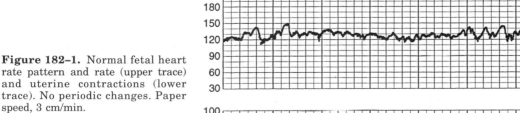
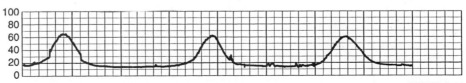

CM161514L.01

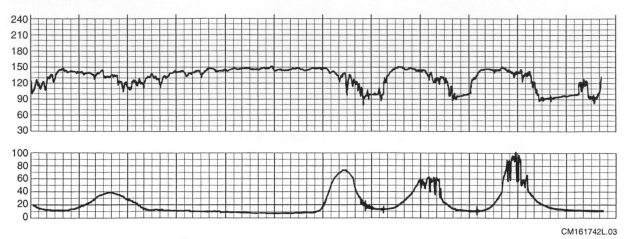

CM161742L.03

Figure 182–2. A previously normal tracing with late decelerations that develop with hypotension. Note that normal variability is maintained. Paper speed, 3 cm/min.

The baseline rate (measured between contractions) is normally 120 to 160 beats/min. Values above or below this range may indicate fetal asphyxia. Baseline variability is normal if the amplitude range is greater than 6 beats/min.

There are three major patterns of fetal heart rate deceleration: early, late, and variable.

Early Decelerations. Early decelerations occur with uterine contractions and are the mirror image of the contraction. They are vagal in origin, and typically less than a 20-beat/min decrease occurs.

Late Decelerations. Late decelerations (Fig. 182–2) occur after termination of the contraction. There are two types of late decelerations. **Reflex late deceleration** occurs when a normally oxygenated fetus experiences a decrease in uterine blood flow and thus insufficient oxygen supply. This results in a transient "late" vagal response due to the circulation time from the placenta to the chemoreceptors. Between contractions, oxygen supply is adequate, and fetal heart rate is normal. This type of late deceleration is accompanied by normal fetal heart rate variability, signifying satisfactory cerebral oxygenation. **Direct myocardial hypoxic depression** occurs with decreased uterine blood flow, with insufficient placental blood to support myocardial function. There is also concomitant vagal activity as chemoreceptors detect low oxygen tension. This type of late deceleration is typically seen with more prolonged asphyxia, preeclampsia, or intrauterine growth retardation. Fetal heart rate variability is decreased or absent, which implies inadequate fetal cerebral and myocardial oxygenation.

Variable Decelerations. Decelerations (Fig. 182–3) vary in duration and appearance but are abrupt in onset and termination. The reflex vagal activity is secondary to insufficient umbilical blood flow from cord compression. Variable decelerations are classified as mild, moderate, or severe depending on the severity of fetal bradycardia and duration of the decelerations.

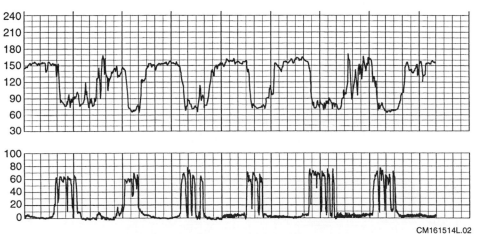

Figure 182–3. Variable decelerations. Note that normal variability is maintained between contractions. Paper speed, 3 cm/min.

CM161514L.02

Suggested References

Barash PG, Cullen BF, Stoelting RK, eds. Clinical Anesthesia. 3rd ed. Philadelphia, Lippincott-Raven, 1997.

Leavett KA. Anesthesia and the Compromised Fetus. In Norris MC, ed. Obstetric Anesthesia. 2nd ed. Philadelphia: Lippincott Williams & Wilkins, 1999:619–640.

Parer JT. Diagnosis and management of fetal asphyxia. In Shnider SM, Levinson G, eds. Anesthesia for Obstetrics. 2nd ed. Baltimore: Williams & Wilkins, 1987:474.

183
Analgesia for Cesarean Section

K.A. Kelly McQueen, M.D.

Cesarean section (C/S) is the most commonly performed operation during pregnancy. Up to 20% of parturients undergo C/S. The anesthetic implications for both mother and fetus are significant and must be carefully considered.

Preoperative Evaluation

Maternal evaluation and surgical consent are essential before anesthesia administration. Along with standard preoperative evaluation, information regarding fetal gestation and pregnancy-related complications should be ascertained. Laboratory studies are obtained as maternal disorders dictate. Preparation for elective, urgent, and emergent C/S includes aspiration prophylaxis and adequate venous access (Table 183–1).

Regional Anesthesia

Subarachnoid block (SAB) and epidural anesthesia (EA) are recommended for elective C/S. When compared with general anesthesia, these techniques provide excellent anesthesia, prevent fetal depression and maternal airway management difficulties, and do not place the mother at risk for aspiration of gastric contents. Local anesthetics, with or without the addition of opioid, may be used for either SAB (Table 183–2) or EA (Table 183–3).

Before initiating neuraxial regional anesthesia, adequate hydration must be given to prevent maternal hypotension and uteroplacental insufficiency. Hypotensive episodes are ideally treated with an **indirect-acting sympathomimetic** (e.g., intravenous ephedrine, titrated to effect).

Regardless of anesthetic technique used, patients should be positioned to provide left uterine displacement to prevent **aortocaval syndrome**.

Emergent or Urgent Cesarean Section

Emergency C/S is a constant threat during labor. An operating room set up for a "crash" induction must always be available. Time is critical to ensure delivery of a healthy fetus. Although general anesthesia is usually the most expedient option for a true emergency situation, regional anesthesia may be a viable option provided that fetal heart rate (FHR) returns to normal after resuscitation efforts (e.g., repositioning, supplemental oxygen, sympathomimetics, intravenous fluids). Communicating these issues to the obstetric team is of paramount importance.

If general anesthesia is required, rapid-sequence induction (Table 183–4) with cricoid pressure should be initiated after sterile abdominal preparation and draping. The surgical team is notified that they can safely proceed as soon as proper endotracheal tube placement is confirmed. Maintenance with low-concentration volatile anesthetic (e.g., isoflurane or sevoflurane), 50% O_2, and N_2O is used until the umbilical cord has been clamped and the neonate is safely delivered. Nondepolarizing muscle relaxants may be given once motor endplate function has recovered from the effects of succinylcholine. After the umbilical cord is clamped, narcotics may be administered with no concern about neonatal respiratory depression. In addition, midazolam is often administered at this time to prevent recall while allowing for a lower dose of volatile anesthetic (i.e., drugs known to relax uterine smooth muscle), thereby decreasing the risk of uterine hypotonia

Table 183–1. Maternal Preparation for Cesarean Section

Type and screen (when indicated)
Large-bore intravenous access (18 or 16 g) × 2
Metoclopramide (Reglan), 10 mg
Sodium citrate (Bicitra), 30 mL

Table 183–2. Drugs for Subarachnoid Block

Bupivacaine, 12 to 15 mg
Fentanyl, 20 µg and/or morphine 0.2–20 mg

Table 183–3. Drugs for Epidural Anesthesia

3% Chloroprocaine, 20 mL
0.5% Bupivacaine, 20 mL
2% Lidocaine*, 20 mL
Fentanyl, 50 μg and/or morphine, 2 mg

*Epinephrine and bicarbonate may be added to lidocaine.

Table 183–4. Rapid-Sequence Induction

Continuous cricoid pressure
Sodium thiopental, 3 mg/kg or propofol, 1 mg/kg
Succinylcholine, 1.5 mg/kg

and persistent uterine bleeding. Following delivery of the placenta, oxytocin (Pitocin, 20 to 40 IU in 1 L of crystalloid solution) may be given to facilitate uterine contractions. If hypotonia persists, Pitocin (as a slow intravenous push) or methylergonovine (Methergine, 0.2 mg intramuscularly) may be given. Both Pitocin and Methergine produce hemodynamic consequences (see Chap. 180).

If the obstetrician is concerned about maternal infection, antibiotics may be given at this time. Time of delivery and APGAR scores should be noted on the anesthetic record. Following surgery, the pa-tient should not be extubated until awake to mini-mize the ongoing risk of aspiration.

Suggested References

Dahl JB, Jeppesen IS, Jorgensen H, et al. Intraoperative and postoperative analgesic efficacy and adverse effects of intrathe-cal opioids in patients undergoing cesarean section with spinal anesthesia. Anesthesiology 1999;91:1919–1927.

Reisner LS, Lin D. Anesthesia for cesarean section. In Chestnut DH, ed. Obstetric Anesthesia: Principles and Practice. 2nd ed. St. Louis: CV Mosby, 1999;465–492.

Shnider SM, Levinson G. Anesthesia for cesarean section. In Shnider SM, Levinson G, eds. Anesthesia for Obstetrics. 3rd ed. Baltimore: Williams & Wilkins, 1993;211–245.

184
Neonatal Resuscitation

Robert V. Johnson, M.D. □ Glenn E. Woodworth, M.D.

At least one person skilled in newborn resuscitation should be present at every birth. Fortunately, most newborns will require only assessment, drying, suctioning, and sometimes bag and mask assistance.

First Steps for Every Newborn

□ Review the maternal history to identify possible risks to the newborn. Is there a risk of sepsis? Is the infant likely to be hypotonic from maternal medications or because of a prolonged labor? Has fetal monitoring predicted a problem? Will the baby be born prematurely?
□ Check the equipment. Do not just assume that it has been stocked properly.
□ Immediately after delivery, place the newborn under radiant heat on a prewarmed mattress. Dry the infant promptly, taking care to remove wet towels from the infant.
□ Next, assess the newborn's response to the ABCs of resuscitation–airway, breathing, and circulation (Fig. 184–1).

Airway

A relatively large cranial occiput and molded head shape (following vaginal delivery) typically hinders placing the newborn in the sniffing position. Placing a rolled washcloth behind the neck or shoulders helps ensure proper positioning.

Suction the mouth, then the nose. If the newborn is sufficiently depressed to require assisted ventilation, or if thick meconium is present in the amniotic fluid, then prompt tracheal intubation is indicated. In the setting of thick meconium, the endotracheal tube is used to facilitate tracheal suctioning.

Once the airway is clear, assess the newborn's breathing. At this point, it is tempting to assess the heart rate, but irrespective of heart rate, if the newborn's color is poor or if breathing efforts seem inadequate, the next step is to assist breathing.

Breathing

If the newborn has good respiratory effort, proceed to checking the heart rate and color. Mask ventilation will be necessary if breathing efforts are poor or absent. You have already stimulated the baby earlier when drying, so further stimulation efforts may only delay ventilatory assistance. Recheck the head position and give several positive pressure breaths by mask. After giving effective breaths at a rate of **40 to 60 breaths/min** for 15 to 30 seconds, assess heart rate.

Circulation

Check the heart rate with a stethoscope or by feeling the base of the umbilical cord. In all cases in which the heart rate is below 100 beats/min, effective positive-pressure ventilation should be initiated or continued.

□ If the heart rate is above 100 beats/min, assess color. If central cyanosis is present, give supplemental oxygen with a FiO_2 of 80% to 100%.
□ If the heart rate is between 60 and 100 beats/min, continue assisting ventilation for another 30 seconds, then recheck the heart rate.
□ If the heart rate now exceeds 80 beats/min or appears to be rapidly increasing, continue positive-pressure ventilation and watch for improvement in heart rate and color and the onset of spontaneous respirations.
□ If the heart rate is remains below 80 beats/min and is not increasing, initiate chest compressions and proceed as described below.
□ If the heart rate is below 60 beats/min, continue assisting ventilation and begin chest compressions at **100 compressions/min**. Recheck the heart rate every 30 seconds. Continue chest compressions until the heart rate exceeds 80 beats/min. If the heart rate remains below 80 beats/min, the infant should be intubated and given an intratracheal dose of epinephrine, and preparations should be made for umbilical venous catheter placement.

Intubation

Indications for intubation include inadequate or absent respiratory effort, the necessity for pro-

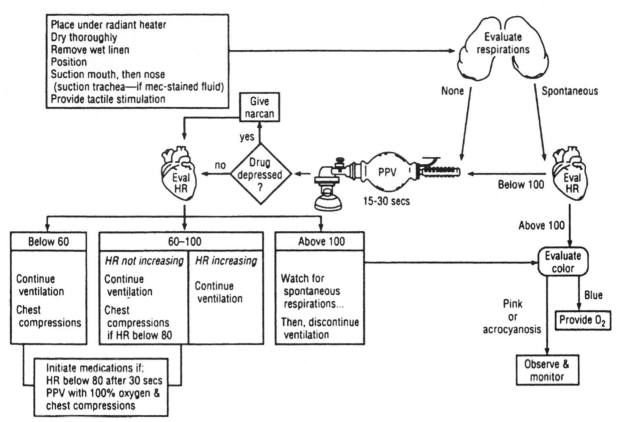

Figure 184–1. An overview of steps in neonatal resuscitation. (From Bloom RS, Cropley C.[1])

longed positive-pressure ventilation, ineffective mask ventilation, the need for repeat tracheal suctioning, or the presence of diaphragmatic hernia. A good tip is to ask for the suction catheter as you begin the intubation attempt. Because you will usually need suctioning for visualization, do not wait until the laryngoscope is in place to realize that you need the suction catheter.

A common tendency is to insert the ET tube too far. The centimeter marking at the lip will usually approximate the baby's weight in kg plus 6 (i.e., a 3-kg baby has an ET tube inserted to 9, at the lips) (Table 184–1).

Medications

If a newborn needs a medication urgently, epinephrine can be given intratracheally. Other medi-

cations will either require parenteral access (typically an umbilical venous line) or are not urgent.

Epinephrine

□ Indications: Asystole or bradycardia with a heart rate below 80 beats/min despite 30 seconds of chest compressions.
□ Dose: 0.01 to 0.03 mg/kg of a 1:10,000 solution (0.1 to 0.3 mL/kg). Repeat every 5 minutes as needed.
□ Route: IV or via endotracheal tube.

Naloxone

□ Indications: Maternal history of narcotics less than 4 hours before delivery and evidence of respiratory depression in the newborn.
□ Dose: 0.1 mg/kg (much lower doses were suggested in the past).
□ Preparations: 0.4 mg/mL (Note that at least two other preparations are available; check the dose before administration.)
□ Route: preferably via IV or endotracheal tube; alternatively, IM or SC.

Bicarbonate

□ Indications: Prolonged arrest not responding to other therapy.

Table 184–1. Approximate Endotracheal Tube Sizes Determined by Weight and Gestational Age

Tube Size	Lip to Midtrachea Length (cm)	Weight (g)	Weeks
2.5	7	<1000	28
3.0	8	1000–2000	28–34
3.5	9	2000–3000	34–38
4.0	10	>3000	>38

□ Dose: 2 mEq/kg of a 0.5 mEq/mL solution delivered no faster than 2 minutes. (The preparation is one-half of the adult concentration.)

Volume Expander

□ Indications: Signs of hypovolemia or acute bleeding. Use normal saline, 5% albumin, lactated Ringer's solution, or type O-negative blood crossmatched with mother.
□ Dose: 10 mL/kg given over 5 to 10 minutes.

Next Steps in Resuscitation

Newborns requiring resuscitation at birth should be subsequently observed and monitored. Final tasks are to document the details of resuscitation in the newborn's chart and arrange for ongoing care in the nursery or intensive care unit.

Typically, such infants will at least be observed with a saturation monitor and have the blood glucose level checked within 30 to 60 minutes following birth. The baby's caregivers will make an assessment of sepsis risk and decide whether antibiotics are indicated.

Selected References

1. Bloom RS, Cropley C. Textbook of Neonatal Resuscitation. Dallas, American Heart Association and the American Academy of Pediatrics, 1994.

Suggested References

Shnider SM, Levinson G. Anesthesia for Obstetrics. 3rd ed. Baltimore, Williams & Wilkins, 1993.

185
Peripartum Hemorrhage

Steven H. Rose, M.D. □ K.A. Kelly McQueen, M.D.

Despite advances in obstetric care and improved diagnostic testing, peripartum hemorrhage remains a leading cause of maternal morbidity and mortality. Severe bleeding is most common in the third trimester of pregnancy and near the time of delivery.

Antepartum Hemorrhage

Severe antepartum hemorrhage is most commonly associated with placenta previa, abruptio placentae, and uterine rupture.

Placenta Previa. Placenta previa is defined as abnormal implantation of the placenta on the lower uterine segment with partial to complete occlusion of the internal cervical os. It is the leading cause of third trimester maternal hemorrhage (1 in 200 pregnancies) and is associated with maternal mortality of up to 0.9%. The multiparous patient is at greater risk, as are patients undergoing repeat cesarean section (C/S). The incidence of recurrence in a subsequent pregnancy is approximately 5%. Other risk factors include older age and multiparity.

Placental Abruption. Placental abruption results from separation of a normally implanted placenta after 20 weeks gestation and before birth. It occurs in 0.2% to 2.4% of pregnant women. Maternal mortality is 1.8% to 2.8%, and fetal mortality may be as high as 50%. Risk factors include hypertensive disorders, high parity, uterine abnormalities, history of previous abruption, and intravenous drug abuse. Bleeding may be revealed (external) or concealed (internal) and varies in severity from mild (<100 mL) to severe (>500 mL).

With intrauterine fetal death, disseminated intravascular coagulation (DIC) may occur within 8 hours. The type of delivery and the timing will depend on the severity. With limited blood loss, vaginal delivery is often possible. If the mother or fetus is in distress, then rapid delivery by C/S is required. In moderate abruptions with fetal death, coagulation must be evaluated before regional anesthetic administration because of the associated risk of DIC.

Uterine Rupture. Uterine rupture is a rare but serious cause of hemorrhage occurring in 0.1% to 0.3% of pregnancies. Risk factors include previous uterine surgery, past history of uterine rupture, abnormal fetal presentation, operative vaginal delivery, use of uterotonic agents, and uterine distention. Maternal mortality approaches 5%, and fetal mortality is as high as 50%. Presenting signs and symptoms include atypical abdominal pain, shoulder pain, vaginal bleeding, uterine tenderness, hypovolemia, and shock.

Anesthetic Management

Anesthetic management includes ensuring the availability of blood and blood products and securing adequate venous access through placement of large-bore central and/or peripheral cannulas. If an emergency cesarean section is required, general anesthesia is usually recommended because of maternal intravascular hypovolemia, positioning problems during regional anesthetic administration, and surgical urgency.

When possible, before C/S all efforts should be made to stabilize the mother while maintaining uterine perfusion pressure (uterine arterial pressure minus uterine venous pressure) and maximizing oxygenation. If time permits, maternal laboratory evaluation, including platelets, prothrombin time, activated partial thromboplastin time, fibrinogen level, and hemoglobin, should be ordered. If maternal hemodynamic status is stable and coagulation status is normal, then regional anesthesia can be used for the urgent C/S.

Postpartum Hemorrhage

The vast majority of cases of severe postpartum hemorrhage occur within a few minutes after delivery. Postpartum hemorrhage is the most common severe hemorrhage in obstetrics and is typically defined as blood loss of 500 mL or more within 24 hours of delivery. Postpartum hemorrhage can be massive and sudden and may require aggressive therapy.

The three most common causes of postpartum hemorrhage are uterine atony, genital tract disruption, and retained placenta and membranes (Table 185–1).

Table 185–1. Causes of Peripartum Hemorrhage

Antepartum Hemorrhage	Postpartum Hemorrhage
Placenta previa	Uterine atony
Placental abruption	Retained placenta
Uterine rupture	Placenta acreta
Vasa previa	Uterine inversion
	Genital trauma

Table 185–2. General Anesthesia for Emergency C/S for Maternal Hemorrhage (see Chapter 183)

Nonparticulate oral antacid
Two large-bore IVs
Replace blood loss with crystalloids, colloids
Blood crossmatched for 2 units
Rapid infusion blood warming device
Preoxygenate
Ongoing fluid resuscitation
Rapid-sequence induction
Provide cricoid pressure
Induction agent:
    Etomidate (0.3 mg/kg)
    Thiopental (3 mg/kg)
    Ketamine (1 mg/kg)
Succinylcholine (1.5 mg/kg)

Uterine Atony. Uterine atony of varying severity commonly occurs after vaginal delivery. Blood loss can be massive and sudden and is sometimes delayed for several hours. Risk factors include multiple births, polyhydramnios, intrauterine manipulation, and retained placenta. Specific treatments include uterine massage and pharmacologic therapy.

Genital Tract Disruption. Genital tract disruption may result in severe postpartum hemorrhage. Lacerations may occur in the vagina, cervix, or body of the uterus. Episiotomy incision is another possible source of bleeding. Vigilance must be maintained after delivery, as blood loss may be delayed.

Retained Placenta and Membranes. The placenta and membranes are retained in about 1% of vaginal deliveries. Treatment usually includes manual exploration of the uterus that may require treatment to provide uterine relaxation. Commonly used agents to facilitate exploration include intravenous nitroglycerin, sedation with ketamine or narcotics, low doses of volatile anesthetics, or induction of general anesthesia.

Treatment of Postpartum Hemorrhage

Treatment is similar to that for antepartum hemorrhage. Early diagnosis and aggressive treatment are important to decrease maternal mortality and morbidity. After the diagnosis is established, large-bore intravenous access should be secured as soon as possible. Preparations should be made for massive transfusion, including adequate supplies of crystalloids, colloids, and blood. Blood warmers should be used to prevent hypothermia. Invasive hemodynamic monitoring, including arterial catheterization and central venous pressure monitoring, should be considered (Table 185–2).

Once circulatory support is established and the above-mentioned conservative means have failed, a **surgical approach** may be necessary to control the bleeding. Surgical approaches include bilateral hypogastric artery ligation (HAL), bilateral ovarian artery ligation, uterine artery ligation, and hysterectomy. In rare cases emergency hysterectomy is required to treat postpartum hemorrhage.

Selected References

1. Mayer DC, Spielman FJ. Antepartum and postpartum hemorrhage. In Chestnut DH, ed. Obstetric Anesthesia Principles and Practice, 2nd ed. St. Louis, Mosby, 1999:725–748.
2. Biehl DR. Antepartum and postpartum hemorrhage. In Shnider SM, Levinson G, eds. Anesthesia for Obstetrics. 3rd ed. Baltimore, Williams & Wilkins, 1993:385–394.

186
Type, Screen, and Crossmatch

Ronald J. Faust, M.D.

Type

Type refers to determining ABO group and Rh type.

□ ABO grouping (Table 186–1) is determined by two methods: directly by mixing patient red blood cells (RBCs) from a patient with reagent antisera or reversing the procedure and mixing patient serum with known A or B cells.
□ Rh typing uses the direct method with reagent anti-D and patient cells.

Screen

Antibody screen describes the detection of abnormal red cell antibodies to clinically significant antigens (Fig. 186–1). There are over 600 RBC antigens, but only a few have been implicated in hemolytic transfusion reactions. Antibodies to D, C, E, c, e, M, N, S, s, Pi, Le^a, Le^b, K, K, Fy^a, Fy^b, JK^a, and JK^b are among those regarded as clinically significant. Anti-A and anti-B are the only naturally occurring antibodies, arising early in infancy in response to A and B substances ubiquitous in nature.

Method. Commercially prepared group O RBCs are used for testing recipient serum (see Fig. 186–1). These cells come from two donors selected to contain between them all blood group antigens capable of causing hemolytic transfusion reactions. Recipient serum is mixed with these cells, centri-

fuged, and then remixed by tapping the tubes to determine whether agglutination has occurred. If no agglutination is observed with either RBC test cell in this "first phase," then the cells are incubated at 20°C and 37°C with and without albumin and other means to enhance the reaction. The entire antibody screen, including the incubation steps, takes 45 minutes. If agglutination is still not observed, then the screen is considered negative and the recipient has no clinically significant abnormal antibodies. The agglutination test is more than 100 years old; it detects a reaction taking place at the molecular level but can be interpreted with only test tubes, a centrifuge, and the necessary reagents.

Antibody Identification

If the screen test result is positive, the recipient's serum is then mixed with a panel of 10 donors' RBCs to identify the antibody(ies) present (Fig. 186–2). These RBCs have been previously typed for all clinically significant antigens. The pattern of

Type and Screen

Type: Recipient cells typed for ABO and Rh antigens

Screen:

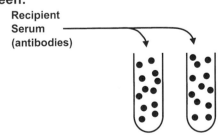

Recipient Serum (antibodies)

Screening red cells are from 2 donors. D, c, E, e, K, Duffy, Kell, Kidd, and all other clinically relevant antigens are known to be present on one or the other's RBCs.

Figure 186–1. The antibody screen is done using patient sera and RBCs selected from two donors commercially. The two donors are known to have (on one or the other) all clinically relevant antigens. See the text for details on the method used.

Table 186–1. ABO Group Frequencies

ABO Group	Frequency (%) in U.S. Population			
	Whites	*Blacks*	*American Indians*	*Orientals*
O	45	49	79	40
A	40	27	16	28
B	11	20	4	27
AB	4	4	<1	5

Adapted from American Association of Blood Banks Technical Manual.[1]

451

Antibody Identification

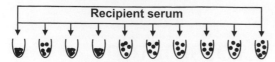

Recipient serum

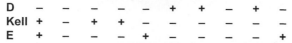

RBCs from 10 donors who have been typed for
all common antigens as below

D	–	–	–	–	–	+	+	–	+	–
Kell	+	–	+	+	–	–	–	–	–	–
E	+	–	–	–	+	–	–	–	–	+

Immediate spin at room temperature ("1st phase")

Enhance RBC antigen-antibody reactions by
incubation at 22 and 37 degrees with and without
albumin and other media to enhance agglutination
(minimum time 45 minutes)

Figure 186–2. Antibody identification is performed by mixing the recipient's serum with RBCs from 10 donors commercially selected and typed for antigens implicated in hemolytic transfusion reactions. The antigen patterns for only D, Kell, and E are marked with + and – for simplicity in this figure. After an immediate spin, the serum and test RBCs are mixed with albumin and other substances and incubated to enhance any antigen-antibody reactions. Agglutination in the first, third, and fourth tubes, as illustrated, would identify anti-Kell antibody in this recipient's serum.

agglutinations in the 10-cell panel is used to identify the unknown antibody in the recipient's serum.

Crossmatch

"Major" and "minor" are outdated terms referring to the crossmatching of recipient serum against donor cells and recipient cells with donor serum, respectively. The minor crossmatch, testing recipient RBCs against donor serum or plasma, is replaced by the antibody screen performed on donor blood. If the patient recently was pregnant or received a transfusion, crossmatch samples should be less than 2 days old to allow detection of any newly developed antibodies. A patient with a recent transfusion occasionally may develop high titer levels of a previously undetectable antibody when his or her immune system has an anamnestic response. A re-

cent transfusion can trigger rapid redevelopment of the antibody.

Both the crossmatch and the antibody screen take at least 45 minutes because of necessary incubation steps. The first phase combines recipient serum and donor cells to test ABO group compatibility at room temperature. It is also effective for M, N, P, and Lewis incompatibilities. This test takes approximately 5 minutes.

The second phase is undertaken at 37°C. Using the products of the first phase, the resulting mixture is incubated in albumin or low ionic strength saline solution, enhancing weak or incomplete antibodies.

The last phase of the crossmatch is the indirect antiglobulin test, in which Coombs' serum is used to detect any antibodies that might be attached to antigens on the RBC wall.

Incompatibility Risk

Considering only incompatibility risk, it is generally accepted that the risk of a hemolytic transfusion reaction from using ABO- and Rh-compatible "first phase" blood is 0.1% if the recipient has never received a transfusion. Risk will rise to 1.0% if the patient had a previous transfusion. Adding a negative antibody screen increases safety to 99.94%. Fully crossmatched blood should carry an incompatibility risk below 0.05%.

Selected References

1. American Association of Blood Banks Technical Manual. 10th ed. Arlington, VA, American Association of Blood Banks, 1990.

Suggested References

Miller RD. Transfusion therapy. In Miller RD, ed. Anesthesia. 5th ed. Philadelphia: Churchill Livingstone, 2000:1613–1644.
Oberman HA, Barnes BA, Friedman BA. The risk of abbreviating the major crossmatch in urgent or massive transfusion. Transfusion 1978;18:137.
Petz LD. The surgeon and the transfusion service: Essentials of compatibility testing, surgical blood ordering, emergency blood needs, and adverse reactions. In Spiess BD, Counts RB, Gould SA. Perioperative Transfusion Medicine. Baltimore: Williams & Wilkins, 1998:45–59.

187
Red Blood Cell Transfusion

Ronald J. Faust, M.D.

The search for an oxygen-carrying blood substitute has continued for decades, but the transfusion of red blood cells (RBCs) continues to be a necessity. Though commonly referred to as "packed" cells, "red blood cells" is the proper terminology for erythrocytes collected and stored in a number of ways.

RBC Collection and Storage

Whole blood is collected as 450-mL aliquots to which 65 mL of anticoagulant preservative is added. RBCs are formed by centrifugation and removal of the majority of platelets and plasma, leaving a 250-mL volume with a 70% to 80% hematocrit level. Storage temperatures of 1°C to 6°C slow glycolysis and bacterial growth. The FDA requires 70% survival of transfused RBCs at 24 hours. Survival at 24 hours predicts a normal cellular life span.

Biochemical changes during RBC storage include progressive acidosis, increasing plasma potassium levels, and decreasing 2,3-diphosphoglycerate (2,3-DPG) levels. These changes occur in whole blood and "packed" RBCs during storage, but after transfusion, the RBC metabolism quickly restores intracellular potassium levels, and intracellular 2,3-DPG becomes normal within a few hours.

RBC Components

Citrate, Phosphate, Dextrose (CPD). This solution is approved for a 21-day storage limit. Citrate acts as an anticoagulant by binding ionic calcium necessary for clot formation. Dextrose is provided as a substrate for glycolysis.

Citrate, Phosphate, Dextrose, Adenine (CPDA). CPDA solution includes adenine for incorporation into adenosine triphosphate (ATP) and extra glucose for prolonged storage. Storage is approved for 35 days.

Deglycerolized RBCs. CPD-preserved RBCs are combined with glycerol to prevent lysis during the freezing process. After thawing, the cells are "deglycerolized" by washing in saline. Advantages include the ability to store rare blood types, fewer febrile reactions because of the decreased leukocyte content, and preservation of 2,3-DPG. Disadvantages include increased cost and a short (24-hour) expiration time after thawing.

Adsol and Neutricel. These additive solutions increase the storage capabilities and decrease the viscosity of stored RBCs. After 35 days of storage, 88% viability is possible with Adsol. After platelets and plasma are removed from RBCs just after collection from the donor, 100 mL of Adsol, containing dextrose, adenine, mannitol, and NaCl, is added to a unit of CPD-preserved RBCs. Saline and mannitol limit lysis to 1% to 2% or less. The viscosity is close to that of whole blood, and no dilution is required. As with other erythrocyte solutions, dilution with lactated Ringer's solution and D_5W is not recommended because of the risks of clotting and hemolysis, respectively.

Indications for RBC Transfusion

Simple formulas and transfusion "triggers" should not be used when the indications for transfusion are considered. This is a medical decision that must be individualized for each patient.[1] Factors taken into account include current hemoglobin level, estimated blood loss, vital signs, the likelihood of ongoing hemorrhage, and the level of risk of myocardial or cerebral ischemia. The dynamic nature of surgical hemorrhage and the likelihood of ongoing hemorrhage necessitate a more aggressive approach to blood replacement at stages of a procedure where blood loss may increase unpredictably.

The inaccuracy of intraoperative blood loss estimates, even by experienced observers, is well substantiated. Although other intraoperative monitoring techniques are very sophisticated, clinical estimation of intravascular blood volume is done only by indirect measures (blood pressure, central venous pressure, heart rate, pulmonary artery occlusion pressure, urine output).

The chronicity of a patient's anemia affects his or her ability to compensate. Patients with chronic anemias increase 2,3-DPG levels to make oxygen transport more efficient; in acute anemia, cardiovascular mechanisms of compensation (e.g., increased cardiac output, heart rate, myocardial oxygen consumption) are more important.

Serial hemoglobin determinations are usually

helpful intraoperatively, although they do not reflect acute changes in intravascular volume and can be misleading in two situations. Overexpansion of intravascular volume with crystalloid or colloid can produce a relatively low hemoglobin level in a hypervolemic patient, possibly leading to overtransfusion. Alternatively, inadequate administration of crystalloids or an excessive diuresis can lead to a normal or high hemoglobin level in a hypovolemic patient.

Myocardial ischemia is often silent and is not always related to the heart rate and blood pressure. Prospective studies have shown a 41% prevalence of postoperative myocardial ischemia in patients with coronary artery disease undergoing noncardiac surgery.[2] Although medical management (β blockade) is most important for most of these patients, anemia could add to their risk of infarction.

Whole-body oxygen transport can be calculated, but the ability to measure oxygen delivery to specific organs is not possible in the intraoperative setting. Even if it were, what would really be necessary would be a way to measure oxygen transport to discrete regions of the myocardium and brain.

Hemodilution and Anemia

A wealth of literature has been published on the merits of hemodilution. Many anecdotal studies support the widely accepted clinical impression that most patients have no adverse effects and no increased risk when their hemoglobin levels decrease to 10 g/dL. Nevertheless, the concept that rheologic changes improve oxygen transport as hemoglobin decreases to 10 g/dL is based on in vivo studies that might not be applicable to the human microcirculation.[1] Although no suggestion of ischemia was made, a 1992 study reported slight decreases in oxygen transport to the brain in normal, mildly hemodiluted volunteers despite increases in cerebral blood flow.[3]

Although otherwise healthy patients can make extraordinary adaptations to severe anemia, there is evidence that those with cardiovascular and cerebrovascular disease have limited ability to compensate for acute anemia below hemoglobin levels of 8 to 10 g/dL. Weisel and colleagues[4] randomized patients scheduled for coronary artery bypass grafting into two groups, one whose mean hemoglobin level was maintained at 12.1 g/dL postoperatively and a second whose hemoglobin was allowed to drift to a mean of 8.9 g/dL. Sensitive measures of myocardial ischemia demonstrated abnormalities of myocardial metabolism in the group with the lower postoperative hemoglobin levels.

Hemodilution is usually studied in anesthetized or resting subjects in whom all factors that might challenge the cardiovascular system are controlled. Metabolic requirements may increase at any time postoperatively because of pain, fever, or physical activity.

A 1997 review found only six randomized clinical trials that studied the effect of transfusion thresholds on outcomes.[5] All but one were thought to be too small to make significant inferences about clinical outcomes; the sixth studied transfusion in patients with sickle cell disease.

Spiess and colleagues[6] reported on the effect of hematocrit level after coronary artery bypass surgery in a large observational study (2202 patients) in 1998. The patients were divided into groups with high (>34%), medium (25% to 33%), and low (<24%) hematocrit levels on entry into postsurgical intensive care. The group with high hematocrit levels had higher rates of myocardial infarction and severe left ventricular dysfunction. Yet it could be said that the patients in this group were actually overtransfused. Mortality was lowest in the group with medium hematocrit levels.

A 1999 multicenter study by Hébert and colleagues[7] prospectively randomized 838 patients entering intensive care units into a restrictive group who were transfused only when their hemoglobin levels dropped below 7 g/dL and a "liberal transfusion strategy" group who were transfused whenever their hemoglobins dropped below 10 g/dL. A higher in-hospital mortality rate was seen in the group with higher hemoglobins. Because many other parameters were not significantly different, it was concluded that the restrictive transfusion strategy was at least as effective as, and possibly superior to, the liberal transfusion strategy in critically ill patients, with the possible exception of patients with acute myocardial infarction and unstable angina.[7]

Recommendations

□ The American Society of Anesthesiologists (ASA) has approved Practice Guidelines for Blood Component Therapy that condemned the use of a single hemoglobin trigger and said that patient risk should determine whether transfusion is indi-

Table 187–1. ASA Practice Guideline: Indications for RBCs

1. Transfusion is rarely indicated when the hemoglobin is above 10 g/dL and almost always indicated when it is below 6 g/dL.
2. Patient risk determines whether intermediate hemoglobin concentrations (6 to 10 g/dL) necessitate transfusion.
3. The use of a single hemoglobin "trigger," failing to consider all important physiologic and surgical factors affecting oxygenation, is not recommended.
4. Autologous techniques and other measures to decrease blood loss may be beneficial.
5. The indication for transfusing autologous RBCs may be more liberal than that for allogeneic RBCs because of the lower (but still significant) risks associated with the former.

From the American Society of Anesthesiologists.[8]

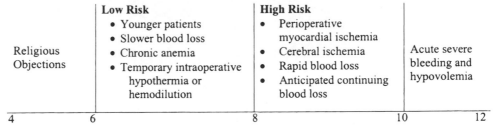

Figure 187–1. Factors affecting the decision whether to transfuse, depicted across a spectrum of severity of anemia. See the text for an explanation.

cated when hemoglobin concentrations are between 6 to 10 g/dL (Table 187–1).[8] Figure 187–1 depicts how patient risks affect the target hemoglobin level or the threshold for transfusion. In patients with severe acute anemia with hemoglobin levels below 6 g/dL, RBCs are withheld only when patients do not consent to transfusion. Low-risk patients with good myocardial reserve can tolerate anemia in the range of 6 to 8 g/dL, as can patients protected by hypothermia and those with chronic anemia. For high-risk patients with acute anemia, transfusion is indicated when the hemoglobin is between 8 and 10 g/dL. The degree of cardiovascular and cerebrovascular disease in the patient influences the medical decision of whether to transfuse for patients in this range. For a patient with hemoglobin above 10 g/dL, acute hypovolemia and hypotension are usually the only indications for transfusion. In acute blood loss and hypovolemia, the hemoglobin can be misleading; restoration of blood volume is more important than hemoglobin concentration in these patients.

Selected References

1. Faust RJ. Perioperative indications for red blood cell transfusion—Has the pendulum swung too far? (Editorial). Mayo Clin Proc 1993;68:512.
2. Mangano DT, Hollenberg M, Fegert G, et al. Perioperative myocardial ischemia in patients undergoing noncardiac surgery. I. Incidence and severity during the 4-day perioperative period. J Am Coll Cardiol 1991;17:843.
3. Hino A, Ueda S, Mizukawa N, et al. Effect of hemodilution on cerebral hemodynamics and oxygen metabolism. Stroke 1992;23:423.
4. Weisel RD, Charlesworth DC, Mickleborough LL, et al. Limitations of blood conservation. J Thorac Cardiovasc Surg 1984;88:26.
5. Hébert PC, Schweitzer I, Calder L, et al. Review of the clinical practice literature on allogeneic red blood cell transfusion. Can Med Assoc J 1997;156:S9–S26.
6. Spiess BD, Ley C, Body SC, et al. Hematocrit value on intensive care unit entry influences the frequency of Q-wave myocardial infarction after coronary artery bypass grafting. J Thorac Cardiovasc Surg 1998;116:460–467.
7. Hébert PC, Wells G, Blajchman MA, et al. A multicenter, randomized clinical trial of transfusion requirements in critical care. N Engl J Med 1999;340:409–417.
8. American Society of Anesthesiologists, Task Force on Blood Component Therapy. Practice guidelines for blood component therapy. Anesthesiology 1996;84:732–747.

188
Massive Transfusion

Scott A. Lockwood, M.D.

Massive transfusion can be defined as the administration of 10 or more units of blood or an amount greater than one blood volume. As blood is stored, it develops a storage lesion that is responsible for many of the complications associated with massive transfusions. During storage, the pH drops, potassium increases, 2,3-diphosphoglycerate (2,3-DPG) decreases, factors V and VIII degrade, platelets are lost, and red blood cells (RBCs) lyse.

Coagulopathies Associated with Massive Transfusion

Large transfusions may be associated with coagulopathies, which can manifest as microvascular bleeding, hematuria, and bleeding from intravenous sites. The differential diagnosis includes dilutional thrombocytopenia; decreased factors V, VIII, and fibrinogen; disseminated intravascular coagulopathy (DIC); preoperative coagulation defects; and hemolytic transfusion reactions. If a coagulopathy is suspected, then the diagnosis should be confirmed with laboratory data, including prothrombin time (PT), activated partial thromboplastin time (APTT), platelet count, fibrin split products, and thromboelastography, if available. These studies may help to differentiate the cause of a coagulopathy when one is clinically evident (Table 188–1 and Fig. 141–2). Elevation of the PT and aPTT by themselves is common during large transfusions; abnormal laboratory values by themselves are not an indication

for prophylactic transfusion of fresh frozen plasma and platelets.

Dilutional thrombocytopenia is the most common cause of abnormal bleeding associated with massive transfusions. In chronic thrombocytopenia, spontaneous bleeding may not occur until the platelet count drops below 10×10^9/L. However, in acute dilutional thrombocytopenia with clinical evidence of a coagulopathy, it is recommended that platelet counts be kept above 100×10^9/L. Abnormal bleeding responds to platelet transfusions; each unit of platelet concentrate usually increases platelet count by about 10,000/unit. Clinical studies have failed to show any efficacy for prophylactic administration of platelets.

Factors V and VIII may be decreased after large transfusions. Factors V and VIII decrease significantly in stored blood. But because only 20% of factor V and 30% of factor VIII are needed for hemostasis, deficiencies of these factors are the cause of bleeding less often than deficiencies of platelets in trauma cases. Prophylactic administration of fresh frozen plasma has been shown to be ineffective in decreasing the incidence of coagulopathies developing during massive transfusions.

Laboratory findings in **DIC** include decreased fibrinogen, thrombocytopenia, prolonged PT and APTT, and the presence of fibrin split products. The maximum amplitude is decreased and the reaction time prolonged on the thromboelastograph. Treatment involves replacing consumed blood products and directly treating the cause of DIC.

Hemolytic transfusion reactions may cause

Table 188–1. Laboratory Evaluation of Intraoperative Coagulopathy

Test	Dilutional Thrombocytopenia	Clotting Factor Deficiencies	Disseminated Intravascular Coagulation	Platelet Function Disorder	Circulating Heparin
Platelet count	Low		Low		
PT, aPTT		High	High		High
Fibrinogen level		Low	Low		
Fibrin split products			Present		
Thromboelastography	Low maximum amplitude	Prolonged reaction time	Prolonged reaction time and low maximum amplitude	Low maximum amplitude	Extremely prolonged reaction time

abnormal bleeding. Cardinal signs in patients under general anesthesia include hemoglobinuria, hypotension, tachycardia, and excessive bleeding or oozing. Clinical complications are caused by renal vascular ischemia and DIC. Laboratory findings include decreased serum haptoglobin, elevated serum and urine hemoglobin, and a positive Coombs test.

Other Complications

Citrate toxicity is caused by accumulation of citrate anticoagulant, which binds calcium and magnesium. Thus, symptoms include those of hypocalcemia, including hypotension, narrow pulse pressure, increased left ventricular end-diastolic pressure and central venous pressure, and a prolonged QT interval on the electrocardiogram (ECG). Hypomagnesemia is often overlooked following massive transfusions and is associated with tachyarrhythmias, torsades de pointes, and refractory ventricular fibrillation. Patients with normal hepatic and renal function who are normothermic and well perfused metabolize citrate rapidly via the Krebs cycle and rarely exhibit toxicity unless blood is transfused very rapidly (>150 mL/min to an adult). Because calcium levels return to pretransfusion levels very quickly after the transfusion is stopped, routine administration of calcium is not recommended. Pediatric patients and those with liver disease and hypothermia are more likely to develop hypocalcemia. ECG changes are not an accurate indication of the need for calcium, but hypocalcemia should be suspected any time that decreased myocardial contractility is suspected during a rapid transfusion.

Acid-base abnormalities, including metabolic acidosis or (more frequently) metabolic alkalosis, may be associated with large transfusions. Blood stored with Adsol anticoagulant preservative solution has a pH of 6.5 after 35 days because of the low pH of the citrate anticoagulant and the progressive erythrocyte metabolism that forms lactic and pyruvic acids. The PCO_2 of stored blood is 150 to 200 mm Hg because of the plastic RBC container's impermeability to CO_2. All of these factors can potentially cause metabolic acidosis. Metabolic alkalosis more commonly results from the conversion of citrate to bicarbonate. Treatment of acid-base abnormalities should be based on frequent arterial blood gas results. Routine administration of bicarbonate is not advised.

Stored blood is associated with progressive reduction of erythrocyte 2,3-DPG, causing a **leftward shift of the oxygen-hemoglobin dissociation curve**. Hypothermia and alkalosis can accentuate this shift, making tissue hypoxia a possibility. However, tissue hypoxia from decreased 2,3-DPG is not considered a significant clinical problem, because 2,3-DPG levels return to normal within hours after RBCs are transfused.

Transfusion of blood products stored at 4°C can rapidly cause hypothermia. This can lead to coagulopathy in itself. If temperature falls to near 30°C, ventricular irritability or cardiac arrest may occur. Postoperative shivering can increase myocardial oxygen consumption by up to 400%. Hypothermia during massive transfusion should be prevented by using blood warmers.

Electrolyte abnormalities are theoretical problems associated with blood transfusions. Potassium is elevated in stored blood (up to 26 mEq/L), causing hyperkalemia if transfused rapidly. However, hyperkalemia is usually not seen for the following reasons: (1) the volume of plasma in each unit of RBCs is small; (2) RBCs quickly regain metabolic activity after transfusion, which activates Na–K pumps to move potassium intracellularly; (3) a dilutional effect occurs with large transfusions; and (4) elevated catecholamine levels draw the ions intracellularly. Hypokalemia is in fact a more common phenomenon associated with large transfusions.

Infection from blood products is a risk with transfusions. Hepatitis C accounts for more than 90% of post-transfusion hepatitis. Each unit of fresh frozen plasma or platelets has the same risk of infection as RBCs. Other infections that can be transmitted through transfusion include human immunodeficiency virus, Epstein-Barr virus, cytomegalovirus, brucellosis, malaria, salmonellosis, and measles (see Chap. 189).

Suggested References

Counts RB, Haisch C, Simon TL, et al. Hemostasis in massively transfused trauma patients. Ann Surg 1979;190:91.

Faust RJ. Transfusion medicine. In Wedel DJ, ed. Orthopedic Anesthesia. New York: Churchill Livingstone, 1993:15.

Kulpmann WR, Rademacher E, Bornscheuer A. Ionized magnesium concentration during liver transplantation, resection of the liver and cardiac surgery. Scand J Clin Lab Invest 1996;56:235–243.

Miller RD. Complications of massive blood transfusions. Anesthesiology 1979;39:82.

Murray DJ, Olson J, Strauss R, et al. Coagulation changes during packed red cell replacement of major blood loss. Anesthesiology 1988;69:839.

Reed RL II, Ciavarella D, Heimbach DM, et al. Prophylactic platelet administration during massive transfusion. Ann Surg 1986;203:40.

189

Infectious Transfusion Risks

Ronald J. Faust, M.D.

Post-transfusion infection rates reached astounding levels in the late 1960s. For example, before the hepatitis B virus (HBV) was identified, the risk of post-transfusion hepatitis was as high as 20%. Non-A, non-B hepatitis infection rates remained at 7% to 11% until this virus was later identified as hepatitis C virus (HCV). Since 1990, routine screening has drastically reduced the risk of HCV infection. Although worrisome, the risk of transfusion-related hepatitis has not triggered public alarm or affected transfusion practices to the extent that acquired immune deficiency syndrome (AIDS) epidemic has done.

Human Immunodeficiency Virus

It is estimated that as many as 30,000 individuals received human immunodeficiency virus (HIV)-positive blood before the screening that began in 1985. Because the viral latency period lasts up to 7 years, most of these persons died of other causes before developing clinical AIDS. Data from the Centers for Disease Control and Prevention cited 8806 transfusion-associated AIDS cases through June 1999.[1] An additional 5243 AIDS cases have been reported in persons with hemophilia and other clotting disorders.

A patient expressing concern about the risk of acquiring AIDS from blood transfusion should be reassured that the current estimated risk is extremely low, approximately 1 in 493,000 (Table 189–1).[2] This is a far lower incidence than many other risks associated with surgery. Unfortunately, it has been impossible to eliminate the risk of transfusion-associated AIDS because of the "window period"

(i.e., the time interval between viral exposure and detectable serologic titer level). This window is currently estimated to be 22 days with HIV antibody testing. Testing for the p24 antigen could reduce the window period to 16 days.

Hepatitis

The frequency of hepatitis is noted in Table 189–1. HBV has an incubation period of 60 to 110 days. Chronic carrier and chronic active states, cirrhosis, and hepatocellular carcinoma may develop in individuals infected with HBV. HBV prophylaxis is achieved using a recombinant DNA vaccine. Although HBV is symptomatic in 50% of individuals infected after transfusion, HCV is symptomatic (often presenting as mild lethargy) in less than 10%. Between 50% and 80% of those infected with HCV become chronic carriers and are predisposed to a high incidence of cirrhosis, liver failure, and hepatoma in later years. Although HBV and HCV are primarily transmitted by contaminated needle or transfusion, hepatitis A virus (HAV) is usually transmitted by oral-fecal contamination. Although rare cases of transfusion-associated HAV have been reported, there is no carrier state for this virus. Delta hepatitis (HDV) requires hepatitis B for its expression. Concomitant infection with HBV and HDV is associated with more severe acute infection and a higher mortality rate. Hepatitis G virus (HGV) may be transmitted in up to 10% of transfusion recipients. Despite a high rate of infection, HGV is typically not associated with clinical or laboratory evidence of hepatitis.[3]

Human T-Cell Lymphotropic Virus

Blood donors are screened for human T-cell lymphotropic virus type I (HTLV-I) and type II (HTLV-II). Type I is associated with chronic degenerative neurologic disease, HTLV-I–associated myelopathy (HAM), tropical spastic paraparesis (TSP), and leukemia.[4] The implications of HTLV-II are less clear.

Table 189–1. Transfusion-Transmitted Viral Risks

Virus	Risk per Unit Transfused	Window Period (Days)
HIV	1:493,000	22*
HBV	1:63,000	59
HCV	1:103,000	82
HTLV-I/II	1:641,000	51

*Depends on the testing method; see the text for an explanation.
Adapted from Schrieber GB et al.[1]

Cytomegalovirus

Cytomegalovirus (CMV) is carried by more than 50% of adults. It is so ubiquitous that routine screening of donated blood products for CMV is not performed. The virus poses a particular risk for immunocompromised recipients, such as low-birth-weight infants and transplant recipients. Besides screening for CMV-negative donors, transmission also can be prevented by using leukocyte-reduction filters, because the CMV virus is transmitted with the white blood cells contained in the stored units of blood.

Sepsis

Post-transfusion sepsis is a potentially lethal complication of blood transfusion. Bacterial contamination of blood components may occur at the time of donation and storage. Platelet concentrates pose the greatest risk (as many as 1 in every 2500 platelet concentrates shows evidence of microbial contamination) because they are stored at room temperature.[5] Some pathogens (e.g., *Yersinia enterocolitica*) grow most rapidly at refrigerated temperatures in an iron-rich medium. In addition to hemolytic and febrile reactions, a spiking fever during or after blood transfusion may also point to sepsis. Sepsis can be a risk even from transfusion of autologous blood; deaths from bacterially contaminated predeposited autologous units have been reported.

The Unknown

Although screening is very effective for the currently known blood-borne pathogens, who knows what might evolve next and move quickly through our global village? A newly emerging agent with a long incubation period or an interval of silent infection might not be detected by the current system for blood donor screening. As Klein[5] has stated, "The chance that such an agent might emerge is small but finite, and it is the patient's perception of risk, not that of the physician, the health insurer, or the framer of health policy that we must balance against statistics involving death, disability, and dollars."

Selected References

1. Centers for Disease Control and Prevention. HIV/AIDS Surveillance Report. 1999;11(1):1–42.
2. Schreiber GB, Busch MP, Kleinman SH, et al. The risk of transfusion-transmitted viral infections. N Engl J Med 1996;334:1685–1690.
3. Alter HJ, Nakatsuji Y, Melpolder J, et al. The incidence of transfusion-associated hepatitis G virus infection and its relation to liver disease. N Engl J Med 1997;336:747–754.
4. ASA Committee on Transfusion Medicine: Questions and Answers About Transfusion Practices. 3rd ed. Park Ridge, IL, American Society of Anesthesiologists, 1998.
5. Klein HG. Transfusion safety: Avoiding unnecessary bloodshed. Mayo Clin Proc 2000;75:5–7.

190
Occupational Transmission of Blood-Borne Pathogens

Linda K. Miller, M.D.

Over the last two decades, occupational transmission of blood-borne pathogens has become one of the most significant hazards to health care workers. Although more than 20 known pathogens may be transmitted, human immunodeficiency virus (HIV), hepatitis B virus (HBV), and hepatitis C virus (HCV) are the pathogens most commonly involved in occupational transmission.

Risk of Occupational Transmission of Blood-Borne Pathogens

The risk of occupational transmission of blood-borne pathogens depends on many variables, the most important of which are the type of exposure and the infectivity of the source of exposure. The prevalence of blood-borne pathogen infections in the patient population, the frequency of exposure to blood-borne pathogens, and the health status of the health care worker are also important. An occupational exposure is defined as skin, eye, mucous membrane, or parenteral contact with blood or other potentially infectious materials.

Type of Exposure

The volume of blood transferred is the most significant predictor of the risk of blood-borne pathogen transmission. The highest-risk exposure incident is that of vascular access procedures involving hollow-core needles; it follows that the larger the bore, the greater the risk. Suture needle percutaneous exposures also carry a high risk for transmission of blood-borne pathogens. Mucous membranes, nonintact skin, and prolonged blood contact with intact skin are considered lower-risk incidents. Depth of the exposure incident is also a determinant of the risk, with deep lacerations and intramuscular needlesticks having the highest risk of transmission of blood-borne pathogens.

Infection in Source of Exposure

Transmission of blood-borne pathogen infection following an occupational exposure also depends on the stage of illness/treatment in the source patient, which affects the concentration of the virus in the blood. Concentrations of HIV, HBV, and HCV in the blood are listed in Table 190–1.

Active hepatitis B infection occurs in 19% to 30% of occupational exposures if hepatitis B antigen is present in the source patient. However, more than 60% of such exposed individuals develop serologic evidence of infection, e.g., antibodies to hepatitis B without other evidence of disease. Transmission of hepatitis B infection is below 6% if hepatitis B antigen is negative, although there is serologic evidence of infection in 23% to 37% of such individuals exposed.

Transmission of hepatitis C has been reported in varying studies to range from 1% to 10% of those individuals exposed. At the present time, the risk is estimated at 2% of those exposed. Although most seroconversions after HCV exposure have been related to parenteral exposures, transmission has occurred after blood splash to the conjunctiva.

HIV transmission rates are 0.3% by percutaneous exposure and 0.1% by mucous membrane exposure in prospective studies. Transmission of HIV after blood contact with skin has not been documented in prospective studies. By June 1999, 55 medical workers had contracted documented occupational transmission of HIV; 75% were nurses and laboratory technicians. Of the 55 cases, 47 had percutaneous exposure, 5 had mucocutaneous exposure, 2 had both percutaneous and mucocutaneous exposures, and 1 had an unknown route of exposure.

Table 190–1. Concentration of Virus in Blood

Pathogen	Viral particles/mL of serum or plasma
HBV	10^2–10^8
HCV	10^0–10^6
HIV	10^0–10^3

Prevalence of Blood-Borne Pathogen Infection

The incidence of HBV, HCV, and HIV in hospitalized patients is listed in Table 190–2.[1] Some populations (e.g., patients in urban emergency departments, individuals with a history of injecting illegal drugs and/or homosexual activities) have a higher prevalence of blood-borne pathogen infection.[1] Individuals who received transfusions and/or transplants before 1992 or hemophiliacs who received clotting factor concentrates before 1987 have a high prevalence of HCV infection.

Frequency of Exposure to Blood-Borne Pathogens

The increased frequency of occupational exposure to blood-borne pathogens will increase the risk of transmission. The frequency of exposure can be reduced by ensuring the use of appropriate personal protective equipment, work practices, and safety devices.

Health of the Health Care Worker

The health care worker's overall health status is an important factor in the immune response to an occupational exposure to a blood-borne pathogen. Increasing age and/or a depressed immune system may increase the risk of infection transmission.

Reducing the Risk of Occupational Transmission of Blood-Borne Pathogens

Most occupational exposures and occupational transmission of blood-borne pathogens are preventable. Prevention depends on HBV vaccination, maintenance of **universal precautions**, safe work practices, use of safety devices, and appropriate management of occupational exposures.

Hepatitis B Vaccine

The war against occupational transmission of blood-borne pathogens is being won, at least against HBV infections. In 1983, the CDC estimated that there were 17,000 new occupationally transmitted HBV infections per year. With the implementation of universal precautions and HBV vaccines in the 1980s, this number has been reduced to 400 new occupationally transmitted infections each year. There has been no evidence of acute, chronic, or clinical infection in individuals who have exhibited serologic evidence of antibody response to the HBV vaccine and have subsequently been occupationally exposed to HBV infections. Studies document a decline in antibody, but the vaccine protection persists for at least 12 years, even with an antibody titer below detectable levels. Anamnestic immune response after HBV exposure is the proposed mechanism of continuing protection against HBV infection despite declining antibody titers. Between 95% and 98% of healthy adults develop protective antibody levels after the series of three doses of HBV vaccine, and no schedule for booster doses of the vaccine has been devised.

Universal Precautions

The concept of universal precautions evolved in the 1970s in dialysis units and dental offices, where a decrease in occupational transmission of HBV infections was documented after implementation of universal precautions. Universal precautions require personal protective equipment (i.e., gloves, gown, mask, eye protection) for every patient. In the surgical setting, double-gloving has been shown to reduce the risk of blood contact by 70%. In addition, wearing vinyl or latex gloves has also been shown to reduce the inoculum volume by up to 50% in the event of a needlestick injury.

Safety Devices

Implementation of safety devices, such as IV connecting systems, safety IV catheters, and shielded syringes, have produced dramatic reductions in needlestick injuries. More than 1000 U.S. patents for injury-preventing medical devices have been granted since 1984. It has been estimated that up to 83% of injuries from hollow-bore needles are potentially preventable by use of safer equipment. Implementation of a safety intravenous catheter system reportedly has produced an 84% reduction in device-specific injury rates.

Management of Exposures

The most important risk-reduction technique after exposure to a possible blood-borne pathogen is immediate back-bleeding and washing of the wound. The exposure must be reported as soon as

Table 190–2. Prevalence of Pathogens in Hospitalized Patients

Pathogen	Prevalence (%)
HBV	2.1–4.7
HCV	0.7–12.7
HIV	0.1–14.5

possible to the occupational health service to facilitate initiation of testing of the source patient and implementation of postexposure management for the health care worker, depending on the type of exposure.

In the event of an occupational exposure of a health care worker to HBV infection, the worker's serologic status must be determined promptly. If the health care worker is unvaccinated or has never had serologic evidence of hepatitis B antibody after vaccination, human hepatitis B immune globulin (HBIG) should be administered within 24 to 48 hours. HBIG is only 60% to 75% effective in preventing HBV infection after exposure, however.

Currently there is no recommendation regarding postexposure prophylaxis for individuals who have occupational exposure to HCV infection.

In the event of exposure to HIV infection or a high-risk exposure, postexposure prophylaxis should be initiated within 1 hour of exposure. In 1995, the CDC published a retrospective study showing that prophylaxis with zidovudine after HIV exposure decreased the risk of acquiring HIV by 80%. In addition, zidovudine administered to pregnant women decreased the vertical transmission of HIV to their infants by 68%. There have been observations that antiretroviral therapy can rapidly reduce viral replication early in HIV infection, and animal studies have shown that earlier treatment of HIV infection is more effective than later treatment. In 1996 the CDC published extensive guidelines for postexposure prophylaxis after occupational exposure to HIV; these were revised in May 1998. Treatment depends on the type of exposure to the health care worker and on previous treatment of the source patient. Because of the HIV infection's increasing resistance to drug therapy, a two- to three-drug regimen is used.

An additional risk is the transmission of blood-borne pathogen infection from the health care worker to the patient. Any exposure of the patient to a health care worker's blood requires investigation of the health care worker's status regarding blood-borne pathogens. Transmission of HBV, HCV, and HIV from health care workers to patients has been reported.

Work Practices

Faulty work practices, such as recapping needles and improperly disposing of needles, are common causes of occupational exposure. However, rules do not stop fatigue and human error, and in the long run, better technology will be needed to prevent occupational exposures.

Selected References

1. Lamphear BP. Trends and patterns in the transmission of blood-borne pathogens to health care workers. Epidemiol Rev 1994;16:437–450.

Suggested References

Ippolito G. Prevention, Management and Chemoprophylaxis of Occupational Exposure to HIV. University of Virginia, Charlottesville, International Health Care Worker Safety Center, 1997.

Kelen GD, Green GB, Purcell RH, et al. Hepatitis B and hepatitis C in emergency department patients. N Engl J Med 1992; 326:1399–1404.

Mahoney FJ. Progress toward elimination of hepatitis B virus transmission among health care workers in the U.S. Arch Int Med 1997;157:2601–2605.

Patterson JM, Novak CB, Mackinnon SE, Patterson GA. Surgeon's concern and practices of protection against blood-borne pathogens. Ann Surg 1998;228(2):266–272.

Public Health Service Guidelines for the Management of Health Care Worker Exposures to HIV and Recommendations for Postexposure Prophylaxis. MMWR, May 15, 1998, 47 (No. RR7).

Recommendations For Prevention and Control of Hepatitis C Virus (HCV) Infection and HCV-Related Chronic Diseases. MMWR, October 16, 1998,47 (No. RR19).

Update: Provisional Public Health Service Recommendations for Chemo-prophylaxis After Occupational Exposure to HIV. MMWR, June 7, 1996;45(22):468–472.

U.S. Department of Labor, Occupational Safety and Health Administration. Occupational Exposure to Blood-borne Pathogens—Final Rule. 56 Fed Reg, 64, 004-64, 1982 (December 6, 1991).

191
Autotransfusion

Ronald J. Faust, M.D.

The acquired immunodeficiency syndrome (AIDS) epidemic that started in the 1980s provided the stimulus for the implementation of autotransfusion as an important part of modern transfusion practice. Techniques that had been available for years became frequently used by health care providers and commonly requested by patients. Three methods of autotransfusion are described:

- Preoperative autologous donation (PAD).
- Acute normovolemic hemodilution (ANH).
- Intraoperative autologous transfusion (IAT).

Preoperative Autologous Donation

PAD is the most simple form of autotransfusion and requires the least equipment. Many studies have shown that it is very underused. When done in properly selected patients, PAD can prevent a very high percentage of allogeneic transfusions.

Longer storage periods for liquid-stored red blood cells (RBCs) allow patients to donate three or more units before elective surgery without the need for RBC freezing. Preoperative donations can be collected from patients at the extremes of age. Reports in the literature describe the use of this technique in patients from age 16 months to 91 years. Autologous blood has also been collected from high-risk patients with cardiovascular and other diseases who were monitored noninvasively in a postanesthesia recovery room during and after donation.

Anemia is usually the limiting factor. Patients are usually given supplemental iron therapy between donations, but studies suggest that they come to surgery more anemic, increasing the likelihood for autologous or allogeneic transfusion. Recombinant human erythropoietin (rHuEPO) was found to be an effective means of increasing the amount of blood that can be collected preoperatively,[1] but its cost may outweigh benefits for most patients.

Cost/benefit ratios must be analyzed for many aspects of autologous transfusion. Like other types of autotransfusion, PAD should be used only when there is a significant chance that the patient will need to be transfused in an upcoming procedure. Specific groups of patients undergoing specific procedures should be identified as candidates to use the technique with minimum wastage. Significant effort and money are spent by patients who choose to donate preoperatively. Those caring for these patients should make certain that they are never given allogeneic blood when autologous components are available.

Acute Normovolemic Hemodilution

The ANH technique lowers a patient's hemoglobin level at the start of surgery so that fewer RBCs are wasted in the blood lost intraoperatively and one or more fresh units of the patient's blood are available when needed. Blood is drawn off from a large-bore intravenous catheter or an arterial line and replaced with crystalloid (3:1 ratio) or colloid (1:1 ratio). The patient is monitored closely for hemodynamic changes while the autologous blood is being collected.

For this technique to obviate the need for allogeneic blood, two to four units must be withdrawn from the patient. This produces a significant shift in blood volume, so vital signs must be monitored closely. Serial hemoglobins should be checked during collection. Careful attention must be given to the mixing of the blood and anticoagulant in the collection bags; if a unit clots, it is wasted, increasing the likelihood that the patient will need allogeneic blood to replace surgical losses.

Although normovolemic hemodilution is widely practiced, few data are available to show that it reduces the need for homologous blood. Computer modeling studies predict that it will not work. If the surgical procedure is completed with minimal blood loss, the hemodilution technique has added significant effort to the anesthesia care and some risk to the patient, with no gain. In a surgical procedure involving high blood loss, allogeneic transfusion (although with fewer units) is often unavoidable. Two prospective randomized controlled studies have been performed on ANH. These showed the technique was as good as, but not superior to, other forms of autologous transfusion.

Intraoperative Autotransfusion

Descriptions of IAT, the intraoperative salvage and reinfusion of blood, can be found in medical writings from the early part of the last century. Many devices are available to collect and filter blood from the wound. More sophisticated equipment can also wash the collected RBCs to remove clots, fat, free hemoglobin, procoagulants, and anticoagulants. The latter devices (e.g., Cell Saver; Haemonetics Corp., Braintree, MA) use a continuous-flow centrifuge to pass saline through RBCs as they are collected. Although cell washing should be the ideal way to purify the collected blood, there is little evidence in the literature suggesting that washed autologous blood is better for the patient than blood that is merely filtered.

Intraoperative salvage is the most expensive type of autotransfusion in terms of equipment and personnel, but it can recover large volumes of blood, making it the only autotransfusion technique that might eliminate the need for allogeneic blood when blood loss is great. The equipment's high cost makes it an inappropriate method when little blood loss is expected. In this situation, the use of canister devices that filter collected blood is preferable.

In older autotransfusion devices, when air was contained in a bag of salvaged cells, it was possible to pump the air into a patient after the blood. Patients died from air embolism. Today's devices have alarms to help prevent this disastrous complication.

Table 191–1 lists the risks and contraindications of intraoperative salvage. The technique is contraindicated in the presence of pus or spilled bowel contents. Although most consider it also contraindicated in the presence of malignancy, one series reported no increase in cancer recurrence when an autotransfusion device was used in patients undergoing radical cystectomy for transitional cell carcinoma of the bladder. Cell washing devices remove platelets and coagulation factors from the salvaged blood, but this should present a problem only when at least one blood volume has been retransfused. Antibiotic irrigants and microfibrillar collagen hemostat (Avitene Hemostat) contraindicate the use of intraoperative salvage.

Significant blood loss occurs through pleural and mediastinal drains after cardiac surgery. In some series of orthopedic procedures (total knee arthroplasty), more blood loss has been reported

Table 191–1. Risks and Contraindications of Intraoperative Blood Salvage

Risks
  Coagulation effects
    Dilutional coagulopathy
    Reinfusion of anticoagulant
  Air embolism
Contraindications
  Pus
  Spilled intestinal contents
  Spread of malignancy (controversial)
  Foreign substances in the wound:
    Antibiotic irrigants
    Microfibrillar collagen hemostat (Avitene)

postoperatively than intraoperatively. Blood can be collected in canister devices that filter blood after orthopedic and cardiothoracic procedures. Cell washing can also be performed during or after collection.

Suggested References

American Society of Anesthesiologists, Task Force on Blood Component Therapy. Practice guidelines for blood component therapy. Anesthesiology 1996;84:732–747.

Birkmeyer JD, Goodnough LT, AuBuchon JP, et al. The cost-effectiveness of preoperative autologous blood donation for total hip and knee replacement. Transfusion 1993;33:544–551.

Bryson GL, Laupacis A, Wells GA. Does acute normovolemic hemodilution reduce perioperative allogeneic transfusion? A meta-analysis. Anesth Analg 1998;86:9–15.

Faust RJ. Ineffectiveness of acute normovolemic hemodilution (Letter to the editor). Anesth Analg 1995;81:660.

Faust RJ. Transfusion medicine. In Wedel DJ, ed. Orthopedic Anesthesia. New York: Churchill Livingstone, 1993:15–53.

Gandini G, Franchini M, Bertuzzo D, et al. Preoperative autologous blood donation by 1073 elderly patients undergoing elective surgery: A safe and effective practice. Transfusion 1999;39:174–178.

Klein HG. Transfusion safety: Avoiding unnecessary bloodshed. Mayo Clin Proc 2000;75:5–7.

Monk TG, Goodnough LT, Brecher ME, et al. Acute normovolemic hemodilution can replace preoperative autologous blood donation as a standard of care for autologous blood procurement in radical prostatectomy. Anesth Analg 1997;85:953–958.

Ness PM, Bourke DL, Walsh PC. A randomized trial of perioperative hemodilution versus transfusion of preoperatively deposited autologous blood in elective surgery. Transfusion 1991;31:225–230.

Ness PM, Walsh PC, Zahurak M, et al. Prostate cancer recurrence in radical surgery patients receiving autologous or homologous blood. Transfusion 1992;32:31–36.

Nuttal GA, Santrach PJ, Oliver WC, et al. Possible guidelines for autologous red blood cell donations before total hip arthroplasty based on the surgical blood order equation. Mayo Clin Proc 2000;75:10–17.

Popovsky MA, Thurer RL, Kuo A. Preoperative autologous blood donation. In Spiess BD, Counts RB, Gould SA, eds. Perioperative Transfusion Medicine. Baltimore: Williams & Wilkins, 1998:111–127.

192
Indications and Risks of Platelet Transfusion

Gregory A. Nuttall, M.D.

Platelets are an essential part of the coagulation process. In their resting form, they circulate in a discoid shape. The peripheral zone of the platelet's membrane, the glycocalyx, is rich in glycoproteins whose heads extend into the extracellular space. The tails of these proteins transduce signals into the submembrane zone, causing intracellular enzymes to induce the physical alterations required for platelet activation. Contractile elements cause the platelet to quickly become more spherical, extending long, spiky pseudopods. The platelet undergoes the fundamental functions of adhesion, aggregation, contraction, and secretion. On the biochemical level, cyclooxygenase converts arachidonic acid (AA) to prostaglandin endoperoxides, which are potent stimuli for further platelet aggregation. Thromboxane synthetase converts AA metabolites to thromboxane A_2, a strong vasoconstrictor and platelet agonist.

Preparation and Storage

Platelet concentrate is prepared by centrifugation of freshly drawn donor blood to separate red cells from platelet-rich plasma (PRP). The PRP is then transferred to a satellite bag aseptically, and the two components are immediately recentrifuged at higher revolutions to separate the platelets from the plasma, which is then squeezed off into another satellite bag, leaving platelet concentrate behind. Each unit of platelet concentrate contains 50 mL of plasma and approximately 5.5×10^{10} platelets.

Platelet concentrate is the preferred source of platelets for transfusion, since they provide a more rapid therapeutic effect with less volume than fresh whole blood or PRP. The platelet count of an adult should increase 5000 to 10,000/mm³ for each unit of platelet concentrate transfused. A standard 170-μm filter is recommended for platelet administration.

Platelets are stored at room temperature on racks, which move slowly to increase mixing of the platelet concentrate with oxygen passing through the wall of each platelet pack. New plastics introduced in the mid-1980s increased the shelf life of platelet concentrate by allowing better gas transfer to the contained cells. Platelets infused within 24 hours of being drawn are viable in the blood for up to 8 days. The normal platelet life span is 9 to 11 days in the blood. However, platelets stored at room temperature acquire a storage lesion that impairs hemostatic function for the first few hours following administration of the platelets.

Alternatively, multiple units of platelets can be drawn from a single donor using pheresis techniques. A continuous flow centrifuge is used to separate platelets from plasma and red cells, which are returned to the donor. Although this technique is more costly, its advantages include decreased infectious risk and the capability of selecting compatible platelet donors for patients with antiplatelet antibodies.

Indications

Table 192–1 summarizes the indications for platelet concentrate listed in the American Society of Anesthesiologists' Guidelines for Perioperative Transfusion Therapy. Patients with abnormal platelet function or thrombocytopenia are likely to benefit from administration of platelet transfusions if the platelet disorder is thought to induce or aggra-

Table 192–1. Indications for Platelet Transfusion

Prophylactic platelet transfusion is ineffective when thrombocytopenia is due to increased platelet destruction.

Platelet transfusion is rarely indicated in surgical patients when the platelet count is $\geq 100 \times 10^9$/L and is usually indicated when the platelet count is $\leq 50 \times 10^9$/L. The determination of whether patients with intermediate platelet counts (50 to 100×10^9/L) require therapy should be based on the risk of bleeding.

Vaginal deliveries or operative procedures ordinarily associated with insignificant blood loss may be undertaken in patients with platelet counts $\leq 50 \times 10^9$/L.

Platelet transfusion may be indicated despite an apparently adequate platelet count if there is known platelet dysfunction and microvascular bleeding.

From the American Society of Anesthesiologists.[1]

vate their bleeding. Platelet counts of less than 10 × 10^9/L often occur in patients receiving chemotherapeutic agents. Platelet transfusions are used to prevent spontaneous intracranial and gastrointestinal hemorrhages in these patients.

For major surgical procedures in thrombocytopenic patients, it is desirable to increase the platelet count to 50 × 10^9/L to 100 × 10^9/L, and prophylactic administration of platelet transfusions is indicated. Prolongation of the bleeding time to twice normal or greater secondary to abnormal platelet function is an indication for transfusion of platelets.

Dilutional thrombocytopenia, the lowering of the platelet count seen in patients receiving large amounts of banked blood, has been long recognized as the most frequent mechanism of coagulopathy in massively transfused patients. However, the majority of patients who require massive transfusion do not develop microvascular bleeding secondary to thrombocytopenia. Therefore, platelet transfusions should not be administered prophylactically unless abnormal microvascular bleeding is evident and thrombocytopenia is present (see Chap. 188).

Patients with immune thrombocytopenic purpura should not receive platelet transfusions unless there is life-threatening bleeding. These patients produce autoantibodies that react against all human platelets, and thus they derive little to no benefit from a platelet transfusion.

Following cardiopulmonary bypass, most patients develop thrombocytopenia and a functional platelet impairment. Although the correlation between platelet counts and the extent of bleeding in these patients is poor, transfusion algorithms using platelet count as an indication for platelet transfusion reduce the number of platelets actually used.

Functional platelet disorders are encountered less frequently than thrombocytopenia. In addition to cardiopulmonary bypass, uremia, liver disease, myeloproliferative disorders, and disproteinemias can cause acquired functional platelet disorders. Drugs that affect cyclooxygenase (aspirin, nonsteroidal anti-inflammatory drugs), theophyllines, tricyclic antidepressants, anesthetics (especially halothane), and some antibiotics cause functional platelet disorders that may or may not become clinically significant. Inherited functional platelet disorders include von Willebrand's disease (which is transported by platelets in addition to being produced by the vascular endothelium), Glanzmann's thrombasthenia, Bernard-Soulier syndrome, gray platelet syndrome, and dense granule deficiency syndrome.

Risks

The major risks associated with platelet transfusion are febrile nonhemolytic transfusion reactions, allergic reactions, sensitization, and transmission of infectious disease. Platelets have HLA antigens on their cell membranes. Sensitization to platelet antigens is common in patients who have received multiple platelet transfusions. Patients who are sensitized to these antigens will rapidly destroy transfused platelets, decreasing the therapeutic effectiveness of the platelet transfusion. Sensitization reactions may also induce respiratory distress and fever. In sensitized patients, only type-specific HLA platelets are effective.

Each unit of platelet concentrate shares the same infectious risk as a unit of red cells, because both are produced from one donor's blood. The viruses transmitted by other blood components are also transmitted by platelets. These viruses include hepatitis virus, human immunodeficiency virus, Epstein-Barr virus, and cytomegalovirus. Syphilis, brucellosis, malaria, and salmonellosis can also be transmitted by platelet concentrate. Although platelet concentrates are drawn from single donors, 6 to 8 units are usually given at a time, increasing the risk of infectious complications. Another concern with platelet transfusions is that bacteria can proliferate in platelet concentrates because they are stored at room temperature; they are often implicated in septic transfusion reactions (see Chap. 189).

Selected References

1. American Society of Anesthesiologists, Task Force on Blood Component Therapy. Practice guidelines for blood component therapy. Anesthesiology 1996:732–747.

Suggested References

American Society of Anesthesiologists. Questions and Answers About Transfusion Practices. 3rd ed. Park Ridge, IL, American Society of Anesthesiologists, 1998.

Faust RJ. Transfusion medicine. In Wedel DJ, ed. Orthopedic Anesthesia. New York: Churchill Livingstone, 1993:15–53.

Faust RJ, Warner MA. Transfusion risks. Int Anesthesiol Clin 1990;28:184.

Murray DJ, Olson J, Strauss R, Tinker JH. Coagulation changes during packed red cell replacement of major blood loss. Anesthesiology 1988;69:839–845.

Rao GHR, Escolar G, White JG. Biochemistry, physiology, and function of platelets stored as concentrates. Transfusion 1993;33:766–778.

Reed RL II, Heimbach DM, Counts RB, et al. Prophylactic platelet administration during massive transfusion: A prospective, randomized, double-blind clinical study. Ann Surg 1986;203:40–48.

Sarkodee-Adoo CB, Kendall JM, Sridhara R, et al. The relationship between the duration of platelet storage and the development of transfusion reactions. Transfusion 1998;38:229–235.

193
Albumin, Hetastarch, and Pentastarch

Edwin H. Rho, M.D. □ Ronald J. Faust, M.D.

The Colloid Controversy

For decades, medical debate has continued over the value of colloid infusion in the perioperative setting. Early colloid advocates argued that it was important to maintain normal colloid osmotic pressure to keep intravascular fluid from passing into the tissues and contributing to pulmonary, cerebral, or subcutaneous edema or ascites in the peritoneum. Albumin was the most widely used colloid until hydroxyethyl starch and pentastarch were developed, although other products, such as dextrans of various molecular sizes, were used as colloids for some indications.

Albumin is available in 5% and 25% concentrations, the latter being useful for normovolemic or hypervolemic patients in the medical setting. The albumin molecule has a tightly wound protein structure that has great heat stability. This allows it to be heated to 60°C for 10 hours during processing—lethal conditions for every possible contaminating cellular life form, including hepatitis viruses and human immunodeficiency virus (HIV). Albumin's origin as one component derived from blood donations has made the product expensive and often produced clinical shortages.

Furthermore, multiple authors have actively studied the importance of albumin in fluid therapy and tried to determine its value in comparison with inexpensive crystalloid fluids. The theory that albumin and other colloids would enable the body to keep more fluid intravascular never held water, figuratively speaking. Colloids were not proved to prevent the extravascular accumulations that lead to edema in the lungs, pleura, brain, abdomen, and soft tissues of critically injured and ill patients. Many sophisticated studies have failed to show a difference in outcome for patients treated aggressively with colloids to enable crystalloid restriction.

The use of hypertonic saline for fluid resuscitation has been investigated. Hypertonic saline is available in a 7.5% concentration. As with colloids, transient increases in intravascular volume occur and may be useful in intravascularly depleted patients. Most studies to date have not shown a statistically significant difference in overall survival of patients. However, hypertonic saline may be beneficial for patients with traumatic brain injury and hypotension.

Nonetheless, colloids are occasionally useful in clinical practice. In the clinical setting, the volume of crystalloid therapy for any given patient that would be interpreted as "too much" is speculative. Yet there is always some level of total intravenous intake that will be embarrassing to those caring for a patient, even if no fluid overload problems are obvious postoperatively. Because they cost slightly less than albumin, the hydroxyethyl starches have become popular colloid choices.

Chemistry

Both hetastarch and pentastarch are composed of chains of glucose molecules to which hydroxyethyl ether groups have been added to retard degradation. The glucose chains are highly branched, being derived from the starch amylopectin. One in 20 glucose monomers branches. Starch chains of various lengths are present in hetastarch, giving it a weight average molecular weight (MW_W) of 450,000. Its number average molecular weight (MW_N) is 69,000; this term describes a simple average of the individual molecular weights and is more closely related to oncotic pressure. Some 80% of hetastarch polymers have molecular weights in the range of 30,000 to 2,400,000. Hetastarch is given as a 6% solution in 0.9% sodium chloride or a lactated electrolyte solution. The chemical and pharmacokinetic properties of hetastarch and pentastarch are listed in Table 193–1.

Pharmacology

The colloidal properties of both hetastarch and pentastarch resemble those of 5% human albumin. Distribution for both is throughout the intravascular space. The principal effect for both following intravenous administration is plasma volume expansion secondary to the colloidal osmotic effect. In hypovolemic patients, both cause a temporary increase in arterial and venous pressures, cardiac index, left ventricular stroke work index, and pulmonary capillary wedge pressure. The effective intravascular half-life is 25.5 hours for 6% hetastarch

Table 193–1. Chemical and Pharmacokinetic Properties of Hetastarch and Pentastarch

	6% Hetastarch	10% Pentastarch
pH	5.5	5.0
MW_W	450,000 (range 10,000–1,000,000)	264,000 (range 150,000–350,000)
MW_N	69,000	63,000
Calculated mosmol	310	326
Molar substitution ratio	0.7	0.45
Intravascular half-life	25.5 h	2.5 h
Renal elimination	Molecules <50,000 daltons are rapidly excreted; <10% detected intravascularly in 2 weeks	Molecules <50,000 daltons are rapidly excreted; are undetectable intravascularly in 1 week
Coagulation effects	↑ PT, APTT, clotting times; may interfere with platelet function	↑ PT, APTT, clotting times; may interfere with platelet function
Other miscellaneous effects	↑ serum indirect bilirubin levels; temporary ↑ in serum amylase	Temporary ↑ in serum amylase

PT, prothrombin time; APTT, activated partial thromboplastin time.

and 2.5 hours for 10% pentastarch. Both substances are eliminated by the kidney. The hydroxyethyl group is not cleared but remains attached to glucose units when excreted. Hetastarch and pentastarch molecules less than 50,000 daltons are rapidly eliminated by the kidneys. However, only 33% of an initial dose of hetastarch is eliminated within 24 hours of administration, compared with approximately 70% of an initial dose of pentastarch. Up to 10% of administered hetastarch can be detected intravascularly after 2 weeks. Pentastarch is undetectable intravascularly 1 week after administration.

Pharmacokinetics

Because of a lower molar substitution ratio (i.e., the number of hydroxyethyl groups/glucose units), pentastarch is more rapidly and completely degraded by circulating amylase than hetastarch. Hetastarch has a very long tissue retention time (a half-life of 10 to 15 days) because the larger molecules are stored in the liver and spleen, where they are slowly degraded enzymatically by amylase. There is a theoretical concern about the possibility of a resulting impairment of reticuloendothelial function caused by hetastarch. Because of this concern, the lower molecular weight pentastarch was developed to minimize this theoretical risk.

Hetastarch and pentastarch do not interfere with blood typing or crossmatching, are stable with fluctuating temperatures, and only rarely cause allergic reactions. Both have been used successfully as an adjunct in leukapheresis by increasing the erythrocyte sedimentation rate to enhance granulocyte yield.

Adverse Effects

Both hetastarch and pentastarch prolong prothrombin time, partial thromboplastin time, and bleeding times when given in large doses. This is most likely secondary to hemodilution. There is some evidence to suggest that platelet function may also be altered by both products. For this reason, the maximum dose is 15 to 20 mL/kg. Although there are case reports of neurosurgical patients developing coagulopathies after large (2 L) doses of hetastarch, its effects on the coagulation system seem clinically insignificant when maximum dose recommendations are not exceeded. Six percent hetastarch may increase the indirect bilirubin serum levels.

Both hetastarch and pentastarch have been reported to produce rare hypersensitivity reactions, such as wheezing and urticaria. However, neither substance has been shown to stimulate antibody formation.

Elevated serum amylase levels have been shown to be a temporary effect of hetastarch and pentastarch administration. However, no association with pancreatitis has been shown.

It is not clear whether prolonged retention of hetastarch in the reticuloendothelial system can cause adverse effects.

Contraindications

Hetastarch and pentastarch are contraindicated in patients with known hypersensitivity to hydroxyethyl starch, with a coagulopathy, with congestive heart failure where volume overload may pose a problem, or with renal disease associated with oliguria or anuria.

Suggested References

Choi PT, Yip G, Quinonez LG, et al. Crystalloids vs. colloids in fluid resuscitation: A systematic review. Crit Care Med 1999;27:200–210.

Claes Y, Van Hemelrijck J, Van Gerven M, et al. Influence of hydroxyethyl starch on coagulation in patients during the perioperative period. Anesth Analg 1992;75:24.

Cucchiara RF, Black S, Michenfelder JD. Clinical Neuroanesthesia. 2nd ed. New York, Churchill Livingstone, 1998.

Cully MD, Larson CP Jr, Silverberg GD. Hetastarch coagulopathy in a neurosurgical patient (letter). Anesthesiology 1987; 66:706.

Engel AK, Losasso TJ, Weglinski MR, et al. Does intraoperative use of hydroxyethyl starch (Hespan) increase the risk of perioperative intracranial hemorrhage (ICH) in patients undergoing intracranial surgery? Anesthesiology 1993;79:A223.

Nolan J: Fluid replacement. Br Med Bull 1999;5:821–843.

Schierhout G, Roberts I. Fluid resuscitation with colloid or crystalloid solutions in critically ill patients: A systematic review of randomised trials. BMJ 1998;16:961–964.

Stoelting RK. Pharmacology and Physiology in Anesthetic Practice. 3rd ed. Philadelphia, JB Lippincott, 1999.

194
Nonhemolytic Transfusion Reactions

C. Thomas Wass, M.D.

Nonhemolytic transfusion reactions (NHTRs) include fever, mild allergic and anaphylactic reactions, transfusion-related acute lung injury (TRALI), and immunomodulation (Table 194–1).[1, 2] Because NHTRs are immune mediated, they can be caused by transfusion of any plasma-containing blood product, including whole blood, red blood cells (RBCs), fresh-frozen plasma, cryoprecipitate, and factor VIII concentrate.

Febrile Reactions

Febrile NHTRs are the most common adverse reaction to blood transfusion. They occur in 5% to 30% of platelet transfusions and approximately 4% of RBC transfusions.[3]

Although the etiology has yet to be fully elucidated, it is hypothesized that recipient alloimmunization (i.e., antibody production in response to a previous transfusion or pregnancy) toward donor white blood cells (WBCs) triggers release of leukocyte-derived pyrogens (e.g., interleukins, cytokines, tumor necrosis factor) that alter the thermoregulatory set point. In addition to recipient alloimmunization, these bioreactive substances are released from donor leukocytes during blood storage. Thus, longer storage periods are associated with a higher frequency of febrile transfusion reactions.[3] Accordingly, WBC reduction before storage (e.g., using leukocyte filtration techniques) prevents or minimizes the likelihood of transfusion-related fever.

If a febrile response occurs, the transfusion must be discontinued or slowed. Bacterial contamination and hemolytic transfusion reaction should be ruled out. Antipyretic drugs may be used prophylactically or to treat febrile NHTRs; however, these medications do not prevent associated symptoms (e.g., chills, rigor, soreness at the transfusion site, headache, nausea, myalgia, chest tightness).

Mild Allergic Reactions

Mild allergic reactions are the second most common transfusion reaction, occurring with a frequency of 1% to 4%.[1] Signs and symptoms include urticarial rash and generalized pruritus. They are caused by IgE-mediated histamine release from mast cells in response to substances (e.g., plasma proteins) found in the transfused blood. Provided evidence of an anaphylactic reaction is lacking, patients may be treated symptomatically with diphenhydramine and the transfusion continued.[1]

Anaphylactic Reactions

Transfusion-related anaphylactic reactions are rare events, occurring in 1 in 20,000 to 47,000 transfusions.[4] Patients experiencing these reactions are typically IgA deficient with circulating anti-IgA that results from either alloimmunization or autoimmunization. Accordingly, transfusion of any plasma-containing blood product may result in an anaphylactic response. Signs, symptoms, and treatment do not differ from other anaphylactic reactions.

The clinical diagnosis of an IgA anaphylactic transfusion reaction requires confirmation of IgA deficiency and the presence of anti-IgA in recipient plasma. These laboratory studies are often time-consuming and may not be readily available. Thus, once this diagnosis is suspected, transfusion should be stopped immediately. If blood transfusion must be continued, IgA-deficient blood products (e.g., blood from donors known to be IgA deficient, or washed or deglycerolized RBCs) should be used.[4]

Table 194–1. Classification of Transfusion Risks

Immune
Nonhemolytic
Febrile
Mild allergic
Anaphylactic
Transfusion-related acute lung injury
Immunomodulation
Hemolytic
Intravascular
Extravascular
Nonimmune
Viral or bacterial infection
Hypervolemia
Electrolyte changes
Coagulopathy
Hypothermia
Citrate toxicity

Both mild allergic and IgA anaphylactic reactions usually begin within 45 minutes after blood transfusion is started, but may be delayed for as long as 1 to 3 hours. Shorter onset times tend to be associated with more severe reactions.[4]

Transfusion-Related Acute Lung Injury

Perioperative pulmonary edema following blood transfusion is often attributed to intravascular volume overload that overwhelms myocardial Frank-Starling forces (i.e., cardiogenic pulmonary edema). In contrast, TRALI is a noncardiogenic form of pulmonary edema that is clinically indistinguishable from adult respiratory distress syndrome (ARDS). TRALI is a diagnosis of exclusion characterized by acute respiratory distress, bilateral pulmonary edema, severe hypoxemia, fever, and hypotension that usually occur within 1 to 6 hours of blood transfusion. The frequency of TRALI is likely underreported; however, it is estimated to be 0.02% per unit transfused.[5]

Because passive transfer of granulocyte antibodies from the donor's plasma to the recipient has been implicated as the etiology in nearly 90% of cases, transfusion of any plasma-containing blood products can cause TRALI. Following transfusion, these antibodies cause pulmonary leukostasis and activation of the complement system. Pulmonary endothelial injury, with subsequent extravasation of protein-laden fluid into adjacent interstitium and alveoli, results from the release of granulocyte-derived proteases, lipid metabolites, and oxygen free-radical species (e.g., superoxide).[5]

Unlike patients with ARDS, who have high morbidity and mortality, most TRALI patients improve clinically, physiologically, and radiographically within 48 to 96 hours.[5] Treatment is supportive, possibly requiring tracheal intubation, oxygenation, and mechanical ventilation.

Immunomodulation

It is widely accepted that blood transfusion can significantly **improve allograft survival** following renal transplantation, yet **worsen tumor recurrence** and mortality rate following resection of many cancers (e.g., breast, colorectal, head and neck, hepatocellular, lung, prostate, renal, soft-tissue sarcoma).[6, 7] In either case, alterations in patient outcome have been attributed to transfusion-related changes in the immune system or immunomodulation. Such an effect may be due to upregulation of humoral immunity (i.e., B-cell function and antibody production), downregulation of cell-mediated immunity (i.e., T-cell function), or both.[6, 7]

Despite improved renal allograft survival in transfused transplant recipients, routine perioperative blood transfusion is not indicated because of the effectiveness and safety of immunosuppressant drugs (e.g., cyclosporin) and concerns about transfusion-related infection.

Selected References

1. Faust RJ. Transfusion medicine. In Wedel DJ, ed. Orthopedic Anesthesia. New York: Churchill Livingstone, 1993:15–53.
2. Dzieczkowski JS, Barrett BB, Nester D, et al. Characterization of reactions after exclusive transfusion of white cell-reduced cellular blood components. Transfusion 1995; 35:20–25.
3. Heddle NM, Klama L, Singer J, et al. The role of the plasma from platelet concentrates in transfusion reactions. N Engl J Med 1994;331:625–628.
4. Sandler S, Mallory D, Malamut D, et al. IgA anaphylactic transfusion reactions. Transfus Med Rev 1995;9:1–8.
5. Popovsky MA, Chaplin HC, Moore SB. Transfusion-related acute lung injury: A neglected, serious complication of hemotherapy. Transfusion 1992;32:589–592.
6. Landers DF, Hill GE, Wong KC, et al. Blood transfusion-induced immunomodulation. Anesth Analg 1996;82:187–204.
7. Klein HG. Immunomodulatory aspects of transfusion. Anesthesiology 1999;91:861–865.

195

Hemolytic Transfusion Reactions

Ronald J. Faust, M.D.

Many adverse reactions are possible when transfusing blood products; however, hemolytic transfusion reaction (HTR) is often regarded as the most serious and potentially life-threatening. HTRs have been reported to occur at various incidences, but a study of 268,000 transfusions at the Mayo Clinic between 1964 and 1973 reported the incidence at 1 in every 6232 transfusions.[1] Mortality rate in this series was 17%, although higher levels have often been reported. A 1984 series reported an incidence of 1 in 35,739 transfusions.[2] Fifty-one percent of 256 transfusion-associated deaths reported to the U.S. Food and Drug Administration between 1976 and 1985 resulted from acute hemolysis following the transfusion of ABO-incompatible blood or plasma.[3]

Etiology

Donor unit red blood cell (RBC) incompatibility with the recipient's blood is the underlying mechanism in this reaction. HTRs are commonly classified as either intravascular hemolysis or extravascular hemolysis. Intravascular hemolysis occurs when antibody-coated RBCs are destroyed by the activation of the complement system. Extravascular hemolysis destroys antibody-coated RBCs via phagocytosis by macrophages in the reticuloendothelial system. In most hemolytic reactions, some RBCs are probably destroyed by both mechanisms.

Intravascular hemolysis (acute HTR) is the most severe type of HTR and is often the result of a clerical error; that is, giving the wrong unit of blood to the patient either by misidentifying the blood unit or the patient. Most hemolytic reactions reported in the 1970s occurred in intensive care units and operating rooms.[4] ABO incompatibility is a frequent cause, although other erythrocytic antigen-antibody systems also may cause acute hemolysis. Anti-C and other antibodies of the Rh group, anti-K (Kell), anti Fya (Duffy), and anti-Jka (Kidd) have also been implicated. Any RBC antibody/antigen reaction that activates complement to C9 results in vasomotor instability, disseminated intravascular coagulation (DIC), and acute renal failure.

Extravascular hemolysis (delayed HTR) is probably underdiagnosed. Hemolysis also occurs extravascularly because of incompatibility involving antigens and antibodies that do not bind complement. Failure to recognize these antibodies at crossmatch is frequently involved. Low titer antibodies can be undetectable, but in the recipient an anamnestic response can follow transfusion, resulting in the buildup of antibodies to the incompatible RBCs several days after the transfusion. The patient develops anemia, mild jaundice, and possibly a fever 1 day or longer after a transfusion. Antibody-coated RBCs are removed in the spleen and other parts of the reticuloendothelial system.

Several factors may predispose to HTR. Females consistently run a higher risk, with the ratio being approximately 3:1. Sensitization through pregnancy is felt to be the responsible mechanism.

Increasing age affects the frequency of HTRs. Older people have an increased likelihood of sensitization from earlier transfusions, and they receive a higher percentage of all transfusions, thus accounting for the higher frequency of HTRs.

Blood products administered on an emergent basis are more likely to lead to HTR. Incomplete crossmatch, large numbers of units, and human error due to pressure on the blood bank and/or the anesthesiologist administering the blood may be responsible.

Pathophysiology

Shock, DIC, and acute renal failure are the three most important pathophysiologic sequelae of HTR. Current thinking stresses the importance of cytokines as biologic mediators of many facets of the reaction. Multiple interleukins, monocyte chemoattractant protein-1, and cytokines, such as tumor necrosis factor, have been implicated as intermediaries in the reaction.[5] Although the literature once held that the acute renal failure seen during HTR might be a consequence of direct toxic effects of hemoglobin on renal tubular cells, current thinking is that the failure is caused by renal vascular ische-

Table 195–1. Signs and Symptoms of Acute Hemolytic Transfusion Reactions

Fever	Nausea
Chills	Flushing
Chest and/or lumbar pain	Dyspnea and respiratory failure
Hypotension[a]	Hemoglobinuria[a]
Tachycardia[a]	Diffuse bleeding[a]

[a]All but these are masked by anesthesia.

Table 195–2. Hemolytic Transfusion Reaction Therapy

1. Stop the blood transfusion
2. Treat hypotension appropriately
   - Crystalloid
   - Dopamine
   - Other compatible blood if necessary
3. Establish the diagnosis with blood bank assistance
   - Repeat clerical check
   - Direct Coombs
   - Repeat grouping, Rh, screen, and crossmatch
   - Serum haptoglobin
4. Treat renal vascular ischemia
   - Crystalloid to keep urine output above $1 \text{ ml} \cdot \text{kg}^{-1} \cdot \text{hr}^{-1}$
   - Furosemide
   - Low-dose dopamine
5. Evaluate and treat DIC
   - Platelet count, APTT, fibrinogen, fibrin split products
   - Platelet concentrate and FFP as indicated

mia secondary to shock and DIC. Many similarities between HTR and the shock state caused by sepsis and endotoxemia have been noted.[5]

Symptomatology

HTR symptomatology is listed in Table 195–1. Fever is the most common symptom; thus, a hemolytic reaction should always be suspected when a patient spikes a fever while receiving blood. Most symptoms are masked by anesthesia, and the first sign might be inappropriate hypotension and tachycardia despite adequate blood replacement. Hemoglobinuria and diffuse bleeding secondary to DIC are late signs of this reaction. Respiratory failure can also occur.

Treatment

Blood bank assistance should be obtained to help confirm or rule out the diagnosis. Table 195–2 lists some important steps with respect to treatment if an HTR is suspected. The transfusion should be stopped immediately. Hypotension should be aggressively treated with fluids, inotropes, or other blood as appropriate. Renal output should be maintained with crystalloids, furosemide, and dopamine as necessary. Component therapy should be used if DIC develops.

Selected References

1. Pineda AA, Brzica SM, Taswell HF. Hemolytic transfusion reaction: Recent experience in a large blood bank. Mayo Clin Proc 1978;53:378.
2. Lichtiger B, Perry-Thornton E. Hemolytic transfusion reactions in oncology patients: Experience in a larger cancer center. J Clin Oncol 1984;2:438.
3. Sazama K. Reports of 355 transfusion-associated deaths: 1976 through 1985. Transfusion 1990;30:583.
4. Myhre BA, Bove JR, Schmidt PJ. Wrong blood—A needless cause of surgical deaths. Anesth Analg 1981;60:777.
5. Capon SM, Goldfinger D. Acute hemolytic transfusion reaction, a paradigm of the systemic inflammatory response: New insights into pathophysiology and treatment. Transfusion 1995;513–520.

Suggested References

Faust RJ, Cucchiara RF, Messick JM Jr. Transfusion medicine and cardiovascular anesthesia. In Tarhan S, ed. Cardiovascular Anesthesia and Postoperative Care. 2nd ed. Chicago: Year Book Medical Publishers, 1989:527.

Goldfinger D. Acute hemolytic transfusion reactions—A fresh look at pathogenesis and considerations regarding therapy. Transfusion 1977;17:85.

Klein HG. Transfusion safety: Avoiding unnecessary bloodshed. Mayo Clin Proc 2000;75:5–7.

196
Sickle Cell Anemia: Anesthetic Implications

Paul J. Hubbell, M.D.

Sickle cell disease (hemoglobin [Hb] SS) occurs in African and American blacks and in some descendants of northern Mediterranean countries. The prevalence in American blacks is 8% to 10%.

There is increased morbidity and mortality with anesthesia and surgery secondary to the sickling of erythrocytes, which occurs in small arterioles at oxygen tensions of 40 to 45 mm Hg.

Sickle cell trait results from Hb genotype AS. It is not as serious and is rarely symptomatic. Erythrocytes sickle at oxygen tensions of 20 to 25 mm Hg.

Pathophysiology

The Hb molecule is a tetramer containing four protein (globin) molecules, each binding one of four hematoporphyrin rings, where oxygen is actually transported (Fig. 196–1). At birth, Hb F predominates, but 97% of an adult's hemoglobin is Hb A. Hemoglobin tetramers differ according to the types of globin subunits they contain (Table 196–1). Sickle cell disease is one of more than 300 inherited abnormalities of hemoglobin synthesis.

In Hb S, a valine is substituted for glutamic acid in the sixth amino acid position of the β-globulin chain. This abnormality causes an internal protein structural deformation that causes sickling on deoxygenation of the hemoglobin molecule. Formation of sickle cells is greater in veins than in arteries (pH-dependent). Hemolytic anemia results from the deformation and altered function, shape, and fluidity of the erythrocyte. Chronically sickled cells are removed by the reticuloendothelial system. Sickling can be reversed by changes in temperature and hemoglobin concentration, and by addition of oxygen or carbon monoxide. Individuals with sickle cell disease (Hb SS) have the following:

- Increased levels of 2,3-diphosphoglycerate.
- A rightward shift of the oxyhemoglobin dissociation curve.
- P_{50} equal to 49.7 mm Hg.
- Oxygen tension of venous blood equal to 44 mm Hg.

The clinical severity of any sickle cell disorder is proportional to the increased viscosity during de-oxygenation and is influenced by the types of hemoglobin in the cell other than genotype S (Table 196–2). Erythrocytes with genotype SS have a life span of 10 to 15 days.

Disease States

Sickle Cell Disease. Individuals with genotype Hb SS have severe repeated vaso-occlusive crises that produce tissue infarction and organ dysfunction. Crises are caused by hypoxemia, acidosis, dehydration, stasis, fever, and infection. With crises, these patients experience pain in the back and abdomen due to massive intrasplenic sickling. Mortal-

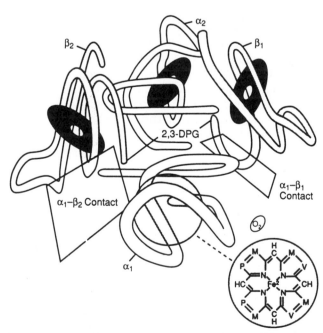

Figure 196–1. Adult hemoglobin molecule with two α- and two β-globin molecules carrying porphyrin rings capable of oxygen transport. In the center of the molecule, 2,3-diphosphoglycerate binds the two β chains together. On the heme molecule: M, methyl; V, vinyl; and P, propionic acid. Hemoglobin S contains an abnormality of the β chains. (From Faust RJ, Cucchiara RF, Messick JM.[1])

Table 196–1. Hemoglobins

Tetramer	Globin Subunits
Hgb A	$\alpha_2 \beta_2$
Hgb A$_2$	$\alpha_2 \delta_2$
Hgb F	$\alpha_2 \gamma_2$
Hgb S	$\alpha_2 S_2$

ity in those without overt organ disease occurs during an acute pain episode or stroke.[3]

Sickle cell disease is often fatal by age 30 because of cardiac and/or renal failure, severe infection, cerebral infarction, or intracerebral hemorrhage. This group also develops decreased total lung capacity and vital capacity and an increased risk of contracting pneumococcal pneumonia. By age 6, many are asplenic secondary to repeated thrombosis. Approximately 50% of patients with sickle anemia live beyond the fifth decade of life. A high level of fetal hemoglobin is predictive of adult life expectancy and is relatively stable throughout life.[3]

Sickle Cell Trait. Those with the Hb AS (trait) genotype are almost always asymptomatic. Their red cells contain less than 50% Hb S. It has been recommended that the actual percentage of Hb S be determined by electrophoresis before patients with sickle cell trait undergo cardiopulmonary bypass.[4] The use of a tourniquet during peripheral surgery or procedures in which temporary arterial occlusion is necessary might present more of a risk than in other patients.

Sickle Cell β Thalassemia. The thalassemias are a group of hemoglobinopathies resulting from inherited defects in the rate of synthesis of one or more of the hemoglobin chains. Early cases were all of Mediterranean origin. Two types of thalassemias, α and β, result from retardation of the synthesis of α and β chains. β thalassemia is a severe disease when homozygous (Cooley's anemia). Although some patients with both α and β thalassemia genes will have very mild disease, the severity depends on the type of β thalassemia gene inherited.

Organ Function

Repeated vaso-occlusive insults lead to compromised organ function. Rigid, deformed sickle cells are easily damaged by the mechanical stress of capillary circulation, causing collection and obstruction to flow.

□ **Cardiopulmonary** changes result in cardiomegaly, hyperdynamic circulation, full pulses, and murmurs. Changes are related to long-term increased cardiac output and decreased arterial Hb saturation due to gradual occlusion of the pulmonary vascular bed. In sickle cell disease, resting arterial oxygen tension is 70 to 90 mm Hg.
□ **Renal** problems include papillary necrosis and nephrotic syndrome, interfering with the ability to concentrate urine.
□ **Hepatic** effects include cirrhosis, jaundice, hepatosplenomegaly, and cholelithiasis.

Diagnosis

Sickle cell anemia can be diagnosed through several means.

□ The **dithionite test** requires one drop of blood and takes 5 minutes. It is based on the insolubility of reduced Hb S at pH below 7.0.
□ **Hb electrophoresis** is used for definitive diagnosis.
□ Glucose-6-phosphate deficiency must be checked in genotype SS and SC patients.

Preoperative Transfusion

Preoperative transfusion and exchange transfusion were once widely recommended for patients with SS disease. The rationale for exchange was that increasing Hb A to close to 50% would decrease the risk of sickling. Modern concerns over the risks

Table 196–2. Usual Findings in Common Sickling Disorders

Condition	Symptomatology	Splenomegaly	Circulating Hb (g/dL)	Sickled Cells	Hb S Present on Electrophoresis	Birth Prevalence of U.S. Blacks (%)
SS disease	+ + + +	0	6–8	Many	90–100% S, remainder F	0.16
S trait	0	0	Normal	0	20–40% S, remainder normal A	8–10
S thalassemia	+ + to + + +	+ +	7–8	Few	65–85% S, remainder A, A$_2$, and F	0.06
SC disease	+ to + +	+ + to + + +	9–11	Few	40–60%, each S and C	0.12
S hereditary persistence of Hb F	0 to +	0	Normal	0	70–80% S, 20–30% F	0.004

Modified from Murphy SB.[2]

of transfusion called this practice into question. Transfusions to correct anemia can be more easily justified, yet some studies have shown no difference in sickle cell–related complication rates between transfused and nontransfused groups (10% vs 8%).[5] A 1993 report cited 54 pediatric patients who underwent 66 elective surgical procedures without preoperative transfusion.[6]

A well-controlled, prospective, randomized multicenter study on preoperative exchange transfusion for patients with SS disease was reported in 1995.[7] Patients undergoing 604 surgical procedures were randomized into two groups. Patients in one group underwent an aggressive regimen of preoperative exchange transfusion to reduce their Hb S level to 30% or less. Those in the other group were merely transfused to correct their anemia, with their Hb raised to 10 g/dL and maintained at that level perioperatively. Although this was achieved with only one unit of blood before surgery in 77% of the group treated conservatively, the adults in the aggressive group required an average of 6.1 units for their exchange transfusions.

Except for transfusion-related complications (14% in the exchanged group vs 7% in the conservative group), the frequency of serious complications was similar in the two groups. About 10% of the exchanged group developed new alloantibodies. Hemolytic transfusion reactions were six times more frequent in that group than in the conservatively transfused group.

The Vichinsky study[7] reported **acute chest syndrome** in 10% of the patients in both groups. The 2 deaths in the 551 patients involved in the study were attributed to this complication. In sickle cell patients, $\dot{V}/\dot{Q}$ mismatch and pulmonary sickling add to the potential for developing pulmonary infarction and infection perioperatively. These patients have a tenfold greater risk of serious perioperative pulmonary complications than that found in the general population.[3]

Anesthetic Management

- Avoid hypoxia, hypercarbia, hypothermia, acidosis, dehydration, and low-flow conditions.
- Avoid premedications causing respiratory depression.
- Increase FIO2 with 100% oxygen by mask in the postoperative period.
- Position the patient to avoid stasis.
- Tourniquet use is relatively contraindicated.
- Maintain 100% arterial oxygen saturation or an arterial oxygen tension greater than 90 mm Hg.
- Provide intravenous hydration and replacement of blood loss.
- Treat atelectasis and pulmonary complications aggressively.
- Monitor acid-base status, renal function, and cardiopulmonary status.

Selected References

1. Faust RJ, Cucchiara RF, Messick JM. Transfusion medicine and cardiovascular anesthesia. In Tarhan S, ed. Cardiovascular Anesthesia and Postoperative Care. 2nd ed. Chicago: Year Book Medical, 1989:527.
2. Murphy SB. Difficulties in sickle cell states. In Orkin FK, Cooperman LH, eds. Complications in Anesthesiology. Philadelphia: JB Lippincott, 1983:476.
3. Platt OS, Brambilla DJ, Rosse WF. Mortality in sickle cell disease. N Engl J Med 1994;330:1639–1644.
4. Murray DJ. Evaluation of the patient with anemia and coagulation disorders. In Rogers MC, Tinker JH, Covino BG, et al, eds. Principles and Practice of Anesthesiology. St. Louis: CV Mosby, 1993:341.
5. Georges RN, McDonald JC, Deitch EA. Preoperative management of sickle cell patients. J La State Med 1992;144:316.
6. Griffin TC, Buchanan GR. Elective surgery in children with sickle cell disease without preoperative blood transfusion. J Pediatr Surg 1993;28:681.
7. Vichinsky EP, Haberkkern CM, Neumayr L, et al. A comparison of conservative and aggressive transfusion regimens in the perioperative management of sickle cell disease. N Engl J Med 1995;333:206–213.

197

Issues in Ambulatory Anesthesia

Brian P. McGlinch, M.D.

Almost 70% of surgery in the United States is performed in the ambulatory setting, where patient discharge the day of surgery is expected. Advances in surgical technology allow procedures with minimal blood loss, fluid shifts, and postoperative discomfort. Newer anesthetic agents are potent and rapidly metabolized, allowing rapid patient awakening without significant associated side effects. The role of the anesthesiologist in ambulatory surgical procedures has expanded into participation in screening, evaluating, and preparing the patient for the given surgical procedure, as well as managing the intraoperative period. Day of surgery delays, cancellations, and unanticipated hospitalizations have significantly decreased in practices where perioperative care of ambulatory surgical patients is managed by an anesthesiologist.

Patient Screening and Evaluation

Patients with American Society of Anesthesiologists physical categories 3 and 4 are not excluded from outpatient procedures as long as their medical conditions are stable, medically managed, and unlikely to be exacerbated by the proposed surgical procedure. In a large retrospective analysis of elderly patients undergoing ambulatory surgical procedures, the 30-day death rates after ambulatory surgical procedures were as low as age-matched controls that did not undergo surgical procedures.[1] Although ambulatory surgery is very safe, not all patients are candidates. Medical conditions listed in Table 197-1 merit hospital admission and medical management during the perioperative period.

A preoperative telephone interview with the patient can determine the presence of significant underlying diseases (e.g., angina, chronic obstructive pulmonary disease, stroke) or special anesthetic concerns (e.g., latex allergy, malignant hyperthermia, a history of difficult intubations) meriting further preoperative evaluation. If the proposed surgery would have a significant impact on the patient's underlying condition, then a more extensive evaluation (e.g., 12-lead electrocardiogram, blood tests, pulmonary function tests) can be performed before the day of surgery to determine whether an ambulatory procedure is appropriate. A preoperative telephone screening also allows confirmation of arrival time, place, and preoperative fasting guidelines (Table 197-2), further reducing day-of-surgery delays and cancellations.

Anesthetic Techniques

Regional Anesthesia

Patients who receive regional anesthesia experience profound analgesia and anesthesia and a lower incidence of postoperative pain, drowsiness, nausea, and vomiting compared with general anesthesia. Small-gauge, pencil-point spinal needles have reduced the risk of postdural puncture headaches. Bupivacaine (0.75%) is associated with prolonged motor blockade and delayed discharge. Hyperbaric lidocaine spinal anesthesia is associated with transient radicular irritation (TRI), which develops 24 hours after a hyperbaric lidocaine spinal and sometimes persists for several days. Dilution of bupivacaine for shorter-duration blocks or lidocaine to reduce the incidence of TRI can result in central neuraxial blockade that is insufficient in either quality or duration for the intended surgical procedures. Lidocaine epidural anesthesia for lower abdominal and lower extremity procedures has been suggested. However, the increased time needed to perform the epidural block and the slower develop-

Table 197-1. Contraindications to Ambulatory Surgery

Serious medical problems that are not adequately managed
Unstable angina
Severe cardiac valvular disease
Reactive airway disease with recent exacerbation meriting hospitalization
Transient ischemic attacks
Brittle diabetes
Morbid obesity
Sickle cell anemia
Obstructive sleep apnea
Ongoing chemical abuse behavior
Children undergoing tonsillectomy for obstructive sleep apnea
Patients with a history of postoperative nausea and vomiting
Patients lacking a responsible adult to provide care the night of surgery

Table 197–2. American Society of Anesthesiologists Summary of Fasting Recommendations to Reduce the Risk of Pulmonary Aspiration[3]

Ingested Material	Minimum Fasting Period
Clear liquids	2 hours
Breast milk	4 hours
Infant formula	6 hours
Nonhuman milk	6 hours
Light meal	6 hours

These guidelines are for otherwise healthy, nonpregnant patients of all ages without underlying conditions that might delay normal gastric emptying. These do not guarantee an empty stomach. Prophylactic use of gastrointestinal stimulants, anticholinergics, histamine-2 receptor blockers, or nonparticulate antacids is not recommended for asymptomatic patients who otherwise are at low risk for pulmonary aspiration.

From the American Society of Anesthesiologists Task Force on Preoperative Fasting.[3]

ment of surgical anesthesia has kept it from gaining widespread use in the ambulatory setting.

Peripheral nerve blockade (e.g., axillary, ankle, popliteal) can be performed quickly with minimal complications. Effective blocks require minimal sedation or analgesia, thereby negating the need for intense postanesthesia recovery care. If ambulation can be facilitated with crutches after a procedure, discharge from the ambulatory facility before resolution of the block is possible.

General Anesthesia

General anesthesia remains the most popular mode of anesthesia delivered for ambulatory surgical procedures; nonetheless, it is associated with an incidence of postoperative nausea and vomiting ranging from 20% to 30%. Propofol is associated with rapid awakening and a low incidence of postoperative nausea and vomiting, making it the preferred intravenous induction agent for ambulatory procedures. Sevoflurane is the agent of choice for inhalation induction. Desflurane and sevoflurane have low solubility characteristics, allowing more rapid patient awakening than under either isoflurane or propofol infusions. Fentanyl is the most commonly used narcotic, but remifentanil is growing in popularity because of its extremely rapid metabolism and prompt awakening. Nonsteroidal anti-inflammatory drugs (e.g., preoperative oral ibuprofen, intravenous ketorolac) are useful in reducing narcotic needs and minimizing side effects perioperatively. Nonsteroidal agents are associated with increased bleeding during head and neck surgery and should be avoided with these cases.

The bispectral index monitor (BIS) (Aspect Medical Systems, Natick, MA) purports to ensure proper anesthetic depth by analyzing electroencephalographic (EEG) data from patients receiving general anesthesia. Use of the BIS monitor may facilitate a reduction in the use of intravenous and volatile anesthetic agents by allowing titration of anesthetic agents to BIS levels associated with loss of patient awareness. Proper titration of anesthetic depth should afford more prompt patient awakening at the end of surgery, allowing the patient to bypass the recovery room.

Recovery Room Issues

The main source for unexpected delayed discharge or hospital admissions following ambulatory surgical procedures is postoperative nausea and vomiting, which occurs in up to 35% of patients undergoing surgery. Nausea and vomiting frequently occurs several hours postoperatively, suggesting a contribution from oral analgesics as well as increased oral intake of fluids and solids by the patient. Prophylactic butyrophenone or serotonin antagonist administration is not uniformly effective but is recommended in highly emetogenic procedures. Factors contributing to postoperative nausea and vomiting are listed in Table 197–3. Common interventions for the treatment of postoperative nausea and vomiting are listed in Table 197–4.

One of the most significant changes likely to affect ambulatory anesthesia practice in the next decade will involve bypassing the recovery room after surgical procedures. When potent, short-acting intravenous and volatile anesthetic agents are used, patients may awaken from anesthesia rapidly with minimal pain, nausea, or hypoventilation, obviating the need for an intensive postoperative monitoring environment. White and colleagues[2] published a proposal for assessing a patient's ability to bypass the postanesthesia care unit by evaluating a number of factors, including consciousness, hemodynamic stability, oxygenation, nausea, and pain. By reducing the number of patients requiring recovery room treatment, nursing resources can be allocated to other areas or reduced. The cost of newer anesthetic agents used in ambulatory settings could be offset by the benefit of reduced recovery room usage.

Table 197–3. Factors Contributing to Increased Postoperative Nausea and Vomiting

Laparoscopic abdominal surgery (highest incidence)
Strabismus eye surgery (dependent on the number of muscles corrected)
Duration of surgery and anesthesia
Female gender and luteal phase (premenstrual/menstrual)
Previous history of postoperative nausea and vomiting or motion sickness
Use of narcotics in any administration mode
Inadequate hydration and postural hypotension
Young age
Large body habitus
Presence of preexisting gastrointestinal conditions

Table 197–4. Interventions for Postoperative Nausea and Vomiting

Medication	IV Dose	Comment
Butyraphenones (droperidol)	10 µg/kg	Dopaminergic antagonism; 20 µg/kg leads to drowsiness. Dysphoric reactions at higher doses. Very effective in adults and children. Given prior to emergence.
Antihistamines (dimenhydrinate)	0.5 mg/kg	Sites of action are the vomiting center and vestibular pathways. Effect persists for up to 24 hours. Does not delay discharge. Given at anesthetic induction.
Serotonin antagonists (ondansetron, granisetron)	4 mg	Serotonin receptor blockade. Lack sedative properties. Lower doses in adults are not effective. Substantial cost precludes its use as a prophylactic agent against PONV when compared with droperidol. Given before emergence.
Glucocorticoids (dexamethasone)	10 mg	Prolonged antiemetic effect. Mechanism of action unknown. Administered at anesthetic induction. Wound healing and blood glucose levels may change at higher doses.

Selected References

1. Warner MA, Shields SE, Chute CG. Major morbidity and mortality within one month of ambulatory surgery and anesthesia. JAMA 1993;270:1437.
2. White PF, Song D. New criteria for fast-tracking after outpatient anesthesia. Anesth Analg 1999;88:1069–1072.
3. American Society of Anesthesiologists Task Force on Preoperative Fasting. Practice guidelines for preoperative fasting and the use of pharmacologic agents to reduce the risk of pulmonary aspiration: Application to healthy patients undergoing elective procedures. Anesthesiology 1999;90:896–905.

198
Positioning

Roy F. Cucchiara, M.D.

It is helpful to remember that the goal is to place the patient in the optimum position to give the surgeon access to the operative field. There may be secondary considerations that restrict the achievement of that goal in a specific operation, and often there are little data on the limits of safety to guide the anesthesiologist and surgeon (both of whom usually share responsibility for the position). The safety of the position must also be balanced against the risk of performing the surgery in a compromising position.

The basic patient positions for surgery are supine, prone, and lateral, with the head down (Trendelenburg's position) or head up (reverse Trendelenburg's). Most other positions are variations on these basic ones. Lithotomy (supine) with the legs elevated and flexed, jackknife (prone and flexed), lateral decubitus (indicates which side is down), beach chair, and sitting are commonly used positioning terms. Diagrams of the various positions can be found in surgery texts.[1, 2]

The most common serious complication of poor positioning is peripheral nerve injury (see Chapters 237 and 238). Common but usually less serious complications relate to the skin. Tape "burns," skin blisters from pressure on surfaces, and skin breakdown from the edges of an unpadded strap are common. **A blister forms either from abrasion of the skin or from ischemia of the skin area.** Abrasions in the operating room are usually shallow enough to heal over without an ulcer. The greatest care must be taken around the face and ears. Although the skin of the face is very vascular and usually heals well, an ischemic area at a fold in the facial tissue can be a serious problem with poor healing, scarring, and possibly even the need for skin grafting. Particular care must be taken with tube tapes and tapes across the head or face to hold the endotracheal tube in position.

Steep Trendelenburg's (head down) position can cause occasional difficulties. Venous engorgement of the face can be impressive, sometimes resulting in marked conjunctival edema. Airway edema can also result, although this is rarely a problem that delays extubation. Pulmonary compliance is reduced from the contents of the abdomen pressing on the diaphragm. This appears to be a transient problem that can be corrected by returning the patient to the supine position. It is reasonable to assume that there might be an increase in interstitial lung water in these patients that could impair diffusion. An unexplained decrease in oxygen saturation is not uncommon. Positive pressure ventilation on resumption of the supine position could be expected to correct this phenomenon fairly quickly. There is a case report of a patient in steep Trendelenburg's position who failed to awaken at the end of the case and was found to have an intracerebral bleed.

The sitting position has many unique benefits and risks (see Chapter 157).

For many cranial nerve and ear, nose, and throat cases, the patient's head is turned to the side to some degree. Cervical bony or disc degeneration or vascular impingement when the head is turned may dictate safe positioning. Only rarely will such a patient have somatosensory evoked potentials monitored to detect spinal cord compromise. The best way to determine the degree of cervical movement that the patient can tolerate is to place the patient in the desired position while awake and check the range of motion carefully before inducing anesthesia. The chin should not be overflexed to the point where there is less than two fingerbreadths between the bone of the chin and the sternal notch; quadriplegia may result. Age should be considered when positioning the patient with the head turned, flexed, or extended. The cervical and vascular degeneration that contribute to problems can begin in middle age and are nearly always present by the sixth decade of life.

In older patients, care must be taken to avoid overflexing the hips, which can cause sciatic nerve injury. Flexion of the neck in patients with severe rheumatoid arthritis may reveal odontoid subluxation, which can narrow the cervical spinal canal. Some have suggested that prolonged prone cases should be performed with the patient's head pinned in a headrest to remove the risk of putting pressure on the eye.

Lumbar laminectomy is a frequently performed procedure in hospitals. It serves as a good example of possible positioning injury (Fig. 198–1). The head is placed either straight down in a foam head holder or turned to the side. The risks to the cranial structures are primarily pressure on the eyes, abrasion of the cornea, or pressure on the delicate structures

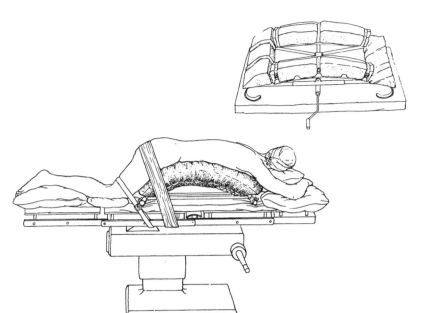

Figure 198–1. The convex saddle frame for spinal operations (Redrawn from Moore DC, Edmonds L. Prone position frame. Surgery 17:276, 1950). Inset: The adjustable Wilson frame for prone position. (From Martin JT, Warner MA.[1])

of the face, such as the lips, nose, and ears. One or both arms are placed on arm boards in the "surrender" position. In some cases, the arms are tucked beneath the arched frame; in others, both arms are placed at the sides. Risks to the arms include pressure on or stretching of the brachial plexus and pressure on the ulnar nerve. Often the brachial plexus can be palpated at the axilla and the shoulder can be maneuvered so as to ensure that the plexus is not under tension or pressure. The anterior iliac crest must be well padded to avoid pressure injury of the lateral femoral cutaneous nerve with subsequent anesthesia of the side of the thigh. If the legs are large, the knees must be padded or even suspended to prevent pressure blisters. The

feet should be free so that the toes are not subjected to supporting the weight of the legs.

In general, our responsibility is to avoid injury to the patient by positioning, even though there are few real guidelines as to how much pressure is safe. Positioning is one of the arts of anesthesia, and its subtleties are best learned through experience.

Selected References

1. Martin JT, Warner MA. Positioning in Anesthesia and Surgery. 3rd ed. Philadelphia, WB Saunders, 1997.
2. Cucchiara RF, Faust RJ. Patient positioning. In Miller RD, ed. Anesthesia. 5th ed. Philadelphia: Churchill Livingstone, 2000:1017–1032.

199
Management of the Difficult Airway

David R. Danielson, M.D.

Managing difficult airways successfully combines forethought, proper equipment, and decisiveness. Concentrating on the first two factors makes the third factor less stressful. A thorough history and physical examination with emphasis on the airway will not reveal every difficult airway but can often avert crisis and prompt the anesthesiologist toward an alternate plan.

Preoperative Evaluation

After any history of a previous difficult intubation has been ruled out through preoperative interview and review of the medical record, three classic bedside tests are recommended.

Tongue Versus Pharyngeal Size. Mallampati and colleagues[1] described grading the relative size of the tongue to the pharynx according to three classes originally. Class II was later subdivided based on whether all of the uvula or only its base can be visualized. Preinduction visualization of the faucial pillars, soft palate, and base of the uvula, with the patient in a sitting position, is used to classify patients according to how well pharyngeal structures can be seen (Fig. 199–1):

◻ Class I: Palate, faucial pillars, entire uvula.
◻ Class II: Palate, faucial pillars, base of uvula.
◻ Class III: Palate, some of the faucial pillars.
◻ Class IV: Palate alone.

Atlanto-Occipital Extension. Mobility of the atlanto-occipital joint enables alignment of the oral, pharyngeal, and laryngeal axes, facilitating mask ventilation and tracheal intubation. Extension of the atlanto-occipital joint can be quantified by observing the angle of the occlusal surface of the upper teeth with respect to horizontal when the upright patient extends the neck; 35 degrees of extension is normal.

Anterior Mandibular Space. This refers to the **thyromental distance**, the distance from the thyroid notch to the mental prominence when the neck is fully extended. A distance of 6 cm in an adult predicts ease of intubation.[2]

None of these classic bedside measures is a definitive predictor of airway ease or difficulty. Evaluation of as many bedside measures as possible to increase the predictive power of the preoperative exam is recommended. Besides the three measures mentioned above, incisor prominence, interincisor distance, width of the palate, temporomandibular joint mobility, and length and thickness of the neck should be evaluated.

Morbid obesity presents increased airway difficulty with respect to increased periglottic tissue, limited neck mobility, and difficult patient positioning. Additionally, obese patients develop rapid oxygen desaturation during apnea. Accordingly, awake fiberoptic intubation should be considered when managing this patient population.

Difficult Airways

By definition, a difficult airway is a clinical situation in which an anesthesiologist experiences difficulty with mask ventilation, direct laryngoscopy, or intubation.[3] The American Society of Anesthesiologists' Difficult Airway Algorithm,[3] as modified by Benumof,[4] is shown in Fig. 199–2. Studying these algorithms ensures having a decision tree in mind **before** airway difficulties are encountered. A recent review[5] estimates that failed intubation occurs in approximately 0.2% of general anesthetics.

In the 1990s, publication of the Difficult Airway Algorithm and emphasis on teaching a multiplicity of airway management techniques became more commonplace. Clinical practice changes have included earlier awakening of patients on encountering a difficult airway, earlier call for assistance, immediate consideration of alternative techniques,

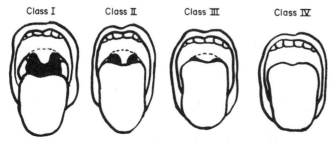

Class I   Class II   Class III   Class IV

Figure 199–1. Mallampati classification of the upper airway. See text for explanation. (Adapted from Mallampati SR, Gatt SP, Gugino LD, et al.[1])

DIFFICULT AIRWAY ALGORITHM

1. Assess the likelihood and clinical impact of basic management problems:

   A. Difficult intubation

   B. Difficult ventilation

   C. Difficulty with patient cooperation or consent

2. Consider the relative merits and feasibility of basic management choices:

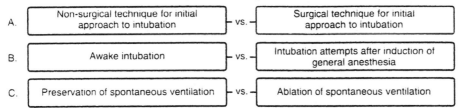

3. Develop primary and alternative strategies:

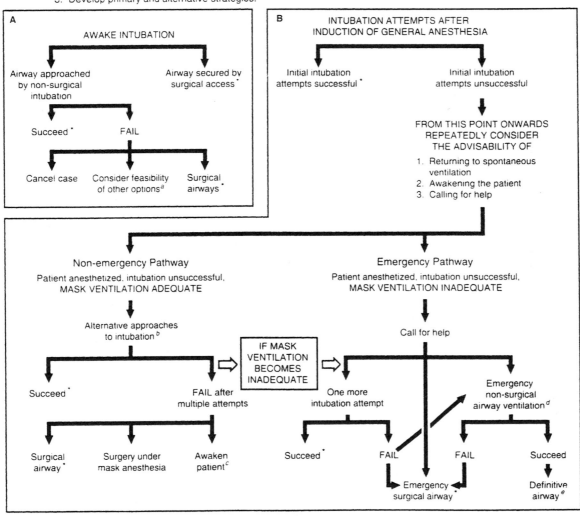

Figure 199–2. ASA Difficult Airway Algorithm. The * denotes that intubation should be confirmed with exhaled CO_2. (A) Other options include, but are not limited to, surgery under mask anesthesia, surgery under local anesthesia infiltration or regional nerve blockade, or intubation attempts after induction of general anesthesia. (B) Alternative approaches to difficult intubation include, but are not limited to, use of different laryngoscope blades, awake intubation, blind oral or nasal intubation, fiberoptic intubation, intubating stylet or tube changer, light wand, retrograde intubation, and surgical airway access. (C) See awake intubation. (D) Options for emergency nonsurgical airway ventilation include, but are not limited to, transtracheal jet ventilation, laryngeal mask ventilation, or esophageal-tracheal combitube ventilation. (E) Options for establishing a definitive airway include, but are not limited to, returning to awake state with spontaneous ventilation, tracheotomy, or endotracheal intubation. (From American Society of Anesthesiologists, Task Force on Management of the Difficult Airway.[3])

and more rapid progression to an "optimal intubation attempt."

Management of the Difficult Airway

Only rarely (e.g., facial or cervical spine trauma, neoplastic disease involving the airway or neck) is a surgical airway the first choice for securing an airway. Usually the elective approach to a difficult airway necessitates familiarity with awake intubation techniques. The key to awake intubation is providing adequate topical anesthesia to the airway and familiarity with required equipment.

Discovery of a difficult airway after the induction of general anesthesia, perhaps in a paralyzed patient, leads to the most stressful arm of the algorithm. Here is where rapid decisions must be made and both equipment and knowledge must be immediately available. This includes multiple intubation aids, such as a light wand, intubating stylet, and fiberoptic bronchoscope. One must always be prepared to manage the airway with transoral supraglottic techniques (e.g., laryngeal mask airway, esophageal-tracheal combitube) as well as techniques involving tracheal instrumentation (transtracheal jet ventilation, tracheostomy). Patient safety depends on planning ahead and progressing rapidly to the next plan when necessary.

The algorithm has been widely accepted and incorporated into training programs with minimal controversy. A notable exception to this involves the arms of the algorithm leading to mask ventilation or regional anesthesia after failed intubation. Significant difference of opinion continues in these areas.

Selected References

1. Mallampati SR, Gatt SP, Gugino LD, et al. A clinical sign to predict difficult tracheal intubation: A prospective study. Can Anaesth Soc J 1985;32:429–434.
2. Benumof J. Management of the difficult adult airway. Anesthesiology 1991;75:1087–1110.
3. American Society of Anesthesiologists, Task Force on Management of the Difficult Airway. Practice guidelines for management of the difficult airway. Anesthesiology 1993;78:597–607.
4. Benumof J. Laryngeal mask airway and the ASA difficult airway algorithm. Anesthesiology 1996;84:686–699.
5. Crosby ET, Cooper RM, Douglas MJ, et al. The unanticipated difficult airway with recommendations for management. Can J Anaesth 1998;45:757–776.

200
Carbon Monoxide Poisoning

John M. Van Erdewyk, M.D.

Carbon monoxide (CO) is a colorless, odorless, tasteless, and nonirritating gas produced by the incomplete combustion of materials containing carbon. Its effects on the oxygen-carrying capacity of blood are profound. CO is responsible for approximately 3500 accidental and suicidal deaths each year in the United States. It is the major cause of death in patients exposed to smoke inhalation from fires. Many more people, however, are exposed to less toxic concentrations.

Pathophysiology

CO is emitted from almost any flame or combustion device. A 3% to 7% concentration is present in the exhaust of internal combustion engines. Much higher concentrations can be generated during the burning of most illuminating and heating gases. Small amounts of CO are present in all individuals, because it is a byproduct of erythrocyte destruction; this level is approximately 1% carboxyhemoglobin. Cigarette smokers often have carboxyhemoglobin levels above 5%.

CO and oxygen both compete for binding with hemoglobin. CO binding results in carboxyhemoglobin, which is incapable of offloading significant quantities of oxygen in tissues. Hemoglobin's affinity for CO is 200 times greater than that for oxygen. At equilibrium, 1 part CO in 1500 parts air will result in 50% conversion of hemoglobin to carboxyhemoglobin. The amount of conversion to carboxyhemoglobin depends on the CO concentration in the air and on the duration of exposure.

Besides decreasing oxygen-carrying capacity, carboxyhemoglobin also interferes with the release of oxygen from oxyhemoglobin (i.e., a leftward shift in the oxyhemoglobin dissociation curve). This further reduces the amount of oxygen available to the tissues and explains why tissue anoxia appears in the CO-poisoned patient at levels of arterial oxyhemoglobin concentrations well tolerated in an anemic patient.

Signs and Symptoms

Signs and symptoms vary depending on the concentration of carboxyhemoglobin present, the tissue oxygen demands, and the hemoglobin concentration.

- Small amounts of CO in the blood may manifest as irritability, headache, nausea or vomiting, confusion, dizziness, visual disturbances, and dyspnea.
- Increasing concentrations may produce respiratory failure, seizures, coma, or death.
- The classic cherry red color of the skin is usually a sign of high CO concentrations in the blood. However, cyanosis may be seen in severe CO poisoning.
- Pulse oximetry overestimates the oxyhemoglobin saturation in the presence of carboxyhemoglobin, because the absorption spectrum is similar. Significant hypoxemia can be present despite oximeter readings above 90%.

Therapy

First, remove the patient from the environment containing CO to prevent further exposure. Next, administer 100% oxygen. Because the binding of CO to hemoglobin is competitive with oxygen, increasing the inspired concentration of oxygen to 100% will cause more oxygen to displace CO from the hemoglobin molecule, shortening the elimination half-life. The half-life of CO elimination can be shortened from 4 hours to 40 minutes by hyperventilation of the lungs with 100% oxygen. Endotracheal intubation and mechanical ventilation may be necessary. Oxygen at 100% will also partially relieve tissue hypoxia by increasing the amount of oxygen dissolved in the plasma. Hyperbaric oxygen therapy is also useful for severe cases. Transfusion of blood or packed cells may be helpful. To decrease tissue oxygen demands, the patient should be sedated. Diuretics and/or steroids may be indicated if the patient develops cerebral edema.

Suggested References

Brown M. ICU: Critical care. In Barash PG, Cullen BF, Stoelting RK, eds. Clinical Anesthesia. 3rd ed. Philadelphia: Lippincott-Raven, 1997:1367–1388.
Stoelting RK, Dierdorf SF. Psychiatric illness and substance abuse. In Stoelting RK, Dierdorf SF, eds. Anesthesia and Co-Existing Disease. 3rd ed. Philadelphia: Churchill Livingstone, 1993:517–538.

201
Anticholinesterase and Anticholinergic Poisoning

David R. Danielson, M.D.

Anesthesiologists are liable to be called to assist in the care of patients with either anticholinesterase or anticholinergic poisoning because of their knowledge of cholinergic pharmacology and physiology and expertise in airway management and intensive care.

Cholinergic Physiology

Acetylcholine (ACh) is the neurotransmitter found at all cholinergic sites, which include:

□ All preganglionic autonomic fibers.
□ All postganglionic parasympathetic fibers (muscarinic sites).
□ The neuromuscular junction (nicotinic sites).

Acetylcholinesterase (AChE) is found in the synaptic cleft of the aforementioned sites. It is responsible for terminating ACh activity in less than 1 millisecond.[1]

Butyrylcholinesterase, also called plasma cholinesterase or pseudocholinesterase:

□ Is encoded by a gene different from that for AChE.
□ Is synthesized by the liver.
□ Has a half-life of approximately 23 hours.
□ Can be used as a marker of liver synthetic function.
□ Is found primarily in plasma (i.e., little or no butyrylcholinesterase is found at the motor endplate).
□ Terminates the action of succinylcholine, mivacurium, and ester local anesthetics by hydrolysis.

Anticholinesterase Poisoning

Anticholinesterase drugs inhibit AChE, thereby increasing ACh at cholinergic sites. Excessive, or toxic, dosing of anticholinesterase drugs results in activation of muscarinic and nicotinic receptors. **Muscarinic** signs and symptoms include those from the mnemonic **SLUDGE** (**s**alivation, **l**acrimation, **u**rination, **d**iaphoresis, **g**astrointestinal upset, and **e**mesis), as well as bronchospasm, bronchorrhea, blurred vision, bradycardia (or tachycardia), hypotension, confusion, and shock.[2] **Nicotinic** effects occur at the neuromuscular junction, where skeletal muscle initially exhibits fasciculation followed by inability to repolarize cell membranes (resulting in weakness or paralysis). Severe reactions, termed **cholinergic crisis**, may lead to ventilatory failure and death within minutes to hours following exposure.[3]

Organophosphates. The most common clinical scenario of anticholinesterase toxicity is insecticide poisoning in agricultural workers. Organophosphate compounds, used either as commercial insecticides or in chemical warfare (e.g., "nerve gases" such as tabun and sarin), are usually applied as aerosols or dusts. These can be **rapidly absorbed through the skin and mucous membranes, or by inhalation**. Organophosphates are also used for medical purposes; for example, **echothiophate** is used to treat glaucoma.

Therapy. When treating organophosphate poisoning, the first line of therapy is **termination of exposure** (e.g., relocating the patient and removing soiled clothing). Pharmacologic intervention includes intravenous **atropine**, 2 to 4 mg (repeated as needed) to reverse muscarinic symptoms. Nicotinic muscle weakness is reversed within a few minutes following intravenous administration of **pralidoxime** (2-PAM), 1 to 2 g over 5 minutes. Pralidoxime is the only oxime commercially available in the United States, although others are available in other countries and through military sources.

Prophylaxis in anticipation of "nerve gas" exposure is usually achieved using **pyridostigmine**.[4] The theory that pyridostigmine will occupy a percentage of receptors, preventing them from binding with the irreversible organophosphates, has been demonstrated in experimental animals. However, data in humans are limited to our experience during the Gulf War. Many Gulf War veterans reported pyridostigmine-induced side effects (e.g., gastrointestinal upset); however, symptoms were generally mild, and combat and daily function were rarely compromised.[5]

Anticholinergic Poisoning

Central anticholinergic effects are biphasic, beginning with central nervous system excitation followed by depression. Signs include fragmentary speech patterns, visual hallucinations, atypical behavior, ataxia, and fever. **Peripheral** anticholinergic effects include decreased saliva, sweat (further contributing to fever), and tearing. Other peripheral symptoms include loss of accommodation, blurred vision, mydriasis, tachycardia, and decreased gastrointestinal motility and urinary bladder tone. The following mnemonic summarizes many central and peripheral effects of anticholinergic poisoning:

□ Hot as a hare—fever.
□ Blind as a bat—loss of accommodation and blurred vision.
□ Dry as a bone—no saliva, sweat, tears.
□ Red as a beet—flushed appearance.
□ Mad as a hatter—CNS excitation, hallucinations, ataxia.

The following botanicals are the best known of the plants that contain atropine, scopolamine, and other antimuscarinic alkaloids:

□ *Datura stramonium* (jimson weed).
□ *Mandragora officinarum* (mandrake).
□ *Hyoscyamus niger* (henbane).
□ *Atropa belladonna* (deadly nightshade).

Clinical Considerations. Common causes of anticholinergic poisoning are eating the seeds or flowers of one of the plants mentioned above or drinking a tea made from one or more of these plants.[6] One historic treatment for asthma was to inhale the smoke from burning jimson weed. The active ingredient in that "folk remedy" was ipratropium, a well-known antimuscarinic bronchodilator.

Therapy. Treatment begins with induced vomiting or gastric lavage plus activated charcoal. **Physostigmine** is the first line of drug therapy, chosen because of its ability to reverse both central (it has a tertiary amine group that readily crosses the blood-brain barrier) and peripheral effects. Possible consequences of the physostigmine administration include hypotension, asystole, and bronchospasm.

Selected References

1. Lefkowitz RJ, Hoffman BB, Taylor P. Neurotransmission. In Hardman JG, Limbird LE, eds. The Pharmacological Basis of Therapeutics. 9th ed. New York: McGraw-Hill, 1996:115.
2. Schneider SM. Mushroom toxicity. In Auerbach PS, ed. Wilderness Medicine: Management of Wilderness and Environmental Emergencies. 3rd ed. St. Louis: CV Mosby, 1995:896–897.
3. Taylor P. Anticholinesterase agents. In Hardman JG, Limbird LE, eds. The Pharmacological Basis of Therapeutics. 9th ed. New York: McGraw-Hill, 1996:161–176.
4. Keeler JR, Hurst CG, Dunn MA. Pyridostigmine used as a nerve agent pretreatment under wartime conditions. JAMA 1991;266:693–695.
5. Welna JO. Personal communication.
6. Brown JH, Taylor P. Muscarinic receptor agonists and antagonists. In Hardman JG, Limbird LE, eds. The Pharmacological Basis of Therapeutics. 9th ed. New York: McGraw-Hill, 1996:154.

202
Malignant Hyperthermia

Denise J. Wedel, M.D.

History

In 1960, Denborough and Lovell reported the first case of anesthesia-induced hypermetabolism in a patient with a familial history of multiple anesthetic deaths during ether administration. The patient survived a halothane-induced malignant hyperthermia (MH) episode. In 1969, Kalow and Britt described a metabolic error of skeletal muscle metabolism noted in patients recovered from MH episodes. This finding formed the scientific basis for modern diagnostic contracture testing. In 1975, Harrison reported the efficacy of dantrolene in treating porcine MH, a treatment that has lowered the mortality rate associated with this rare problem from as high as 80% to below 10%.[1]

Incidence and Mortality

The incidence of MH reportedly ranges from 1:4500 to 1:60,000 general anesthetics (geographic variation is related to the gene prevalence). Approximately 50% of MH-susceptible individuals have had a previous triggering anesthetic without developing MH. MH is rare in infants, and incidence decreases after age 50 years, with males more commonly affected than females. The reasons for these variations are not understood.

MH has been clearly associated with central core disease. MH-like symptoms have been associated with other neuromuscular disorders such as Duchenne's muscular dystrophy; nontriggering anesthesia is recommended for these patients. Association with other conditions such as myotonia, sudden infant death syndrome (SIDS), neuroleptic malignant syndrome (NMS), and sudden death in adults is controversial.

Genetics of MH

Most families have an autosomal dominant pattern of inheritance with variable expression. The rate of spontaneous mutation is unknown but is probably less than 10%. Recent reports suggest that more than one gene may be involved.

A single gene mutation responsible for MH has been identified in the swine model (ryanodine receptor). The ryanodine receptor is a protein that comprises the calcium release channel in the skeletal muscle sarcoplasmic reticulum, a site shown to be defective in MH-susceptible swine. Unfortunately, human MH is far more complicated genetically. More than 20 mutations have been reported in humans, some isolated to a single family. Only about 50% of the known mutations are situated on the ryanodine receptor, and several genes have been implicated. Thus, a single preoperative genetic screening test in humans is unlikely.

Clinical Presentation

Onset of clinical signs can be acute and fulminant or delayed. MH can occur at any time during the anesthetic and has been reported to occur as late as 24 hours postoperatively.

Trismus or masseter muscle spasm following inhalation induction and succinylcholine is associated with an approximately 50% incidence of MH diagnosed by contracture testing. Trismus is often not associated with signs of a fulminant MH episode; however, patients must be closely observed for evidence of hypermetabolism as well as rhabdomyolysis. The presence of whole body rigidity or signs of hypermetabolism following trismus increases the risk of MH susceptibility as a cause, as does a peak creatine phosphokinase (CK) level exceeding 25,000 IU/L postoperatively.

Clinical signs and symptoms reflect a state of highly increased metabolism. The onset of hyperthermia is often delayed (Table 202–1). The earliest signs of MH include increased end-tidal CO_2 levels, tachycardia, and tachypnea (in an unparalyzed patient).

Table 202–1. Clinical Signs of Malignant Hyperthermia

Increased temperature	Increased sympathetic activity
Tachypnea	Tachycardia
Rhabdomyolysis	Dysrhythmias
Metabolic/respiratory acidosis	Sweating
Rigidity (75% humans)	Hypertension

Supportive laboratory tests for confirmation of MH diagnosis include:

□ Elevated end-tidal CO_2.
□ Blood gas analysis: mixed venous, arterial, or venous samples will show a metabolic acidosis.
□ Elevated serum creatine phosphokinase (CK): draw every 6 hours for 24 hours.
□ Myoglobin in serum and urine.
□ Increased serum K^+, Ca^{2+}, lactate.

Triggers include:

□ All potent volatile anesthetics.
□ Succinylcholine.
□ Potassium, reported to cause retriggering in a patient treated for MH.

Safe anesthetic agents include nitrous oxide, etomidate, ketamine, propofol, all narcotics, **all** local anesthetics, all barbiturates, and all nondepolarizing muscle relaxants. Agents used for reversal of muscle relaxants are also safe.

Mechanism. Exposure to triggering anesthetics causes decreased control of intracellular calcium, resulting in release of free unbound ionized Ca^{2+} from storage sites. The calcium pumps attempt to restore homeostasis, which results in ATP utilization, increased aerobic and anaerobic metabolism, and a runaway metabolic state. Rigidity occurs when unbound myofibrillar Ca^{2+} approaches the contractile threshold.

Treatment. Discontinue triggers immediately and hyperventilate with 100% oxygen.

Dantrolene should be given early and rapidly when MH is suspected in a dosage of 2 mg/kg intravenously (IV), repeated every 5 minutes to effect or to a maximum of 10 mg/kg (this limit may be exceeded if necessary). After successful treatment, dantrolene is continued at 1 mg/kg IV every 6 hours for 24 to 48 hours to prevent recrudescence of symptoms. Calcium channel blockers should not be given in the presence of dantrolene, because myocardial depression has been demonstrated in swine. Treatment efficacy is monitored with arterial blood gases, serum CK, and vital signs.

Symptomatic treatment includes, as appropriate:

□ Cooling (avoid hypothermia).
□ Antiarrhythmics.
□ Management of hyperkalemia with insulin and glucose.
□ Diuretics: mannitol, lasix.
□ Sodium bicarbonate.

Anesthesia for MH-Susceptible Patients

Pretreatment with dantrolene is not recommended. Choose nontriggering anesthetic agents. Prepare the machine by removing vaporizers (if possible) and replacing rubber hoses and soda lime. Flush with high-flow air or oxygen (10 L/min) for 10 minutes.

Monitoring should include all standard monitors with an emphasis on end-tidal CO_2, oxygen saturation, and core temperature (skin monitors may not reflect core changes). Arterial and central venous pressures should be monitored only if indicated by the surgical procedure or the patient's medical condition.

Evaluation of Susceptibility

Patients are referred for evaluation for a number of reasons:

□ Unexplained intraoperative death in family members.
□ History of adverse anesthetic event (e.g., trismus).
□ Perioperative fever.
□ Idiopathic elevated CK levels.
□ History of rhabdomyolysis.
□ Associated myopathies (e.g., central core disease).

A serum CK level is often obtained in patients suspected of being susceptible to MH. This value is elevated in approximately 70% of affected individuals.

The muscle biopsy contracture testing is the only reliable diagnostic test for MH. Muscle is tested with caffeine and halothane alone, or in combination, and contracture responses are measured. This test has been standardized in European and North American laboratories.

The Malignant Hyperthermia Association of the United States (MHAUS, 39 East State St., P.O. Box 1069, Sherburne, NY 13460-1069) is a lay organization that provides support for patients and physicians. It publishes books, pamphlets, and a quarterly newsletter at nominal costs, and sponsors a 24-hour hotline (1-800-MHHYPER) to provide assistance to physicians managing MH-susceptible patients or treating acute MH episodes. Information can also be obtained at www.MHAUS.org.

Selected References

1. Kolb ME, Horne ML, Martz R. Dantrolene in human malignant hyperthermia. Anesthesiology 1982;56:254–262.

Suggested References

Gronert GA, Schulman SR, Mott J. Malignant hyperthermia. In Miller RD, ed. Anesthesia. 3rd ed. New York: Churchill Livingstone, 1990:935.

Hogan K, Couch F, Powers PA, et al. A cysteine-for-arginine substitution (R614C) in the human skeletal muscle calcium release channel cosegregates with malignant hyperthermia. Anesth Analg 1992;75:441–448.

Morgan KG, Bryant SH. The mechanism of action of dantrolene sodium. J Pharmacol Exp Ther 1977;201:138–147.

203
Myasthenia Gravis and Lambert-Eaton Myasthenic Syndrome

Claude A. Vachon, M.D.

Myasthenia gravis (MG) is an autoimmune disease of the neuromuscular junction characterized by weakness of voluntary skeletal muscles, with muscles innervated by the cranial nerves most frequently involved. The incidence of MG is approximately 3:100,000, with 1:20,000 in the adult population. It has been classified by symptomatology: Class I, ocular symptoms only; Class IIA, mild generalized symptoms; Class IIB, moderate generalized symptoms with some bulbar symptoms; Class III, acute and severe bulbar symptoms; and Class IV, severe disease with marked bulbar symptoms. Clinical presentations are also grouped according to age (Table 203–1).

Mechanism

MG is caused by a decrease in acetylcholine receptors (AChRs) at the neuromuscular junction. It is considered an autoimmune disease, with 70% to 90% of patients found to have circulating antibodies to AChRs. These antibodies are thought to reduce the number of AChRs in three ways: competitive blockade of receptors by blocking access to the receptor, increasing degradation of the receptor, and complement-mediated lysis of the receptor and muscular end-plate of the neuromuscular junction. These factors result in a motor end-plate with decreased surface area and decreased functional AChRs (Fig. 203–1).

Therapy

Therapy for MG usually involves administration of an anticholinesterase, such as pyridostigmine, that increases the amount of acetylcholine available at the neuromuscular junction by blocking cholinesterase activity. Patients with MG will often also receive immunosuppression therapy with a steroid, azathioprine, or cyclosporine. Thymectomy is performed to treat MG for its effect in reducing the antibody levels, although the mechanism by which this produces benefits is still uncertain. Plasmapheresis and intravenous immune globulin are used to treat acute myasthenic exacerbations.

Anesthetic Implications

Preoperative Evaluation. The duration, severity, and treatment of MG are all important fac-

Table 203–1. Clinical Presentations of Myasthenia Gravis

	Etiology	Onset	Sex	Thymus	Course
Neonatal myasthenia	Passage of antibodies from myasthenic mothers across the placenta	Neonatal	Both sexes	Normal	Transient
Congenital myasthenia	Congenital endplate pathology genetic, autosomal recessive	0–2 years	Male>female	Normal	Nonfluctuating, compatible with long survival
Juvenile myasthenia	Autoimmune disorder	2–20 years	Female>male (4:1)	Hyperplasia	Slowly progressive, tendency to relapse and remission
Adult myasthenia	Autoimmune disorder	20–40 years	Female>male	Hyperplasia>thymoma	Maximum severity within 3–5 years
Elderly myasthenia	Autoimmune disorder	>40 years	Male>female	Thymoma (benign or locally invasive)	Rapid progress, higher mortality

From Baraka A.[1]

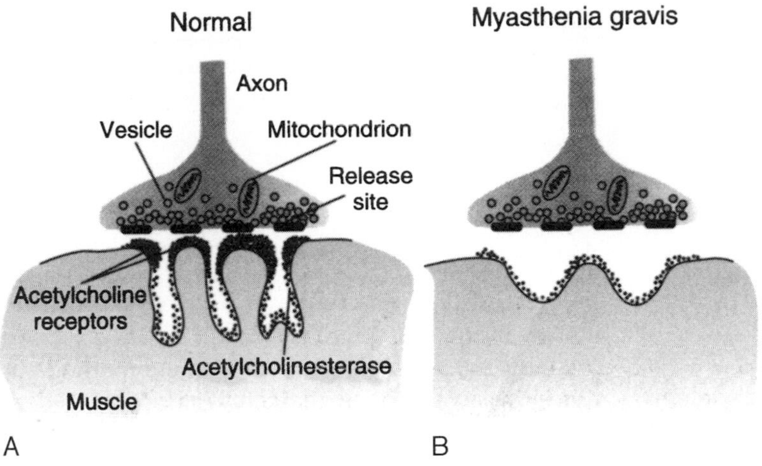

Figure 203–1. Normal *(A)* and myasthenic *(B)* neuromuscular junctions. In neuromuscular junctions, vesicles release acetylcholine at specialized release sites of the nerve terminal. Acetylcholine crosses the synaptic space to reach receptors that are concentrated at the peaks of junctional folds. Acetylcholinesterase in the clefts rapidly terminates transmission by hydrolyzing acetylcholine. The myasthenic junction has reduced numbers of acetylcholine receptors, simplified synaptic folds, a widened synaptic space, and a normal nerve terminal. (From Drachman DB.[2])

tors to assess. Some practitioners will omit or reduce the morning dose of pyridostigmine on the day of surgery, which could alter the effects of neuromuscular blockade. Patients with MG are also more sensitive to the respiratory depressant effects of narcotics and anxiolytics, having reduced respiratory reserve. These drugs should be avoided or used judiciously with careful monitoring. The presence of a thymoma requires all of the usual airway management precautions for an anterior mediastinal mass.

Neuromuscular Relaxants. Patients with MG are very sensitive to nondepolarizing muscle relaxants (NDMRs), often requiring as little as one-tenth the normal dose. This extreme sensitivity has been described in patients with minimal disease, patients in clinical remission, and patients with undiagnosed MG. Long-acting NDMRs should be avoided. Very careful neuromuscular monitoring is warranted during NDMR therapy in patients with MG.

Patients with MG have a relative resistance to depolarizing muscle relaxants, with unpredictable responses because of decreased AChR. Required doses of succinylcholine are usually two to three times normal, with the possibility of prolonged activity.

Volatile Agents. Inhalation anesthetic agents cause muscle relaxation in normal patients but cause profound muscle relaxation in myasthenic patients.

Intravenous Anesthetics. IV anesthetics (thiopental and propofol) have not been shown to have any undesirable effects on myasthenic patients. Narcotics can create respiratory distress in patients with little respiratory reserve.

Regional Anesthetics. Many practitioners prefer regional anesthesia in myasthenic patients, because it allows one to avoid using NDMRs. However, concern for affecting accessory respiratory muscles in patients who may have decreased func-

tion warrants careful dosage. Also, ester-type local anesthetics should be avoided because they are degraded by pseudocholinesterase, which is affected by the anticholinesterase therapy.

Postoperative Management. There are several risk factors that help assess the potential for postoperative ventilatory insufficiency. These include (1) duration of MG greater than 6 years; (2) a history of other chronic respiratory disease; (3) a pyridostigmine dose above 750 mg/day; and (4) preoperative vital capacity below 2.9 L. Other postoperative concerns that arise are myasthenic crisis, cholinergic crisis (both of which could occur with changes in anticholinesterase treatment perioperatively) and residual effects of anesthesia. Postoperative pain control with epidural analgesia has also been shown to help maintain respiratory function.

Lambert-Eaton Myasthenic Syndrome

Lambert-Eaton myasthenic syndrome (LEMS) is a rare disorder of neuromuscular transmission most often associated with carcinoma of the lung, especially oat cell carcinoma of the bronchus. Antibody-mediated destruction of presynaptic voltage gated calcium channels leads to deficient release of acetylcholine at the neuromuscular junction, causing muscle weakness. It is often confused with MG (Table 203–2), but the skeletal muscle weakness associated with LEMS is not reliably reversed with anticholinesterases or corticosteroids. Furthermore, exercise improves, rather than reduces, muscle strength in this condition. Patients with LEMS are very sensitive to the effects of both depolarizing and nondepolarizing muscle relaxants. The potential for LEMS should be considered in patients with known or probable carcinoma, especially of the lung.

Table 203–2. Comparison of Lambert-Eaton Myasthenic Syndrome and Myasthenia Gravis

	Lambert-Eaton Myasthenic Syndrome	Myasthenia Gravis
Manifestations	Proximal limb weakness (legs > arms)	Extraocular, bulbar, and facial muscle weakness
	Exercise improves strength	Fatigue with exercise
	Muscle pain common	Muscle pain uncommon
	Reflexes absent or decreased	Reflexes normal
Gender	Male > female	Female > male
Coexisting pathology	Small cell carcinoma of the lung	Thymoma
Response to muscle relaxant	Sensitive to succinylcholine and nondepolarizing muscle relaxants	Resistant to succinylcholine
		Sensitive to nondepolarizing muscle relaxant
	Poor response to anticholinesterase	Good response to anticholinesterases

From Stoelting RK, Dierdorf SF.[3]

Selected References

1. Baraka A. Anaesthesia and myasthenia gravis. Can J Anaesth 1992;39:476–486.
2. Drachman DB. Medical progress: Myasthenia gravis. NEJM 1994;330:1797–1810.
3. Stoelting RK, Dierdorf SF, eds. Anesthesia and Co-Existing Disease. 3rd ed. New York, Churchill Livingstone, 1993.

Suggested References

Farag E, Barsoum S, Spagnuolo S, et al. Anesthesia and muscle disease. Am J Anesthesiol 2000;27:491–501.
Krucylak PE, Naunheim KS. Preoperative preparation and anesthetic management of patients with myasthenia gravis. Sem Thorac Cardiovasc Surg 1999;11:47–53.

204
Anesthesia for Myotonic Dystrophy

Joseph J. Sandor, M.D.

Myotonias are characterized by delayed muscle relaxation following contraction. **Myotonic dystrophy** is the most common of the triad of myotonias, which also includes **myotonia congenita** and **paramyotonia**.

□ Myotonic dystrophy is transmitted as an autosomal dominant disorder, with expression occurring in the second or third decade of life.
□ An abnormality in the intracellular ATP system that fails to return calcium to the sarcoplasmic reticulum is the theoretical pathologic mechanism of the contracture.
□ Contractures are not relieved by nondepolarizing muscle relaxants, regional anesthesia, or deep anesthesia; however, infiltration of local anesthetics into involved muscle may produce relaxation.
□ Depression of rapid sodium flux into muscle cells by phenytoin, procainamide, quinine, tocainide, or mexiletine may alleviate contracture by delaying membrane excitability.

Coexisting Organ System Dysfunction

Patients may feature the triad of frontal baldness, mental retardation, and cataract formation. Other common features may include gonadal atrophy, facial weakness, ptosis, dysarthria, wasting of neck musculature, and inability to relax grip.

Cardiac involvement may include structural and functional abnormalities.

□ **Mitral valve prolapse** occurs in 20% of affected individuals.
□ Progressive deterioration of the His-Purkinje system may lead to **arrhythmias**. Sudden death is usually related to abrupt onset of **atrioventricular block**.
□ Involvement of cardiac muscle may produce **cardiomyopathy**.

Pulmonary pathophysiology also may be both structural and functional.

□ Pulmonary function testing reveals a **restrictive lung disease** pattern.
□ **Ventilatory responses** to hypoxia and hypercarbia are impaired.

□ Patients are predisposed to **pneumonia** as a result of reduced lung volumes and ineffective cough mechanisms.

Gastrointestinal abnormalities that predispose these patients to gastric content aspiration include gastric atony, intestinal hypermotility, and pharyngeal muscle weakness with impaired airway protection.

Endocrine abnormalities may manifest as diabetes mellitus, thyroid dysfunction, adrenal dysfunction, and gonadal atrophy.

Pregnancy exacerbates myotonic dystrophy, probably secondary to elevated progesterone levels. There is also a high incidence of obstetric complications seen, including

□ Polyhydramnios.
□ Premature onset of labor.
□ Breech presentation.
□ Uterine atony.
□ Retained placenta.
□ Postpartum hemorrhage.
□ Impaired cervical dilation.

Anesthetic Management

Preoperative evaluation should focus on cardiac conduction abnormalities, pulmonary function, cardiac reserve, and the patient's ability to protect the airway.

Preoperative medication might include oral antacids and metoclopramide. These patients have an increased sensitivity to preoperative sedative medications, and these should be avoided, if possible.

Patients with congenital myotonia have an increased sensitivity to intravenous (IV) induction **agents**; thus, these should be used cautiously and titrated to effect. Etomidate may cause myoclonus and precipitate contractures.

Depolarizing neuromuscular blockade is to be avoided because it produces an exaggerated contracture. **Succinylcholine**-induced fasciculation can lead to contractures severe enough to impair ventilation. Because of impaired airway protective mechanisms, placement of a cuffed endotracheal tube is recommended.

- **Endotracheal intubation** can be performed awake or as a rapid-sequence induction with **cricoid pressure** along with a reduced dose of IV induction agent.
- **Neuromuscular blockade** might not be needed to facilitate intubation.

Maintenance of anesthesia is best achieved with a balance of inhalation agent, opioid, and neuromuscular blocking agents.

- Halothane may augment cardiac conduction abnormalities and should be avoided.
- Exaggerated myocardial depression may result from use of isoflurane or enflurane, but cautious use may minimize these effects and obviate the need for IV neuromuscular blocking agents.
- Exaggerated respiratory depressant effects from narcotics used for anesthetic maintenance should be anticipated. Use of short-acting opioids (fentanyl, alfentanil) for supplemental analgesia is recommended.
- If neuromuscular blockade is needed, careful titration of shorter-acting agents (vecuronium, atracurium) is guided by the use of a peripheral nerve stimulator.
- Use of an anticholinesterase agent for neuromuscular blockade reversal could theoretically precipitate myoclonus because of acetylcholine-facilitated depolarization at the neuromuscular junction. Use of short-acting neuromuscular blockers may eliminate the need for pharmacologic reversal.
- Monitoring should include electrocardiogram, blood pressure measurement, anesthetic gas analysis, pulse oximetry, and neuromuscular blockade monitor.
- Ambient room temperature should be kept warm to avoid shivering, which can precipitate contractures.
- Extubation should be performed when the patient is fully awake.
- Postoperative analgesia can be provided by local injection of local anesthetics, peripheral nerve blocks, and epidural opioid administration.

Suggested References

Anderson BJ, Brown TC. Congenital myotonic dystrophy in children: A review of ten years' experience. Anaesth Intensive Care 1989;17:320–324.

Azar I. The response of patients with neuromuscular disorders to muscle relaxants: A review. Anesthesiology 1984;61:173–187.

Dierdorf SF. Anesthesia for patients with rare and co-existing diseases. In Barash PG, Cullen BF, Stoelting RK, eds. Clinical Anesthesia. 3rd ed. Philadelphia: JB Lippincott, 1997:461–88.

Farag E, Barsoum S, Spagnuolo S, et al. Anesthesia and muscle disease. Am J Anesthesiol 2000;27:491–501.

Hageman AT, Gabreels FJ, Liem KD, et al. Congenital myotonic dystrophy: A report on thirteen cases and a review of the literature. J Neurol Sci 1993;115:95–101.

Stoelting RK, Dierdorf SF. Anesthesia and Co-Existing Disease. 3rd ed. New York, Churchill Livingstone, 1993.

Webb D, Muir I, Faulkner J, et al. Myotonia dystrophia: obstetric complications. Am J Obstet Gynecol 1978;132:265–270.

205
Anesthesia for Patients with Epilepsy

Margaret R. Weglinski, M.D.

Epilepsy is a common disorder. From epidemiologic studies, it can be extrapolated that at the time of the 1990 census approximately 1.65 million individuals in the United States were subject to recurrent seizures. This figure does not include those patients in whom convulsions complicate febrile and other intercurrent illnesses or injuries. More than two-thirds of all seizure disorders begin in childhood (most in the first year of life). In the practice of pediatric neurology, epilepsy is the most common disorder, and in adults it is surpassed only by cerebral vascular disorders. It has been estimated that in the United States, nearly 1% of persons will have epilepsy by age 20.

Adams and colleagues[1] define epilepsy as "an intermittent derangement of the nervous system due presumably to a sudden, excessive, disorderly discharge of cerebral neurons." They go on to say that "the discharge results in an almost instantaneous disturbance of sensation, loss of consciousness, impairment of psychic function, convulsive movements, or some combination thereof."[1]

Classification of Seizures

Seizures are divided into two types, based mainly on the clinical form of the seizure and its electroencephalographic (EEG) features (Table 205–1): partial, in which a localized or focal onset occurs, and generalized, in which the seizures appear to begin bilaterally. Partial seizures are classified as simple when consciousness is retained and complex when consciousness is disturbed. Simple partial seizures are further divided according to their main clinical manifestations: motor, sensory, autonomic, or psychic. There are two types of generalized seizures: convulsive and nonconvulsive. Tonic-clonic (grand mal) seizure is the common convulsive type. The brief loss of consciousness or absence (petit mal) is the most common nonconvulsive generalized seizure.

Antiepileptic Drug Therapy

The use of anticonvulsant medications is the most important aspect of epilepsy treatment. Approximately two-thirds of all patients with epilepsy experience complete or almost complete seizure control with the use of antiepileptic drugs; an additional 20% to 25% experience a significant reduction in frequency and severity of attacks. The most commonly used drugs are listed in Table 205–2, along with their dosages, serum half-lives, effective blood levels, and therapeutic indications.

Antiepileptic Drugs and Anesthetic Care. The most pertinent interaction between antiepileptic drugs and anesthetic agents involves the use of nondepolarizing muscle relaxants in patients chronically taking such enzyme-inducting anticonvulsants as phenytoin, carbamazepine, and phenobarbital. These patients can be resistant to the effects of neuromuscular blocking agents. They also require higher doses of fentanyl to maintain a compa-

Table 205–1. International Classification of Epileptic Seizures

I. Generalized seizures (bilaterally symmetrical and without local onset)
  A. Tonic, clonic, or tonic-clonic (grand mal)
  B. Absence (petit mal)
    1. Simple—loss of consciousness only
    2. Complex—with brief tonic, clonic, or automatic movements
  C. Lennox-Gastaut syndrome
  D. Juvenile myoclonic epilepsy
  E. Infantile spasms (West syndrome)
  F. Atonic (astatic, akinetic) seizures (sometimes with myoclonic jerks)
II. Partial, or focal, seizures (seizures beginning locally)
  A. Simple (without loss of consciousness)
    1. Motor (tonic, clonic, tonic-clonic; jacksonian; benign childhood epilepsy; epilepsia partialis continua)
    2. Somatosensory or special sensory (visual, auditory, olfactory, gustatory, vertiginous)
    3. Autonomic
    4. Psychic
  B. Complex (with impaired consciousness)
    1. Beginning as simple partial seizures and progressing to impairment of consciousness
    2. With impairment of consciousness at onset
III. Special epileptic syndromes
  A. Myoclonus and myoclonic seizures
  B. Reflex epilepsy
  C. Acquired aphasia with convulsive disorder
  D. Febrile and other seizures of infancy and childhood
  E. Hysterical seizures

From Adams RD, Victor M, and Ropper AH.[1]

Table 205–2. Common Antiepileptic Drugs

Generic Name	Trade Name	Usual Daily Dosage		Principal Therapeutic Indications	Serum Half-Life (hours)	Effective Blood Level[a] (µg/mL)
		Children	Adults (mg)			
Phenobarbital	Luminal	3–5 mg/kg (8 mg/kg in infants)	60–200	Tonic-clonic seizures; simple and complex partial seizures; absence	96 ± 12	15–35
Phenytoin	Dilantin	4–7 mg/kg	300–400	Tonic-clonic seizures; simple and complex partial seizures	24 ± 12	10–20
Carbamazepine	Tegretol	20–30 mg/kg	600–1200	Tonic-clonic seizures; complex partial seizures	12 ± 4	4–12
Primidone	Mysoline	10–25 mg/kg	750–1500	Tonic-clonic seizures; simple and complex partial seizures	10 ± 2	5–12
Ethosuximide	Zarontin	20–40 mg/kg	750–1500	Absence	50 ± 6	50–100
Methsuximide	Celontin	10–20 mg/kg	500–1000	Absence	40 ± 6	40–100
Diazepam	Valium	0.15–2 mg/kg (intravenously)	10–150	Status epilepticus		
Lorazepam	Ativan	0.03–0.22 mg/kg (intravenously)		Status epilepticus		
ACTH		40–60 units/day		Infantile spasms		
Valproate	Depakote	30–60 mg/kg	1000–3000	Absence and myoclonic seizures; as an adjunctive drug in tonic clonic and complex partial seizures	8 ± 2	50–100
Clonazepam	Klonopin	0.01–0.2 mg/kg	1.5–20	Absence; myoclonus	18–50	0.01–0.07

[a]Average trough values.
From Adams RD, Victor M, and Ropper AH.[1]

rable level of anesthesia. It is not known why resistance develops to neuromuscular blocking agents and opioids in these patients, but possible explanations include changes in the number of receptors, interactions with endogenous neurotransmitters, and alterations in drug metabolism.

Antiepileptic drugs with significant hematologic or hepatic toxicity can also influence anesthetic management. Anticonvulsant therapy can produce biochemical abnormalities in liver function (γ-glutamyl transpeptidase, alkaline phosphatase, and alanine aminotransferase). These alterations are not symptomatic and are not believed to be clinically significant. Valproate can cause a dose-dependent thrombocytopenia as well as a coagulopathy via intrinsic factors. Valproate's effect on hemostasis is most reliably monitored via the platelet count and other studies. Carbamazepine metabolism is inhibited by erythromycin and cimetidine, leading to increased blood levels and toxicity.

Surgery for Epilepsy

Failure to control seizures with medication occurs in 10% to 20% of patients with epilepsy. Although there is no precise definition of intractable epilepsy, considerations include seizure frequency, seizure type, severity of attacks, and impact on quality of life. It is also essential to verify that the proper drugs have been used in the correct amounts. Complex partial seizures are more resistant to medical treatment than tonic-clonic or other common forms of epilepsy. Surgery is neither simpler nor safer than medication and thus should not be considered an alternative to medical treatment. If it is determined that the patient indeed has intractable epilepsy, then surgery should be considered.

Patient Selection. The most favorable candidates for surgery are those with complex partial seizures, a unilateral temporal lobe focus, normal intelligence quotient, high level of motivation, no diffuse brain damage, seizures that were uncontrolled by medication for more than 4 years, and a seizure focus that is resectable without causing major neurologic deficits. Characteristics associated with the most improvement psychosocially after surgical control of seizures are age under 30 years, good family support preoperatively, and a low degree of psychopathology.

The primary aim of the evaluation and preparation of the patient for surgery is to locate the discharging seizure focus. This requires a careful analysis of clinical and EEG findings, often including those obtained by telemetry and the use of stereotactic or subdural strip electrodes. Table 205–3 lists the various tests that may be included in the evaluation of a potential epilepsy surgery candidate.

Surgery: Goals, Approaches, Results, Complications. It has been estimated that approximately 40% of all patients with partial epilepsy are candidates for surgical treatment. The main objective of epilepsy surgery is to abolish or reduce the frequency of seizures without cognitive or neurological deficits and without aggravation of psychiatric symptoms. The most commonly performed procedure is temporal lobectomy, followed by procedures of less proven value, such as hemispherectomy and section of the corpus callosum.

Table 205–3. Clinical Evaluation of Epilepsy Surgery Candidates

Scalp/sphenoidal interictal EEG
Video, scalp/sphenoidal telemetry
Neuropsychologic testing
Neuroradiologic testing (CT scan, angiography)
Positron computed tomography scan of cerebral glucose metabolism
Magnetic resonance imaging
Video and stereoelectroencephalography telemetry
After discharge thresholds
Intracarotid amobarbital (Wada test)
Thiopental study

From Crandall PH, Rausch R, and Engel J Jr.

Anterior temporal lobectomy successfully stops complex partial seizures in 60% to 80% of surgical patients, but anticonvulsant medication may still be needed postoperatively to fully suppress seizure activity. Mortality following temporal lobectomy is approximately 1% and is most commonly attributed to postoperative hemorrhage, infarction, pulmonary complications, and sudden death. Morbidity is approximately 2% and includes such complications as hemiparesis, visual field deficits, cranial nerve palsy (oculomotor and/or facial nerve), infection, aphasia, memory deficits, and psychiatric deterioration.

For patients with medically refractory seizures and for whom surgery is not an option or is unsuccessful, chronic intermittent stimulation of the vagus nerve via implantation of a vagal nerve stimulator is an alternative treatment.

In the early postoperative period after craniotomy for epilepsy, special considerations include the management of anticonvulsant drugs and of early postoperative seizures. The combination of the stress of surgery and anesthesia and the antibiotics and steroids routinely administered with craniotomies often has dramatic and rather unpredictable effects on serum anticonvulsant drug levels in the first postoperative week. These oscillations in antiepileptic drug levels, as well as alterations in cortical excitability from operative exposure, are likely factors contributing to the occurrence of early postoperative seizures. Several studies suggest that these early seizures may have no correlation with eventual outcome.

Anesthetic Techniques. Epilepsy surgery may be performed in the awake and cooperative but sedated patient. Pain control is achieved with the use of local anesthesia and intravenous opioids. The patient may be sedated with barbiturates or propofol in the initial stages of the procedure; these agents are then withheld during functional mapping and electrocorticography. Several anesthetic agents (e.g., etomidate, methohexital, and alfentanil) have been found to activate spikes or spike-burst suppression during electrocorticography and thus aid in the localization of epileptic foci.

General anesthesia is also used for epilepsy surgery, with its goal being to exert a minimal impact on electrocerebral activity and hence be able to observe electrocorticographic spike activity. The most commonly used anesthetic agents are isoflurane, nitrous oxide, fentanyl, sufentanil, alfentanil, and droperidol. No premedications are administered before induction with thiopental and fentanyl. Excellent intraoperative electrophysiologic studies can be obtained using these agents. Isoflurane is usually discontinued and activating drugs may be added just before electrical recording. Despite this fairly light anesthesia, patients rarely have intraoperative recall.

Selected References

1. Adams RD, Victor M, Ropper AH. Epilepsy and other seizure disorders. In Principles of Neurology. 6th ed. New York: McGraw-Hill, 1997:313–343.
2. Crandall PH, Rausch R, Engel J Jr. Preoperative indicators for optimal surgical outcome for temporal lobe epilepsy. In Wieser HG, Elger CE, eds. Presurgical Evaluation of Epileptics: Basics, Techniques, Implications. Berlin: Springer-Verlag, 1987:325.

Suggested References

Kofke WA, Tempelhoff R, Dasheiff RM. Anesthetic implications of epilepsy, status epilepticus, and epilepsy surgery. J Neurosurg Anesthesiol 1997;9:349–372.
Ornstein E, Matteo RS, Schwartz AE, et al. The effect of phenytoin on the magnitude and duration of neuromuscular block following atracurium or vecuronium. Anesthesiology 1987;67:191–196.
Tempelhoff R, Modica PA, Spitznagel EL Jr. Anticonvulsant therapy increases fentanyl requirements during anaesthesia for craniotomy. Can J Anaesth 1990;37:327–332.

206
Morbid Obesity and Anesthesia

Stephen T. Gott, M.D.

Obesity is the most common nutritional disorder in the industrialized world. Approximately 34 million Americans are classified as obese (more than 20% above ideal body weight). Morbid obesity is defined as body weight greater than twice the ideal weight. The body mass index (BMI) is the ratio of weight (kg) to height^2 (m^2). A ratio between 26 and 29 is classified as overweight; a ratio greater than or equal to 30 is obese.

Obese patients present with an increased anesthetic risk because of technical difficulties and physiologic changes. They also tend to have associated disorders that complicate their anesthetic management, such as hypertension, impaired pulmonary function, coronary artery disease, non–insulin-dependent diabetes mellitus, cancer, and renal and gastrointestinal abnormalities.

Cardiovascular Function

Obesity causes a proportional increase in circulating blood volume, plasma volume, and cardiac output. Cardiac output increases by 0.1 L/min for each kilogram of adipose tissue perfused. This increase in volume perfused increases afterload. Preload is also increased secondary to increased systemic and pulmonary blood volume. This results in elevated right atrial, pulmonary artery, and pulmonary capillary wedge pressures. Moderate hypertension is present in 50% of morbidly obese patients, and severe hypertension is seen in 5% to 10% of them. The incidence rate of coronary artery disease in morbidly obese individuals is double that in the nonobese population. Increased afterload, decreased oxygen supply, and coronary artery disease can lead to left ventricular hypertrophy and failure. Right ventricular hypertrophy and failure may result from chronic hypoxemia, hypercarbia, polycythemia, and pulmonary hypertension (pickwickian syndrome).

Respiratory Function

Obesity causes a proportional increase in oxygen consumption and carbon dioxide (CO$_2$) production secondary to fat metabolism. These patients require increased energy expenditures to maintain the high minute volume needed to achieve normocarbia in the presence of reduced chest wall compliance and increased CO$_2$ production. Lung compliance is usually normal. Obesity causes restrictive lung disease. In the upright position, both expiratory reserve volume and functional residual capacity are reduced, which may lead to ventilation/perfusion mismatching if tidal volumes fall within the closing capacity. This is exacerbated in the supine position (Fig. 206–1). In the healthy obese individual, forced vital capacity, forced expiratory volume in 1 second, and peak expiratory flow rate are usually normal.

Pickwickian Syndrome

The **pickwickian syndrome**, named by Burwell in 1956, is also known as the obesity-hypoventilation syndrome. The term stems from the Charles Dickens' portrayal of Joe, the fat, somnolent, red-faced boy in the *Posthumous Papers of the Pickwick Club*, written in 1837.

The syndrome is estimated to occur in 8% of the obese population. Body weight is typically over 130

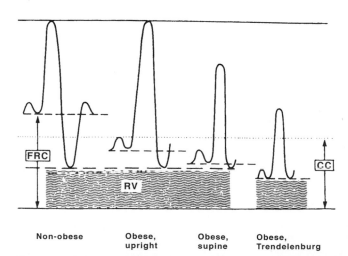

| Non-obese | Obese, upright | Obese, supine | Obese, Trendelenburg |

Figure 206–1. Effect of position changes on various lung volumes in a nonobese and a morbidly obese subject. FRC, functional residual capacity; RV, residual volume; CC, closing capacity. (From Vaughan RW, Vaughan MS.[1])

kg and, in most cases, a very rapid increase in weight has occurred.

Symptomatology. The hallmarks of this condition are alveolar hypoventilation, hypersomnia, and obesity. Hypoventilation leads to respiratory acidosis, arterial hypoxemia, and polycythemia. Chronic hypoxemia and polycythemia are thought to cause the pulmonary vascular changes in this syndrome, including marked pulmonary hypertension, right axis deviation on electrocardiogram, and evidence of right ventricular hypertrophy or cor pulmonale in extreme cases. Complications from immobility include pulmonary emboli and pneumonia.

Obstructive sleep apnea may occur with this syndrome. Obesity and sleep-induced relaxation of the pharyngeal musculature are thought to cause intermittent upper airway obstruction. Obstruction leads to hypoxemia and hypercapnia, which results in arousal and the return of normal respiration. Repeated awakening at night can lead to daytime hypersomnolence.

Etiology. The cause of the pickwickian syndrome is not clear. It is thought to be a disorder of the regulation of ventilation by the respiratory control centers of the central nervous system and/or inability of the muscles of respiration to respond to neural impulses. Patients with this syndrome show blunted ventilatory responses to hypercapnia and hypoxia and often develop hypercapnia and hypoxemia from decreased basal ventilation.

Metabolic, Renal, and Hepatic Function

Obesity is associated with insulin resistance. There is a marked increase in adult-onset diabetes mellitus in the obese population. These patients may exhibit elevated cholesterol, triglyceride, and liver transaminase serum levels. During efforts to lose weight, there is a potential for fluid and electrolyte imbalances from extreme dieting and laxative and diuretic use or abuse. Halothane hepatitis is epidemiologically associated with obesity. There is increased metabolism of halothane through reductive pathways, which may predispose to this condition. However, there is no evidence that halothane causes more hepatocellular damage than other anesthetic agents, as measured by postoperative SGOT and SGPT levels.

Gastrointestinal Function

Some 90% of morbidly obese patients have a gastric volume greater than 25 mL and a pH below 2.5. These factors are associated with more severe lung parenchymal damage should aspiration of gastric contents occur. Because of the increased abdominal wall mass, intra-abdominal pressure is elevated, and these patients have an increased incidence of diaphragmatic hernia. Because of these factors, obese individuals are at a greater risk for aspiration pneumonitis.

There is a threefold increase in the incidence rate of gallbladder and biliary tract disease in obese patients.

Pharmacokinetics

Highly lipophilic drugs, such as thiopental and benzodiazepines, have an increased volume of distribution and longer elimination half-life in obese patients than in nonobese patients, but similar clearance rates. The action of fat-soluble volatile agents is not prolonged in obesity, however. Hydrophilic drugs have similar volumes of distribution, elimination half-lives, and clearances in obese and nonobese individuals. Because of higher pseudocholinesterase levels in the obese individuals, larger doses of succinylcholine may be required.

Management of Anesthesia

Preoperative considerations include the following:

□ **Cardiovascular**: Evaluate for right and/or left ventricular failure, hypertension, and coronary artery disease.
□ **Respiratory**: Evaluate for airway abnormalities and nocturnal airway obstruction. Spirometry and arterial blood gases may help predict pre-, peri-, and postoperative respiratory complications.
□ **Metabolic, renal, hepatic**: Serum glucose, electrolytes, liver function tests, and creatinine are used as a preoperative baseline.
□ **Gastrointestinal**: Consider the use of metoclopramide or an H_2 blocker.
□ **Miscellaneous**: Venous access may require central line placement or a cutdown. A large blood pressure cuff may be necessary. Direct arterial line pressure measurement may be more accurate than noninvasive measures. Monitoring of neuromuscular blockade may show a decreased response from surface electrodes due to overlying fat.

Anesthetic Technique

General. For general anesthesia, the following measures apply.

□ **Airway management**: Increased soft tissue and decreased mandibular and cervical mobility may necessitate awake fiberoptic intubation. In morbidly obese patients, excessive soft tissue surrounding the upper airway tends to block any view past the tip of the laryngoscope blade, making direct laryngoscopy difficult, if not impossible. Mask ventilation is also more difficult.

□ **Induction**: There is an accelerated rate of rise in alveolar concentration with volatile agents and a rapid arterial oxygen desaturation with intubation secondary to a reduced functional residual capacity.

□ **Maintenance**: Increased reductive metabolism of halothane and the theoretical risk of halothane hepatitis discourage its use. When ventilation is adequate and a high inspired oxygen level is not needed, nitrous oxide is useful because of its lipid insolubility. Respiratory compromise occurs because of anesthetic-induced decreases in functional residual capacity. Positioning and the operative site can also influence respiratory function. Mechanical ventilation with large tidal volumes and positive end-expiratory pressure (if there is no hemodynamic compromise) can be used to improve ventilation-perfusion matching.

Regional. Spinal and epidural anesthesia may be technically difficult because of excessive subcutaneous tissue. There is a decreased anesthetic requirement for epidural local anesthetics. This is because of decreased epidural space volume secondary to increased intra-abdominal pressure, which dilates the epidural veins. There is a relatively high incidence rate of preexisting mechanical back pain in obese patients.

Postoperative Considerations

Obese patients have increased postoperative morbidity and mortality. Atelectasis, pneumonia, thrombophlebitis, pulmonary embolism, wound infection, and dehiscence are more common in obese than in nonobese postoperative patients.

Selected References

1. Vaughan RW, Vaughan MS. Anesthetic management of patients with massive obesity. In Utting JE, Brown BR, Jr, eds. General Anesthesia. London: Butterworths, 1989:749.

Suggested References

Buckley FP. Anesthesia and obesity and gastrointestinal disorders. In Barash PG, Cullen BF, Stoelting RK, eds. Clinical Anesthesia. 3rd ed. Philadelphia: JB Lippincott, 1997:975–990.
Roizen MF. Anesthetic implications of concurrent diseases. In Miller RD, ed. Anesthesia. 5th ed. New York: Churchill Livingstone, 2000:903–1016.
Stoelting RK, Dierdorf SE. Anesthesia and Co-Existing Disease. 3rd ed. New York, Churchill Livingstone, 1993.

207
Anesthetic Implications of Thyrotoxicosis and Thyroid Storm

Michael L. Bishop, M.D.

Thyrotoxicosis (hyperthyroidism) is a constellation of signs and symptoms resulting from biochemical alterations caused by the hypersecretion of thyroid hormones. These hormones exert influences on nuclear, ribosomal, and mitochondrial functions. Low concentrations of thyroid hormones produce an increase in the oxidative process without markedly influencing energy transfer; however, high concentrations result in uncoupling of oxidative phosphorylation. Heat production is increased because of the increased oxidative state as well as the decreased efficiency of energy conversion. Profuse sweating, peripheral vasodilation, and tachycardia are compensatory mechanisms for dissipating the excess heat. Other signs and symptoms related to the hypermetabolic state include weight loss; increased appetite; increased oxygen consumption; muscle wasting and weakness, especially in the proximal muscle groups; warm, moist skin; and heat intolerance.

In addition to tachycardia, cardiac manifestations include arrhythmias, increased cardiac output, cardiomegaly, heart failure, pulmonary edema, peripheral edema, and mitral valve prolapse. The increase in cardiac output is greater than that required by the hypermetabolic state and probably results from vasodilation of the circulatory beds supplying muscle and skin. There may be electrocardiogram changes consistent with left ventricular hypertrophy. The cardiac abnormalities are generally resistant to the cardiac glycosides. The "apathetic" form of hyperthyroidism seen in patients over age 60 has predominantly cardiac manifestations. In this age group, unexplained atrial fibrillation may be the first sign of hyperthyroidism. Although catecholamine levels are normal, there is a question of sensitization of existing adrenergic receptors or an increased number of receptors caused by the excess of thyroid hormones.

Other abnormalities seen in thyrotoxicosis include mild anemia, thrombocytopenia, bone loss, increased alkaline phosphatase, hypercalcemia, menstrual irregularities, diarrhea, insomnia, fatigue, nervousness, emotional lability, hyperpigmentation, vitiligo, pretibial myxedema, alopecia, pruritus, and a fine tremor. Ocular manifestations include exophthalmus from an infiltrative process involving the retrobulbar fat and eyelids, lid lag, and involvement of the extraocular muscles, cornea, and optic nerve.

Preparation for Surgery

Patients should be rendered euthyroid including control of the hyperkinetic cardiovascular system before proceeding with anything but emergency surgery. An acceptable resting heart rate is a reliable indicator of adequate treatment.[1]

The traditional preoperative preparation involves administration of antithyroid drugs for 2–3 months before the expected date of surgery to inhibit thyroid hormone synthesis. Medication should be continued through the morning of surgery. Propylthiouracil (300 mg/day) is most commonly used because it inhibits not only hormone synthesis, but also peripheral conversion of T_4 to T_3. Alternatively, methimazole (30 to 60 mg/day) may be used. In addition, saturated potassium iodide solution (10 drops/day) is added starting 10 days preoperatively. The use of iodine causes a transient decrease in the synthesis and secretion of thyroid hormones, a phenomenon known as the Wolff-Chaikoff effect. It also reduces vascularity and hyperplasia of the overactive gland. Patients treated for longer than 2 weeks exhibit a slow return to pretreatment status. It is important to note that an occasional patient may exhibit exacerbation of thyrotoxicosis with the use of iodine. Lithium carbonate (300 mg/day) may be used in place of potassium iodide (iodine allergy). The antithyroid drug and potassium iodide (or lithium carbonate) may be stopped postoperatively.

The newer method of preoperative preparation includes the use of β-blocking drugs and an iodide alone for 7–14 days preoperatively, allowing for a shorter preparation period. This method shrinks the thyroid gland and treats symptoms, but it may fail to correct abnormalities in left ventricular function. The dose of potassium iodide is as described above. Propranolol (80 mg or more every 8 hours) is most commonly used, but at least one group of authors[2] advocate using nadolol (160 mg/day), because its longer half-life allows once-a-day dosing and provides more stable perioperative levels. In addition, the clearance of nadolol is not increased by hyperthyroidism, as is the clearance of propranolol. β-blockers and potassium iodide must be given through the morning of surgery. The β-blockers should be continued for at least 7 days postoperatively, because of the long half-life of thyroid hormones.

Management of Anesthesia

Anticholinergics should be avoided because of interference with sweating as well as a potential increase in heart rate. The induction agent of choice is thiopental because of its inherent antithyroid activity. Ketamine should not be used, because of its tendency to stimulate the sympathetic nervous system. Succinylcholine or nondepolarizing relaxants that produce no significant cardiac effects can be safely used for endotracheal intubation.

During maintenance of anesthesia, increased cardiac output and temperature will result in an increased MAC for the volatile agents. High doses of narcotics would be required to provide adequate inhibition of the sympathetic nervous system. Muscle relaxation with nondepolarizing agents with minimal cardiac effects is preferable. A prolonged response to nondepolarizing agents may occur in patients with preexisting muscle weakness. Hypercarbia will cause stimulation of the sympathetic nervous system and thus should be avoided.

Treatment of hypotension is best achieved with the use of a direct-acting agent such as phenylephrine, rather than agents such as ephedrine, which act in part by an indirect mechanism. β-blockade is essential during the perioperative period.

Spinal and epidural anesthesia provide blockade of the sympathetic nervous system; however, this advantage is partially offset by the potential need to treat hypotension. Epinephrine should not be routinely added to the local anesthetic solution.

Temperature monitoring is essential. A cooling blanket should be available. Volume deficits and electrolyte abnormalities should be corrected. Patients with exophthalmus are particularly prone to corneal injury.

Special Considerations in Pregnancy

Chronic use of iodine in the pregnant patient is contraindicated, because fetal goiter and hypothyroidism may result. Antithyroid drugs cross the placenta; however, small doses (e.g., propylthiouracil (50–100 mg/day) can be administered to the mother with minimal risk to the fetus. The use of propranolol in pregnancy is controversial because of its association with intrauterine growth retardation, low Apgar scores, and fetal bradycardia and hypoglycemia. Thyrotoxicosis of pregnancy is usually mild and often improves in the second and third trimesters. Surgery after the first trimester may be an acceptable alternative to medical management for this problem. Following delivery, the mother and neonate must be evaluated for both hypo- and hyperthyroid states.

Thyroid Storm

Thyroid storm is a severe exacerbation of thyrotoxicosis resulting from the sudden release of thyroid hormones into the circulation. It may occur after rapid withdrawal of iodine therapy, with diabetic ketoacidosis, infection, trauma to or vigorous palpation of the thyroid gland, radioactive iodine therapy, or ether anesthesia. A reduction in thyroid-binding globulin can also occur after surgery or other stress and results in increased levels of free thyroid hormones in the blood. Thyroid storm usually occurs 6–18 hours postoperatively, but may also occur intraoperatively. Its onset is usually sudden. Duration of the storm averages 3 days. Manifestations include hyperthermia, tachycardia, congestive heart failure, dehydration, hyperglycemia, changes in consciousness, shock, and death.

Treatment involves diagnosis and management of the underlying cause. Supportive therapy includes infusion of iced intravenous solutions and the use of a cooling blanket. Aspirin should not be used, because it may displace thyroid hormones from carrier proteins. Digitalis may not be effective in treating associated congestive heart failure. Antithyroid drugs, such as propylthiouracil (600–1,000 mg) or methimazole (60–100 mg orally or via a nasogastric tube), can inhibit thyroid hormone synthesis within an hour. This may be followed by propylthiouracil (200–400 mg orally every 8 hr). An hour after the administration of an antithyroid drug, an iodide, such as saturated potassium iodide (30 drops by mouth each day) or sodium iodide (500–1,000 mg IV every 8 hr), may be given. Propranolol (1–2 mg IV every minute) as required to slow the heart rate below 90 beats/min, to a total dose of 10 mg, can be given to treat the cardiac and psychomotor manifestations. Thereafter, it may be given orally (20–120 mg every 4–8 hr). Hydrocortisone (100–200 mg IV every 8 hr) has been reported to increase survival.

Selected References

1. Stoelting RK, Dierdorf SF. Endocrine disease. In Stoelting RK, Dierdorf SF, eds. Anesthesia and Co-Existing Disease. 3rd ed. New York: Churchill Livingstone, 1993:339.
2. Hamilton WF, Forrest AL, Gunn A, et al. Beta-adrenoceptor blockade and anesthesia for thyroidectomy. Anaesthesia 1984;39:335–342.

Suggested References

Benumof JL. Anesthesia and Uncommon Diseases. 4th ed. Philadelphia, W B Saunders, 1998.

Feek CM, Sawers JSA, Irvine WJ, et al. Combination of potassium iodide and propranolol in preparation of patients with Graves' disease for thyroid surgery. N Engl J Med 1980; 302:883–885.

Mackin JF, Canary JJ, Pittman CS. Thyroid storm and its management. N Engl J Med 1974;291:1396–1398.

Stehling LC. Anesthetic management of the patient with hyperthyroidism. Anesthesiology 1974;41:585–595.

208
Anesthesia for Patients with Chronic Renal Failure

Joseph J. Sandor, M.D.

The anesthetic approach to the patient with chronic renal failure (CRF) must consider coexisting organ system pathology as well as the pharmacokinetics and dynamics of anesthetic agents in CRF patients. Various disease entities may lead to CRF, including chronic glomerulonephritis, tubulointerstitial diseases, diabetes mellitus, and polycystic kidney. No abnormalities in laboratory tests of renal function appear until 60% of nephrons are destroyed. When normal functioning nephrons are reduced to 10% or 40%, the patient may also show signs of renal compromise (decreased concentrating ability and impaired excretion of acid loads). Obvious signs of renal failure (hyperkalemia, acidosis, uremia, anemia, hyperphosphatemia) occur when fewer than 10% of normally functioning glomeruli remain.

Uremic Syndrome

The **uremic syndrome** is a **dialysis-dependent** renal failure with widespread involvement of other organ systems.

□ Hematologic abnormalities include a normochromic, normocytic anemia. CRF patients typically have hemoglobin values of 5 to 8 mg/dL. The anemia results from decreased erythropoietin levels, increased red blood cell membrane fragility, and increased bleeding tendency (gastrointestinal, genitourinary). The resulting decreased oxygen-carrying capacity is compensated for by increased tissue oxygen delivery (i.e., increased cardiac output, decreased viscosity, increased 2,3-diphosphoglycerate).

□ Coagulopathy is primarily from decreased platelet adhesiveness, thought to be secondary to metabolic acidosis. Creatinine levels above 6 mg/dL are necessary before platelet function decreases. Coexisting liver disease and heparinization from dialysis also contribute to clotting abnormalities.

□ Autonomic nervous system dysfunction causes patients with CRF to be essentially unresponsive to hypotension induced by anesthetic drugs. Although patients may have fluid overload, they respond to induction as if they are hypovolemic. Other central nervous system (CNS) symptoms include fatigue, irritability, depression, seizures, and uremia-induced peripheral neuropathy, especially of the median and peroneal nerves.

□ Common electrolyte abnormalities include hyperkalemia, hypermagnesemia, hyperphosphatemia, and hypocalcemia. Metabolic acidosis is common. Hyperkalemia may be exacerbated by infection, acidosis, tissue trauma, and blood transfusion. Elective surgery should usually be postponed for patients with K^+ levels above 5.5 to 6 mEq/L. If emergency surgery is needed, hyperkalemia may be treated with glucose/insulin infusion and hyperventilation to drive K^+ into the cells, HCO_3^- to buffer the metabolic acidosis resulting in $H^+ - K^+$ exchange across the cell membrane, and $CaCl_2$ to treat the cardiac arrhythmias induced by hyperkalemia.

□ CRF patients have an increased incidence of coronary artery disease. In addition, they often have chronic hypertension, cardiomegaly, uremic cardiomyopathy, congestive heart failure, left ventricular hypertrophy, and pleural or pericardial effusions.

□ The risk of pulmonary aspiration is high because of increased gastric volumes and delayed gastric emptying.

□ Coexisting hepatic dysfunction may alter the response to drugs administered in the perioperative period.

□ Increased susceptibility to infectious agents is noted in CRF with sepsis being the most common cause of death in these patients. CRF patients have a high incidence of viral hepatitis.

Preoperative Evaluation

Preoperative evaluation should focus on the degree of renal impairment, exercise tolerance, neurologic dysfunction, blood pressure, location of shunts or fistulae, and frequency and date of last dialysis. Laboratory tests of importance include electrolytes, creatinine, albumin, hemoglobin, prothrombin time, partial thromboplastin time, platelet count, and bleeding time or thromboelastograph. The electrocardiogram and chest radiograph should be reviewed.

Monitoring

In addition to standard monitors, patients with severe renal failure scheduled for major surgical procedures or procedures with large volume requirements merit consideration for central venous and pulmonary artery pressure monitoring. The anesthesiologist is also responsible for proper patient positioning, avoiding compression of arteriovenous shunts. Pathologic fractures have an increased incidence in patients with coexisting renal osteodystrophy.

Anesthetic Management

Uremic patients manifest increased sedation in response to benzodiazepines. Narcotic-induced respiratory depression may be prolonged with morphine use because excretion of morphine glucuronides is reduced. The use of short-acting narcotics is appropriate. Because of hypoalbuminemia and reduced protein binding, doses of barbiturates and etomidate should be reduced and titrated to effect. Succinylcholine may be used safely if serum K^+ is not elevated. Dialysis treatment will lower serum cholinesterase levels and thus produce a prolonged response to succinylcholine. Pancuronium has a prolonged elimination half-life in uremic patients. Atracurium and vecuronium may be safely used. Because of ester hydrolysis and Hofmann degradation, there is little if any difference in the kinetics of atracurium between normal patients and those with CRF.

Halogenated volatile agents have the advantages of allowing use of high F_iO_2 and facilitation of neuromuscular blockade. Halothane should be avoided because of the higher incidence of liver abnormalities in CRF patients. Enflurane's metabolism was shown to produce inorganic fluoride, which can lead to high-output renal failure in high concentrations. Isoflurane, sevoflurane, and desflurane can be used for anesthetic maintenance in patients with any degree of renal impairment. Hyperventilation shifts the oxygen-hemoglobin dissociation curve to the left (alkalosis). Slow respiratory rates allow sufficient venous return to the heart. Although it contains only 4 mEq K/L, lactated Ringer's solution might be best avoided.

Although neuromuscular blocking drugs may have prolonged half-lives, anticholinesterase agents also have elimination kinetics prolonged by at least 100%.

The duration of action of local anesthetics used in regional blocks may be diminished by 40% because of increases in cardiac output and decreases in pH. In addition, coagulation abnormalities may preclude the use of regional anesthetic techniques.

Postoperative considerations include the potential for exaggerated CNS depression, electrolyte abnormalities, and compromised tissue oxygenation. Hypertension may be treated with hydralazine, labetalol, or nitroprusside. Fluid overload is best managed by dialysis.

Suggested References

Malhotra V, Diwan S. Anesthesia and the renal and genitourinary systems. In Miller RD, ed. Anesthesia. 5th ed. Philadelphia: Churchill Livingstone, 2000:1934–1959.

Monk TG, Weldon BC. The renal system and anesthesia for urologic surgery. In Barash PG, Cullen BF, Stoelting RK, eds. Clinical Anesthesia. 3rd ed. Philadelphia: Lippincott-Raven, 1997:945–973.

Stoelting RK, Dierdorf SF. Anesthesia and Co-Existing Disease. 3rd ed. New York, Churchill Livingstone, 1993.

209
Anesthesia for Patients with Carcinoid Tumors

Michelle A. O. Kinney, M.D. □ Mary Ellen Warner, M.D.

Carcinoid Tumors

Carcinoid tumors are the most common gastrointestinal endocrine tumor, with an incidence of 15:1 million per year. These tumors are found most commonly in the appendix, ileum, and rectum and less commonly in the pancreas, ovaries, and lungs. Carcinoid tumors arise from enterochromaffin tissues and thus may release various vasoactive substances (e.g., histamine, serotonin, kallikreins). Clinical symptoms of carcinoid syndrome (Table 209–1)[1] will manifest when the quantity of vasoactive substances surpasses hepatic metabolic capability. Also, symptoms occur when hepatic metastases are present. Alternatively, bronchial or ovarian carcinoid tumors do not drain into the portal venous system, and their vasoactive secretions are not inactivated by the liver.

Anesthetic Management

Preoperative Anesthetic Management. Octreotide acetate (Fig. 209–1) is a long-acting analogue of the naturally occurring peptide somatostatin. It inhibits release of serotonin, gastrin, vasoactive intestinal peptide, secretin, motilin, and pancreatic polypeptide. The usual preoperative dose of octreotide is 50 to 300 μg, but there is no ceiling dose, and IV bolus injections of 1000 μg have been given without complications. Acute octreotide administration has no significant side effects. Octreotide can be administered intravenously or subcutaneously, depending on the desired time of onset and duration. Intravenous administration results in peak serum concentrations within approximately 3 minutes. Subcutaneous injections of octreotide result in peak concentrations 30 to 60 minutes after injection, with a plasma half-life of 113 minutes. The biologic duration of effect may be as long as 12 hours.

Octreotide is also now available as a once-monthly intramuscular (IM) slow-release preparation. Patients on the IM dose who need surgery may have high sustained levels of octreotide. Nonetheless, these patients may still require subcutaneous or intravenous octreotide in the perioperative period.

Preoperative sedation may be administered to avoid sympathetic stimulation, which could result in a carcinoid crisis. The presence of hypovolemia, electrolyte abnormalities, and right-sided cardiac

Table 209–1. Signs and Symptoms of Carcinoid Syndrome

Bronchoconstriction
Episodic cutaneous flushing or cyanosis
Chronic abdominal pain and diarrhea
Hemodynamic instability
Tricuspid regurgitation and/or pulmonic stenosis
Premature atrial beats and supraventricular tachydysrhythmias
Venous telangiectasia
Hepatomegaly
Hyperglycemia
Decreased plasma albumin concentrations

Modified from Stoelting RK, Dierdorf SF.[1]

Somatostatin-14

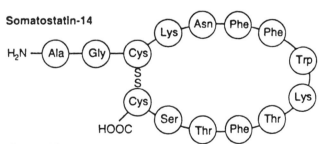

Octreotide

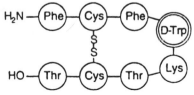

Figure 209–1. Structures of somatostatin-14 and octreotide. The double circle denotes the substitution of D-tryptophan for the naturally occurring L-tryptophan. This substitution inhibits peptide degradation and prolongs serum half-life. (From Kaplan LM.[2])

valvular lesions should be ascertained. Left-sided cardiac valves are usually spared from carcinoid-related abnormalities, which reflects the ability of the pulmonary parenchyma to inactivate vasoactive substances.

Intraoperative Anesthetic Management. Gentle surgical skin preparation to avoid tumor compression is advised. Consider avoiding histamine-releasing drugs, although these drugs have been used without complications. β-Adrenergic agonists have been shown to stimulate the release of vasoactive substances; however, phenylephrine, amrinone, and calcium chloride can be safely used.

Octreotide should be readily available for immediate treatment of carcinoid symptoms intraoperatively. Administer octreotide whenever carcinoid symptoms (e.g., bronchospasm, unexpected hypotension, facial flushing) occur, along with volume infusion and phenylephrine as needed. The usual intraoperative IV **bolus** dose for carcinoid symptoms is 50 to 300 μg and may need to be repeated. The total intraoperative dose of octreotide administered may reach 4000 μg, although this is uncommon.

Postoperative Management. The humoral effects of metastatic carcinoid lesions are usually not eliminated by surgery. Thus, octreotide should be continued if the patient was using it preoperatively.

Selected References

1. Stoelting RK, Dierdorf SF. Diseases of the gastrointestinal system. In Stoelting RK, Dierdorf SF, eds. Anesthesia and Co-Existing Disease. 3rd ed. New York: Churchill Livingstone, 1993:277–287.
2. Kaplan LM. Endocrine tumors of the gastrointestinal tract and pancreas. In Fauci AS, Braunwald E, Isselbacher KJ, et al, eds. Harrison's Principles of Internal Medicine. 14th ed. New York: McGraw-Hill, 1998:584–591.

Suggested References

Mason RA, Steane PA. Carcinoid syndrome: Its relevance to the anaesthetist. Anaesthesia 1976;31:228–242.
Roizen MF, Fleisher LA. Essence of Anesthesia Practice. Philadelphia, WB Saunders, 1997;64:360.
Veall GRQ, Peacock JE, Bax NDS, et al. Review of the anaesthetic management of 21 patients undergoing laparotomy for carcinoid syndrome. Br J Anaesth 1994;72:335–341.

210
Extracorporeal Shock Wave Lithotripsy

Christopher J. Jankowski, M.D.

Most renal and ureteral calculi are amenable to extracorporeal shock wave lithotripsy (ESWL). Since its introduction in 1980, ESWL has become the treatment of choice for urinary calculi. ESWL is effective and provides obvious advantages over open surgical treatment. It can be an outpatient procedure and is associated with minimal morbidity and reduced costs.

Technical Aspects

The shock wave lithotriptor consists of the following components: a shock source, a focusing device, a coupling medium, and a system for localizing stones. Spark plug generators produce shock waves at energies from 16 to 24 kV, leading to pressures of approximately 1000 bar at the target focus. The focusing device is an elliptical reflector, and the coupling medium is water. Early lithotriptors, such as the Dornier HM-3, required the patient to be submerged in a water bath (Fig. 210–1). The water bath permits transmission of the shock waves and serves as a coupling medium. Other models transmit the shock waves to patients via a shock tube. A "water cushion" serves as a coupling medium and

eliminates the need to immerse the patient. Fluoroscopy or ultrasound is used to localize and target the stones.

Physiological Effects of Water Immersion

Cardiovascular. Water immersion causes significant and variable alterations in cardiovascular physiology. Peripheral venous compression increases central blood volume and can increase cardiac filling pressures. However, some patients become hypotensive despite increased central volume, because of peripheral arterial vasodilation caused by the warm water bath. Further, some authors report increases in peripheral vascular resistance, mean arterial pressure, and decreases in cardiac output during general anesthesia with water immersion.

Respiratory. The work of breathing increases with water immersion. Respirations can become rapid and shallow, making ventilation/perfusion mismatch and hypoxemia more likely. Functional residual capacity and vital capacity decrease by

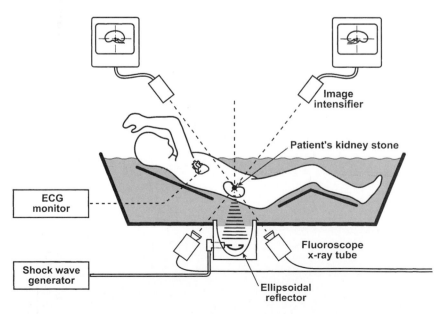

Figure 210–1. A patient positioned in the Dornier HM-3 lithotriptor. (Reprinted with permission from Hunter PT II. The physics and geometry pertinent to ESWL. In Riehle RA Jr, Newman RC, eds. Principles of Extracorporeal Shock Wave Lithotripsy. New York: Churchill Livingstone, 1987.)

20% to 30% because of decreased chest wall compliance. Pulmonary blood flow increases.

Renal. Antidiuretic hormone and prostaglandin levels decrease, leading to diuresis, natriuresis, and kaliuresis.

Temperature. The water bath should be maintained at 35.8 to 37.5°C to avoid hypothermia and hyperthermia. Water temperature should be checked before immersion and monitored throughout the procedure.

Contraindications. Pregnancy, coagulopathy, and active, untreated urinary tract infections are absolute contraindications for ESWL. Obesity, renal artery or aortic calcifications and aneurysms, renal insufficiency, complete urinary tract obstruction distal to the stone, and multiple staghorn calculi are relative contraindications. It may be difficult to properly position patients who are less than 48 inches tall.

Lithotripsy can be safely performed in patients with pectorally placed pacemakers. The pacemaker should be interrogated before and after the procedure. A programming device should be available to switch the device to a nondemand mode should the shocks interfere with pacemaker function. Alternate modes of pacing should also be available. Treatment begins with the lowest possible shock intensity, and the energy is gradually increased while pacemaker function is monitored.

An automatic implantable cardiac defibrillator (AICD) generally is considered a contraindication for ESWL. However, recent evidence suggests that ESWL may be performed in patients with AICDs if the device is contralateral to the side of the procedure, turned off during the procedure, and reactivated and interrogated following the procedure.

Complications. Mortality is less than 0.02%. Renal failure has been reported but is rare; however, bilateral procedures are avoided for this reason. Most patients experience some hematuria because of renal parenchymal damage after ESWL. Approximately 0.5% of patients develop subcapsular hematomas. Bleeding requiring transfusion is rare. Fever may occur, especially in the presence of infected stones and active urinary tract infection. Stone fragments can also cause urinary tract obstruction. If the shock waves are not aimed properly, damage to other organs may occur. Pulmonary contusions and hemorrhage, pancreatitis, and gastrointestinal erosions have been described. Animal studies have shown that ESWL can cause bony fractures.

Cardiac arrhythmias occur in 10% to 14% of patients. These may result from mechanical stress placed on the conducting system by the shock waves.

Premature atrial and ventricular complexes, supraventricular and ventricular tachycardias, and atrial fibrillation have been reported. They usually resolve at the conclusion of the procedure and rarely require treatment.

Anesthetic Management

Various anesthetic techniques have been used for ESWL, including general anesthesia, neuraxial blocks, flank infiltration with and without intercostal blocks, and conscious sedation. Older lithotriptors deliver higher-energy shock waves, cause more pain, and require general or neuraxial anesthesia. A sensory level of T6 is required for neuraxial anesthesia. Epidural anesthesia is commonly used in this setting. It allows patients to assist with positioning and reduces the potential for injury. Spinal anesthesia is associated with a higher incidence of hypotension than epidural anesthesia in this setting. However, general anesthesia may be associated with more rapid early recovery than epidural anesthesia. Newer equipment delivers lower-energy shock waves, producing less pain; thus, conscious sedation may be an acceptable approach.

Suggested References

Behnia R, Shanks CA, Ovassapian A, et al. Hemodynamic responses associated with lithotripsy. Anesth Analg 1987;66:354–356.

Cooper D, Wilkoff B, Masterson M, et al. Effects of extracorporeal shock wave lithotripsy on cardiac pacemakers and its safety in patients with implanted cardiac pacemakers. Pacing Clin Electrophysiol 1988;11:1607–1616.

Malhotra V, Diwan S. Anesthesia and the renal and genitourinary systems. In Miller RD, ed. Anesthesia. 5th ed. Philadelphia: Churchill Livingstone, 2000:1934–1959.

Monk TG, Weldon BC. The renal system and anesthesia for urologic surgery. In Barash PG, Cullen BF, Stoelting RK, eds. Clinical Anesthesia. 3rd ed. Philadelphia: Lippincott-Raven, 1996:945–973.

Richardson MG, Dooley JW. The effects of general versus epidural anesthesia for outpatient extracorporeal shock wave lithotripsy. Anesth Analg 1998;86:1214–1218.

Streem SB. Contemporary clinical practice of shock wave lithotripsy: A reevaluation of contraindications. J Urol 1997;157:1197–1203.

Vassolas G, Roth RA, Venditti FJ Jr. Effect of extracorporeal shock wave lithotripsy on implantable cardioverter. Pacing Clin Electrophysiol 1993;16:1245–1248.

Weber W, Bach P, Wildgans H, et al. Anesthetic considerations in patients with cardiac pacemakers undergoing extracorporeal shock wave lithotripsy. Anesth Analg 1988;67:S251.

211
Anesthesia for Laryngeal Surgery

Gurinder Vasdev, M.D. □ Barry A. Harrison, M.D.

Indications for laryngeal surgery are grouped into three broad categories: acquired, congenital (Table 211–1), and traumatic. With the advent of antibiotics, infectious causes have decreased substantially in the United States. Key issues for the safe provision of anesthesia include **anticipating** a difficult airway and being familiar with the American Society of Anesthesiologist's **Difficult Airway Algorithm** (see Fig. 199–2) and **specialized airway equipment**.

Airway Anatomy and Physiology

The human larynx has three basic functions: protection, respiration, and phonation. These are achieved through a complex system of neuronal innervation. The **internal branch of the superior laryngeal nerve** provides ipsilateral sensation to the supraglottic (i.e., above the true vocal folds) larynx. Below the vocal cords, ipsilateral sensation is supplied by the **recurrent laryngeal nerve**. The posterior half of the vocal cords has the highest density of touch receptors. This is important during fiberoptic intubation when regional or topical anesthesia is used. Stimulation of epiglottic water-sensitive chemoreceptors causes slowed respiration with increased tidal volume, resulting in increased laryngeal airflow. This centrally mediated response appears to be more active in children and is a mechanism by which humidification improves breathing during partial airway obstruction (i.e., slow, large tidal volume breathing decreases turbulent airflow).

The **recurrent laryngeal nerve** provides the motor supply to all intrinsic laryngeal muscles except the cricothyroid muscle. The **cricothyroid**

Table 211–1. Congenital Causes of Laryngeal Pathology

Atresia
Laryngomalacia
Congenital laryngeal paralysis
Congenital subglottic stenosis
Laryngeal web
Congenital hemangiomas
Lymphangiomas
Laryngotracheoesophageal cleft

muscle receives motor innervation from the external branch of the **superior laryngeal nerve**. The actions of each muscle are summarized in Figure 211–1. Nerve trauma offers little chance of effective reinnervation with good laryngeal function.

Phonation is produced by fundamental tone formation in the larynx. This is modified by the resonating chambers of the upper airway. Frequency is determined by isotonic contraction of the cricothyroid muscles. Pitch is determined by changes in the length of the cords and in subglottic pressure.

Direct Laryngoscopy

Direct laryngoscopy is used for subglottic and tracheal examinations with or without biopsies. Preexisting cardiac disease accounts for 1.5% to 4% of perioperative mortality in this patient population. Vocal cord surgery requiring injection of Teflon, gelatin, botulinum toxin type A, or steroid can be performed with conscious sedation, but may require general anesthesia.

Preoperative airway assessment can include physical examination, direct and indirect laryngoscopy, computed tomography (CT), and magnetic resonance imaging (MRI). If airway patency is questionable, then either awake fiberoptic intubation or tracheotomy should be performed under local anesthesia. Premedication with an antisialagogue is beneficial. In surgical procedures requiring general anesthesia, induction can be achieved with either spontaneous ventilation (using a nonirritating volatile anesthetic) or intravenous medications. Topical application of local anesthetic can decrease general anesthetic requirements. Oxygenation is maintained using one of the following techniques:

□ Apneic oxygenation. Patients are hyperventilated with 100% oxygen. The surgeon is then allowed airway access in 3- to 5-minute epochs or until desaturation occurs. Carbon dioxide monitoring is not possible with this technique; accordingly, hypercapnia is a potential problem.
□ Side-port jet ventilation. **Air is entrained** by the **Venturi effect** when a 30- to 50-psi blast from the jet ventilator insufflates the airway. A properly placed jet allows visualization of chest wall

510

laryngeal edema, and laryngospasm are major risks associated with direct laryngoscopy. As modern technology evolves, direct laryngoscopy may be replaced by indirect methods.

Microlaryngoscopy

This technique involves placement of a rigid laryngoscope. Tissue visualization is enhanced using an operating microscope. Anesthesia for this procedure includes use of short-acting general anesthetics and muscle relaxants. Oxygenation is achieved using the same techniques as described for direct laryngoscopy.

High-Frequency Ventilation

In the early 1980s, high-frequency ventilation was used for laryngeal and tracheal surgery. Major advantages include use of a small ETT and minimal chest wall excursion. Problems with barotrauma, humidification, necrotizing tracheobronchitis, and bronchospasm have limited this method's clinical usefulness. Additionally, it offers little advantage over conventional methods of ventilation for laryngeal surgery.

Laryngectomy

Laryngeal carcinoma accounts for 2% to 3% of all malignancies. Tobacco, alcohol, radiotherapy, and herpes simplex viral infection have been implicated as risk factors. Patients are predominantly males over age 50 years. Laryngeal carcinoma occurs in supraglottic (30%), glottic (60%), and subglottic (10%) forms. Most laryngeal tumors can be treated with radiation therapy alone, whereas others require partial or complete laryngectomy.

Careful preoperative patient assessment is vital, because these patients often have significant comorbid disease (e.g., chronic obstructive lung disease, coronary artery disease, congestive heart failure, hypertension, nicotine dependence, and alcohol abuse). Liver function should be evaluated in patients with a significant history of alcohol intake.

The airway is often secured using awake techniques with conscious sedation (e.g., fiberoptic intubation or tracheostomy). Type of anesthesia (i.e., awake versus general anesthesia) is determined by airway anatomy, severity of comorbid diseases, and patient and care team preference. Arterial line monitoring is helpful, especially when the neck dissection involves the area around the carotid sinus. Additionally, it provides access for laboratory work (e.g., obtaining serial hemoglobin concentrations), which is essential during surgical procedures associated with large blood loss (e.g., total laryngectomy

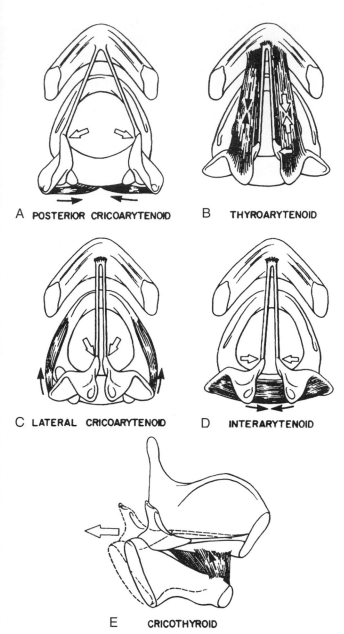

Figure 211–1. Laryngoscopic view of the intrinsic muscles responsible for activating vocal cord position. (From Sasaki CT, Weaver EM.[1])

A POSTERIOR CRICOARYTENOID

B THYROARYTENOID

C LATERAL CRICOARYTENOID

D INTERARYTENOID

E CRICOTHYROID

movement. During jet ventilation, inhaled anesthesia is not possible; intravenous anesthesia is best suited for this oxygenation technique.

□ Microlaryngeal tubes. Microlaryngeal tubes are 3.5 to 4 mm OD endotracheal tubes (ETTs) that require stylet-guided placement. General anesthesia should be maintained with short-acting medications, because emergence can be challenging.

□ Insufflation in a spontaneously breathing patient.

Regardless of the technique used, dental injury can occur. Patients with difficult airways are at particular risk. ENT surgeons often use dental guards to reduce the risk of injury during direct laryngoscopy. Postsurgical hemoptysis, obstruction, with neck dissection). If a central line is indicated, it can be placed via the subclavian route, or a long line can be inserted from the antecubital space. Perioperative complications include air embolism, hypertension, parathyroid and cranial nerve dysfunction, and facial edema. A nasogastric tube is helpful in the postoperative period for both gastric drainage and postoperative feeding.

Laryngeal and Tracheal Trauma

Laryngeal or tracheal trauma is seen in approximately 1 in 43,000 emergency department admissions. Clinical signs include hoarseness, tenderness, hemoptysis, subcutaneous emphysema, respiratory distress (e.g., stridor), dysphagia, and hemoptysis.

Recommendations for securing the airway include:

□ Presence of an ENT surgeon.
□ Operating room setting.
□ If the airway is stable, oral intubation under general anesthesia with either rapid sequence or inhaled induction.

□ If the airway is unstable, the laryngeal mucosa is disrupted, or there is a laryngoskeletal fracture on CT scan, awake fiberoptic intubation or awake tracheostomy under local anesthesia.
□ Inhaled induction of anesthesia followed by orotracheal intubation may be necessary in confused or uncooperative patients, even in the presence of a risk for aspiration.

Selected References

1. Sasaki CT, Weaver EM. Physiology of the larynx. Am J Med 1997;103:9S–18S.

Suggested References

Bastian RW, Delsupehe KG. Indirect larynx and pharynx surgery: A replacement for direct laryngoscopy. Laryngoscope 1996;106:1280–1286.
Biro P, Eyrich G, Rohling RG. The efficiency of CO_2 elimination during high-frequency jet ventilation for laryngeal microsurgery. Anesth Analg 1998;87:180–184.
Donlon JV Jr. Anesthesia for eye, ear, nose, and throat surgery. In Miller RD, ed. Anesthesia. 5th ed. Philadelphia: Churchill Livingstone, 2000:2173–2198.
O'Connor PJ, Russell JD, Moriarty DC. Anesthetic implications of laryngeal trauma. Anesth Analg 1998;87:1283–1284.

212
Anesthesia for Bronchoscopy

Barry A. Harrison, M.D. □ Gurinder Vasdev, M.D.

The rigid bronchoscope is a metal tube with a light source and eyepiece used to examine and gain access to the major airways. Bronchoscopy is usually performed under general anesthesia with controlled ventilation to remove foreign bodies from the trachea, to control massive hemoptysis, to perform laser procedures, and to provide airway dilation. The rigid bronchoscope provides excellent illumination, but its use is limited to the major airways. Gustav Killian first described it in 1898.

In 1968, fiberoptics were used to fashion the first flexible bronchoscope. Today, the flexible bronchoscope is used extensively to examine the tracheobronchial tree. Patients are usually sedated and the airway anesthetized with a local anesthetic. Ventilation is usually spontaneous but occasionally needs to be controlled. Although the fiberoptic bronchoscope provides excellent access to the tracheobronchial tree, its size limits the procedures that it can perform.

Clinical Bronchoscopy

The indications for bronchoscopy are outlined in Table 212–1. Concurrent medical problems increase the risks associated with the procedure (Table 212–2). Patients with reactive airway disease have an increased incidence of bronchospasm during bronchoscopy. Similarly, patients with restrictive ventilatory defects (e.g., interstitial lung disease) may experience significant hypoxia. Patients with lung cancer undergoing bronchoscopy commonly have other comorbidities, such as central airway obstruction, SVC obstruction, metastatic lesions (bone, brain, liver), or electrolyte imbalance (hyponatremia and hypercalcemia).

Patients with recent myocardial infarction, unstable angina, and refractory arrhythmias may undergo bronchoscopy without significant complications. The risk of postoperative bleeding is increased with pulmonary hypertension, elevated blood urea (>30 mg/dL), chronic renal disease, and aspirin ingestion.

A complete history and physical examination will facilitate patient care during and after bronchoscopy. A preoperative chest radiograph is mandatory; other investigations (e.g., CBC, electrolyte panel,

coagulation studies) are performed as indicated. Pulmonary function testing provides information on the type of ventilatory defect (restrictive or obstructive), its severity, and the degree of reversibility with treatment. If respiratory failure is suspected or the patient is on domiciliary oxygen, arterial blood gas analysis is indicated.

Anesthesia for Bronchoscopy

Preoperative Preparation

Anesthesia and risks are discussed with a fasted (more than 6 hours) patient, then an antisialagogue (either atropine 0.4 to 0.8 mg or glycopyrrolate 0.1 to 0.2 mg) is administered IM or IV 40 minutes before the procedure. Aerosolized bronchodilators,

Table 212–1. Indications for Bronchoscopy

Therapeutic	Diagnostic
Removal of:	Identify:
• Foreign body	• Source of hemorrhage (patient with hemoptysis)
• Secretions	• Source of unexplained chronic cough
Control of hemorrhage	Assess
Treatment of endobronchial obstruction	• Airway anatomy
	• Airway function
• Thermal lasers	• Tracheobronchial mucosa
• Photodynamic therapy	• Peribronchial structures
• Brachytherapy	
	Brush
Airway dilation	
	• Mucosa, lung parenchyma, cytology
• Rigid scope dilation	• Protective brush for quantitative bacteriological culture
• Stent placement	
• Balloon dilation	
	Biopsy
Closure of bronchopleural fistula	
	• Bronchial wall
	• Transbronchial lung biopsy
	• Transbronchial lymph node biopsy
	Lavage
	• Qualitative for inflammatory cells, neutrophils
	• Quantitative for bacteria

Table 212–2. Complications of Bronchoscopy

General	Local
Hypoxemia:	Dental and facial trauma
• Sedation/anesthetic	Hemorrhage
• Methemoglobinemia	Bronchospasm
	Pneumothorax
Hypercarbia	Airway obstruction
• Sedation/anesthetic	• Tumor
• Inadequate ventilation	• Blood
	• Secretions
Cardiovascular—cardiac arrhythmias	Peripheral airway obstruction
Awareness and recall	• Asthma
Neurological—seizures	• Chronic bronchitis
	• Emphysema
Cardiac arrest and death	Airway perforation

β2-agonists, and anticholinergic agents are administered to patients with reactive airway disease. Corticosteroids are indicated during an exacerbation of reactive airway disease. The American Heart Association recommends SBE prophylaxis for rigid bronchoscopy, but not for flexible bronchoscopy. Previous endocarditis, prosthetic heart valve, and surgically corrected cardiac shunt are exceptions requiring prophylaxis. IV heparin should be discontinued 6 hours before the procedure and platelets transfused as necessary to maintain platelet levels greater than $50 \times 10^9/L$.

Sedation

ASA Guidelines for monitoring must be followed. Incremental midazolam (0.5 to 1.0 mg) or diazepam (1 to 2 mg) is administered IV to achieve conscious sedation. IV opioids act synergistically with benzodiazepines to provide sedation, suppress airway reflexes, and potentiate respiratory depression. Fentanyl, sufentanil, alfentanil, and remifentanil are suitable opiate choices. Propofol can be used as a sedative agent; it is titrated in doses of 10 mg to provide conscious sedation and suppress the cough reflex. Significant hypotension and apnea may result from excessive drug administration; thus a balanced technique is advisable.

Local Anesthesia for the Upper Airway for Flexible Fiberoptic Bronchoscopy

In a 70-kg adult, the bronchoscope alone occupies less than 20% of the tracheal lumen, allowing for adequate oxygenation. However, in some patients, the suction channel may be used to supplement oxygen.

Sensory innervation of the upper airway is described in Table 212–3. Topical anesthesia and/or nerve blocks are used to anesthetize the upper airway; 2% lidocaine liquid or gel is commonly used because of its wider safety margin, fast onset, and prolonged duration of action. The maximum safe dose is 4 mg/kg. Toxicity depends on blood levels, and the rate of absorption. The alveoli have the maximum absorption rate.

The following methods are used for anesthetizing the nasopharyngeal mucosa when nasal intubation is necessary:

□ Phenylephrine or cocaine is used for vasoconstriction.
□ 2% lidocaine spray.
□ 4% viscous lidocaine soaked pledgets placed in the nares.

Oropharyngeal anesthesia can be achieved by:

□ Gargled 2% viscous lidocaine.
□ Nebulized 2% lidocaine solution (95% effective when nebulized for 10 minutes).
□ Superior laryngeal nerve blocks.
□ Directly spraying the larynx while using a mirror with the patient sitting.
□ Transtracheal injection.
□ Topical anesthesia of the larynx and trachea with lidocaine injected through the suction port.

One or a combination of these techniques provide satisfactory anesthesia of the upper airway. If persistent gag reflex prevents bronchoscopy, then bilateral glossopharyngeal nerve blocks are indicated. Using a tonsillar needle, 3 mL of 2% lidocaine is injected into the midpoint of the posterior tonsillar pillar to a depth of 1 cm. This will effectively block the submucosa pressoreceptors at the posterior aspect of the tongue. This block is always performed after superior laryngeal nerve block, because significant pharyngeal muscle and tongue relaxation may result, precipitating respiratory obstruction.

General Anesthesia for Rigid Bronchoscopy

The induction technique is chosen based on airway assessment findings. Awake intubation is planned for an anticipated difficult airway. If awake

Table 212–3. Sensory Innervation of the Upper Airway

Anatomical Structure	Nerve Supply
Nose	Trigeminal V, ophthalmic V1, maxillary V2
Tongue	
• Anterior	Trigeminal V, lingual V3
• Posterior	Glossopharyngeal IX
Pharynx	
• Nasal	Trigeminal V, maxillary branch V2
• Oral	Glossopharyngeal IX
Larynx	Vagus X, internal laryngeal branch
Vocal cords	Vagus X, internal laryngeal branch
Trachea	Vagus X, internal laryngeal branch

intubation is not feasible, a graduated inhalation induction technique with halothane or sevoflurane is a safe alternative. An intravenous induction technique is used if no airway difficulty is anticipated.

Except when a ventilating rigid bronchoscope is used, the total intravenous anesthetic (TIVA) technique is used. The pharmacokinetics of propofol, with its fast onset and offset plus its profound suppression of airway reflexes, is an ideal choice. Because bronchoscopy increases mean arterial pressure (by 30%), heart rate (by 43%), cardiac index (by 28%), and pulmonary artery occlusion pressure (by 26%), the administration of a potent opioid is necessary. Fentanyl and sufentanil can be given intermittently, or alfentanil and remifentanil can be given as a continuous infusion following a loading dose.

Muscle relaxation is essential for successful bronchoscopy. This can be achieved by a nondepolarizing, short- to median-acting agent (e.g., rocuronium) or alternatively with a succinylcholine drip. Eaton-Lambert syndrome, a neuromuscular disorder associated with small-cell lung neoplasms, increases the sensitivity of these patients to both depolarizing and nondepolarizing neuromuscular relaxants.

In a bronchoscopy procedure of short duration, **apneic oxygenation** with intermittent ventilation is both easy and effective. After induction of anesthesia and neuromuscular blockade, the patient is denitrogenated with 100% oxygen and a catheter passed through the vocal cords to lie just above the main carina. Oxygen at 6 L/min is insufflated via the catheter throughout the procedure. Although oxygenation is satisfactory, arterial carbon dioxide tension increases by an average of 3 mm Hg per minute (a range of 1 to 6 mm Hg). Intermittent periods of ventilation may be necessary to prevent acidosis. The side arm to the rigid bronchoscope can be used to enable ventilation and anesthesia using a volatile anesthetic agent.

When the rigid ventilating bronchoscopy technique is used for prolonged, complicated procedures, hypoxemia and hypercapnia may develop from inadequate ventilation, especially during the times when the proximal end is open to pass instruments.

The Sanders jet injector technique, another common method, uses the Venturi principle, in which gas (FIO_2 0.20 to 1.0) under high pressure (50 psi) is directed through a long metal tube with a small orifice near the end of the bronchoscope or laryngoscope. The jet entrains gas from the open outlet, maintaining ventilation. Maintaining adequate ventilation and oxygenation is often difficult in patients with low lung compliance due to intrinsic lung disease or obesity. Because expiration is passive and the gas is injected under high pressure, significant barotrauma may result unless the upper airway is patent.

General Anesthesia: Flexible Fiberoptic Bronchoscopy

A 7.5-mm ID endotracheal tube (ETT) is needed to allow passage of the larger fiberoptic bronchoscope. The resultant decrease in airway cross-sectional area often necessitates assisted ventilation and supplemental oxygen. A closed system is achieved with a self-sealing rubber diaphragm in the elbow connector. Adequate expiration prevents barotrauma. As in rigid bronchoscopy, either a total intravenous technique or an inhalation technique can be used. Use of topical local anesthesia in the airway before general anesthesia will decrease the level of anesthesia needed.

Removal of an Inhaled Foreign Body

The typical case is a young child who has aspirated a peanut or other small object. Anesthesia-related problems in this situation involve the challenges posed by a nonfasted, distressed child. Atropine is administered for its vagolytic and anti-sialagogue effect. Induction is aimed at reducing patient distress, to avoid disrupting the foreign body which could cause asphyxia. Either systemic ketamine or an inhalation technique with sevoflurane can be used. After induction, the aim is to keep the patient spontaneously breathing to prevent further dislodgment of the foreign body. If neuromuscular blockade is necessary, then ample time is allowed for expiration, to prevent excessive barotrauma from a ball valve effect of the foreign body. Although the foreign body usually lodges in the right main stem bronchi allowing for adequate oxygenation and ventilation, it may detach when it is being removed and obstruct the lumen of the trachea. In this instance the solution is to push the foreign body distally to the bronchi to relieve the tracheal obstruction. Postprocedure mucosal edema may cause obstruction; thus corticosteroids are administered prophylactically.

Management of Massive Hemoptysis

Massive hemoptysis (>600 mL of blood/24 hr) is a rare but life-threatening crisis. The immediate therapy is correction of hypoxia by placing an ETT and administering 100% O_2. IV fluid resuscitation is indicated to correct hypovolemia. A rigid ventilating bronchoscope locates the source of bleeding and allows adequate aspiration of the clotted blood, the instillation of iced cold saline and vasoconstrictors, and, if necessary, the placement of a bronchial blocker to isolate the remaining lung. The jet ventilation technique is inappropriate, because the gas under high pressure is dry and will cause the blood to solidify, exacerbating the obstruction and hypoxemia.

Malignant Airway Obstruction: Lasers and Stents

Rigid bronchoscopy is often used for the application of lasers to treat bronchogenic cancer in major bronchi, followed by placement of prosthesis or stents to hold the airway open. If there is obstruction of trachea and bronchi, then a spontaneous inhalation technique is important with a test of positive pressure ventilation once the patient has been adequately anesthetized. The rigid bronchoscope is then introduced, and the nose and mouth are packed. During laser firing, it is important to decrease the F_{IO_2} as low as possible with air to minimize the possibility of airway fires. Obstruction of the airway from necrotic tissue and excessive bleeding can precipitate hypoxia, requiring laser cessation, 100% O_2, and vigorous suction.

Complications/Outcomes Associated with Bronchoscopy

A mortality rate below 0.1%, major complications in less than 1.5% of cases, and minor complications in leas than 6.5% of cases have been reported. Significantly, 50% of the complications are from premedication, general anesthetic, and local anesthetic agents. Because rigid bronchoscopy is usually carried out under total intravenous anesthesia, awareness is a recognized complication.

Bronchoscopy-induced hemodynamic changes include increased myocardial oxygen demand and the risk of myocardial ischemia. Hypoxemia predisposes to cardiac arrhythmias and ST segment changes, whereas coronary artery disease does not increase the risk for arrhythmias. Hypoxemia and hypercarbia contribute greatly to the cardiovascular complications associated with bronchoscopy. Severe hypoxemia and hypercarbia may also produce seizures, but these are usually associated with local anesthetic toxicity.

Summary

During bronchoscopy, the airway is at constant risk for obstruction and loss of ventilation. It is important to remember that a flexible bronchoscope is never an airway, whereas a rigid bronchoscope may be. Complications can result in hypoxemia and hypercarbia, leading to cardiovascular complications and collapse. The airway is shared, and with it the complications are also shared by the anesthesiologist and bronchoscopist. Good communication, cooperation, and meticulous attention to details of monitoring, most importantly pulse oximetry, will help ensure a safe outcome.

Selected References

1. Prakash UBS. Bronchoscopy. New York: Raven Press, 1994.
2. Benumof JL. Anesthesia for Thoracic Surgery. 2nd ed. Philadelphia: WB Saunders, 1995.
3. Marshall BE, Longnecker DE, Fairley HB. Anesthesia for Thoracic Procedures. Boston: Blackwell Scientific, 1988.
4. Latto IP, Vaughan RS. Difficulties in Tracheal Intubation. 2nd ed. London: WB Saunders, 1997.

213
Anesthesia for Patients with Diabetes Mellitus

Joseph J. Sandor, M.D.

Diabetes mellitus is classified as **type I** (juvenile onset, insulin-dependent, ketosis prone) or **type II** (non–insulin-dependent, maturity onset). **Type I** diabetes usually appears before age 16 years and requires exogenous insulin administration to prevent ketosis. Ophthalmic, cardiovascular, renal, and neurologic complications are likely. Although **type II** diabetics may require exogenous insulin, they are not prone to ketosis.

Complications of Diabetes

Complications of diabetes include ketoacidosis, neuropathies, atherosclerosis, microangiopathies, delayed wound healing, and increased susceptibility to infection. Segmental demyelination leads to the development of peripheral neuropathies. Autonomic dysfunction may manifest as orthostatic hypotension, resting tachycardia, and loss of beat-to-beat variability in heart rate. Parasympathetic cardiac dysfunction is more prevalent than sympathetic cardiac dysfunction, with bradycardia unresponsive to atropine. Interference with autonomic control of ventilation may lead to enhanced sensitivity to the respiratory depressant effects of barbiturates, benzodiazepines, and narcotics. Other manifestations of autonomic dysfunction include gastroparesis, bladder dysfunction, diarrhea, painless myocardial ischemia, and unexplained cardiac arrest.

Diabetic patients may have accelerated coronary artery disease. Myocardial ischemia, cerebral ischemia, and peripheral vascular disease are twice as common than in nondiabetics. Hypertension and cardiomyopathy also occur with increased frequency. Microangiopathy develops most frequently in the retinas and kidneys. Renal involvement manifests as proteinuria and elevated serum creatinine.

Preoperative Assessment

Preoperative assessment of the diabetic patient should determine the adequacy of blood glucose control and confirm the absence of ketoacidosis. Signs and symptoms of myocardial dysfunction, cerebral ischemia, hypertension, and renal disease should be sought. Juvenile onset diabetic patients may be of short stature with limited joint mobility. Adult-onset diabetic patients are often obese. In both circumstances, difficulty with airway management should be anticipated.

Management of Blood Glucose Intraoperatively

Close control of glucose throughout life has become an important goal for diabetic patients, because it is thought to reduce the development of the diabetic complications discussed earlier. In the perioperative period, it is important to guard against the development of severe hypoglycemia in fasting, anesthetized diabetic patients. Alternatively, mild hyperglycemia can increase risk even when glucose levels causing diuresis and diabetic coma are avoided. It has been clearly established that hyperglycemia increases the risk of neurologic injury when the brain suffers an ischemic insult. These insults are not uncommon in the perioperative period through embolic or low-flow mechanisms.

Thus the anesthesiologist has two important goals during surgery for the diabetic patient. First, hypoglycemia is prevented by monitoring serum glucose levels. Exogenous glucose can be provided when needed as a standard glucose administration of 5 to 10 g/hr (100 to 200 mL/hr of D_5NS). Second, severe hyperglycemia and ketoacidosis must be prevented. This is accomplished by providing exogenous insulin to maintain blood glucose between 100 and 150 mg/dL.

- If the diabetic patient takes oral hypoglycemic agents, these should be continued until the evening before surgery.
- If the surgical procedure is short and the patient is relatively unstressed, insulin supplementation may not be needed. Preoperative and postoperative serum glucose levels should be determined.
- If the patient takes insulin, three approaches to

glucose control are used. First, the usual morning dose is decreased and the patient receives intermediate-acting insulin (one-fourth to one-half the usual dose). Serum glucose levels are checked regularly, and regular insulin is administered as needed. A second approach is to administer regular insulin on a sliding scale based on frequent serum glucose determinations. The third approach is to administer a continuous infusion of low-dose insulin at 1 unit/hr (7 to 10 units of regular insulin added to 1 L of D_5NS and run at 75 to 100 mL/h), adjusted according to frequent serum glucose determinations.

Management of Anesthesia

The anesthesiologist must determine in advance the types of physiologic monitoring to be used during anesthesia. Electrocardiography, blood pressure, oximetry, temperature, and respiratory gas analysis are essential. Arterial cannulation provides easy access for frequent sampling of blood for glucose, electrolytes, and arterial blood gases. These patients are at risk for aspiration of gastric contents. Metoclopramide and antacid regimens should be considered before anesthesia induction. Rapid-sequence administration of induction agents should be performed and the trachea protected with a cuffed tube. Patients taking oral hypoglycemic agents show enhanced effects of barbiturates and anticoagulants. In addition, attention to the patient's intraoperative positioning is important, because injuries to the limbs and nerves are more likely in diabetic individuals because of their increased vulnerability to ischemia from pressure and stretch injuries.

Coexisting cardiac disease may make these patients more susceptible to the myocardial depressant effects of volatile agents used for anesthetic maintenance. However, the choice of anesthetic technique is less important than the institution of an appropriate monitoring plan during anesthesia. If regional anesthesia is used, consideration must be given to the high incidence rate of peripheral neuropathies.

Suggested References

Firestone LL, Lebowitz PW, Cork CE. Clinical Anesthesia Procedures of the Massachusetts General Hospital. 5th ed. Boston, Little, Brown, 1998.

Graf G, Rosenbaum S. Anesthesia and the endocrine system. In Barash DG, Cullen BF, Stoelting RK, eds. Clinical Anesthesia. 2nd ed. Philadelphia: JB Lippincott, 1992:1237.

McAnulty GR, Robertshaw HJ, Hall GM. Anaesthetic management of patients with diabetes mellitus. Br J Anaesth 2000;85:80–90.

Stoelting RK, Dierdorf SF. Anesthesia and Co-existing Disease. 3rd ed. New York, Churchill Livingstone, 1993.

214
Hyperosmolar Coma

Paul E. Stensrud, M.D.

The syndrome of hyperglycemia, dehydration, and coma in older patients with mild-to-moderate diabetes mellitus was first described in 1957 by Sament and Schwartz.[1] Despite increased awareness of the syndrome, now termed **hyperosmolar hyperglycemic nonketotic coma (HHNC)**, the reported mortality rate is as high as 50%.[2]

Pathophysiology

The development of HHNC may involve three components[3]:

□ Relative insulin deficiency results in hyperglycemia.
□ Renal insufficiency, whether chronic or acute, interferes with the patient's ability to excrete the glucose load.
□ Impaired thirst mechanisms prevent the patient from responding appropriately to the intravascular volume depletion.

Unlike in diabetic ketoacidosis (DKA), in HHNC ketosis does not develop. Hepatic insulin levels are higher than plasma levels in HHNC patients, perhaps allowing metabolism of the free fatty acids. HHNC patients have lower baseline plasma levels of free fatty acids. The marked hyperosmolarity secondary to extreme levels of hyperglycemia further inhibits free fatty acid release, which may further reduce susceptibility to ketosis. Hyperglycemia leads to an osmotic diuresis and intravascular volume depletion. Combined with limited fluid intake (secondary to impaired thirst sensation [stroke, central nervous system depressants, age] and the inability to respond adequately to thirst [trauma, burns]) leads to hemoconcentration. Prerenal azotemia and further elevation of glucose and osmolarity develop, and shock ensues. Coma develops when plasma osmolarity exceeds 350 mosmol/kg.[2–4]

Clinical Manifestations

Patients suffering from HHNC tend to be elderly, although the syndrome has been reported in all age groups. There may be a history of mild non–insulin-dependent diabetes mellitus (NIDDM), and many patients have underlying renal or cardiovascular disease, which may complicate the management of HHNC. However, two-thirds of HHNC patients have no history of diabetes mellitus and require no subsequent insulin therapy.[4] Acute medical events (CVA, myocardial infarction, infection), which elevate glucose as a stress response, or drugs which inhibit insulin release (thiazides, dilantin, β blockers, immunosuppressants, and cimetidine) may precipitate HHNC. Administration of hypertonic glucose solutions, such as parenteral nutrition solutions, may also precipitate HHNC. Patients with NIDDM undergoing cardiopulmonary bypass may develop the hyperglycemia characteristic of this syndrome.[6]

Early signs and symptoms of HHNC include fever, tachycardia, and hypotension. Patients may present with tremors and fasciculations, disorientation, or coma. Seizures are noted in up to one-third of HHNC patients.[3]

Diagnosis is based on the demonstration of hyperglycemia and hyperosmolarity in the absence of ketosis. Typical features include the following:[2–5]

□ **Hyperglycemia,** with glucose level greater than 600 mg/dL (higher than in DKA).
□ **Hyperosmolarity,** greater than 330 mosmol/kg.
□ Serum and urine ketones absent or minimal.
□ Arterial pH normal unless lactic acidosis supervenes due to shock.
□ **Hypovolemia** secondary to hemoconcentration.
□ **Osmotic diuresis,** usually associated with **hypokalemia**.
□ Central nervous system dysfunction.

In addition, prerenal azotemia develops secondary to the osmotic diuresis and attendant volume depletion, and the blood urea nitrogen/creatinine ratio often exceeds 30:1. Serum sodium is usually normal. The laboratory sodium value must be corrected to compensate for the dilutional effect of the osmotically active glucose (sodium decreases 1.6 mEq/L for each 100-mg/dL increase in glucose).[3]

Other causes of hyperosmolarity, grouped into three major categories,[6] are listed in Table 214–1.

Therapy

The best therapy is prevention, as the mortality rate continues to be high. Susceptible patients

Table 214–1. Differential Diagnosis of HHNC

Pure water loss
    Primary hypodipsia
    Hyperthermia
    Diabetes insipidus
Hypertonic water loss
    Burns
    Diarrhea
    Vomiting
    Bowel obstruction
    Osmotic diuresis
Hypertonic fluid excess
    Administration of sodium bicarbonate
    Administration of hypertonic sodium chloride
    Administration of mannitol

should be carefully monitored with regard to fluid and glucose status. Definitive therapy after treatment of the initiating event includes intravenous fluids, insulin, and potassium administration.

□ **Intravenous fluid** administration is the mainstay of treatment. Typically, 6 to 8 L of fluid are needed in the first 12 hours. One-half normal saline is the most commonly recommended solution for fluid resuscitation in HHNC,[2] although normal saline has been recommended as the initial fluid administered to rapidly expand the intravascular volume in severely hypovolemic patients.[3]

□ Intravenous fluids alone will reduce glucose levels, but insulin administration will facilitate more rapid glucose control. Regular insulin, 10 to 30 units, is given initially, and glucose levels are monitored closely. A target glucose level of 300 mg/L is maintained for 24 hours to avoid potential cerebral edema.[2–4]

□ Electrolytes should be monitored closely. **Hypokalemia** is likely, especially with rapid fluid replacement and insulin administration.[3]

Complications

Hypotension results from intravascular volume depletion and glucose shifts to the intracellular compartment, with consequent further osmotic depletion of the extracellular compartment. Large amounts of intravenous fluids may need to be rapidly administered, and the patient should be continuously monitored.

Cerebral edema occurs during precipitous falls in blood glucose levels. In response to the extreme hyperglycemia, the brain accumulates idiogenic osmoles (e.g., glucose, polyols, free amino acids) to prevent cerebral osmotic dehydration. As the movement of these osmoles across the blood-brain barrier is very slow relative to water, rapid reduction in plasma glucose leaves the brain hyperosmolar relative to plasma, leading to the development of an osmotic cerebral edema. For this reason, plasma glucose should be decreased to only 300 mg/dL in the first 24 hours, and then gradually returned to normal levels.[7]

Selected References

1. Sament S, Schwartz MB. Severe diabetic stupor without ketosis. South Afr Med J 1957:31:893.
2. Nathan DM. Diabetes mellitus. In Rubenstein E, Federman DD, eds. Scientific American Medicine. New York: Scientific American, 1993;21:9.
3. Rossini AA, Mordes JP. The diabetic coma. In Rippi VM, Irwin RS, Alpert JS, et al., eds. Intensive Care Medicine. Boston: Little, Brown, 1985:792.
4. Stoelting RK, Dierdorf SF. Anesthesia and Co-Existing Disease. 3rd ed. New York: Churchill Livingstone, 1993:346.
5. Hirsch IB, Magill JB, Cryer PE, et al. Perioperative management of surgical patients with diabetes mellitus. Anesthesiology 1991;74:346–359.
6. Geheb MA. Clinical approach to the hyperosmolar patient. Crit Care Clin 1987;5:797–815.
7. Cutler RWP. Metabolic and nutritional disorders. In Rubenstein E, Federman DD, eds. Scientific American Medicine. New York: Scientific American, 1993;VII:11.

215
Anesthesia for Patients with Hepatocellular Disease

Joseph J. Sandor, M.D.

Knowledge of the varied physiologic functions of the liver allows for anticipation of potential problems when patients with hepatocellular disease present for surgery. The liver is responsible for:

□ Glucose homeostasis (gluconeogenesis, glycogenesis, glycogenolysis, insulin degradation).
□ Albumin formation ($t_{1/2}$ approximately 23 days; plasma oncotic pressure, drug binding).
□ Protein formation (clotting factors, gamma globulin, plasma cholinesterase).
□ Vitamin storage and synthesis (A, D, B_{12}).
□ Drug and hormone metabolism.
□ Lipid metabolism.
□ Storage and filtration of blood (clearance of the degradation products of fibrinolysis, wastes, bacteria).
□ Bile formation and excretion (absorption of fat-soluble vitamins A, D, E, and K).

Patients with hepatocellular disease may manifest altered **perioperative coagulation disorders**, **altered drug pharmacokinetics** and **pharmacodynamics**, and hypoglycemia. In addition, underlying liver disease makes hepatocytes more vulnerable to hypoxia, which may cause **centrilobular necrosis** if hepatic blood flow is decreased.

Acute Hepatic Failure

Central nervous system manifestations of acute hepatic failure include **encephalopathy**, altered levels of consciousness, and hyperventilation from increased serum levels of ammonia and other toxic metabolites. **Hypoglycemia** may result from impaired gluconeogenesis, depleted glycogen stores, and reduced insulin degradation. **Cardiac output is increased** from reduced systemic vascular resistance and increased arteriovenous (AV) shunting. Intrapulmonary shunting may produce **hypoxemia**. Patients often have coexisting renal disease (including renal failure) and are more susceptible to infection. Of the proteins synthesized by the liver, coagulation factor VII has one of the shortest half-lives ($t_{1/2}$ approximately 6 hours). Accordingly,

the prothrombin time (PT) provides valuable information as to acute changes in hepatic function.

Surgery should be performed only in an emergency. Fresh frozen plasma can be given preoperatively to correct coagulation abnormalities. Because of decreased metabolism, anesthetic requirements are significantly reduced. Barbiturate and narcotic effects are prolonged. Plasma cholinesterase levels may be decreased, but are usually adequate ($t_{1/2}$ approximately 14 days), so that succinylcholine can be used without significantly prolonging apnea. Serum glucose should be monitored to confirm the absence of hypoglycemia. Blood transfusion can produce **citrate toxicity** if large amounts of blood products are administered rapidly.

These patients are vulnerable to **hypotension, hypoxemia, acidosis, hypokalemia, hypocalcemia,** and **hypomagnesemia.** Large-bore intravenous lines should be placed, and hemodynamics should be managed with appropriate invasive monitoring.

Chronic Liver Disease

Anesthetic management of patients with chronic liver disease is dictated by the degree of cirrhosis-induced **extrahepatic complications.**

□ Cardiovascular abnormalities include increased cardiac output, increased intravascular volume, decreased viscosity, increased AV shunting, congestive heart failure, and cardiomyopathy (e.g., ethanol-induced dilated cardiomyopathy).
□ Arterial hypoxemia results from intrapulmonary AV shunting, ventilation/perfusion mismatch, and recurrent pneumonia.
□ Hypoglycemia in the perioperative period should be anticipated.
□ Increased incidence of cholestasis and cholelithiasis increases susceptibility to cholecystitis and pancreatitis.
□ Peptic ulcer disease occurs twice as often as in patients without liver disease. These patients also may have gastroesophageal reflux and intestinal hypomotility.

- □ Portal hypertension (causing varices and spleno-megaly) and impaired coagulation from thrombo-cytopenia, factor deficiencies, disseminated intra-vascular coagulation, and **fibrinolysis** place these patients at risk for sudden massive bleeding.
- □ Renal disease may coexist with chronic liver disease.
- □ Hepatic encephalopathy and peripheral neuropathy from nutritional deficiencies may occur.

Anesthesia for Patients with Cirrhosis

Preoperative evaluation should screen for extra-hepatic manifestations of chronic liver failure. Laboratory evaluation includes arterial blood gases (ABGs), hemoglobin concentration (Hb), platelet count, coagulation studies, chemistry panel, albumin, and glucose. Adequate blood components should be available for transfusion. Supplemental glucose may be necessary. If no bleeding or clotting abnormalities exist, then regional anesthesia may be selected.

Benzodiazepines and narcotics should be used cautiously because of altered metabolism. To reduce the risk of aspirating gastric contents, H_2 antagonists, nonparticulate antacids, and metoclopramide can be given before induction.

Along with routine monitors, an intra-arterial catheter should be inserted to monitor perioperative blood pressure, ABGs, electrolytes, Hb, and glucose. Central venous pressure and pulmonary artery monitoring aids perioperative fluid management. If surgery is likely to be associated with massive blood loss, then intraoperative monitoring of coagulation status is recommended. A peripheral nerve stimulator should be used if neuromuscular blockade is needed.

Rapid-sequence induction or awake intubation facilitates airway protection from aspiration. Doses of induction agents (thiopental, etomidate) should be reduced because of coexisting hypoalbuminemia or cardiomyopathy. In patients with liver disease, the hepatic arteries contribute a much greater proportion of blood to total hepatic blood flow. Thus, decreases in mean arterial pressure should be avoided to prevent hepatocellular hypoxia. Avoiding light anesthesia, hypoxia, hypercarbia, and excessive positive-pressure ventilation prevents increased splanchnic vascular resistance. Using halogenated volatile agents allows for higher F_iO_2. Isoflurane and desflurane, which undergo minimal metabolism, are frequently recommended. The MAC of isoflurane may be increased secondary to the increased phospholipid content of brain tissue. Renal function is maintained with fluids and diuretics as necessary. Postoperative analgesic requirements are usually reduced.

Suggested References

Maze M, Bass NM. Anesthesia and the hepatobiliary system. In Miller RD, ed. Anesthesia. 5th ed. Philadelphia: Churchill Livingstone, 2000:1960–1972.

Rogers EL. Evaluation of the patient with liver disease. In Rogers MC, Tinker JH, Covino BG, et al, eds. Principles and Practice of Anesthesiology. St. Louis: Mosby, 1993:311–339.

Stoelting RK. Liver and the gastrointestinal tract. In Stoelting RK, ed. Pharmacology and Physiology in Anesthetic Practice. 3rd ed. Philadelphia: Lippincott-Raven, 1999:736–747.

Stoelting RK, Dierdorf SF. Disease of the liver and biliary tract. In Stoelting RK, Dierdorf SF, eds. Anesthesia and Co-Existing Disease. 3rd ed. New York: Churchill Livingstone, 1993:251–275.

216
Acute and Chronic Alcoholism and Anesthesia

Frank D. Crowl, M.D.

Ethyl alcohol (ethanol, ETOH) is an addictive central nervous system (CNS) depressant. There are an estimated 12 million alcoholics in the United States. Chronic and acute exposure to alcohol can affect multiple organ systems. Alcoholic deaths have been attributed to cardiac arrhythmias, cardiomyopathy, cirrhosis, bleeding from gastritis or esophageal varices, hepatitis, malnutrition, pancreatitis, and psychiatric disorders.

Metabolism

ETOH is metabolized as follows:

$$\text{ethanol} \xrightarrow[\text{NAD} \rightarrow \text{NADH}]{\text{alchohol dehydrogenase}}$$

$$\text{acetaldehyde} \xrightarrow[\text{NAD} \rightarrow \text{NADH}]{\text{acetaldehyde dehydrogenase}}$$

$$CO_2 + H_2O + \text{acetate}$$

□ The rate-limiting step in ETOH metabolism is intake. An intake of 20 mL/h exceeds the metabolic capacity.
□ ETOH is highly diffusible, with rapid distribution to all aqueous compartments. The liver metabolizes 90%, and the remaining 10% is eliminated by diffusing directly in the lungs or kidneys.

Central Nervous System Effects

The central nervous system (CNS) effects of alcohol depend on the serum concentration as follows:

□ At 50 mg/100 mL, effects include depression of higher cortical centers, disinhibition, increased emotional excitability, decreased mental activity, and impaired judgment.
□ At 150 mg/100 mL, emotional imbalance, slurred speech, and ataxia are seen.
□ At above 350 mg/100 mL, the patient may exhibit lethargy, stupor, and coma. Death may result from cardiac or respiratory depression, or aspiration-related asphyxia.

Chronic Alcoholism

Alcoholic liver disease progresses in stages. **Initially, elevated liver transaminases** (e.g., AST, ALT) and increased mean red cell transfer volume may be the only clues to the presence of parenchymal damage. **Fatty liver disease** (manifesting as hepatomegaly) is an early finding that will resolve if ETOH ingestion is stopped. With continued intake, **alcoholic hepatitis** ensues (overall survival is 56% at 5 years). Alcoholic hepatitis carries an increased nonsurgical mortality between 25% and 60% per year. **Cirrhosis** and **portal hypertension** are the final sequelae of alcoholic liver disease (40% 5-year mortality rate).

Alcoholic Cirrhosis

Abnormalities associated with alcoholic cirrhosis include the following:

□ **Nutritional**: Decreased albumin, megaloblastic anemia requiring B_{12} and folate replacement, decreased vitamin K absorption, and hypoglycemia (decreased gluconeogenesis, decreased glycogen stores).
□ **Cardiovascular**: Hyperdynamic increased cardiac output, arteriovenous (AV) shunting, increased intravascular volume, decreased blood viscosity secondary to anemia, cardiomyopathy, and congestive heart failure.
□ **Pulmonary**: Hypoxia secondary to extrinsic restrictive lung disease resulting from ascites-induced cephalad displacement of the diaphragm, right-to-left shunting secondary to portal vein hypertension, intrapulmonary AV shunting, and pneumonia secondary to decreased pulmonary phagocytic activity or aspiration of gastric contents.
□ **Gastrointestinal**: Fetor hepaticus (peculiar breath odor), anemia, portal vein hypertension, gastroesophageal varices, increased incidence of cholelithiasis and pancreatitis, peptic ulcer disease, decreased gastroesophageal sphincter tone, and splenomegaly.

□ **CNS**: Asterixis and encephalopathy.
□ **Hematologic**: Coagulopathy from decreased synthesis of clotting factors (except factor VIII), resulting in increased prothrombin time and activated partial thromboplastin time. ETOH suppresses platelet function and survival (splenic sequestration), and enhances fibrinolysis.
□ **Renal**: Decreased renal blood flow, decreased glomerular filtration rate, increased renin, angiotensin, and aldosterone. Abrupt oliguria with concomitant cirrhosis (hepatorenal syndrome) is associated with 60% mortality.
□ **Immunologic**: Suppressed immune defense mechanisms.

Anesthetic Management of Alcoholic Patients

Patients with alcoholic cirrhosis may exhibit an unpredictable response to induction of general anesthesia. For example, cross-tolerance with barbiturates has been reported. Accordingly, barbiturate dose may need to be increased. However, if the patient's nutritional status is poor, a decrease in serum albumin may increase the amount of free drug and potentiate the drug's myocardial depressant effect. Chronic alcoholics are at **risk for aspiration** of gastric contents for the following reasons: increased gastric acid secretion, decreased gastric motility, ascites-induced changes in the gastroesophageal junction angle, and increased intragastric pressure. **Plasma cholinesterase** synthesis may be **decreased** in cirrhotic patients, although prolonged apnea after succinylcholine would usually not be noticeable clinically.

Minimal alveolar concentration **(MAC)** is decreased following **acute ETOH ingestion**. In contrast, MAC is **increased in chronic alcoholics**. Patients with alcoholic cardiomyopathy may be exquisitely sensitive to the myocardial depressant effects of anesthetic drugs. Opioids and benzodiazepines may also have prolonged half-lives because of impaired hepatic biotransformation.

Alcoholics may appear **resistant to nondepolarizing muscle relaxants**. D-Tubocurarine and pancuronium have been shown to bind to both albumin and gamma globulin at a ratio of 1:1.5. Gamma globulin production is markedly increased in cirrhotic patients. This results in decreased free fraction of drug, which necessitates increased initial doses of muscle relaxant. Increased volume of distribution is also reflected in prolonged elimination half-lives of the long-acting nondepolarizing muscle

relaxants. Elimination half-lives of vecuronium (in doses below 0.1 mg/kg), atracurium, and cisatracurium are unaffected by hepatic disease.

Regional anesthesia may be used in patients with chronic alcoholism. Relative contraindications include coagulopathy, peripheral neuropathy, and decreased intravascular volume.

Monitoring should include periodic monitoring of neuromuscular blockade, measurement of urine output, periodic measurement of serum glucose, and electrolytes.

Postoperative problems include poor wound healing, bleeding, infection, and hepatic dysfunction.

Delirium Tremens

Onset of **delirium tremens** typically occurs 48 to 72 hours after cessation of drinking.

□ Signs and symptoms include tremulousness, disorientation, hallucinations, autonomic hyperactivity (diaphoresis, hyperpyrexia, tachycardia, and hypertension), and grand mal seizures.
□ Laboratory findings include hypomagnesemia, hypokalemia, and respiratory alkalosis.
□ Treatment includes benzodiazepines, possibly accompanied by supplemental thiamine, magnesium, and potassium.

Disulfiram (Antabuse)

Disulfiram blocks the conversion of acetaldehyde by **acetaldehyde dehydrogenase**. With alcohol ingestion, acetaldehyde levels increase rapidly and cause nausea, vomiting, tearing, and potential bronchoconstriction and cardiac arrhythmias. The **half-life** of disulfiram is **1 to 2 weeks**. Disulfiram can **inhibit** the enzyme (**dopamine-β-hydroxylase**) necessary for conversion of dopamine to norepinephrine, resulting in perioperative hypotension, potentiation of benzodiazepines, and drowsiness.

Suggested References

Bruce DL. Alcoholism and anesthesia. Anesth Analg 1983;62:84–96.
Stoelting RK, Dierdorf SF. Diseases of the liver and biliary tract. In Stoelting RK, Dierdorf SF, eds. Anesthesia and Co-Existing Disease. 3rd ed. New York: Churchill Livingstone, 1993:251–275.
Wyngaarden JB, Smith LH Jr, Bennett JC. Cecil Textbook of Medicine. 19th ed. Philadelphia: WB Saunders, 1992.

217
Anesthesia for Liver Transplantation

James Y. Findlay, M.B. Ch.B., F.R.C.A.

Liver transplantation is a well-accepted (more than 4000 transplants performed in 125 centers in 1998) therapy for end-stage liver disease. The number of liver transplantations has been limited only by the number of suitable donor livers available. By splitting donor livers, some surgeons are now able to offer the procedure to more adult and pediatric patients.

Liver transplantation presents a challenge to the anesthesiologist, because, in addition to the operative complexity, most patients begin with greatly altered physiology because of their hepatic disease.

Preoperative Evaluation

Table 217–1 lists relevant physiologic consequences of liver failure. A thorough cardiac assessment includes echocardiography to determine baseline cardiac function and pulmonary artery pressures. Arterial blood gases are obtained, along with routine studies and coagulation testing.

Intraoperative Management

Anesthesia

Induction of anesthesia may be achieved using any of the commonly used agents. Rapid-sequence induction is often performed because of concerns about increased intragastric pressures and the threat of aspiration pneumonitis. Maintenance is typically achieved using inhaled anesthetics (e.g., isoflurane) and short-acting IV opioids (e.g., fentanyl). Neuromuscular blockade is maintained with nondepolarizing medications that are not dependent on hepatic elimination (e.g., cisatracurium).

Table 217–2 lists the monitoring commonly done during hepatic transplantation. A "stat lab" in close proximity to the operating room is used for the rapid analysis of blood gases, electrolytes, glucose, and coagulation status. Many centers use thromboelastography (TEG) to provide a rapid assessment of coagulation.

Adequate large-bore venous access is essential because of the potential for sudden, massive hemorrhage. This must be obtained in the upper body, because the procedure involves inferior vena cava (IVC) obstruction. This access is also required for the return of blood if veno-veno bypass is used (see below). At least one, often two, 8 French or larger catheters are inserted peripherally or centrally. A rapid infusion pump capable of delivering up to 1.5 L/min of blood or fluids warmed to 37°C is connected to the cannula. Red blood cell salvage is usually used. The blood bank should be able to quickly provide large quantities of blood products.

The large surgical incisions and prolonged operating times make hypothermia a potential problem. Fluid warmers and forced-air convective warming blankets can help prevent or minimize perioperative hypothermia.

Transplant Procedure

Initial dissection and hepatectomy can result in significant blood loss from friable collateral blood

Table 217–1. Pathophysiologic Changes Associated with Liver Failure

Organ System	Physiologic Effect
Cardiovascular	Hyperdynamic circulation High cardiac output Low resistance Pulmonary hypertension[a]
Respiratory	Hypoxia Restrictive pattern (ascites) Intrapulmonary shunting (hepatopulmonary syndrome)
Hematologic	Coagulopathy Decreased factor synthesis Thrombocytopenia Anemia
CNS	Hepatic encephalopathy Cerebral edema (fulminant failure)
Renal	Hepatorenal syndrome Hyponatremia

[a]Rare, but associated with poor outcome.

Table 217–2. Intraoperative Monitoring During Liver Transplantation

ECG
Pulse oximetry
Temperature
Arterial catheter (radial or brachial)
Pulmonary artery catheter
Transesophageal echocardiography (in some centers)

vessels. Excision of the liver involves clamping and dividing the hepatic vasculature (including the IVC). The resulting loss of venous return to the heart can cause cardiovascular collapse. To overcome this, veno-veno bypass may be necessary. This involves cannulation of portal and femoral veins. Blood is drained into a reservoir and returned to an upper body large bore cannula via a roller pump. An alternative surgical approach, the "piggy-back" technique, excises the liver using a "side-bite" of the IVC (i.e., partial IVC occlusion), allowing venous return to continue during surgery.

Once venous anastomosis to the graft is complete, the liver is flushed with blood, and the IVC clamp is released (i.e., recirculation). This causes an abrupt increase in serum potassium and acid load, resulting in ECG changes, hypotension, and cardiac arrhythmias. Intravenous calcium chloride antagonizes potassium-induced myocardial changes. Vasopressors, inotropes, and sodium bicarbonate may be needed for cardiovascular support. Air embolism is also a possibility.

Postreperfusion syndrome may be seen after recirculation. This involves decreased systemic vascular resistance, increased cardiac output, and hypotension. This syndrome typically resolves spontaneously within 30 minutes, but may require aggressive hemodynamic support. The final stage of transplantation involves hepatic artery anastomosis and a biliary drainage procedure.

Intraoperative coagulation management is often challenging (Fig. 217–1). Most patients are thrombocytopenic because of sequestration and destruction of platelets in the liver and spleen. Adequate replacement is essential because platelets are required for functional clotting. Low levels of soluble coagulation factors from decreased synthesis also need to be replaced with fresh frozen plasma (FFP).

After recirculation, uncontrolled fibrinolysis can occur, necessitating large quantities of cryoprecipi-

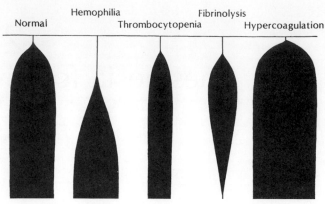

Figure 217–1. Normal and abnormal thromboelastograph patterns. Hemophilia is an example of factor deficiency.

tate and FFP. Antifibrinolytics (e.g., ϵ-aminocaproic acid, aprotinin) may be useful. Transfusion of large quantities of blood products may be associated with citrate toxicity, resulting in decreased levels of ionized calcium. This manifests clinically as prolonged Q–T interval on the ECG, hypotension, skeletal muscle weakness, and laryngospasm. Accordingly, ionized calcium should be checked often and replaced as needed.

At the conclusion of surgery, the patient is transferred to the intensive care unit for postoperative management.

Suggested References

Carton EG, Plevak DJ, Kranner PW, et al. Perioperative care of the liver transplant patient: Part II. Anesth Analg 1994;78:382–399.

Klinck JR. Liver transplantation: Anesthesia. In Klinck JR, Lindop MJ, eds. Anesthesia and Intensive Care for Organ Transplantation. London: Chapman and Hall, 1998:169–199.

Ramsay MAE, Swygert TH. Anesthesia for liver transplantation. In Busuttil RW, Klintmalm GB, eds. Transplantation of the Liver. Philadelphia: WB Saunders, 1996:419–433.

218
Anesthesia for Tubal Ligation

Scott A. Gammel, M.D.

Tubal ligations are performed using either local, general, or regional anesthesia. They are done either as an interval (not postpartum) procedure or as an immediate postpartum procedure.

Interval Tubal Ligations

Laparoscopy is the most common surgical approach for this procedure. Anesthetic considerations include pneumoperitoneum, head-down positioning with related cardiovascular and pulmonary physiologic changes, and rapid recovery.

Pneumoperitoneum is performed via a needle inserted at the lower margin of the umbilicus (a relatively avascular and thin portion of the abdominal wall). An incorrectly placed needle can insufflate the abdominal wall, retroperitoneum, mesentery, omentum, or bowel. **Carbon dioxide** (CO_2) is the gas of choice because it is highly soluble and rapidly absorbed postoperatively. CO_2 also provides a margin of safety if injected intravascularly. **Nitrous oxide** (N_2O) is less soluble and is not eliminated as quickly, but is associated with less peritoneal and diaphragmatic irritation (and postoperative shoulder pain), which is especially helpful when local anesthesia is used.

Head-down (Trendelenburg's) positioning is associated with brachial plexus injury. This is the most common injury in this position, a result of clavicular compression of nerve roots from shoulder rests. Steep Trendelenburg's positioning requires endotracheal intubation, and tube position should be checked because the mediastinum may shift cephalad, leading to mainstem intubation.

Cardiovascular changes result from increased intra-abdominal pressure. When greater than 30 mm Hg, this causes significant decreases in central venous, arterial, and pulse pressures and a small decrease in cardiac output secondary to decreased venous return, increased peripheral resistance, and elevated peak inspiratory pressures. At 20 mm Hg, circulatory stimulation with elevated arterial and central venous pressures, tachycardia, hypercarbia, and decreased pH may be seen. There is a high incidence of premature ventricular contractions when CO_2 is used to insufflate during spontaneous ventilation and with the use of halothane. This inci-

dence is greatly reduced by mechanical ventilation. Vagally mediated bradycardia or asystole can also occur; prophylactic glycopyrrolate is often used.

Respiratory changes include decreased vital capacity, decreased functional residual capacity, increased blood volume, and decreased pulmonary compliance, which can lead to postoperative atelectasis. A significant increase in arterial CO_2 and decrease in pH occur during general anesthesia when CO_2 is used for insufflation, because of absorption from the pneumoperitoneum. Spontaneous ventilation can also lead to significant hypercarbia.

Other complications include hemorrhage (accounting for almost one-half of complications), gas embolism, pneumothorax, pneumomediastinum, and mesenteric ischemia.

Anesthetic Techniques

Local Anesthesia. Although it is not commonly used for laparoscopy, local anesthesia for tubal ligation has been associated with shorter anesthesia and recovery times (albeit not statistically significant) than general anesthesia, and less likelihood of intraoperative hypertension, hypotension, or tachycardia. There was less nausea and vomiting and other postoperative complications. It was also less expensive. Success of local anesthesia is dependent on patient selection, intraoperative communication with the patient, gentle surgeons, and use of N_2O for insufflation to avoid diaphragm irritation. For periumbilical anesthesia, 10 mL of 2% chloroprocaine can be used. Through the inserted laparoscope, 20 mL of 0.5% bupivacaine or 12 mL of 2% lidocaine is sprayed on tubes from fimbriae to uterus.

General Anesthesia. Common postoperative complications of general anesthesia are abdominal and shoulder pain and nausea and vomiting.

□ It has been shown that metoclopramide (10 to 20 mg IV 15 to 30 minutes before induction) and droperidol (0.5 to 1.0 mg 3 to 6 minutes before induction) are synergistic in decreasing nausea, vomiting, and recovery time. Droperidol by itself (0.625 to 2.15 mg) after intubation is an effective antiemetic for outpatient tubal ligation and shorter recovery room time. Ondansetron (4 or 8 mg IV) before induction also significantly reduces the incidence of postoperative nausea and vomiting.[1]

□ After intravenous induction, oxygen, N_2O, and a volatile anesthetic are used to maintain anesthesia. This is supplemented with short-acting narcotics and muscle relaxants.

□ Narcotic requirements postoperatively, vomiting, and overnight hospital stay were reduced by dropping 5 mL of 1% etidocaine on each fallopian tube before banding. Using etidocaine instead of bupivacaine produced a significant decrease in postoperative pain.

Regional Anesthesia (Spinal or Epidural). Regional anesthesia is not often used for interval tubal sterilization. The block may take too long to develop, and the complication of spinal headache is more likely in this patient group; also, spontaneous ventilation, especially with steep head-down positions, is difficult. However, the incidence of nausea and vomiting is less than one-eighth of that associated with general anesthesia.

Postpartum Tubal Sterilization

Although it has been common practice to wait 8 hours postpartum before inducing general anesthesia (because of the risk of maternal aspiration), there is no proven safe delivery-to-surgery interval; all groups studied had pHs below 2.5 and/or gastric volumes above 25 mL. Additional complications associated with postpartum tubal sterilization include increased risk of infection and episiotomy breakdown secondary to increased abdominal pressure. It is recommended that if a patient has any associated medical or obstetrical problems, surgery should be postponed for 6 months.

Anesthetic Techniques

Recommended considerations for general anesthesia include checking preoperative hemoglobin, because it is difficult to determine blood loss at delivery.

□ Wait 8 hours postdelivery; keep the patient NPO, and consider preoperative antacids and/or metoclopramide.

□ Perform rapid-sequence induction with endotracheal intubation. Use N_2O as the primary volatile agent, avoiding high concentrations of other volatile agents because of uterine artery bleeding. Supplement with a short-acting narcotic and muscle relaxant or use succinylcholine infusion (which is highly ionized, and thus little is found in breast milk). It is not known whether any of the stereoisomers of mivacurium are secreted in breast milk; thus mivacurium infusion should be done cautiously.

□ Remember that MAC is reduced in the postpartum period for 24 to 36 hours, with a gradual return to normal by 72 hours.[2]

□ Ventilation should be controlled; blood pressure should be frequently measured during insufflation of the abdomen.

□ Extubate when the patient is fully awake and relaxants are reversed; recovery in the lateral position is ideal.

Regional anesthesia for postpartum tubal sterilizations entails routine considerations for regional anesthesia, as well as precautions related to the differences in potency at term and postpartum.

□ When compared with parturients, patients 36 to 48 hours postpartum require an increased anesthetic dose via continuous spinal anesthesia to achieve the same level. Cardiovascular changes are markedly decreased in postpartum patients. There is a faster onset, higher level, and longer duration of spinal anesthesia in term patients than in young gynecological patients. There is also a progressive decline in duration of block during the first 3 days postpartum.

□ Starting 18 hours postpartum, there is a progressive decrease in dermatomal spread of epidural anesthesia compared to that in patients given epidurals for cesarean section. At 36 hours postpartum, there is no significant difference in spread in nonpregnant patients. Reactivation of labor epidural catheters is reliable for 24 hours.[3]

□ A T4 block provides excellent operating conditions and pain relief. A T10 block may be inadequate, especially if it is difficult to mobilize the uterus during surgery.

Selected References

1. McKenzie R, Kovac A, O'Conner T, et al. Comparison of ondansetron versus placebo to prevent postoperative nausea vomiting in women undergoing ambulatory gynecologic surgery. Anesthesiology 1993;78:21–28.
2. Chan MT, Gin T. Postpartum changes in the minimum alveolar concentration of isoflurane. Anesthesiology 1995;82:1360–1363.
3. Goodman EJ, Dumas SD. The rate of successful reactivation of labor epidural catheters for postpartum tubal ligation surgery. Reg Anesth Pain Manage 1998;23:258–261.

Suggested References

Abouleish E. Postpartum tubal ligation requires more bupivacaine for spinal anesthesia than does cesarean section. Anesth Analg 1986;65:897.
Hanley ES. Anesthesia for laparoscopic surgery. Surg Clin North Am 1992;72:1013.
McKenzie R. Postoperative pain after laparoscopic sterilization (Letter). Anaesthesia 1989;44:450.
Peterson HB, Hulka JF, Spielman FJ, et al. Local versus general anesthesia for laparoscopic sterilization: A randomized study. Obstet Gynecol 1987;70:6.
Shnider SM, Levinson G, eds. Anesthesia for Obstetrics. 3rd ed. Baltimore: Williams & Wilkins, 1993.
Spielman FG. Laparoscopic surgery. Probl Anesth 1989;3:1.

219
Complications of Transurethral Resection of the Prostate

Stephen T. Gott, M.D.

Transurethral resection of the prostate (TURP) is one of the most common surgical procedures performed in males over age 60. TURP is the definitive therapy for benign prostatic hypertrophy when symptomatic obstruction of urinary outflow occurs. Major complications occur in 2.5% to 20% of TURP patients, and perioperative mortality rates of 0.5% to 6% have been reported.

Operative Procedure

The operation is performed under direct vision through a modified cystoscope (resectoscope) with an electrically energized wire loop. Bleeding is controlled with a coagulating current. Continuous irrigation is used to distend the bladder and to remove blood and dissected prostatic tissue. Because the prostate contains large venous sinuses, it is inevitable that irrigating solution will be absorbed into the vascular system. The volume absorbed depends on three factors:

- **Hydrostatic pressure**, determined by the height of the irrigating fluid above the patient. Prostate venous sinuses have a pressure of approximately 10 mm Hg.
- **Duration of resection and experience of the surgeon**. Approximately 10 to 30 mL of irrigating solution is absorbed per minute of resection time.
- The number and size of the opened venous sinuses.

Irrigation Solutions

The choice of irrigating fluid depends on its optical properties, osmolarity, potential for inducing hemolysis, degree of ionization, and cost.

- **Distilled water** was used in the past because of its low cost and least interference with visibility, but has been abandoned because of its potential for inducing marked dilutional hyponatremia and intravascular red blood cell hemolysis.

- **Lactated Ringer's and normal saline** solutions have also been abandoned, because they are highly ionized and promote current dispersion from the resectoscope.
- **Glycine (1.5%)** is low in cost, is nonelectrolytic, and is only slightly hypo-osmolar. If large amounts are absorbed, transient blindness and encephalopathy can evolve, as well as potential complications associated with increased fluid load.
- **Sorbitol (2.7%) and mannitol (0.54%) (Cytal)** has the advantage of being nonelectrolytic, isosmolar, and is rapidly cleared from the plasma. Disadvantages are relative cost and the potential for complications resulting from increased fluid load.

Complications

TURP Syndrome. TURP syndrome may occur at any time perioperatively. Under regional anesthesia, the patient will often complain of headache, dizziness, confusion, and shortness of breath. Restlessness often ensues, with elevated blood pressure and bradycardia. Without prompt treatment, seizures, hypertension, and cardiac arrest may follow. Under general anesthesia, TURP syndrome may be difficult to diagnose until late when the presenting signs may include an unexplained rise and fall in blood pressure, respiratory arrest, and severe refractory bradycardia. These signs and symptoms are frequently seen in the patient with preexisting compromised myocardial function with the inability to handle the increased intravascular absorption of the irrigating solution.

- **Circulatory overload** depends on cardiovascular status, amount and rapidity of absorption of irrigating solution, and amount of surgical blood loss.
- **Dilutional hyponatremia** associated with TURP is a hypervolemic hyponatremia representing excess total body water with normal total body sodium. If serum sodium concentrations fall below 120 mEq/L, signs and symptoms of water

intoxication may develop. This should be treated with hypertonic 3.5% saline at a rate below 100 mL/hr, allowing the most rapid correction of plasma sodium concentration. The volume of distribution of sodium equals total body water, so free water excess can be estimated from the following formula

$$\text{Total body water} = \text{weight in kg} \times 0.6$$

From this, an estimation of the mEq of Na^+ necessary to normalize the plasma sodium concentration can be obtained:

$$\text{Sodium deficit} = (140 - \text{observed plasma Na}) \times (\text{total body water})$$

Hypertonic 3.5% saline contains 598 mEq of Na^+/L and should be administered no faster than 100 mL/hr. Once the symptoms have abated (or sodium concentration rises above 120 mEq/L), the hypertonic saline should be stopped and Lasix (furosemide, 40 to 60 mg IV) administered to aid free water excretion by the kidneys. Frequent serum sodium measurements should be obtained. Too-rapid correction of hyponatremia can cause seizures, central pontine myelinolysis, and permanent brain damage.

□ **Glycine toxicity** usually manifests as visual disturbances and transient blindness, but may also include other signs and symptoms seen in TURP syndrome. The mechanism of action may be attributed to glycine acting as an inhibitory neurotransmitter, because it has a distribution similar to that of γ-aminobutyric acid in the retina, spinal cord, and brain stem.
□ **Ammonia toxicity.** Ammonia is a major byproduct of glycine metabolism. Hyperammonemia usually manifests with nausea and vomiting, followed by encephalopathy.

Blood Loss. Assessment of blood loss is difficult during TURP because of dilution with irrigation fluid. The usual hemodynamic responses to blood loss are not reliable because of increased circulating volume from the irrigating solution. The amount of blood loss is proportional to the vascularity of the prostate, the surgeon's experience, length of the operation, and the weight of the prostate gland resected. Continuous postoperative bleeding may indicate a coagulopathy, as patients undergoing TURP have a higher incidence of fibrinolysis. Dilutional thrombocytopenia should also be considered in the differential diagnosis.

Hypothermia. Hypothermia could be another cause of confusion in the elderly patient. Intraoperative hypothermia has not been shown to be influenced by anesthetic technique.

Bacteremia. Despite preoperative intravenous antibiotics, bacteremia commonly occurs after TURP. Sudden cardiovascular collapse after TURP may be a manifestation of septicemia.

Perforation of Bladder or Urethra with Extravasation. Bladder perforation may be extraperitoneal or intraperitoneal.

□ **Extraperitoneal** (most common). In the awake patient, perforation may present as pain in the periumbilical, inguinal, or suprapubic region.
□ **Intraperitoneal.** Perforation is usually through the bladder wall. Pain may be generalized to the upper abdomen or referred from the diaphragm to the shoulder. Other signs and symptoms include pallor, sweating, nausea, vomiting, shortness of breath, abdominal rigidity, hypotension, and hypertension.

Prevention of Complications

Optimizing the patient's preoperative state is essential to proper anesthetic management, because TURP is generally an elective procedure. Minimizing absorption of the irrigating solution can reduce the risk of complications. Risks can be reduced by limiting the duration of surgery, using isosmotic solutions, limiting the depth of dissection, and limiting the pressure of irrigating solution (60 cm H_2O is suggested). Use of spinal anesthesia should promote earlier detection of complications.

Suggested References

Malhotra V, Divan S. Anesthesia and the renal and genitourinary systems. In Miller RD, ed. Anesthesia. Vol. 2. 5th ed. Philadelphia: Churchill Livingstone, 2000:1934–1959.

Monk TG, Weldon BC. The renal system and anesthesia for urologic surgery. In Barash PG, Cullen BF, Stoelting RK, eds. Clinical Anesthesia. 3rd ed. Philadelphia: Lippincott-Raven, 1997:945–974.

220
Anesthesia for Electroconvulsive Therapy

Joseph J. Sandor, M.D.

Convulsive therapy for psychiatric disorders has been used since 1934. Electroconvulsive therapy (ECT), modified over the years to incorporate monitoring, intravenous anesthetic drugs, neuromuscular blockade, and supplemental oxygen, is both safe and effective for the treatment of **endogenous depression** in patients who:

- Have failed to respond to an adequate course of antidepressant drugs.
- May be jeopardized by drug side effects.
- Suffer from severe melancholia.
- Are suicidal.

Mechanism of Action

Seizures induced by ECT are similar to grand mal seizures. A 2- to 3-second **latent phase** is followed by a **tonic phase** lasting 10 to 12 seconds, then a **clonic phase** of 30 to 50 seconds. Both the duration of individual seizures and cumulative seizure time correlate with clinical improvement. The number of treatments is determined by the patient's clinical response.

The physiologic mechanisms responsible for the therapeutic benefit are unknown. Current theories include:

- Changes in blood-brain barrier permeability.
- Regional cerebral blood flow changes and electrolyte changes.
- Changes in neurometabolic activity.
- Acute discharges of neuroendocrine units (e.g., adrenocorticotropic hormone [ACTH], prolactin, hypothalamic peptides).
- Changes in ion transport, neurotransmitters, and biogenic amines.
- Stimulation of β-adrenergic receptors.

Physiologic Response

The **cardiovascular response** to ECT is secondary to **autonomic nervous system** discharge. **Parasympathetic** discharge is immediate and may cause asystole, bradycardia, premature ventricular contractions, hypotension, and ventricular escape. **Sympathetic** discharge then follows within seconds, possibly manifesting as increased heart rate, PVCs, bigeminy, trigeminy, sinus tachycardia, and severe hypertension. A marked increase in myocardial oxygen consumption frequently occurs.

An initial constriction of cerebral vessels is followed by increased cerebral blood flow (1.5 to 7 times baseline) from increased cerebral oxygen consumption and elevated blood pressure. Preoxygenation is used to prevent cerebral hypoxia.

The neuroendocrine response to ECT is manifested by increased levels of ACTH, cortisol, and catecholamines. The effects on glucose levels vary; thus, diabetics should have their glucose levels closely monitored post-ECT.

Miscellaneous effects of ECT of importance to the anesthesiologist include increased intragastric pressure and **increased intraocular pressure**.

Morbidity and Mortality Rates

The mortality risk from ECT is 0.03%. Other complications include transient arrhythmias (10% to 40%), gastric aspiration (2.5%), and musculoskeletal disorder (0.4%), including fractures. In addition, post-ECT complications may include pulmonary edema, headache, memory disturbance, and agitation.

Relative contraindications to ECT include:

- Angina pectoris.
- Congestive heart failure.
- Chronic obstructive pulmonary disease.
- Thrombophlebitis.
- High-risk pregnancy.
- Pacemakers.
- Severe osteoporosis.
- Glaucoma.
- Retinal detachment.

Absolute contraindications to ECT include:

- Recent myocardial infarction.
- Recent stroke.

□ Intracranial mass.
□ Pheochromocytoma.

Anesthetic Management

Preoperative assessment should document cardiopulmonary and neurologic status, risk of gastrointestinal reflux, and history of earlier drug therapy. Ideally, monoamine oxidase inhibitors and tricyclic antidepressants should be discontinued 2 weeks before ECT. Patients receiving lithium therapy may exhibit delayed awakening, memory loss, and confusion postictally. Lithium may interfere with success of ECT.

Monitoring should include (at a minimum) electrocardiography, blood pressure, and pulse oximetry. Patients should be adequately preoxygenated after intravenous access is established.

Pharmacologic intervention before ECT may include:

□ Antacids (sodium citrate and/or H_2 antagonists) and metoclopramide to reduce risks of aspiration of gastric contents.
□ Methohexital, thiopental, or etomidate for hypnosis. Propofol has been effective for this purpose, but it shortens the convulsive period in comparison to methohexital.

□ Succinylcholine (0.5 mg/kg) for muscle relaxation; smaller doses may not provide protection from musculoskeletal injuries, increasing the risk of fractures, whereas larger doses may produce prolonged apnea and interfere with detection of the motor seizure.
□ Anticholinergics to modify the parasympathetic response. Glycopyrrolate, which causes less tachycardia and central nervous system confusion, is preferred.
□ Various agents to blunt the sympathetic response. These may include sodium nitroprusside, hydralazine, clonidine, nitroglycerin ointment, β-blockers, and lidocaine. Esmolol in bolus doses of 2 to 3 mg/kghas proven to be effective.

Suggested References

Avramov MN, Husain MM, White PF. The comparative effects of methohexital, propofol, and etomidate for electroconvulsive therapy. Anesth Analg 1995;81:596–602.

Gaines GY, Rees DI. Electroconvulsive therapy and anesthetic considerations. Anesth Analg 1986;65:1345–1356.

Rampton AJ, Griffin RM, Stuart CS, et al. Comparison of methohexital and propofol for electroconvulsive therapy: Effects on hemodynamic responses and seizure duration. Anesthesiology 1989;70:412–417.

Selvin BI. Electroconvulsive therapy—1987. Anesthesiology 1987;67:367–385.

Stoelting RK, Dierdorf ST. Anesthesia and Co-Existing Disease. 3rd ed. New York: Churchill Livingstone, 1993.

221
Anesthesia for MRI

Margaret R. Weglinski, M.D.

Magnetic resonance imaging (MRI) is a diagnostic technique that uses electromagnetic fields—static, gradient, and radiofrequency—to perform noninvasive imaging. Over the past decade, MRI has become one of the most important advances in diagnostic imaging since the x-ray. Because of improvements in the type of magnetic resonance images available, it appears that the utility of MRI will continue to grow and its applications will continue to expand.

Clinical Uses

MRI offers several advantages over other imaging modalities. It provides multiplane images and excellent spatial resolution, is not affected by bony artifact, does not employ ionizing radiation, and requires little patient preparation. It is especially useful for evaluating the central nervous system (e.g., posterior fossa tumors, cerebral infarction, head trauma, dementia, and intracranial infections). It is also used to evaluate the spinal canal, cardiac chambers, traumatic muscle and ligament injuries, and intrathoracic and intra-abdominal disorders.

Indications for Anesthesia Involvement

To obtain magnetic resonance images free of movement artifacts, patients must remain motionless for periods of up to 2 hours. This is impossible for young children and difficult for adults with painful conditions, movement disorders, claustrophobia, and mental illness. Some patients have serious medical problems or traumatic injuries that require intensive monitoring. It is primarily the requirement for a motionless patient that makes the services of an anesthesiologist essential to ensure that these patients receive a high-quality scan in a safe and efficient manner.

Hazards of MRI

Problems common to any anesthetizing location outside of the operating room are also applicable to the MRI suite. These include the remoteness of the location, the lack of trained personnel to assist in the event of an emergency, and the minimal consideration given to anesthetic requirements in the design of the area, such as lack of pipeline gases, suction, and waste gas exhaust capabilities. Problems that are unique to the MRI suite stem from the limitations imposed by the powerful magnetic field of the imager and the physical structure of the magnet bore itself. The strength of the static magnetic field of most MRI units ranges from 0.5 to 1.5 tesla, with increasing strength associated with better spatial resolution. The problems associated with the strong magnetic fields and radiofrequency pulses of the MRI scanner can be divided into five categories:

- Any object near the scanner that contains ferromagnetic material may launch toward the magnet with considerable and possibly lethal force, risking injury to the patient or others in the room. These objects include scissors, laryngoscopes, stylets, stethoscopes, gas cylinders, transport carts, and even anesthesia machines. Of equal concern is the effect of the magnetic field on in vivo metals contained in pacemakers, automatic implanted cardiac defibrillators, cochlear implants, and some cerebrovascular clips. When exposed to a strong magnetic field, these items present a risk of dislodgment, hemorrhage, or motile injury to adjacent vulnerable structures (e.g., brain).
- Most electronic monitoring devices and anesthesia equipment do not function properly when located near the magnet; thus alternate specially adapted monitors and equipment must be used or, if possible, shielded and positioned as far from the magnet bore as possible.
- Metal objects or electronic monitors can produce radiofrequency waves that interfere with the image generated by the MRI scanner, resulting in degraded nondiagnostic images.
- Radiofrequency energy produced by the scanner can be absorbed by tissue or other objects and result in localized heating, particularly in a large metal prosthesis. The clinical impression is that these thermal effects are not great enough to cause tissue damage and are well tolerated.
- The magnetic field gradients produce a loud bang-

ing sound (65 to 95 dB) that not only makes it extremely difficult to monitor heart sounds via an esophageal or precordial stethoscope but also can be associated with temporary or permanent hearing loss after the MRI examination. For this reason, the patient and all health care personnel in the MRI room should wear ear plugs.

Anesthetic Technique

Sedation and general anesthesia have both been effectively used for patients undergoing MRI scans and any anesthetic technique is acceptable. The fact that the patient is essentially out of sight and out of reach when they are in the magnet bore makes access to the airway impossible. Many anesthesiologists prefer to use general anesthesia with endotracheal intubation or placement of a laryngeal mask airway to avoid problems with hypoventilation and airway obstruction in heavily sedated patients. Although MRI or MRA (magnetic resonance angiography) is often chosen because of its noninvasive advantages to other studies, the general anesthesia that some patients need to complete an MRI should prompt reconsideration as to the relative safety of other studies (such as angiography) that could be accomplished with only monitored anesthesia care.

Whatever technique is chosen, preparation for and induction of anesthesia is best completed outside of the MRI unit, where the effects of the magnet on the laryngoscope and other anesthesia equipment and monitors do not present a problem. Wire spiral endotracheal tubes cannot be used, because they can degrade the image. Intravenous lines and ventilator hoses should include long extensions. Infusion pumps cannot be brought near the MRI unit, thus patients lacking cardiovascular stability who are dependent on infusions of vasoactive medications for hemodynamic support are not candidates for MRI scanning.

Monitoring and Equipment

Most of the standards of care adopted by the American Society of Anesthesiologists can be met in the MRI suite with varying amounts of difficulty. General guidelines are as follows:

□ Direct access and visualization of the patient during imaging is limited, making accurate patient monitoring essential.

□ MRI-compatible monitors should be placed to minimize magnetic pull from the scanner by securely mounting the devices and placing them at least 5 to 8 feet from the magnet bore.

□ The high radiofrequency power used in magnetic resonance scanning presents the risk of excessive heat at the monitoring sites and subsequent radiofrequency current burns. Burns have been reported with the use of ECG pads, standard pulse oximeter leads, and temperature monitoring.

□ The electrocardiogram is distorted by both the radiofrequency energy and static magnetic fields, possibly rendering it useless.

□ Physiologic monitors may interfere with MRI quality. Each new piece of equipment should be evaluated individually on the basis of both its ability to function in the MRI suite and its effect on MRI quality.

Resuscitation

For most MRI scanners, the time required to decrease the magnetic field to a normal level is 3 to 20 minutes. It then takes 3 to 4 days to restore the magnetic field to a superconductive level, costing thousands of dollars to replenish the liquid nitrogen and helium. Therefore, the magnetic field is deactivated in only the most dire emergencies. Patients should be quickly removed from the MRI room to initiate resuscitation.

Suggested References

Forbes RB. Anesthesia for nonsurgical procedures. In Longnecker DE, Tinker JH, Morgan GE Jr, eds. Principles and Practice of Anesthesiology. 2nd ed. St. Louis: Mosby, 1998;2287–2301.

Jorgensen NH, Messick JM Jr, Gray J, et al. ASA monitoring standards and magnetic resonance imaging. Anesth Analg 1994;79:1141–1147.

Kanal E, Shellock FG. Patient monitoring during clinical MR imaging. Radiology 1992;185:623–629.

Kanal E, Shellock FG, Talagala L. Safety considerations in MR imaging. Radiology 1990;176:593–606.

Patteson SK, Chesney JT. Anesthetic management for magnetic resonance imaging: Problems and solutions. Anesth Analg 1992;74:121–128.

222
Strabismus Surgery

Thomas J. Christopherson, M.D.

Malignant Hyperthermia

In the past, there was great concern regarding a possible association between muscle surgery (e.g., strabismus surgery) and malignant hyperthermia.[1] Currently, most agree that the **incidence of malignant hyperthermia is not increased** in patients undergoing strabismus surgery where succinylcholine (SCh) is used to facilitate tracheal intubation. Nonetheless, due to concerns of unrecognized muscular dystrophy in children, SCh is rarely used when managing this patient population.

Oculocardiac Reflex

Strabismus surgery has the well-known propensity to trigger the **oculocardiac reflex** (see Chap. 223). This **trigeminovagal reflex** presents most commonly as bradycardia, although atrial premature contractions, junctional rhythms, ventricular premature contractions, and asystole have all been described during episodes of extraocular muscle traction and during direct globe compression. **Prophylactic intramuscular atropine probably has no effect in preventing** this reflex, but intravenous atropine (0.02 mg/kg) can provide a vagolytic effect during bradycardic episodes. Atropine should be used with caution, however, because more serious and prolonged arrhythmias may occur secondary to atropine administration. Thus, if arrhythmias occur during strabismus repair, (1) ask the surgeon to immediately release eye muscle stimulation, (2) deepen general anesthesia and ensure adequate ventilation, and (3) use intravenous atropine cautiously, realizing the potential for more serious arrhythmias.

Uninterpretable Forced Duction Test

In determining a surgical therapeutic plan for strabismus patients, ophthalmologists often find the forced duction test (FDT) to be helpful. By grasping the sclera of the anesthetized eye with forceps, the surgeon can determine whether the strabismus is secondary to a paretic muscle or to a restrictive force that prevents adequate eye motion. SCh directly **interferes with the FDT test for up to 20 minutes**. France and colleagues[2] suggest that the FDT test can ideally be performed on anesthetized patients (1) during mask inhalation with subsequent use of SCh for tracheal intubation, (2) after tracheal intubation using a nondepolarizing neuromuscular relaxant, and (3) after intubation under deep anesthesia in which no neuromuscular relaxant was used.

Increased Incidence of Postoperative Nausea and Vomiting

Vomiting after strabismus repair is common. Avoiding narcotic premedications and using a potent antiemetic such as ondansetron (50 μg/kg) significantly decreases the frequency and severity of postoperative vomiting.[3] Droperidol (9 to 20 μg/kg) has also been used effectively 30 minutes before terminating surgery.

Increased Myoglobinemia

Intermittent administration of SCh causes a fourfold increase in the incidence rate of myoglobinemia in strabismus patients compared with general surgical patients.[3] Perhaps this also is a sign of latent muscle disturbance.

Selected References

1. Lewandowski KB. Strabismus as a possible sign of subclinical muscle dystrophy predisposing to rhabdomyolysis and myoglobinuria: A study of an affected family. Can Anaesth Soc J 1982;29:372–376.
2. France NK, France TD, Woodburn JD, et al. Succinylcholine alteration of the forced duction test. Ophthalmology 1980;87:1282–1287.
3. Watcha MF, Bras PJ, Cieslak GD, et al. The dose-response relationship of odansetron in preventing postoperative emesis in pediatric patients undergoing ambulatory surgery. Anesthesiology 1995;82:47–52.

223
Oculocardiac Reflex

Brian C. Kerr, M.D.

The oculocardiac reflex (OCR) was first described by Aschner and Dagnini in 1908.

Anatomy

The **afferent limb is trigeminal**, and **the efferent limb is vagal**. Specifically, **afferent impulses** travel via short and long ciliary nerves to the ciliary ganglion. From here, afferent information is sent to the gasserian ganglion via the ophthalmic branch of the trigeminal nerve. **Efferent impulses** leave the brain stem by way of the vagus nerve.

Triggering Stimuli

This reflex is triggered by traction on extraocular muscles (especially the medial rectus), direct pressure on the globe, ocular manipulation, and ocular pain. It may also be elicited by retrobulbar block, ocular trauma, and manipulation of tissue remaining in the orbital apex after enucleation. The OCR seems to fatigue with repeated manipulation.

Manifestations

The **most common manifestation of the OCR is sinus bradycardia**. Other cardiac arrhythmias include ectopic beats, junctional rhythms, atrioventricular blockade, ventricular bigeminy, multifocal premature ventricular contractions, wandering pacemaker, ventricular tachycardia, and asystole.

Prevalence

The reported prevalence is highly variable, ranging from 16% to 82%. Children and young adults undergoing eye muscle surgery under general anesthesia are the most susceptible to the OCR. Additionally, hypoxemia, hypercarbia, and acidosis increase the incidence and severity of the problem.

Intraoperative Management

The OCR may occur during local or general anesthesia. Retrobulbar block may help prevent arrhythmias by blocking the afferent limb of the reflex arc. However, the injection of anesthetic may itself stimulate the OCR.

If a cardiac arrhythmia appears, the initial course of action is to notify the surgeon that orbital stimulation should be halted. Next, the depth of anesthesia and adequacy of ventilation and oxygenation are optimized. Commonly, heart rate and rhythm will return to baseline within 20 seconds after these measures. However, if the initial cardiac arrhythmia is serious or if the reflex recurs, intravenous atropine should be given in 0.02 mg/kg increments (smaller doses may have no effect, or a paradoxical effect, worsening bradycardia) until resolution is achieved.

During pediatric strabismus surgery, many advocate administration of intravenous atropine (0.02 mg/kg) or glycopyrrolate (0.01 mg/kg) before the extraocular muscles are manipulated. Glycopyrrolate may be associated with less tachycardia than atropine, but has a slower onset of action.

Postoperative Management

Onset time may be variable. For example, following retrobulbar block, the OCR may appear immediately or as much as 1.5 hours after an uncomplicated block. Retrobulbar hemorrhage can also result in delayed OCR as persistent bleeding gradually increases periocular pressure. Therefore, careful monitoring should continue for several hours after a suspected or known retrobulbar hemorrhage.

Suggested References

Donlon JV Jr. Anesthesia for eye, ear, nose, and throat surgery. In Miller RD, ed. Anesthesia. 5th ed. Philadelphia: Churchill Livingstone, 2000:2173–2198.

McGoldrick KE. Anesthesia and the eye. In Barash PG, Cullen BF, Stoelting RK, eds. Clinical Anesthesia. 3rd ed. Philadelphia: Lippincott-Raven, 1997:911–928.

McGoldrick KE, Feitl ME, Krupin T. Neural blockade for ophthalmologic surgery. In Cousins MJ, Bridenbaugh PO, eds. Neural Blockade in Clinical Anesthesia and Management of Pain. 3rd ed. Philadelphia: Lippincott-Raven, 1998:533–556.

224
Anesthesia for Drug Abusers

Daniel J. Janik, M.D.

Illicit drug use is a major problem in the United States. Patients often abuse more than one substance simultaneously (i.e., polydrug abuse). Chronic "recreational" drug use can cause **physical dependence** (i.e., a condition in which withdrawal symptoms occur when the abused drug is withheld) and **tolerance** (i.e., the need for progressively larger doses to achieve the desired effect). **Abuse potential** correlates closely with euphoric potential. It is generally accepted that the perioperative period is **not** an appropriate time to attempt withdrawal. Rather, it is better to provide the patient with his or her usual maintenance dose preoperatively and delay withdrawal until the stress of surgery has abated.

Narcotics

Narcotics (e.g., heroin, morphine, meperidine, buprenorphine, fentanyl) are administered via oral, subcutaneous, intranasal, and intravenous routes. Chronic abuse affects several major organ systems. Common complications include cellulitis, abscess formation, thrombophlebitis, subacute bacterial endocarditis, atelectasis, pneumonia, acute pulmonary edema, pulmonary emboli, pulmonary hypertension, mild anemia, adrenal suppression, sclerosing glomerulonephritis, tetanus, hepatitis, acquired immunodeficiency syndrome, acute transverse neuritis, anaphylaxis, and death from overdose. Abuse potential of the narcotics correlates well with μ-receptor activity. If an addict's dose and time schedule for maintenance is known, then it should be continued during the procedure and into recovery.

If an addict shows signs of respiratory depression, narcotic premedication should be avoided. General, regional, or local anesthesia may be used. Perioperative hypotension may result from adrenal suppression. For abusers successfully withdrawn from opioids before surgery, butorphanol and nalbuphine are good analgesic choices. However, effective doses of potent μ–agonists should not be deleted from the therapeutic armamentarium, because underdosing can result in pain, anxiety, and drug craving. Opioid antagonists (e.g., naloxone) should be avoided.

Barbiturates and Benzodiazepines

Barbiturates and benzodiazepines are central nervous system (CNS) depressants that exert their pharmacologic affect by stimulating γ-aminobutyric acid (GABA) receptors. Chronic barbiturate or benzodiazepine use does not cause major organ changes like those seen in narcotic addicts; however, **hepatic enzyme induction** does occur. Accordingly, intravenous anesthetic requirements may be increased in the perioperative period. Additionally, **acute intoxication decreases** the minimum alveolar concentration **(MAC)** of inhaled anesthetics, whereas **chronic use increases MAC**. In chronic abusers, abrupt withdrawal increases CNS irritability, resulting in anxiety, delirium, seizures, trauma, postural hypotension, tachycardia, abdominal cramping, and nausea. Treatment of abstinence syndrome includes titration of barbiturates or benzodiazepines until symptoms resolve. Sufficient preoperative sedation should prevent abstinence syndrome. In the setting of overdose, nasogastric lavage and urine alkalinization are useful to speed clearance of the drug. Patients taking warfarin drugs require increased doses to maintain therapeutic anticoagulation.

Glue

Some teenagers sniff glue or other solvents (e.g., spray paint) to experience excitation, euphoria, vertigo, and hallucinations. Many solvents cause stupor, encephalopathy, coma, seizures, hepatic and renal damage, hematopoietic derangements, muscle weakness and rhabdomyolysis, nausea, vomiting, hyperchloremia, hypokalemia, hypophosphatemia, pulmonary edema, and cardiac arrhythmias.

Hallucinogens

LSD, psilocybin, and mescaline cause CNS excitation, sensory distortion, delusions, altered mood, depersonalization, hallucinations, and euphoria. Autonomic effects, mediated via the hypothalamus, include tachycardia, hypertension, mydriasis, piloerection, fever, hyperglycemia, salivation, lacrimation, nausea, vomiting, occasional seizures, and, rarely, prolonged psychotic reactions. LSD has both analgesic and anticholinesterase properties. The stress of surgery or general anesthesia can initiate a "flashback." Psychotic effects can be treated with chlorpromazine, barbiturates, chlordiazepoxide, or diazepam. Premedication should control anxiety or panic. There may be little need for narcotics preoperatively. Tachycardia and hypertension can be controlled with α- and β-blockers. General anesthesia is acceptable, and regional anesthesia may be possible if the patient is cooperative.

Amphetamines

Amphetamines stimulate the CNS, causing euphoria, increased performance, and hallucinations. Amphetamine intoxication appears to augment narcotic-mediated analgesia. Amphetamines stimulate α- and β-receptors, release catecholamines in the CNS, and inhibit reuptake of catecholamines into adrenergic nerve endings. Sympathetic effects include tachycardia, hypertension, diaphoresis, flushing, palpitations, headache, convulsions, nausea, vomiting, fever, arrhythmias, myocardial infarction, and cardiomyopathy. Extremely high doses may cause toxic delirium, coma, cerebral hemorrhage, or circulatory collapse. Toxicity may be treated with chlorpromazine or haloperidol, α-blockers or direct vasodilators, and β-blockers. Intravenous hydration, gastric lavage, and acidification of urine promote excretion. **Acute amphetamine administration increases MAC, whereas chronic use may decrease MAC.** Chronic users respond poorly to indirect-acting vasopressors; thus treatment of hypotension may require direct-acting catecholamines (e.g., epinephrine).

Cocaine

Cocaine is the most popular illegal drug in the United States. It is an **ester local anesthetic** that, when applied topically to nasal mucosa, smoked, or injected, stimulates dopaminergic neurons in the CNS and inhibits the reuptake of norepinephrine in sympathetic nerve endings. Cocaine is a CNS stimulant that causes euphoria, excitement, hallucinations with paranoid ideation, and aggressive behavior. Autonomic effects include vasoconstriction, hypertension, tachycardia, ventricular arrhythmias, mydriasis, hyperglycemia, hyperpyrexia, tremor, and seizures. Cocaine may also be associated with angina, cardiomyopathy, subacute

bacterial endocarditis, chronic productive cough with black sputum, decreased carbon monoxide-diffusing capacity, pulmonary edema, or abruptio placenta. Death may result from cerebral hemorrhage, myocardial infarction, or cardiac arrhythmia. Absence of prenatal care is the single most important predictor of cocaine abuse among parturients.

Anesthesia for cocaine abusers should include adequate preoperative sedation with barbiturates, benzodiazepines, and haloperidol and control of the autonomic nervous system. **Acute cocaine intoxication increases MAC.** Volatile anesthetics or regional techniques are acceptable for patients intoxicated with cocaine. Ketamine, gallamine, and pancuronium should be avoided.

Phencyclidine

Phencyclidine (PCP) is a cyclohexylamine that is well absorbed by all routes of administration and causes euphoria, amnesia, paresthesias, distortions of body image, psychosis, and agitated delirium. With high doses, a cataleptic (dissociative) state will occur. Nystagmus is usually present. Laryngeal and gag reflexes remain present; laryngospasm may occur. PCP can block the reuptake of norepinephrine and serotonin, and tachycardia and hypertension occur. PCP can **inhibit pseudocholinesterase**; however, prolonged apnea following succinylcholine administration typically does not occur. Cerebral hemorrhage, rhabdomyolysis, and renal failure have been reported. Acidification of the urine (ammonium chloride, 1 g PO) and nasogastric suction will increase PCP clearance. Seizures may be treated with barbiturates, benzodiazepines, or phenytoin. General anesthesia may be preferable in these patients because of their propensity for violent behavior. Cataleptic patients may not require anesthesia, but good airway control is essential.

Suggested References

Kain ZN, Mayes LC, Ferris CA, et al. Cocaine-abusing parturients undergoing cesarean section. A cohort study. Anesthesiology 1996;85:1028–1035.

Kain ZN, Rimar S, Barash PG. Cocaine abuse in the parturient and effects on the fetus and neonate. Anesth Analg 1993; 77:835–845.

Stoelting RK, Dierdorf SF. Psychiatric illness and substance abuse. In Stoelting RK, Dierdorf SF, eds. Anesthesia and Co-Existing Disease. 3rd ed. New York: Churchill Livingstone, 1999:517–538.

Wood PR, Soni N. Anaesthesia for substance abuse. Anaesthesia 1989;44:672–680.

Zacny JP, Galinkin JL. Psychotropic drugs used in anesthesia practice. Abuse liability and epidemiology of abuse. Anesthesiology 1999;90:269–288.

225
Chemical Dependency in Anesthesia Personnel

Keith H. Berge, M.D.

Chemical dependence is a devastating disease that must be recognized before it can be treated. In most cases, the addict is the last to acknowledge the problem. Thus, it is imperative that we, the friends, colleagues, and relatives, gain a clear understanding of the disease before we are confronted with it.[1]

Chemical dependency, especially narcotic addiction, is an occupational hazard for anesthesia providers. This is presumably because of the ready access to highly potent synthetic narcotics used in anesthetic practice. Narcotic abuse in anesthesia personnel typically occurs in the workplace. Tragically, there are many reports of anesthesia providers suffering severe morbidity (e.g., anoxic encephalopathy) or mortality from an overdose of self-administered narcotics.

In an effort to better define the dangers and incidence of chemical dependency in operating room personnel (specifically, anesthesiologists and residents training in anesthesiology, hereafter referred to simply as anesthesiologists), the American Society of Anesthesiologists (ASA) Committee on Occupational Health of Operating Room Personnel has developed an ongoing yearly prospective linear study of anesthesia personnel with chemical dependency. In addition, this Committee has recently published an excellent handbook (also available in full-text format from the ASA website) concerning chemical dependency in anesthesiologists. ASA survey data suggest an incidence of chemical dependency of 0.5% per year of anesthesia training or practice.[1] No similar published data exists defining the incidence in nurse anesthesia personnel.

Although anesthesiologists are at risk to develop addiction to the same licit (e.g., ethanol) and illicit drugs (e.g., cocaine) as society at large, the "drug of choice" for anesthesiologists undergoing rehabilitation for chemical abuse in a 1983 study was typically fentanyl or meperidine, although more recent evidence suggests that sufentanil has replaced meperidine as a common drug of abuse.[2, 3]

Fentanyl, available as a street drug ("China white") is considered by addiction medicine specialists to have an addictive potential similar to that of "crack" cocaine. It carries the risk of extremely rapid addiction (Fig. 225–1). This is in contrast to ethanol or even narcotics such as morphine or meperidine, for which a longer period of abuse is typically required before psychological and physical addiction result.

Recognizing Impairment in a Colleague

Chemical dependency threatens the career and possibly the life of an impaired colleague and those under their care. Therefore, it is imperative that telltale signs of addiction be recognized and treated, not ignored (Table 225–1). These signs, typically subtle, may not be apparent in the workplace until the addictive illness is relatively far advanced. Instead, the afflicted individual may appear to function well in the workplace while his or her family and social functioning may be in a state of chaos. In the case of narcotic addiction, this may be an attempt to preserve both career and access to the needed drug. It is interesting to note that although the incidence of narcotic abuse by anesthetic care

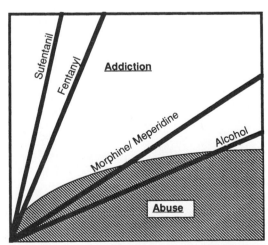

Figure 225–1. Time course of addiction. Dependence on alcohol develops over years, whereas sufentanil or fentanyl addiction develops quickly after a very short period of abuse. (Adapted from Arnold WP III.[3])

Table 225–1. Signs of Chemical Abuse in an Anesthesia Colleague

1. Unusual behavior, mood swings, periods of depression, anger and irritability, alternating with periods of euphoria.
2. "Signing out" unusual and increasing quantities of narcotics.
3. Reclusive behavior.
4. Frequent bathroom breaks.
5. Frequently relieving others.
6. Volunteering to clean rooms, volunteering for extra call, or spending off-duty hours at the hospital.
7. Wearing long sleeves to hide needle marks.
8. Patients arriving in recovery room with pain out of proportion to the amount of narcotic charted as given during their case.
9. Evidence of withdrawal including agitation, tremors, and diaphoresis.

providers, even while on duty, is known to occur with distressing frequency, documented harm to patients by impaired caregivers is rare.[4]

Intervention

Confronting an impaired colleague is extremely stressful and unpleasant. The intervention process is greatly facilitated if a departmental policy is in place outlining procedures to follow regarding intervention, evaluation, and the option of reentry into the workplace after treatment.[5] If sufficient evidence exists to suggest that a colleague is indeed chemically impaired or addicted, it is imperative that this physician be evaluated by a qualified addiction medicine specialist. Because denial is a hallmark of addiction, those responsible for the intervention should not attempt to judge the presence or absence of addiction by the response of the suspected colleague. Rather, the purpose of the session should simply be to notify the colleague that he or she must submit to an evaluation by a qualified specialist. Prior arrangements should be made to facilitate immediate evaluation, and the colleague should be physically escorted to the evaluation, recognizing the potential for self-inflicted harm. If reasonable suspicion exists for chemical dependence, then an evaluation can be demanded. It is not necessary to achieve the higher legal standard of clear and convincing evidence.

Risk of Relapse

Although the potential for long-term recovery from addiction to ethanol or benzodiazepines is good, the risk of relapse into abuse is high for the narcotic-addicted physician in recovery. The rate of relapse into narcotic abuse has been reported to be between 14% and 70%.[6,7] In 1993, eight anesthesiologists died from substance abuse, five of them from fentanyl overdose. For these reasons, whether or not an anesthesiologist in recovery from narcotic abuse should be allowed to reenter the clinical practice of anesthesiology is controversial. If reentry is undertaken, it is typically associated with an intensive aftercare program mandated by each state. Components of this program usually include random drug screening, active participation in support groups such as Alcoholics Anonymous or NarcAnon, and prolonged witnessed use of antagonists such as naltrexone for those with a history of narcotic abuse or disulfiram for those with a history of ethanol abuse.

Selected References

1. American Society of Anesthesiologists, Task Force on Chemical Dependence of the Committee on Occupational Health of Operating Room Personnel. Chemical dependence in anesthesiologists: What you need to know when you need to know it. Park Ridge, IL, American Society of Anesthesiologists, 1998.
2. Ward CF, Ward GC, Saidman LJ. Drug abuse in anesthesia training programs. JAMA 1983;250:922.
3. Arnold WP III. Environmental safety including chemical dependency. In Miller RD, ed. Anesthesia. 5th ed. Philadelphia: Churchill Livingstone, 2000:2701–2717.
4. Sivarajan M, Posner KL, Caplan RA, et al. Substance abuse among anesthesiologists: I. Anesthesiology 1994;80:704.
5. American Society of Anesthesiologists. Chemical Dependence Guidelines for Department of Anesthesiology. Park Ridge, IL, American Society of Anesthesiologists, 1991.
6. Menk EJ, Baumgarten RK, Kingsley CP, et al. Success of reentry into anesthesiology training programs by residents with a history of substance abuse. JAMA 1990;263:3060.
7. Pelton C, Ikeda RM. The California Physicians Diversion Program's experience with recovery anesthesiologists. J Psychoactive Drugs 1991;23:427.

226
Medical Ethics

Keith H. Berge, M.D.

Medical practice is a complex undertaking, fraught with ambiguity and uncertainty. A clinician is often forced to choose between alternate courses of action when there is little in the way of guidance for his or her actions. How, then, is a decision to be reached in the face of such ambiguity, especially if the decision creates a moral conflict for the physician? While medical ethics focus on the "oughts" and "shoulds" of patient care, the study of medical ethics will usually fail to reveal a single "right" course of action. However, clarification of the relevant issues of the case at hand will often allow for a decision to be reached in a manner that is not capricious or based on a visceral reaction to the clinical facts.

Medical ethics have been a part of the practice of medicine for ages. Perhaps the most famous code of ethics is the Oath of Hippocrates, which states many of the principles that still guide the modern-day physician. As modern medical practice has evolved, many ethical dilemmas have become manifest as a result of advances in technology. This has forced a rapid evolution in medical ethics from the relatively simplistic codes that have guided the "virtuous" physician for centuries. Hand-in-hand with this evolution has been an evolution in the laws regarding a vast array of complex biomedical issues, such as assisted suicide and euthanasia, abortion, surrogate motherhood, genetic testing of minors, withdrawal of artificial nutrition and hydration, and allocation of scarce resources. No broad consensus exists on most of these topics, reflecting the wide range of values within our pluralistic society.

Principles of Medical Ethics

The principles of autonomy, beneficence, nonmaleficence, and justice, expounded on at length by Beachamps and Childress, are cornerstones of current ethical writings.[1]

Autonomy. Autonomy is derived from the Greek roots *autos* (self) and *nomos* (rule, governance, or law). The autonomous person retains personal rule of the self while remaining free from both controlling interferences by others and personal limitations, such as coercion or inadequate understanding, that prevent meaningful choice.[1] For example,

courts and medical ethicists have long agreed that any patient with the capacity to understand the consequences of their actions has the right to reject any medical care, even "life-saving" care, for themselves.

Beneficence. Beneficence is an obligation to help others further their important and legitimate interests.[1] This requires the removal of harm as well as the provision of benefit and an effort to balance the benefits and harms of alternate plans of action so as to maximize the benefit. An example of this is the obligation for a physician to render emergency assistance when necessary.

Nonmaleficence. Nonmaleficence is an obligation to not inflict evil or harm on others, and associated with the maxim *primum non nocere*, "above all, do no harm." The Hippocratic oath addresses the duty to both nonmaleficence and beneficence with the statement, "I will use treatment to help the sick according to my ability and judgment, but I will never use it to injure or wrong them."

Justice. Justice is giving to each their due. This principle has been focused in medical ethics to address just distribution of medical resources. In other words, what characteristics, if any, give one person or group of people an entitlement to more health care opportunities than others?[1] The principle of justice lies at the very heart of the debate regarding health care reform. That is, if it is now necessary to do less than everything for some people, on what basis do we choose who gets less and how much does each of us "deserve?"

There is no societal consensus as to the hierarchical ordering of these principles, and yet altering the priority of the principles can lead to dramatically different, and yet equally "ethical," solutions to an ethical dilemma. As such, only a naive person will look to these principles for absolute answers to an ethical dilemma. How, then, is one to bring any order from such seeming chaos? What is needed is common sense and an orderly approach.

A Method of Resolving an Ethical Dilemma

As proposed by Jonsen et al[2] and outlined only briefly here, an ethical dilemma can be approached in much the same way as a routine patient history. The familiar chief complaint, history of the present illness, past medical history, and review of systems are replaced with analogous historical features. Ethical features in a clinical case include (1) medical indications (risk:benefit), (2) patient preferences, (3) quality of life, and (4) the contextual features surrounding the case, such as social, economic, legal, and administrative features. Most difficult and ambiguous patient care situations become easier to manage once the issues have been clarified.

Ethical Dilemmas Encountered in Anesthesia Practice

Most of the common ethical dilemmas encountered by the anesthesiologist in the operating room or the intensive care unit are primarily questions of the limits of patient autonomy. Examples of such dilemmas include, for example, the Jehovah's Witness patient who refuses a potentially life-saving blood transfusion despite full disclosure of the risks and benefits of a decision. Another example would be the patient who demands to retain a DNR status throughout the perioperative period. Excellent reviews of these two topics can be found in the recent literature.[3–5] In both of these circumstances, and indeed in any circumstance in which a competent adult rejects medical intervention for himself, the courts have been consistent in requiring that the patient's wishes be honored.

Further complexity is introduced into these already difficult situations when these decisions are being either made or related by a surrogate decision maker (e.g., a spouse or family member) on behalf of an incompetent patient. Reflecting growing societal interest and concern brought about by recent court decisions in so-called "right-to-die" cases, such as that of Nancy Cruzan, Congress enacted the Patient Self-Determination Act in 1991 in an effort to increase the use of advance directives. "Living wills" and "durable powers of attorney" are ways for a patient to give advance directives for care in the event that the patient might become incompetent. A **living will** can be difficult to use because its terms can be difficult to define and interpret and the conditions can change at various stages of an illness. What do "extraordinary measures" mean for this patient? No mechanical ventilation was requested, but wouldn't the patient want to be ventilated until he regains consciousness after this anesthetic?

Durable power of attorney can be more workable in that decisions can be made by an appointed relative, spouse, or friend in an ongoing fashion as judged by conditions at the time. These documents,

Table 226–1. Clinical Criteria for Brain Death in Adults

Normothermia (T ≥ 35°C, T ≤ 39°C).
Absence of drugs which depress the CNS.
Absence of neuromuscular blockade.
The cause of coma should be established.
Absent brain stem reflexes:[a]
 • Fixed pupils.
 • Absent corneal reflex.
 • Absent vestibulo-ocular reflex (cold caloric test).
 • Absence of respiratory effort during apnea testing.
Supporting tests are not required but should be documented if performed:
 • Cerebral angiography.
 • Transcranial Doppler.
 • Radionuclide brain scan.
 • Electroencephalogram.
 • Magnetic resonance imaging angiography.

[a]Spinal cord reflexes may be preserved in the brain-dead patient.

in general, are legally binding and obligate the treating physicians to honor the requests contained therein.

In situations where honoring patient autonomy would create a moral dilemma for the treating physician, if no acceptable compromise position can be reached with reasoned discussion (not coercion), then the physician's only options are to either honor the patient's requests or to withdraw from the care of that patient. The physician who in such a circumstance chooses to simply impose his or her values on a patient does so at the potential risk of both civil and criminal penalties.

Another example of a potential ethical conflict encountered by anesthesiologists is the brain-dead patient presenting for organ procurement. In such cases, it is imperative that the medical record reflect the diagnostic tests used to determine brain death and the results of such tests. A checklist to ensure adequate documentation is given in Table 226–1.

The study of ethics allows the physician to better recognize that not all people share common beliefs and values, and to accept that a well-informed patient with decision-making capacity is the person most capable of determining the "right" course of action for him or her.

Selected References

1. Beachamp TL, Childress JF. Principles of Biomedical Ethics. 3rd ed. New York: Oxford University Press, 1989.
2. Jonsen AR, Siegler M, Winslade WJ. Clinical Ethics. 3rd ed. New York: McGraw-Hill, 1992.
3. Truog RD. "Do-not-resuscitate" orders during anesthesia and surgery. Anesthesiology 1991;74:606–608.
4. Benson KT. The Jehovah's Witness patient: Considerations for the anesthesiologist. Anesth Analg 1989;69:647–656.
5. Truog RD, Waisel DB, Burns JP. DNR in the OR: A goal-directed approach. Anesthesiology 1999;90:289–295.

227
Awareness Under Anesthesia

Theresia L. Lee, M.D.

In the early 1900s, intraoperative awareness in a patient undergoing nitrous oxide/oxygen anesthesia was reported. Interest in intraoperative awareness, especially with nitrous oxide/oxygen anesthetics, resurged in the 1950s, after the use of muscle relaxants became commonplace. Even after the introduction of volatile anesthetics, intraoperative awareness continues to be a problem.

Although the molecular mechanism for the abolition of awareness by general anesthesia is unknown, one theory holds that general anesthesia interferes not only with sensory inputs but also the consolidation of unstable short-term memory into stable long-term memory storage.

The memory process involves acquisition (perceiving the information), storage (keeping the information), and retrieval (bringing the information out of storage). Memory is quantal and can be expressed in mnemons (unit of memory).

A weak engram (a stable, physical memory trace in the brain) has only a few mnemons, and a strong engram has many mnemons. Engrams follow a gradual pattern of growth and decay. Recall is not all-or-none (i.e., weak engrams have a subthreshold of mnemons and cannot be recalled unless the threshold is lowered by hypnosis or administration of certain drugs). Cherkin and Harroun[1] suggested that increasing depth of anesthesia decreases the number of mnemons formed by a given information input, decreasing the probability of the engram's being above threshold.

Prevalence

The prevalence of awareness under anesthesia varies (Table 227–1).

- In the American Society of Anesthesiologists Closed Claims Project database, 1.7% of 4183 medicolegal closed claims were related to awareness.
- The use of intraoperative relaxants and opioids and no use of volatile agents were more common in patients with awareness.
- Because anesthetic concentrations that block awareness are lower than those that prevent motor responses, inadequately anesthetized patients can communicate awareness by movement if they are not paralyzed.
- In cardiac surgery, the incidence is increased, especially if a pure high-dose narcotic technique is used, and in the young. A 2-mg/kg dose of morphine administered to healthy volunteers did not reliably induce unconsciousness. A 6- to 7-μg/kg dose of fentanyl resulted in visual amnesia in only 50% of patients.
- Patients informed of the risk of intraoperative recall appear to have a higher rate of reported recall.
- Patients undergoing emergency surgery for trauma have a high incidence of awareness (11% to 43%).[2] Shock and severe injury do not guarantee amnesia; the incidence of awareness is highest in those most lightly anesthetized. In one study, 4 of 51 patients undergoing emergency surgery reported that awareness was their worst hospital experience.[2] **Midazolam, ketamine,** and **scopolamine** are effective in preventing awareness in patients whose hypovolemia does not allow the use of adequate levels of other anesthetics.

Periods at Risk for Awareness

Patients are at risk for awareness during various periods:

- Preoperatively, when a nondepolarizing muscle relaxant is given before succinylcholine is administered. Occasionally, patients develop substantial muscle relaxation in these cases. Patients may recall "awake" intubation even after sedation via intravenous benzodiazepines.
- During intubation after induction. There are reports of recall from a return of consciousness while the patient is still in a relaxed state from the muscle relaxant.
- Intraoperatively, from light anesthesia. Note that

Table 227–1. Prevalence of Awareness

0.2% to 0.4% in non-OB and noncardiac surgery
0.4% during cesarean section
1.5% during cardiac surgery
11% to 43% in major trauma

□ the wake-up test used in scoliosis surgery is tolerated well.
□ Postoperatively, from muscle relaxants used without sufficient sedation.

Monitoring for Awareness

There are several methods of monitoring for awareness:

□ EEG does not reliably detect awareness. Power spectrum analysis may help by demonstrating a decrease in total power of the EEG or a shift to high-frequency (18 to 30 Hz) activity during arousal.
□ Pulse volume plethysmography may show vasoconstriction with insufficient anesthetic.
□ The isolated forearm technique is reportedly a useful method for awareness monitoring during cesarean section procedures. This technique involves inflating a contralateral blood pressure cuff above arterial pressure before injecting succinylcholine. The patient may retain the use of that arm to follow commands if aware.
□ Clinical signs may suggest arousal, but not necessarily recall of intraoperative events. Clinical signs of light anesthesia (e.g., decreased chest compliance, bronchospasm, swallowing, sweating, lacrimation, hypertension, tachycardia, eye movement) are absent in most cases.[3] Lower esophageal contractility (both frequency and intensity) declines with general anesthesia. Measurement of esophageal contractions has been used to assess the depth of anesthesia.
□ The BIS monitor has been proposed as a method of monitoring for awareness.

Prevention of Awareness

Ways to prevent awareness include the following:

□ Vigilance and meticulous attention to detail when giving anesthesia are the practical ways to prevent awareness (Table 227–2).

Table 227–2. Equipment Problems Leading To Awareness

Empty vaporizers
Malfunctioning, misprogrammed, or misloaded drug pumps
Syringe swaps
Tubing disconnects
Infiltrated IVs

□ Use of volatile anesthetics decreases the risk of awareness.
□ Because hearing is the last sense lost after induction and the first to return on emergence from general anesthesia, conversation should be minimal and/or supportive in the operating room.
□ If awareness occurs, the anesthesiologist should openly discuss intraoperative events with the patient, document the incident, apologize, and offer psychiatric support when appropriate.

Selected References

1. Cherkin A, Harroun P. Anesthesia and memory processes. Anesthesiology 1971;34:469.
2. Bogetz MS, Katz JA. Recall of surgery for major trauma. Anesthesiology 1984;61:6.
3. Domino KB, Posner KL, Caplan RA, et al. Awareness during anesthesia. Anesthesiology 1999;90:1053–10.

Suggested References

Baraka A, Louis F, Noueihid R, et al. Awareness following different techniques of general anesthesia for caesarean section. Br J Anaesth 1989;62:645.
Bonke B, Fitch W, Millar K, eds. Memory Awareness in Anesthesia. Berwyn, PA: Swets and Zeittinger, 1990.
Bovill JG, Sebel PS, Stanley TH. Opioid analgesics in anesthesia: With special reference to their use in cardiovascular anesthesia. Anesthesiology 1984;61:731–755.
Ghoneim MM. Awareness during anesthesia. Anesthesiology 2000;92:597–602.
Ghoneim MM, Meivaldt SP. Benzodiazepines and human memory: A review. Anesthesiology 1990;72:926–998.
Lyons G, Macdonald R. Awareness during caesarean section. Anaesthesia 1991;46:62.

228
Eye Complications

Margaret R. Weglinski, M.D.

Anesthesia-related eye injuries are relatively uncommon but are given a high degree of priority because the eye is one of the major sense organs. An analysis of eye injury claims against anesthesiologists published in 1992 as part of the American Society of Anesthesiologists Closed Claims Project found that 3% of all claims in the database were for eye injury.[1] The frequency of payment for eye injury claims was significantly higher than that for non–eye injury claims (70% vs. 56%). However, the median cost of eye injury claims was significantly less than that for other claims ($24,000 vs. $95,000).

Corneal Abrasion

The most commonly reported eye complication following general anesthesia is corneal abrasion. The prevalence varies depending on the methods used to detect it, ranging from 44% (in patients whose eyes were not taped and partly open during anesthesia and whose corneal epithelium was stained with fluorescein postoperatively)[2] to 0.17% (assessed by clinical symptoms in patients whose eyes were taped closed during anesthesia).[3] The mechanism of injury leading to corneal abrasion is generally unknown but is believed to be related to direct trauma to the cornea from face masks, surgical drapes, fingers, or other foreign objects that inadvertently contact the eye. Another possible cause, although unproved, may be decreased basal tear production due to general anesthesia. In two different studies of corneal abrasion, a specific cause of injury could be determined in only 20% of the cases.[1, 4] Because the mechanism of corneal abrasion is poorly understood, it is difficult to formulate preventive strategies likely to decrease the risk of injury. However, a review of the literature reveals several recurring themes that appear to support the following recommendations:

- Tape the patient's eyes closed immediately after induction of anesthesia (do not wait until after intubation). Studies show that if the patient's eyes are taped closed, no extra protection is achieved by using eye ointment.
- Beware of foreign objects coming into contact with the patient's eyes during intubation (e.g.,

stethoscope draped around anesthesiologist's neck, identification badge clipped to chest pocket, loose watchband, bracelet).
- Place the pulse oximeter on the patient's fourth or fifth finger. The patient is less likely to rub the eyes with these fingers.

If a corneal abrasion is suspected postoperatively (the patient complains of pain, photophobia, and/or a foreign body sensation in the eye), promptly obtain an ophthalmology consult. The diagnosis is confirmed by fluorescein staining of the cornea. Treatment involves patching the eye and applying antibiotic ointment. Most abrasions heal within 1 or 2 days without permanent sequelae.

Ischemic Optic Neuropathy

Although postoperative visual loss can result from pressure-related eye injuries associated with positioning, in recent years the most frequently reported cause of permanent postoperative visual loss is ischemic optic neuropathy (ION).[5] The mechanism is infarction of the optic nerve(s) in a watershed area of their vascular supply. The association of hemorrhage, shock, and blindness was reportedly noted by Hippocrates. ION has been reported after cardiopulmonary bypass, spinal surgery, and many other types of surgical procedures. All age groups are affected, and many patients do not have predisposing factors, such as vascular disease, diabetes, or hypertension.

Anatomy. The optic nerve comprises four sections (Fig. 228–1): anterior (or intraocular), posterior (or intraorbital), intracanalicular, and intracranial. Postoperative visual loss is associated with decreased oxygen supply from various causes and is characterized as either anterior ischemic optic neuropathy or posterior ischemic optic neuropathy. This classification is based on the fact that these sections of the optic nerve have different blood supplies, different risk factors for infarction, and different clinical scenarios. Other vascular etiologies of postoperative visual loss include cortical blindness (visual loss associated with the optic radiation and occipital cortex), central retinal artery occlusion, and obstruction of venous drainage from the eye.

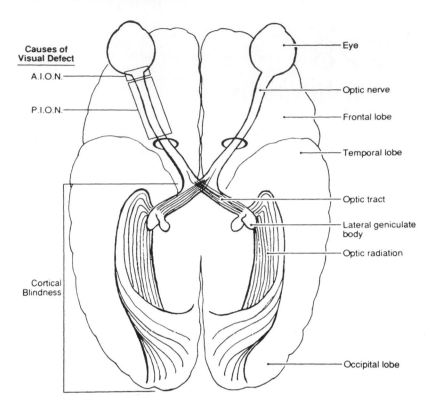

Causes of Visual Defect

A.I.O.N.

P.I.O.N.

Cortical Blindness

Eye

Optic nerve

Frontal lobe

Temporal lobe

Optic tract

Lateral geniculate body

Optic radiation

Occipital lobe

Figure 228–1. Diagram of the visual pathway at the base of the brain. The sites of the more common causes of postoperative visual loss are shown on the left side. AION, anterior ischemic optic neuropathy; PION, posterior ischemic optic neuropathy. (From Williams EL, Hart WM Jr, Tempelhoff R.[5])

Risk Factors. The cause of ischemic optic neuropathy is not well understood but probably is multifactorial: severe hypotension and anemia in combination with at least one other factor (e.g., venous obstruction, infection, etc.). One series of case reports suggests that although severe anemia alone may not cause ischemic optic neuropathy, an episode of hypotension in an already anemic patient may predispose to vision loss.[6] This possibility has led to concerns about guidelines for transfusion practice published by multiple organizations. Their suggestions of hemoglobin concentrations of 8 and 7 g/dL as transfusion trigger points are thought to possibly expose patients to a higher risk of ischemic optic neuropathy. This is particularly relevant for patients undergoing extensive surgeries, who have a increased risk of blood loss and hypotension.

Diagnosis and Treatment. The patient may note loss of vision immediately on awakening or within several days, depending on the postoperative level of confusion and/or lethargy. Ischemic optic neuropathy may occur in one or both eyes; about 50% of cases are bilateral. The extent of visual loss is variable, as is the nature of the deficit. Ophthalmoscopic examination may reveal swelling of the optic disc or a normal-appearing optic disc. In all cases, the optic disc eventually becomes pale. As soon as the diagnosis is suspected, ophthalmologic consultation should be obtained.

Although ischemic optic neuropathy has a poor prognosis, administration of osmotic diuretics and high-dose steroids in the first 48 hours after the ischemic insult may assist the anterior optic nerve's residual circulation and decrease the nerve fiber edema. In patients with nonarteritic anterior ischemic optic neuropathy, surgical optic nerve decompression has been found to be ineffective and in some cases has exacerbated the visual deficit. Other measures, such as maintenance of normal to slightly increased mean arterial pressure and normal hematocrit level, appear to be logical and may offer some therapeutic benefit.

Prevention. Obvious safeguards include avoiding external pressure on the ocular globe intraoperatively and minimizing micro- and macroemboli during cardiopulmonary bypass. Additional precautions focus on the frequent association between postoperative visual loss and decreases in blood pressure and hematocrit.

Selected References

1. Gild WM, Posner KL, Caplan RA, et al. Eye injuries associated with anesthesia: A closed claims analysis. Anesthesiology 1992;76:204–208.
2. Batra YK, Bali IM. Corneal abrasions during general anesthesia. Anesth Analg 1977;56:363–365.
3. Cucchiara RF, Black S. Corneal abrasion during anesthesia and surgery. Anesthesiology 1988;69:978–979.
4. Roth S, Thisted RA, Erickson JP, et al. Eye injuries after nonocular surgery: A study of 60,965 anesthetics from 1988 to 1992. Anesthesiology 1996;85:1020–1027.
5. Williams EL, Hart WM Jr, Tempelhoff R. Postoperative ischemic optic neuropathy. Anesth Analg 1995;80:1018–1029.
6. Brown RH, Schauble JF, Miller NR. Anemia and hypotension as contributors to perioperative loss of vision. Anesthesiology 1994;80:222–226.

229
Complications of Endotracheal Intubation

Scott A. Eskuri, M.D.

Standards for endotracheal tube (ETT) design, testing, and manufacturing have been established by the American National Standards Institute and the American Society for Testing and Materials. Polyvinyl chloride is currently the most commonly used ETT material. Its ability to soften at body temperature decreases pressure on laryngotracheal mucosa; however, this device is still a poor substitute for the human larynx. Complications of ETT intubation can be divided into those occurring during intubation, while the ETT is in place, and after extubation.

Intubation

Eye and Facial Soft Tissue. Contusions or lacerations of the upper and lower lip can occur secondary to trauma from the laryngoscope blade or ETT. Corneal abrasions may also occur when an instrument (e.g., wristwatch) or the intubating arm or sleeve brushes the eye.

Tooth Trauma. Dental injuries are the most common causes of anesthesia-related malpractice claims (30% to 40%). The incidence of perioperative dental injury ranges from 1 in 150 to 1 in 1500, with 75% of injuries occurring during intubation (25% with emergence). Care must be taken to recover all pieces of a broken tooth to prevent aspiration. If an entire tooth is dislodged, it should be promptly reimplanted and dental consultation obtained.

Cervical Spine Injury. Increased potential exists for spine injury in trauma patients, osteogenesis imperfecta, severe osteoporosis, rheumatoid arthritis, Down's syndrome, Morquio's syndrome, and lytic bone lesions.

Laryngeal and Pharyngeal Trauma. Minor trauma, including lacerations, vocal cord paralysis, subluxation of arytenoids, and vocal cord hematoma, can occur in up to 6% of intubations. Long-term sequelae are unusual.

Airway Reflexes. Stimulation of pharyngeal and/or laryngeal mucosa results in laryngovagal-mediated reflexes, such as laryngospasm, broncho- spasm, bradycardia, and arrhythmias. Sympathetic activation can cause hypertension and tachycardia. In addition, tactile stimulation can cause cough, straining, or vomiting. This can lend to increased intraocular and intracranial pressure. Aspiration can occur before ETT intubation.

Esophageal Intubation. Unrecognized esophageal intubation is the most disastrous complication. Many methods are used to assess correct position; however, the "gold standard" is to confirm the presence of expired carbon dioxide.

Endobronchial Intubation. Complications in this category may be more difficult to detect but may be minor if underlying pulmonary function is good. A simple rule of thumb that results in correct positioning in nearly 100% of adults is to place the tube 23 cm from the teeth in males and 21 cm in females. In children, advance the tip 2 to 3 cm beyond the cords or use the following formula:

$$\text{Length (cm)} = 12 + \frac{\text{age}}{2}$$

Tracheal or Bronchial Rupture. Risk factors include stylets protruding from the end of the ETT, excessive force during intubation, and multiple attempts at intubation. Chest drainage and open surgical repair may be required.

Endotracheal Tube in Place

Excessive Leak or Resistance. Choice of a proper-sized tube is necessary in adults and critical in children. In pediatric patients older than 1 year, tube diameter can be determined by the following formula:

$$\text{ETT size (mm)} = 4 + \frac{\text{age in years}}{4}$$

Obstruction. ETT obstruction is caused by external force (most commonly, the patient biting down), internal obstruction, or tube abnormalities. Kinking and cuff obstruction can occur; however, lumen obstruction (e.g., secretions, blood, tumor, foreign body) is more common. Clearing with irrigation and suction is indicated, and replacing the ETT may be necessary.

Migration. Head flexion and extension can advance and withdraw (respectively) the ETT by 2 cm. This can lend to endobronchial intubation or tracheal extubation.

Mucosal Ulceration or Necrosis. Mucosal ulceration can occur anteriorly on the trachea where the ETT tip lies. Necrosis can be induced if mucosal blood flow is impeded (cuff pressures greater than 25 mm Hg).

Ignition. ETT ignition may occur during laser surgery.

Dehydration/Hypothermia. These complications may occur in nonhumidified, nonwarmed gas delivery systems. Dehydration causes thickened secretions and decreased ciliary function, increasing the risk of postoperative pulmonary complications.

Nasal Alar Necrosis. Nasal alar necrosis can be prevented by careful ETT positioning.

Sinusitis. The prevalence of clinically significant sinusitis is 2% to 20% in those nasotracheally intubated for more than 5 days.

Miscellaneous. Airway reflexes, unintentional extubation, tracheal perforation (with subsequent tracheal esophageal fistula), aspiration, and nasal or oral excoriation may occur.

Immediate Postextubation

Supraglottic, Glottic, Subglottic Edema. This is the most significant complication (morbidity/mortality rate) in the early postextubation period. It is most common in pediatric patients; however, adults with an allergic response to lubricant on plastic may develop stridor. In pediatric patients, the strongest predictor of postextubation stridor is the absence of an air leak at 30 cm H_2O. The use of intravenous steroids and/or racemic epinephrine nebulizers is advocated, but proof of their efficacy is not conclusive.

Laryngeal Dysfunction. Immediately after extubation, patients frequently have difficulty protecting their airway. The incidence of aspiration is highest after prolonged intubation; the risk declines with time after extubation.

Sore Throat. A high prevalence of sore throat has been reported (up to 90%). Risk factors for postextubation sore throat or hoarseness include large ETT, female gender, and use of lubricant.

Vocal Cord Paralysis. Vocal cord paralysis may be secondary to surgical trauma of the vagus or recurrent laryngeal nerves. However, it is also postulated that pressure from the ETT cuff could compress the recurrent laryngeal nerve against the thyroid lamina.

Miscellaneous. Laryngospasm, bronchospasm, acute sialadenopathy ("surgical mumps"), sore jaw, dysphonia, or tracheal collapse may occur.

Delayed Complications

Mucosal Lesions. In patients intubated for more than 1 week, 67% had vocal cord ulcerations. Most lesions resolved within 8 weeks. Laryngeal ulcers may occur as quickly as 6 hours, but most heal without sequelae. Laryngeal granulomas and polyps occur in 1 in 150 to 250 cases of prolonged intubation. These usually require surgical excision.

Laryngeal or Tracheal Stenosis. The risk of this rare complication is lowered by the use of high-volume, low-pressure ETT cuffs. If laryngeal or tracheal stenosis does occur, surgical correction is usually required.

Cricoid Abscess. Cricoid abscess is an extremely rare complication that develops in the retrocricoid region after mucosal injury and secondary bacterial invasion.

Vocal Cord Paralysis. The cause of vocal cord paralysis is unknown. However, direct trauma and/or pressure or a local reaction to ethylene-oxide sterilized ETT may contribute to the occurrence of this complication.

Suggested References

McCulloch TM, Bishop MJ. Complications of translaryngeal intubation. Clin Chest Med 1991;12:507.

Stone DJ, Gel TJ. Airway management. In Miller RD, ed. Anesthesia. 3rd ed. Philadelphia: Churchill Livingstone, 1991:1265.

230
Pulmonary Embolism: Etiology, Diagnosis, and Treatment

David O. Warner, M.D.

Etiology and Risk Factors

Most pulmonary emboli (PE) arise from deep venous thrombosis (DVT) in the lower extremities; symptomatic PE occurs in approximately 30% of DVT patients. Risk factors for DVT include venous stasis, damage of the vasculature, and alterations in blood coagulation. These conditions are frequently present in the perioperative period, and PE may be responsible for up to 20% of postoperative deaths. Two-thirds of deaths from PTE occur within the first 2 hours of occurrence; hence prompt diagnosis and therapy are essential.

The risk of PE depends primarily on the age of the patient and the type of surgery. Patients younger than 40 years are at low risk, whereas older patients undergoing more extensive procedures have a higher risk. Patients at highest risk include those with a history of DVT, patients with hip or pelvic fractures, patients undergoing major lower extremity orthopedic procedures, and patients with neoplasms undergoing major pelvic or abdominal surgeries. The incidence of fatal PE may approach 4% in this group without prophylaxis. Other conditions that may increase risk include obesity, acute myocardial infarction, prolonged immobilization, major trauma, oral contraceptive use, pregnancy, and congestive heart failure.

Diagnosis

The clinical diagnosis of PE remains problematic, especially in the postoperative patient.

Signs and Symptoms. Findings include dyspnea (present in 80% of patients with angiographically documented PE), pleuritic chest pain with or without a pleural friction rub on auscultation, hemoptysis, tachypnea, cough, wheezing, and fever (higher than 38°C). Major emboli may cause syncope and cardiovascular collapse. However, these signs and symptoms may be unreliable in the postoperative period because of the many other conditions that may cause them.

Laboratory Studies. The electrocardiogram is normal in most patients aside from tachycardia; findings may include right bundle branch block and T-wave inversion. The chest roentgenogram may show atelectasis, pleural effusion (usually small and unilateral), infiltrates, an elevated hemidiaphragm, and an enlarged pulmonary artery; however, the roentgenogram is often normal. Larger emboli cause hypoxemia (with a widened $(A - a)O_2$ difference) and hypocarbia; however, arterial blood gas values may be normal.

Ventilation/Perfusion ($\dot{V}/\dot{Q}$) Scans. PE should cause a regional defect in perfusion without a regional defect in ventilation (V/Q mismatch). The most useful scan is a normal one, which nearly excludes the diagnosis of PE. However, scans in postoperative patients, especially those at high risk, are often abnormal even in the absence of PE because of atelectasis, infection, and other postoperative complications. The frequency of false-positive studies may range up to 50% for intermediate or low-probability scans, and is at least 10% even for high-probability studies.

Pulmonary Angiography. Pulmonary angiography remains the standard for the diagnosis of PE, although false-negative and false-positive results are possible. Mortality is approximately 0.2% and morbidity is approximately 5%; the risk increases in patients with elevated pulmonary artery pressures. Pulmonary angiography is mandatory before treatment with such methods as an inferior vena cava filter, embolectomy, thrombolytic therapy, or anticoagulation after major surgery.

Other Imaging Studies. New modes of CT and MRI scanning are under investigation, with some modes showing good specificity and sensitivity compared with angiography, especially in patients with large-vessel PE. Their exact place in the diagnostic approach remains to be determined.

Diagnosis of DVT. Evidence of DVT should be sought and used in concert with other diagnostic methods to increase the sensitivity and specificity of PE diagnosis. However, some patients with PE have no clinical evidence of DVT, so that the absence of detectable DVT does not exclude the diagnosis of PE. Currently, duplex ultrasound with manual compression of the vessels is most commonly used and is most reliable in the thigh. It appears to be more useful than traditional impedance plethysmography. Contrast venography still represents the standard for diagnosis, especially when ultrasound results are technically poor or equivocal.

Prophylaxis

Prophylactic measures may decrease the risk of perioperative PE by tenfold or more.

Anticoagulation. Anticoagulation regimens instituted before and continued for at least a week after surgery reduce (but do not eliminate) the perioperative risk of DVT and PE. Because of their more predictable pharmacokinetic and pharmacodynamic properties, low molecular weight heparins have gained popularity as prophylactic agents, administered typically by subcutaneous injection without laboratory monitoring.

Compression Devices. Compression devices provide either continuous (stockings) or intermittent (pneumatic cuffs) pressure to the lower extremities and are effective in reducing the incidence of perioperative DVT. Combination with anticoagulants may provide additive effects.

Treatment

Heparin. Unfractionated intravenous heparin is usually the initial pharmacologic therapy when not contraindicated, ameliorating mediator-induced pulmonary vasoconstriction and further thrombin activity. In uncomplicated cases, heparin is continued for 7 to 10 days, then tapered while coumarin therapy is instituted. Treatment with low molecular weight heparin is under investigation.

Supportive Therapies. Supplemental oxygen is usually indicated. Mechanical ventilation is reserved for massive emboli. Vasopressors may be needed to maintain cardiac output and perfusion pressures after massive PE; dopamine, dobutamine, and norepinephrine have been recommended. Vasodilators are not effective in increasing pulmonary blood flow and are not recommended.

Inferior Vena Caval Procedures. The most common inferior vena caval procedure is the transvenous placement of filters through the femoral vein. This procedure has low mortality and is suitable for postoperative patients but does nothing to treat the existing PE and is not complete protection against recurrence.

Thrombolytic Therapy. Thrombolytic therapy is usually reserved for massive PE with significant cor pulmonale and hemodynamic compromise. Streptokinase (antigenic but inexpensive), urokinase (nonantigenic but expensive), and tissue plasminogen activator are currently approved for use in PE. The major complication is bleeding (approximately 15%); thus, this technique has limited applicability in patients with recent major surgery.

Pulmonary Embolectomy. The indications for pulmonary embolectomy are similar to those for thrombolytic therapy. With the advent of thrombolytic therapy, controversy has arisen regarding the choice between embolectomy and thrombolytic therapy, with no clear resolution of the question. The mortality from this procedure ranges from 10% to more than 80%, depending on the indications used for surgery. The institution of partial cardiopulmonary bypass before embolectomy may improve survival. Unfortunately, it may be difficult to obtain the angiographic proof desirable before either instituting thrombolytic therapy or proceeding with pulmonary embolectomy. Newer imaging studies such as spiral CT scanning may be useful in this setting.

Suggested References

Dehring DJ, Arens JF. Pulmonary thromboembolism: Disease recognition and patient management. Anesthesiology 1990; 73:146–164.

Hyers TM. Venous thromboembolism. Am J Resp Crit Care Med 1999;159:1.

Sasahara AA, Sharma GV, Barsamian EM, et al. Pulmonary thromboembolism: Diagnosis and treatment. JAMA 1983; 249:2945.

231
Intraoperative Wheezing: Etiology and Treatment

Mary M. Rajala, M.D.

Wheezing is caused by turbulence from gases passing through narrowed anatomic passages. In addition to bronchospasm from asthma, bronchitis, or COPD, there are multiple etiologies for ventilatory obstruction, including mechanical obstruction, accumulation of secretions, mucosal edema, light anesthesia, cardiopulmonary causes, allergic responses, infection, or inflammation (Table 231–1). Most (80%) of the resistance to flow in airways occurs in the large central airways. The remaining 20% of airway resistance is from the peripheral bronchioles. Thus, large changes in caliber of small-caliber airways may result in small changes in resistance, making it a clinically silent area. A history of recent (within 3 weeks) upper respiratory infection (especially in patients with obstructive airway disease), recent smoking, sputum or cough, chronic bronchitis, or asthma are all pertinent in predicting intraoperative wheezing.

Mechanisms

Stimulation of the cholinergic system and subsequent bronchiolar constriction can result in wheezing when the airway is irritated, such as when intubation is undertaken in a hyperreflexic airway or during inadequate anesthetic depth for the level of surgical stimulation.

Wheezing may indicate the presence of **bronchospastic disease**—asthma, chronic obstructive pulmonary disease, chronic bronchitis, or cystic fibrosis. Aspiration pneumonitis, pulmonary edema, or pneumothorax may also trigger bronchospasm. Numerous factors may provoke an attack in patients with bronchospastic disease, including exercise, cold air, allergens, respiratory infections, emotional factors, β-adrenergic blockade, and the use of a prostaglandin inhibitor, such as aspirin. The immunologic component to asthma is well recognized and includes immunoglobulin E antibody fixed to mast cells and basophils, which release immune mediators on challenge with specific antigens. In children, allergy is an important component in reactive airway disease, whereas in adults irritant reflexes are a more important cause. The immune mediators include serotonin, prostaglandins (PGD_2, PGF_2, thromboxane A_2) leukotrienes (LTC_4, LTD_4, LTE_4), kinin, and perhaps histamine (H_1). Prostaglandins are produced from arachidonic acid by the cyclooxygenase pathway and are potent mast cell mediators causing bronchospasm. Leukotrienes are synthesized after mast cell activation from metabolism of arachidonic acid via the lipooxygenase pathway. Kinin, produced by mast cells and basophils, can cause bronchoconstriction. In addition, thromboxane B_2, a metabolite of thromboxane A_2 produced by polymorphonuclear leukocytes and mast cells, may cause pulmonary hypertension. These mediators may cause mucosal edema and excessive secretions, as well as bronchoconstriction.

Table 231–1. Causes of Ventilatory Obstruction

Airway disease
  Asthma
  Bronchitis
  COPD
  Cystic fibrosis
  Tumors of the larynx or pharynx
  Foreign body
  Bronchiectasis
  Tracheomalacia
  Laryngeal edema or infection
Bronchoconstriction during anesthesia
  Airway manipulation
  Endotracheal intubation
  Endobronchial intubation
  Carinal pressure from endotracheal tube
  Light anesthesia
  Secretions in large airways
  Aspiration of stomach contents
  Infection, pneumonia
  Pulmonary edema
  Negative pressure pulmonary edema
  Pulmonary embolus
  Pneumothorax
  Allergens
  Anaphylaxis, anaphylactoid reactions
  Drug reactions from histamine release, antagonism
  Carcinoid tumors
Mechanical obstruction
  Kinked ETT
  Secretions in ETT
  Obstructed ETT

Histamine release may occur with administration of anesthetic drugs, including curare, atracurium, or mivacurium. Administered rapidly or in large doses (as in induction and airway manipulation), these drugs are associated with increased risk of bronchoconstriction. The muscarinic action of cholinesterase inhibitors used for reversal may precipitate bronchospasm. In these cases prudence suggests using larger than usual doses of atropine (>1.0 mg), or glycopyrrolate (>0.5 mg) to minimize potential bronchospasm in patients who are actively wheezing.

Bronchospasm may result from an **anaphylactic** or **anaphylactoid reaction**. Accompanying signs include hypotension, periorbital and airway edema, urticaria, tachycardia, and arrhythmias. Antibiotics, transfusions, and intravenous contrast agents can be suspected if followed by wheezing.

Rarely, **carcinoid tumors** may cause bronchospasm. Serotonin (5-hydroxytryptamine [5-HT]) secreted by carcinoid tumors causes bronchoconstriction, which can accompany the hypotension, diarrhea, flushing, and valvular heart disease of carcinoid syndrome. Conventional treatment for bronchospasm is not helpful and may actually provoke bronchospasm in these patients. Therefore, most recommendations are targeted toward preventing tumor substance release. Somatostatin analogue (Sandostatin) can be used in 100- to 600-μg intravenous doses to prevent or treat carcinoid crisis. In addition to blocking the release of pituitary growth hormone and thyrotropin, somatostatin analogue reduces hormonal and exocrine secretions from the gut. It has become the therapy of choice for preoperative, intraoperative, and postoperative management of carcinoid crises.

Anesthetic care involves avoiding histamine-releasing agents (morphine, curare), succinylcholine, indirect or direct-acting catecholamines, and extremes of blood pressure to decrease the release of 5-HT from carcinoid tumors. Succinylcholine is thought to provoke release by increasing abdominal pressure and compressing the tumor, not by intrinsic releasing properties. In addition to bronchospasm, one must be ready to deal with decreased peripheral resistance, hypotension, and hypertension intraoperatively in patients with carcinoid tumors.

Treatment

Treatment should be directed toward the etiology of bronchospasm. Prophylaxis should be entertained in patients with known reactive airway disease. Patients with history of disease should take their prescribed inhalers preoperatively. Because etiology in children is more frequently due to allergens, mediator inhibitors and anti-inflammatory medications are important in prevention. In adults, reducing or reversing irritant reflexes should be the goal.

In true bronchospasm, volatile anesthetics will depress airway reactivity and bronchoconstriction, causing bronchiolar smooth muscle relaxation. Volatile agents are useful for treating bronchospasm by increasing anesthetic depth but this may be difficult to accomplish in acute bronchospasm because of ventilation/perfusion mismatch. All potent inhalation agents have been shown to decrease airway reactivity and bronchoconstriction, probably by a direct relaxation of bronchial smooth muscle and by attenuating parasympathetic constrictive airway reflexes. Bronchodilators, whether they be β-2 agonists or anticholinergic drugs may be given as metered aerosols or as hand-held nebulizers. A more complete discussion of bronchodilators is located in Chapter 73.

Certain anesthetic drugs leave the airway reflexes largely intact. Thiopental may be associated with bronchospasm if other drugs are not used to blunt the effect or adequate depth of anesthesia is not achieved before airway manipulation. Both propofol and ketamine offer advantages in patients with history of bronchospasm. Propofol reduces airway resistance in patients with asthma and chronic obstructive disease. Ketamine helps protect against irritant reflexes, although it increases secretions from salivary and tracheobronchial mucus glands. This is related to its sympathomimetic properties and may be abolished by blockade.

β-2 antagonists (labetolol, esmolol) may increase the risk of bronchoconstriction but have been used without untoward effects when used to treat hypertension. Anecdotal reports exist of bronchoconstriction in patients with reactive airway disease, although controlled studies show no untoward effect after use of two specific antagonists.

Lidocaine (1 to 2 mg/kg) IV during induction is effective in preventing bronchoconstriction during airway manipulation or treating acute intraoperative bronchoconstriction. It blocks vagal afferent nerves. It is as effective given intravenously as topically.

Extubation while under deep anesthesia in a patient with wheezing is not safe. Despite the rationale of reducing bronchospasm, it exposes the patient to residual anesthetic effects, including ventilation/perfusion mismatch. Additional medications, such as lidocaine, sympathomimetics, anticholinergics, or anxiolytics, may be needed to afford better tolerance of maintained inhibitors and any necessary ventilatory support.

Suggested References

Gal TJ. Bronchospasm. In Gravenstein N, Kirby R, eds. Complications in Anesthesiology. 2nd ed. Philadelphia: Lippincott-Raven, 1996:199–211.

Marsh HM, Martin JK Jr, Kvols LK, et al. Carcinoid crisis during anesthesia: Successful treatment with a somatostatin analogue. Anesthesiology 1987;66:89–91.

Peruzzi WT. Evaluation, preparation, and management of the patient with respiratory disease. In Schwartz, ed. Refresher Courses in Anesthesiology. Vol. 26. Philadelphia: Lippincott Williams & Wilkins, 1998:137–151.

Stoelting RK, Dierdorf SF. Anesthesia and Co-Existing Disease. 3rd ed. New York: Churchill Livingstone, 1993.

Wilson JD, Braunwald E, Isselbacher KJ, et al, eds. Harrison's Principles of Internal Medicine. 12th ed. New York: McGraw-Hill, 1991.

232
Evaluation of Prolonged Postoperative Arousal

Mary M. Rajala, M.D.

Recovery from anesthesia has no exact end point. Wakefulness requires diffuse cortical activation via the reticular formation in the brain stem. The reticular activating system mediates cortical arousal and the focus of attention elicited by afferent sensory stimuli. After general anesthesia (GA), there is a continuum of arousal with ability to follow commands returning before the ability to converse rationally. Delayed awakening after GA has multiple possible etiologies that can be broadly classified as pharmacologic, metabolic, and neurologic (Table 232–1). Certain operations, such as coronary artery bypass and open ventricle procedures, correlate with high risk of neurologic impairment. A patient with delayed arousal must be approached in a systematic fashion, using clinical findings, past medical history, and laboratory evaluation to diagnose the most likely etiology and appropriate treatment.

Pharmacologic Causes

Rate of emergence correlates with timing, half-life, and total dose of anesthetic as well as individual responses due to biovariability. Residual effects of preoperative medication, sedatives, and anesthetic agents are the most frequently cited etiology for delayed awakening after general anesthesia. Multiple drug effects may result in a relative overdose. Volatile agents may be implicated when high concentrations are delivered for long periods without tapering at the end of the case. Hypoventilation slows emergence, prolonging recovery.

Narcotics cause respiratory depression by decreasing the response to hypercarbia, resulting in hypoventilation and subsequent decreased clearance of volatile agents. Benzodiazepines, droperidol, scopolamine, and ketamine, when given as part of the anesthetic, may potentiate other general anesthetic agents, prolonging arousal. These effects may be more pronounced with large doses, when such agents are administered shortly before emergence, or when there is delayed absorption (e.g., oral or rectal dosage). Large doses of barbiturates or benzodiazepines may overwhelm lean tissue distribution

and subsequent metabolism in the liver, prolonging anesthetic effects. Monoamine oxidase inhibitors potentiate the effects of narcotics, barbiturates, and sedatives by an unknown mechanism.

When muscle relaxants are not fully reversed, muscle weakness may result in hypoventilation, hypercarbia, and incomplete washout of volatile an-

Table 232–1. Causes of Delayed Postoperative Arousal

Pharmacologic causes
  Residual drugs, overdose
    Premedications
    Induction agents
    Anesthetic agents
    Muscle relaxants
    Decreased metabolism, excretion, or protein binding
  Increased sensitivity to drugs
    Age
    Drug interactions
    Underlying renal, hepatic disease
    Biologic variability
    Hypothermia
Metabolic causes
  Liver disease
  Kidney disease
  Hypothyroidism
  Adrenal insufficiency
  Hypoxemia
  Hypercapnia
  Hypoglycemia
  Hyperosmolar hyperglycemic nonketotic coma
  Hyponatremia
  Other electrolyte abnormalities
  Sepsis
  Malignant hyperthermia
Neurologic causes
  Hypoperfusion
    Low cardiac output, occlusive cerebrovascular disease
    Embolism
      Thrombus
      Paradoxical air embolus
      Intraoperative retraction, resection
  Hyperperfusion
    Intracerebral hemorrhage
  Elevated intracranial pressure
    Sub- or epidural hematoma
    Cerebral edema
    Pneumocephalus
  Differential awakening
  Undetected head injury

esthetics. Acidosis, hypermagnesemia, and certain drugs (furosemide, clindamycin, gentamicin, neomycin) accentuate muscle relaxant effects and may interfere with reversal.

Low cardiac output or hypovolemia may cause inadequate perfusion of pulmonary, renal, and liver beds, affecting metabolism and excretion. Decreased protein binding of anesthetics may occur through hypoproteinemia or competition with other drugs (e.g., intravenous contrast dyes, sodium acetrizoate, sulfadimethoxine) for binding sites.

Decreased liver metabolism of anesthetic agents occurs in malnutrition, at extremes of age, through immature or decreased enzyme activity, in the presence of hypothermia (below 33°C), or in simultaneous administration of multiple drugs dependent on liver microsomal detoxification (e.g., ethanol or barbiturates). Ketamine administration in patients with liver dysfunction delays anesthetic emergence. Patients with liver disease and a history of hepatic coma develop central nervous system (CNS) depression following small amounts of morphine. Cimetidine may also cause mental status changes in such patients. Although reported in animals with hepatectomy or liver damage, increased sensitivity to barbiturates has not been demonstrated in humans.

Renal failure and azotemia correlate with increased sensitivity to hypnotics, possibly because of changes in permeability of the blood-brain barrier. Delayed emergence may also be attributed to renal effects on acid-base status, decreased protein binding, delayed or reduced excretion, or electrolyte changes.

Mental status changes occur with cerebrospinal fluid (CSF) pH below 7.25. During acute hypercapnia, CNS depression is more severe, because the hydrogen ion crosses the blood-brain barrier more quickly than bicarbonate.

Increased central sensitivity to anesthesia is a diagnosis of exclusion. Any anesthetic may cause central respiratory depression. Biologic variability in sensitivity follows a bell-shaped gaussian distribution. Anesthetic requirements diminish with age, hypothyroidism, and hypothermia. The mechanisms suggested for hypothermia-induced CNS depression include cold narcosis, increased solubility of volatile agents, and reduced rate of biotransformation.

Metabolic Disturbances

Numerous systemic metabolic disturbances result in CNS depression and may be difficult to distinguish from residual anesthetic effects. Hypoxia and hypercapnia result in metabolic encephalopathy. In addition, one may encounter elevated sensitivity to CNS depressants in the presence of a metabolic encephalopathy. Certain endocrine disorders are associated with altered anesthetic emergence. The decrease in anesthetic requirement with **hypothyroidism** has already been mentioned. **Adrenal**

insufficiency is associated with prolonged unconsciousness after anesthesia.

Postoperative hypoglycemia can occur in diabetics given insulin or chlorpropamide preoperatively. The stress of anesthesia and surgery generally causes increased blood glucose. However, hypoglycemia may occur after manipulation of insulin-producing tumors and retroperitoneal carcinomas or in patients with severe liver disease who have decreased gluconeogenesis.

Hyperosmolar hyperglycemic nonketotic coma (HHNK) can also cause delayed anesthetic emergence. This condition is associated with severe sepsis, pancreatitis, pneumonia, uremia, burns, and administration of hypertonic solutions or mannitol.

Electrolyte disorders may cause postoperative coma. Hypo-osmolality, as seen in hyponatremia, often results from dilution after absorption of large volumes of hypotonic fluids (e.g., absorption of fluid during transurethral resection of the prostate) or from the syndrome of inappropriate antidiuretic hormone secretion. Other electrolyte abnormalities to consider include hypercalcemia, hypocalcemia, and hypomagnesemia.

Neurologic Injury

Delayed arousal after anesthesia may be due to cerebral hypoperfusion or hyperperfusion, hypoxia, elevated intracranial pressure (ICP), cerebral hemorrhage, or undetected head injury (in a trauma patient).

Cerebral **hypoperfusion** may be caused by reduced cardiac output, obstruction to flow or decreased systemic vascular resistance. Hypotension occurring perioperatively may result in cerebral ischemia and stroke and is more frequent in patients with preoperative cerebrovascular disease. Thromboembolic events may occur in patients undergoing cardiac, vascular, and invasive neck procedures, or in patients with atrial fibrillation or hypercoagulable states. Venous air embolus can occur in cases where the surgical site is higher than the heart. Even small amounts of air are dangerous in patients with right-to-left cardiac shunts. This can occur in a patient with a probe-patent foramen ovale. Arterial compression from retraction or improper positioning of the head and neck are other causes of hypoperfusion. Decreased systemic vascular resistance due to shock may also cause cerebral hypotension.

Hypertension is a frequent cause of cerebral **hyperperfusion** which may lead to stroke via hemorrhage. ICP may increase from hyperperfusion, intracerebral or subdural hemorrhage or hematoma, cerebral edema, pneumocephalus, and malfunctioning shunt or drain.

Differential awakening presents as hemiplegia or other focal signs on awakening; the neurologic deficits resolve over a period of minutes. In theory, focal areas of underperfused or previously injured brain tissue may have trapping or increased sensitivity to anesthetic agents.

Suggested References

Black S, Enneking FK, Cucchiara RF. Failure to awaken after general anesthesia due to cerebrovascular events. J Neurosurg Anesthesiol 1998;10:10–15.

Denlinger, JK. Prolonged emergence and failure to regain consciousness. In Gravenstein N, Kirby RR, eds. Complications in Anesthesiology. Philadelphia: Lippincott-Raven, 1996:441–451.

Feeley TW, Macario A. The postanesthesia care unit. In Miller RD, ed. Anesthesia. 5th ed. New York: Churchill Livingstone, 2000:2302–2322.

Gronert GA, Messick JM, Cucchiara RF, et al. Paradoxical air embolism from a patent foramen ovale. Anesthesiology 1979;50:548–549.

Oliver SB, Cucchiara RF, Warner MA, et al. Unexpected focal neurologic deficit from anesthesia: A report of three cases. Anesthesiology 1987;67:823–826.

233
Postoperative Nausea and Vomiting

John M. Van Erdewyk, M.D.

The vomiting center of the brain is in the reticular formation of the medulla at the level of the olivary nuclei. Various impulses transmitted by afferent fibers of the sympathetic and parasympathetic nervous system initiate the process of vomiting (Fig. 233–1). The motor impulses that initiate vomiting are carried in cranial nerves V, VII, IX, X, and XII to the upper gastrointestinal tract and through the cervical and thoracic nerves to the diaphragm and abdominal muscles.

Predisposing Factors

The incidence of postoperative nausea and vomiting (PONV) varies depending on numerous factors, but it occurs in a significant percentage of patients after receiving anesthesia. Factors that seem to increase the risk of PONV include:

- Female gender (probably estrogen-related).
- Obesity.
- Age (younger patients have a higher risk).
- Predisposition to nausea or history of postoperative emesis.
- Certain anesthetic agents.
- Pain, hypotension, or hypoglycemia in the postoperative period.
- Type of surgery. Middle ear manipulation, ophthalmologic procedures (especially strabismus surgery), peritoneal irritation, gastrointestinal trauma, or surgery that results in blood in the stomach are all associated with higher incidence rates of PONV.

In addition to nausea and vomiting being an unpleasant problem for the patient and the postoperative staff, it can lead to delayed discharge, significant increases in hospital costs, and be a cause of more significant morbidity. Autonomic effects can include tachycardia, bradycardia, hypotension, or hypertension. (The risk of hypertension is increased in patients with intracranial, ocular, or cardiovascular disorder.) Disruption of suture lines, aspiration, and prolonged hospitalization are also adverse effects. PONV is the leading cause of unexpected hospital admission after outpatient surgery.

Certain anesthetic agents and techniques seem to lead to an increased incidence of postoperative nausea and vomiting.

- **Opioids** produce nausea and vomiting by stimulating the chemoreceptor trigger zone (CTZ), which activates the vomiting center. Morphine-like drugs have been shown to increase vestibular sensitivity so that emesis is more common in ambulatory patients than in recumbent patients. All clinically useful opioids will produce nausea and vomiting, and at equianalgesic doses the incidence is similar among the different opioids.[2] High-dose opioids can depress the CTZ-stimulating effect, reducing the incidence of nausea. Opioids used for postoperative analgesia can also cause nausea and vomiting attributed incorrectly to the anesthetic.
- **Nitrous oxide** (N_2O) has been implicated in increasing the incidence of PONV. The proposed mechanism is dilation of the bowel and/or an increase in middle ear pressure by N_2O. Other studies, however, report no increased incidence of PONV when using N_2O. N_2O continues to be used frequently, even in outpatient surgery.
- **Supplemental oxygen** reduces PONV in some groups of patients. In 1999 Grief and colleagues[3] reported that supplemental oxygen reduced the incidence of PONV in 231 patients undergoing colon resection. Patients were randomized to groups maintained on either 30% or 80% oxygen with nitrogen and isoflurane intraoperatively; the incidence of PONV was reduced from 30% in the patients given 30% oxygen to 17% in the group given 80% oxygen. One postulated mechanism for this was decreased regional intestinal hypoxia leading to decreased serotonin release. Dopamine release from the carotid bodies is known to be inversely related to PO_2; dopamine is known to stimulate the CTZ.[3]
- The three main **volatile agents**—isoflurane, enflurane, and halothane—are associated with postoperative nausea and vomiting; however, they have a decreased incidence as compared to opioids.
- Of the **intravenous induction agents**, propofol is associated with less PONV than thiopental or methohexital. Benzodiazepines and ketamine appear to have a relatively low incidence of PONV

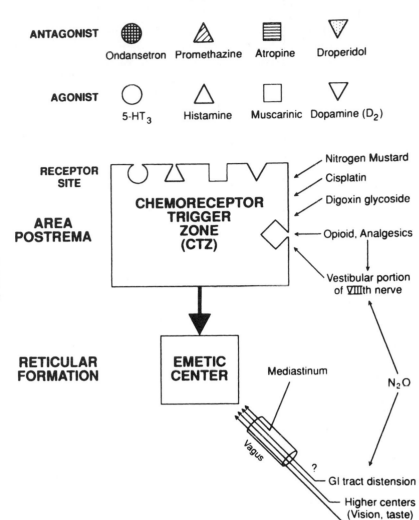

Figure 233–1. The chemoreceptor trigger zone and the emetic center with the agonist and antagonist sites of action of various anesthesia-related agents and stimuli. (From Watcha MF and White PF.[1])

(approximately 0% to 15%); however, etomidate seems to have a greater incidence than average.

□ Nausea and vomiting may also occur during **regional blockade**, possibly from hypotension, cerebral hypoxia, or adjuvant medications used for sedation. The local anesthetic-induced sympathectomy and resulting unopposed vagal activity may also contribute. Atropine may be useful but does not always prevent nausea.

Prevention

A number of drugs have been used intraoperatively or preoperatively in an attempt to lower the incidence of PONV (Table 233–1). Studies have shown the effectiveness of single and combination drug therapies. In patients who are morbidly obese, have hiatal hernias, or in pregnant patients, prophylactic therapy is used to decrease the risk of aspiration, as well as decrease postoperative nausea and vomiting.

Therapy

Although certain anesthetic agents have a decreased incidence of nausea and vomiting, no anesthetic technique can be guaranteed to eliminate this problem postoperatively. Use of agents associated with a lower incidence, if possible, should help decrease the risk of postoperative nausea and vomiting, especially in patients known to be susceptible.

Table 233–1. Drugs Used to Decrease Postoperative Nausea and Vomiting

Drug	Dose
Propofol	10–20 mg IV
Metoclopramide	10–20 mg IV
Odansetron	4 mg IV
Droperidol	0.63–1.25 mg IV
Cimetidine	300 mg IV or PO
Ranitidine	150 mg PO or 50 mg IV
Scopolamine	1.5 mg transdermally
Dexamethasone	4 mg IV

Treatment should initially be directed at evaluating and treating any underlying causes such as hypoxia, hypotension, hypoglycemia, or pain. Keeping the patient supine and avoiding sudden movements should also help. Antiemetics should be administered as necessary (see Chap. 70).

Selected References

1. Watcha MF, White PF. Postoperative nausea and vomiting: Its etiology, treatment, and prevention. Anesthesiology 1992;77:162–184.
2. Moyers JR. Preoperative medication. In Barash PG, Cullen BF, Stoelting RK, eds. Clinical Anesthesia. 3rd ed. Philadelphia: JB Lippincott, 1997:519.
3. Grief R, Laciny S, Rapf B, et al. Supplemental oxygen reduces the incidence of postoperative nausea and vomiting. Anesthesiology 1999;91:1246–1252.

Suggested References

Stoelting RK. Pharmacology and Physiology in Anesthetic Practice. Philadelphia, JB Lippincott, 1987.
van Vlymen JM, White PF. Outpatient anesthesia. In Miller RD, ed. Anesthesia. 5th ed. New York: Churchill Livingstone, 2000:2213–2240.

234
Latex Allergy

Beth A. Elliott, M.D.

Latex-containing materials are ubiquitous in to-day's health care environment. Following the recommendation by the Centers for Disease Control for universal precautions in 1987, the demand for and use of latex gloves increased dramatically (from 800 million to 20 billion annually). Whether the result of increased glove use or abnormally high levels of residual latex antigens in the gloves, the increase in latex allergies among health care workers and patients is of great concern.

What is Latex?

Latex is derived from the milky sap of the rubber tree, *Hevea brasiliensis*, harvested primarily in Malaysia, Indonesia, and Thailand. Approximately 90% of the latex is used in the production of "dry" rubber for tires; the remaining 10% is used in the manufacture of "dipped" products such as gloves, condoms, and balloons. During the manufacturing process, a variety of chemicals are added (e.g., stabilizers, antioxidants, accelerators) to give the rubber the desired characteristics. Once formed, the rubber products are then vulcanized, cured with heat and sulfur at a temperature of 130°C for 5 to 30 minutes. For latex gloves, a series of leaching baths are used to rid the gloves of residual water-soluble proteins and excess additives.

Antigenic proteins constitute up to 3.0% of the final latex product. Antigen levels are typically much higher in "dipped" latex products than in "dry" ones, but can vary as much as 1000-fold among lots of gloves by the same manufacturer and as much as 3000-fold among manufacturers. These latex proteins (allergens) are water-soluble and can be eluted during contact with moist surfaces (mucous membranes, peritoneal surfaces, and normal skin moisture). Latex allergens also adsorb onto the powder inside gloves. When donned or discarded, these powders disperse into the air and are inhaled by those nearby.

Clinical Manifestations

Irritant contact dermatitis produces a dry, scaly irritation of the skin, typically on the hands. This problem is the most common work-related reaction to rubber products (80%). The reaction results from direct irritation by latex and residual chemicals used in the manufacturing process and is exacerbated by frequent hand washing and use of irritant surgical soaps. This reaction is not immune mediated and can be prevented with simple barrier protection or use of a nonlatex alternative.

Allergic contact dermatitis is another common problem associated with exposure to latex products. A red vesicular rash typically appears within 6 to 72 hours after contact. The reaction is a **type IV cell-mediated** immune response to low molecular weight accelerators and antioxidants in the rubber product. Antibodies are not involved in type IV reactions. The diagnosis is based on clinical history and on the morphology and distribution of skin lesions. Patch testing confirms the diagnosis. Use of a glove liner or nonlatex alternative should be preventive.

The first case of **type I IgE-mediated** immediate hypersensitivity reaction to latex was reported in the German literature in 1927. The second case was not reported until 1979. As of 1997, the FDA database contained more than 2300 reports of allergic reactions involving latex products, including 225 cases of anaphylaxis, 53 cardiac arrests, and 17 deaths.

Contact urticaria (hives) is the most common manifestation of IgE-mediated latex allergy. Symptoms appear within 10 to 15 minutes after contact and include itching, redness, and wheal and flare reactions at the site of contact.

Rhinitis and asthma may follow airborne exposure. One study of latex-sensitive individuals found that 51% had experienced rhinitis and 31% dyspnea. Another found a 73% prevalence of rhinoconjunctivitis and a 27% prevalence of asthma. Most latex-sensitive people are atopic and may have a history of seasonal allergic asthma, which may delay the diagnosis.

Anaphylaxis is a life-threatening condition triggered by the interaction between allergen and IgE antibodies attached to mast cells and basophils. Antibodies are formed after the initial exposure. On subsequent exposure, the allergen cross-links two IgE molecules, resulting in degranulation of the cell and the release of a host of factors (e.g., histamine, leukotrienes, and prostaglandins) responsible for the anaphylactic response. Capillary dilation, increased vascular permeability, bronchoconstriction, hypotension, edema, clotting defects, and hypoxemia are common manifestations of anaphylaxis. Anaphylactic reactions to latex may be delayed for as long as 60 minutes after exposure. The delay is thought to be related to the time needed for sufficient antigen to be eluted from surgical gloves and absorbed into the body. When recognized and treated early, there is a good prognosis. Persistent hypotension and bronchospasm may require continued treatment. Intensive care monitoring is warranted for 24 to 48 hours, because relapses may occur every 1 to 8 hours in 20% of cases.

Risk Factors for Latex Allergy

Anyone with frequent exposure to latex-containing materials is at risk for the development of latex allergy. The prevalence in the general population has been thought to be less than 1%, but may be somewhat higher in those with a history of atopy. A recent sampling of 1000 blood donors found a 6.4% incidence of IgE antibodies to latex, with 2.3% strongly positive.

Occupational exposure increases the likelihood of allergy. For example, the incidence is 5% to 17% in health care providers and 11% in latex manufacturing workers.

Although latex allergy was originally associated with spina bifida (where the incidence approaches 28% to 67%), it has recently come to light that any patient with congenital abnormalities (particularly neuraxial or urogenital) requiring multiple surgical procedures, indwelling catheters, or personal care using latex gloves is at high risk for developing significant latex allergies. Several reports have noted an association between latex allergy and allergy to various fruits and nuts, most commonly bananas, avocados, kiwi fruit, and chestnuts.

Treatment

Individuals with contact dermatitis should avoid unnecessary exposure to latex products. Vinyl and neoprene gloves are available in sterile and nonsterile packaging. Barrier creams and cotton glove liners are alternative methods to limit further exposure. It should be noted that chronic open sores on the hands are a potential site of exposure and sensitization, which can lead to later type I (immediate) hypersensitivity reactions. As many as 79% of individuals with type I hypersensitivity previously had type IV skin eruptions.

IgE-mediated allergic reactions extend across a spectrum of rhinoconjunctivitis to severe, life-threatening anaphylaxis. Elimination of further exposure to the antigen should be one of the first steps when responding to an acute problem. Airway management, volume resuscitation, and catecholamine therapy (epinephrine) remain mainstays of therapy for anaphylaxis.

Endotracheal intubation and mechanical ventilation may be required in cases of significant laryngeal edema, bronchospasm, pulmonary edema, and $\dot{V}/\dot{Q}$ mismatch. As much as 20% to 40% of the intravascular volume may be lost from acute transcapillary leakage during anaphylactic reactions. Combined with peripheral vasodilation, this can result in severe hypotension. Fulminant noncardiogenic pulmonary edema, pulmonary hypertension, and right-sided heart failure frequently complicate the clinical picture.

Pharmacologic therapy for anaphylaxis is aimed at inhibiting further mediator release, providing competitive blockade of receptors interacting with mediators already released, reversing the end-organ effects of physiologically active substances, and inhibiting the recruitment and migration of other inflammatory cells.

Antihistamines and steroids probably have little effect in acute management, but may help attenuate late-phase reactions and secondary inflammatory responses.

Prevention

Unlike in patients with a history of anaphylactoid reactions to IV contrast dye, in latex-sensitive patients pretreatment with antihistamines, steroids, and catecholamines will not prevent IgE-mediated anaphylaxis.

Careful preoperative questioning of those patients in high-risk groups for latex sensitivity should be done routinely. Patients with spina bifida and congenital urogenital abnormalities are at such high risk for latex allergy that they should completely avoid latex exposure from birth.

A totally latex-free environment is ideal but is achieved only in some hospitals. Recent efforts have focused on creating "latex-safe" environments. If possible, surgical procedures involving latex-sensitive patients should be scheduled as "first cases" with all latex-containing materials removed the preceding night. Airborne particles containing latex allergens can remain suspended in air for up to 5 hours. A cart containing nonlatex alternative supplies should be available. Regardless of precautions taken to prevent latex exposure, operating personnel should be prepared to treat anaphylaxis in all latex-sensitive patients.

Work environments in which latex gloves are used frequently should make an effort to eliminate

high-allergen products from their inventory to decrease the likelihood of sensitization of employees.

Suggested References
Eon B, Papazian L, Gouin F. Management of anaphylactic and
anaphylactoid reactions during anesthesia. Clin Rev Allergy
1991;9:415–429.

Moneret-Vautrin DA, Laxenaire MC. Anaphylactic and anaphylactoid reactions. Clinical presentation. Clin Rev Allergy
1991;9:249–258.

Porri F, Pradal M, Lemiere C, et al. Association between latex
sensitization and repeated latex exposure in children. Anesthesiology 1997;86:599–602.

Slater JE. Latex allergy. J Allergy Clin Immunol 1994;94:139–
149.

Yunginger JW. Natural rubber latex allergy. In Middleton E, ed.
Allergy: Principles and Practice. 5th ed. St. Louis: Mosby, 1998.

235
Medical Legal Principles: Medical Negligence

Ann E. Decker, J.D.

A medical negligence or malpractice lawsuit is a civil action commenced by a patient or an authorized representative on behalf of the patient seeking monetary damages for injuries claimed to have resulted from negligent treatment. Medical negligence is the most common threat of liability faced by physicians in the United States.

Elements of Malpractice Actions

Patients recover money from a physician if they can prove that the physician's conduct fell below accepted norms and that the conduct caused injury. It is not enough that a patient suffered a complication or was injured as a result of medical care; the patient must show negligence by the physician.

To recover damages, a patient has the burden of proving that a deviation from the standard of care occurred and that the injury was directly caused by that deviation. A preponderance of the evidence must support the allegations, and proof must be to a "reasonable degree of medical certainty." To prove a deviation from the standard of care, it must be shown that an anesthesiologist failed to use that amount of care and skill commonly exercised by other anesthesiologists with similar training and experience under the same circumstances. Physicians are not negligent if they elect to pursue one of several recognized courses of treatment, provided that a respectable minority of physicians accepts the course of treatment. In addition, reasonable medical judgment, even if in error, is not malpractice.

The standard of care is most often proved by expert testimony. A physician sued for medical malpractice has the right to a jury trial. Jurors are usually unable to evaluate whether medical care is appropriate. The physicians and expert explain the medicine to assist the jury in reaching a conclusion. The expert witness generally has credentials and experience like those of the physician on trial and testifies as to whether the physician acted in accordance with the usual and customary practice. The stringency of the rules on expert qualifications vary by state.

The standard of care may also be established by a variety of other means, including medical treatises or guidelines written by professional organizations, policies of the hospital in which care was provided, and recommendations of drug and device manufacturers. Out-of-court statements by physicians (such as statements to the patient or other colleagues) or documents may constitute admissions against interest and may also be introduced as evidence of a deviation from the standard of care.

If a deviation from the standard of care can be proven, then some type of injury must also be proven. Generally, at least some physical injury is necessary. Damages may be awarded to compensate for lost income, past or future medical expenses, and for other less tangible elements of an injury, such as pain and suffering and embarrassment.

Finally, a patient must prove that the anesthesiologist's deviation from the standard of care proximately caused injury and that the injury was not caused by an underlying disease process. An anesthesiologist's negligent conduct may be a legal cause of harm if it is a substantial factor in bringing about the injury.

Types of Claims Against Anesthesia Personnel

A nationwide study of closed malpractice claims by the Committee on Professional Liability of the American Society of Anesthesiologists provides important information about the types of claims against anesthesia personnel. The study, initiated in 1984, set out to collect information from insurance companies about closed claims related to events leading to anesthesia-related injury. The Closed Claims Project has gathered information from companies that insure approximately 14,500 of the 23,000 anesthesiologists practicing in the United States. Numerous references have been published from the data about specific types of anesthetic injuries and resultant malpractice claims, giving a broad-based rather than an anecdotal picture. In general, the types of injuries that result in malpractice claims against anesthesia personnel include dental injury, nerve injury, and death or brain injury caused by either respiratory or cardiac events.

Lack of Informed Consent

Courts have long recognized that patients have a right to consent to medical treatment. A patient may allege that no consent was given for a procedure and seek damages for battery. More often, however, patients allege lack of informed consent or negligent nondisclosure. A physician has a legal obligation to advise the patient of certain risks associated with medical care, as well as available alternatives. There are two standards by which a physician may be judged to determine whether this legal obligation is met. Some states require a physician to provide information that a reasonable patient would deem significant; others require disclosure of the risks and alternatives that a reasonable physician would have disclosed under similar circumstances. Liability is then based on whether the physician failed to disclose a risk that should have been disclosed, and whether that risk occurred.

The Process

Medical malpractice lawsuits are formally commenced by filing or service of a summons and complaint. Notification of the claim may occur before formal commencement of a lawsuit and may come in the form of a letter or formal notice. Individuals as well as corporations may be named as defendants. The lawsuit must be commenced within the statute of limitations, a time period that varies by state. If the lawsuit continues, pretrial discovery occurs in the form of either depositions or written documentation. A relatively small percentage of cases are tried; most are either settled or dismissed. If a trial occurs, a jury is generally charged with determining the facts, and the presiding judge is responsible for determining the applicable law.

Managing Legal Risk

Practicing within accepted standards is the best defense against malpractice liability. Good communication among health care providers and with the patient is critical. Documentation is an essential part of a risk management strategy and should be comprehensive, accurate, objective, and timely. Inadvertent admissions against interest should be avoided. The most common forms of admissions against interest are self-criticism or criticism of colleagues after an adverse outcome and speculation about the cause of an event before all of the facts are known. Guidelines and policies should be realistic and written to allow for emergencies.

Suggested References

Caplan RA. Professional liability: What's ahead? ASA Newsletter 1996;60(6):6–9.

Cheney FW. The American Society of Anesthesiologists Closed Claims Project: What have we learned, how has it affected practice, and how will it affect practice in the future. Anesthesiology 1999;91:552–556.

Lobe TE. Medical Malpractice: A Physician's Guide. New York: McGraw-Hill, 1995.

Sandbar SS, Gibofsky A, Firestone MH, et al. Legal Medicine. 4th ed. St. Louis: Mosby, 1998.

236

Perioperative Pulmonary Aspiration

Mark A. Warner, M.D.

Recent studies suggest that perioperative pulmonary aspiration is an infrequent event (approximately 1:3000 general anesthetics), but its impact on individual patients can be devastating. Patients who appear to have the greatest risk of severe pulmonary morbidity or death after aspiration are those who are sick (American Society of Anesthesiologists physical classification 3 or greater) and elderly. As a general rule, children have less morbidity from pulmonary aspiration.

Importance of Pulmonary Aspiration

Five large studies from 1970 to 2000 have documented the overall frequency of perioperative pulmonary aspiration to be approximately 1:3000. Fortunately, not all patients who aspirate develop respiratory sequelae. The frequency of pulmonary complications and mortality as a consequence of aspiration are shown in Table 236–1. Although the frequency of death from pulmonary aspiration is very low, the rate of death in patients who have a clearly documented perioperative aspiration perioperatively is quite high (5%).

Based on the information in Table 236–1, if similar mortality rates were to be found within the

United States in general, approximately 200 deaths from perioperative pulmonary aspiration would be expected each year. In our largest institutions (i.e., those that perform as many as 50,000 general anesthetics annually), there would be only 1 death from pulmonary aspiration every 18 months. By applying the numbers (1 death per 75,000 general anesthetics) to individual practice settings, an idea of the anticipated frequency of this event can be derived.

Serious morbidity and considerable costs are associated with pulmonary aspiration that does not result in death. Approximately 25% of patients who aspirate gastric contents perioperatively require intensive care support. About 10% of those who aspirate need mechanical ventilation support for more than 24 hours.

Pulmonary Aspiration in Children

The rate of perioperative pulmonary aspiration in children is similar to that in adults, but children rarely die from this event. Their outcomes after aspiration tend to be better and their recoveries seem to be quicker. The children at highest risk for aspiration and serious morbidity are those under age 1 year with gastrointestinal ileus.

Use of Medications and Preoperative Fasting

Medications used to decrease gastric contents and/or acidity clearly work as advertised. However, no data suggest that the use of these medications decreases the risk of pulmonary aspiration. Many anesthesia organizations around the world have developed guidelines to decrease the risk of perioperative aspiration, and all are similar. The recommendations of the American Society of Anesthesiologists for medications and fasting are given in Tables 236–2 and 236–3, respectively. Although no routine use of any of the commonly used medications is recommended, they may be useful when the anticipated risk of pulmonary aspiration is high.

Table 236–1. Risk of Aspiration-Associated Pulmonary Complications and Death After General Anesthesia by ASA Physical Status Classification

ASA Physical Status Classification	Pulmonary Complications*	Death†
I	1/39,865 (1:39,865)	0
II	2/87,471 (1:43,735)	0
III	7/78,714 (1:11,245)	1/78,714 (1:78,714)
IV and V	3/9438 (1:3146)	2/9438 (1:4719)
Total	13/215,488	3/215,488 (1:71,829)

*Pulmonary complications include adult respiratory distress syndrome, pneumonitis, or pneumonia (with or without positive viral or bacterial identification).

†Death from aspiration-associated pulmonary complications within 6 months of aspiration.

From Warner MA, Anesthesiology 1993;78:56–62.

Table 236–2. Summary of 1999 ASA Task Force Pharmacologic Recommendations to Reduce the Risk of Pulmonary Aspiration

Drug Type and Common Examples	Recommendation
Gastrointestinal stimulants	No routine use
Metoclopramide	
Gastric acid secretion blockers	No routine use
Cimetidine	
Famotidine	
Ranitidine	
Omeprazole	
Lansoprazole	
Antacids	No routine use
Sodium citrate	
Sodium bicarbonate	
Magnesium trisilicate	
Antiemetics	No routine use
Droperidol	
Ondansetron	
Anticholinergics	No use
Atropine	
Scopolamine	
Glycopyrrolate	
Combinations of the medications above	No routine use

Occurrence of Aspiration in the Perioperative Period

Although aspiration may occur at any time (including immediately before anesthesia induction), it is most common during tracheal intubation and extubation. A common factor found in patients who aspirate when an endotracheal tube is being used is inadequate muscle relaxation. Laryngoscopy in an inadequately paralyzed patient may cause the patient to gag and vomit. The same sequence occurs during extubation in a patient who is either weak or not alert and nonresponsive. There is insufficient information on the effectiveness of laryngeal mask airways to prevent aspiration, but there are case

Table 236–3. Summary of 1999 ASA Task Force Fasting Recommendations to Reduce the Risk of Pulmonary Aspiration*

Ingested Material	Minimum Fasting Period† (h)
Clear liquids‡	2
Breast milk	4
Infant formula	6
Nonhuman milk§	6
Light meal¶	6

*These recommendations apply to healthy patients who are undergoing elective procedures. They are not intended for women in labor. Following the Guidelines does not guarantee complete gastric emptying.

†The fasting periods noted above apply to all ages.

‡Examples of clear liquids include water, fruit juices without pulp, carbonated beverages, clear tea, and black coffee.

§Since nonhuman milk is similar to solids in gastric emptying time, the amount ingested must be considered when determining an appropriate fasting period.

¶A light meal typically consists of toast and clear liquids. Meals that include fried or fatty foods or meat may prolong gastric emptying time. Both the amount and type of foods ingested must be considered when determining an appropriate fasting period.

reports of aspiration with their use in both high-risk and low-risk patients.

Management of Perioperative Pulmonary Aspiration

Patients who aspirate require supportive care. Careful suctioning of aspirated material is useful to decrease the volume remaining in the lungs, but lavage with saline is discouraged, because it may increase the spread of aspirate. If particulate material is present, bronchoscopy should be performed to prevent bronchial obstruction. Prophylactic use of antibiotics or steroids has been ineffective in decreasing the frequency of pneumonia or lung inflammation or improving outcomes. Respiratory support is provided as needed.

The severity of pulmonary aspiration and its consequences vary widely. Scant amounts of aspirated gastric contents may have little impact on the lungs, whereas large volumes of aspirate may immediately impair oxygenation. Patients who aspirate small volumes perioperatively and who are asymptomatic during the first 2 postoperative hours are unlikely to develop respiratory sequelae. Therefore, it is reasonable to discharge asymptomatic patients to regular postoperative nursing units or even home with little risk of delayed development of respiratory symptoms.

Conclusion

Pulmonary aspiration is an infrequent perioperative event, occurring at a rate of approximately 1 per 3000 children and adult patients undergoing general anesthesia. This rate varies dramatically between patients, with those who are sicker and undergoing emergency procedures having the highest rate of aspiration. Approximately 25% of patients who aspirate gastric contents during the perioperative period develop significant respiratory complications. The overall mortality rate from pulmonary aspiration after aspiration is 5%, and death occurs primarily in adults; children rarely die after perioperative aspiration. The routine use of preoperative medications to reduce the risk of pulmonary aspiration does not appear to be warranted. Preoperative fasting guidelines suggest decreased fasting periods, especially for clear liquids.

Suggested References

American Society of Anesthesiologists, Task Force on Preoperative Fasting. Practice guidelines for preoperative fasting and the use of pharmacologic agents to reduce the risk of pulmonary aspiration: Application to healthy patients undergoing elective procedures. Anesthesiology 1999;90:896–905.

Kluger MT, Short TG. Aspiration during anaesthesia: A review of 133 cases from the Australian anaesthetic incident monitoring study (AIMS). Anaesthesia 1999;54:19–26.

Warner, MA. Is pulmonary aspiration still an important problem in anesthesia? Curr Opin Anesthesiol 2000;13:215–218.

237
Perioperative Neuropathies in the Upper Extremities

Mark A. Warner, M.D.

Any nerve that passes into the upper extremity may sustain an injury or convert from an abnormal but asymptomatic state to a symptomatic state during the perioperative period. Of the major nerve structures of the upper extremity, the ulnar nerve and brachial plexus nerves are the most prone to becoming symptomatic, leading to major disability during the perioperative period.

Ulnar Neuropathy

Typically, anesthesia-related ulnar nerve injury is thought to be associated with external nerve compression or stretch caused by malpositioning during the intraoperative period. Although this implication may be true for some patients, three findings suggest that other factors may contribute. First, male gender (various reports suggest that 70% to 90% of patients who develop this problem are male), high body mass index ($\geq$38), and prolonged bed rest are associated with ulnar neuropathies. Second, many patients with perioperative ulnar neuropathies

have a high incidence rate of contralateral ulnar nerve conduction dysfunction. This finding suggests that many of these patients likely have asymptomatic but abnormal ulnar nerves before anesthetic induction, and that these abnormal nerves may become symptomatic during the perioperative period. Finally, many patients do not notice or complain of ulnar nerve symptoms until more than 48 hours after their surgical procedures.

Perioperative ulnar neuropathy may be caused by factors other than improper patient positioning during surgery. Elbow flexion, especially to greater than 110°, can tighten the cubital tunnel retinaculum and directly compress the ulnar nerve (Figs. 237–1 and 237–2).

External compression of the ulnar nerve in the absence of elbow flexion also may damage the nerve. Although compression within the bony groove posterior to the medial epicondyle may be possible, the

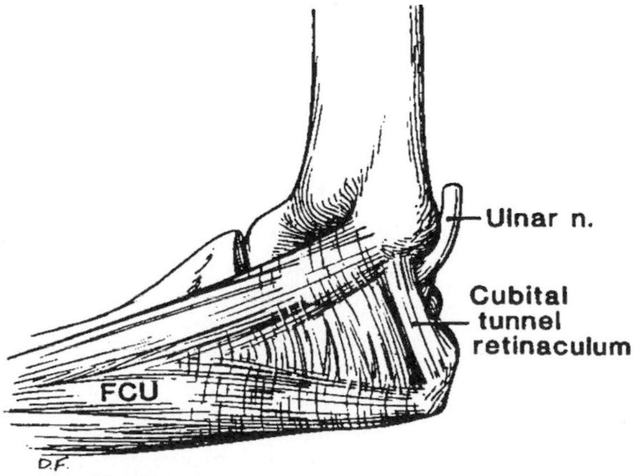

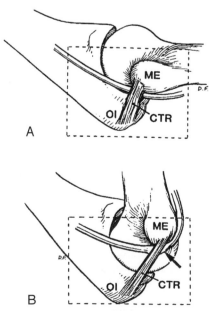

Figure 237–1. The proximal edge of the roof of the cubital tunnel is formed by a retinaculum that originates on the medial epicondyle and inserts on the olecranon. It is distinct from the aponeurosis of the flexor carpi ulnaris (FCU) with which its distal margin blends. (From O'Driscoll SW, Horii E, Carmichael SW, et al.[1])

Figure 237–2. In this medial-to-lateral view of the right elbow, the cubital tunnel retinaculum (CTR) is lax in extension (A) as it stretches from the medial epicondyle (ME) to the olecranon (Ol). The retinaculum tightens in flexion (B) and can compress the ulnar nerve (arrow). (From O'Driscoll SW, Horii E, Carmichael SW, et al.[1])

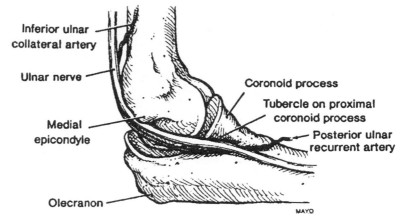

Figure 237-3. The ulnar nerve and its primary blood supply in the proximal forearm, the posterior ulnar recurrent artery, are very superficial and appear to be susceptible to compression from external pressure as they pass posteriomedially to the tubercle of the coronoid process. The tubercle is larger in men than women, and the adipose layer in this area is thinner in men. (From Warner MA.[2])

ulnar nerve is usually deep and well protected from external compression. Forearm rotation, especially pronation, can increase pressure in the postcondylar groove; thus it seems reasonable to position the patient's forearms in a neutral or supinated position. External compression of the ulnar nerve may occur distal to the medial epicondyle, where the nerve and its associated artery are more superficial (Fig. 237-3).

Brachial Plexus Neuropathy

Brachial plexus neuropathies may masquerade as ulnar neuropathies or be associated with symptoms that suggest injuries to other nerve structures. Most often, perioperative brachial plexus neuropathies are associated with median sternotomy. This neuropathy often involves stretching or compression of the brachial plexus during sternal separation. Other potential mechanisms of injury include direct trauma from fractured first ribs. Brachial plexus nerve injury during sternal retraction is most common during internal mammary artery dissection. The mechanism is assumed to be asymmet-

rical retraction of the rib cage. In general, brachial plexus neuropathy does not appear to be related to a patient's arm position or to padding during the sternotomy and related procedures.

The brachial plexus is vulnerable to stretching in a patient positioned prone (Fig. 237-4). Stretching of the brachial plexus, especially its lower trunks, is most likely when the head is turned to the contralateral side, the ipsilateral shoulder is abducted, and the ipsilateral elbow is bent. Although this position is commonly used during surgical procedures and the frequency of perioperative brachial plexus neuropathy is low, it would appear to be prudent to place the arms at the patient's side whenever possible, to decrease the risk of brachial plexus stretching.

Preventing and Caring for Upper Extremity Neuropathies

Suggestions for padding and positioning upper extremities and managing perioperative neuropathies are described in Chapter 238.

Figure 237-4. Sources of potential injury to the brachial plexus and its peripheral components in a pronated patient. Head position stretching plexus against anchors in shoulder (A). Closure of retroclavicular space by chest support with arms at side; neurovascular bundle trapped against first rib (B). Head of humerus thrust into neurovascular bundle if arm and axilla are not relaxed (C). Compression of ulnar nerve in cubital tunnel (D). Area of vulnerability of radial nerve to compression above elbow (E). (From Martin JT.[3])

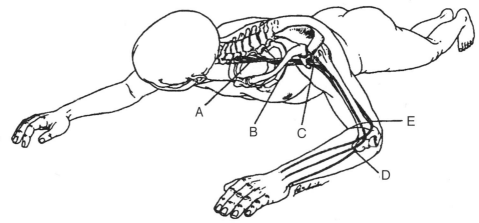

Selected References

1. O'Driscoll SW, Horii E, Carmichael SW, et al. The cubital tunnel and ulnar neuropathy. J Bone Joint Surg 1991;73:613–617.
2. Warner MA. Perioperative neuropathies. Mayo Clin Proc 1998;73:567–574.
3. Martin JT. The ventral decubitus (prone) positions. In Martin JT, Warner MA, eds. Positioning in Anesthesia and Surgery. 3rd ed. Philadelphia: WB Saunders, 1997;155–195.

Suggested References

American Society of Anesthesiologists, Task Force on Prevention of Perioperative Neuropathies. Practice guidelines for the prevention of perioperative neuropathies. Anesthesiology 2000;92:1168–1182.

Contreras MG, Warner MA, Charboneau WJ, et al. The anatomy of the ulnar nerve at the elbow: Potential relationship of acute ulnar neuropathy to gender differences. Clin Anat 1998;11:372–378.

Prielipp RC, Morell RC, Walker FO, et al. Ulnar nerve pressure: Influence of arm position and relationship to somatosensory evoked potentials. Anesthesiology 1999;91:335–336.

Vahl CF, Carl I, Muller-Vahl H, et al. Brachial plexus injury after cardiac surgery. The role of internal artery preparation: A prospective study of 1000 consecutive patients. J Thorac Cardiovasc Surg 1991;102:724–729.

238
Perioperative Neuropathies in the Lower Extremities

Mark A. Warner, M.D.

Although neuropathies of the lower extremities may occur in a variety of patient postures, most of these occur in patients undergoing procedures while placed in a lithotomy position. These neuropathies often have been considered to be preventable and to occur because of poor intraoperative care (e.g., improper positioning or padding) or judgment (e.g., excessively prolonged use of lithotomy position). This perception has significant impact on the outcomes of medicolegal cases involving these types of problems.

Risk Factors

A number of studies have suggested that many factors other than improper intraoperative care may contribute to the risk of lower extremity nerve injury. The neuropathies most frequently associated with major disability involve the common peroneal, sciatic, and femoral nerves. Specific patient characteristics contribute to the risk of neuropathy and suggest that not all neuropathies should be assumed to be the result of improper positioning. These include extremes of body weight (both low and high body mass indexes) and prolonged duration in lithotomy. In both retrospective and prospective studies, the longer that anesthetized patients are maintained in lithotomy positions, the greater their risk of developing a neuropathy.

Outcomes

Fortunately, most lower extremity neuropathies are mild and resolve spontaneously. The obturator, lateral femoral cutaneous, peroneal, sciatic, and femoral nerves can all become dysfunctional, but the peroneal, sciatic, and femoral are the most likely to have loss of motor capability. In contrast to upper extremity neuropathies, especially those involving the ulnar nerve, most lower extremity neuropathies are symptomatic immediately after the analgesic effects of anesthesia are dissipated. This contrast suggests that the etiology for periop-erative lower extremity neuropathies occurs intra-operatively whereas the etiology for ulnar neuropathy appears to occur most frequently in the postoperative period.

Motor dysfunction of lower extremity nerves can be severe, leading to footdrop and other gait abnormalities. Approximately 50% of patients who develop a motor neuropathy after surgery regain full motor function within 6 months. However, few patients with residual motor dysfunction at 6 months exhibit further improvement thereafter.

Specific Lower Extremity Neuropathies

Common Peroneal Neuropathy. The common peroneal nerve is very superficial as it wraps around the head of the fibula. Because it is quite exposed at this level, it may be easily compressed and injured. Although direct compression of the common peroneal nerve by leg holders commonly has been considered the primary mechanism of injury in peroneal neuropathy, the superficial branch of the common peroneal nerve (sensory only) may be affected distal to the fibular head.

Sciatic Neuropathy. The same forces that contribute to stretch injuries of the hamstring group muscles (e.g., biceps femoris muscle) may stretch the sciatic nerve. Simultaneous hyperflexion of the hip and extension of the knee will stretch and possibly injure the sciatic nerve. This set of actions can occur during the establishment and maintenance of a lithotomy position. A patient in a lithotomy position may passively shift toward the caudal end of an operating table when placed in a head-up posture or be actively shifted caudally by a member of the operating team in an attempt to obtain increased exposure of the perineum.

Femoral Neuropathy. Neuropathies involving the femoral nerve and its cutaneous branches often are considered to result from improper placement of abdominal wall retractors and direct compression of the nerve. When related to retractors, the assumption is that retractors place continuous pressure on the iliopsoas muscle and either stretch the nerve or cause it to become ischemic by occluding the external iliac artery or penetrating vessels of the nerve as it passes through the muscle.

Obturator Neuropathy. The obturator nerve passes through the pelvis, where it may be stretched or compressed by surgical retractors placed deep below the pelvic brim. Excessive abduction of the thigh at the hip beyond comfortable limits may stretch the nerve. In general, obturator neuropathies involve sensory loss, although motor dysfunction of the adductor muscles of the thigh has been reported. These sensory neuropathies are usually transient, lasting 1 to 6 weeks.

Lateral Femoral Cutaneous Neuropathy. Unlike the other lower extremity nerves, the lateral femoral cutaneous nerve is sensory only. The nerve has a varied course; in many patients, small branches of the nerve perforate the inguinal ligament. Hyperflexion of the hip onto the abdomen may increase pressure within the inguinal ligament and compress these sensory branches. In addition, direct pressure can be applied to the nerve during a surgical procedure. Like obturator neuropathies, most of these are transient.

Practical Considerations for Upper and Lower Extremity Neuropathies

Efforts to prevent perioperative neuropathies are frequently debated, and there often is confusion on how to manage a neuropathy once it has occurred. In general, there are no data to support recommendations on any of these issues.

Padding Exposed Peripheral Nerves. Many types of padding materials are advocated to protect exposed peripheral nerves. They often consist of cloth (e.g., blankets and towels), foam sponges (e.g., egg crate foam), and gel pads. There are no data to suggest that any of these materials is more effective than any other or that any is better than no padding at all. Positioning and padding of exposed peripheral nerves should prevent their stretch beyond normally tolerated limits while awake, avoid their direct compression, if possible, and distribute any compressive forces that must be placed on them over as large an area as possible.

Prolonged Duration in One Position.

Prolonged duration in one position appears to increase the risk of neuropathy and other integumentary damage. It would appear prudent to limit the time that any patient spends in one position as much as possible. Intermittent movement of the limbs or head during the intraoperative period is occasionally possible but may increase the risk of various other problems, including but not limited to endotracheal tube dislodgment, corneal abrasion, or movement of an extremity into a suboptimal position.

What to Do if a Patient Develops a Neuropathy. Although each situation is unique and requires careful assessment, the following guidelines suggest a basic course of action that will lead to appropriate care:

□ Is the neuropathy sensory or motor? Sensory lesions are more frequently transient than motor lesions. If the symptoms are numbness and/or tingling only, then it may be appropriate to inform the patient that many of these neuropathies will resolve during the first 5 days. The patient should be instructed to avoid postures that might compress or stretch the involved nerve. Arrangements should be made for frequent contact with the patient. A call to alert a neurologist would be appropriate, and if the symptoms still persist on postoperative day 5, the neurologist should be consulted.

□ If the neuropathy has a motor component, a neurologist should be consulted immediately. Electromyographic studies may be needed to assess the location of any acute lesion. This knowledge may direct an appropriate treatment plan. The studies may also demonstrate chronic abnormalities of the nerve or, if applicable, the contralateral nerve.

Suggested References

American Society of Anesthesiologists, Task Force on the Prevention of Perioperative Neuropathies. Practice guidelines for the prevention of perioperative neuropathies. Anesthesiology 2000;92:1168–1182.

Cheney FW, Domino KB, Caplan RA, et al. Nerve injury associated with anesthesia. Anesthesiology 1999;90:1062–1069.

Warner MA. Perioperative neuropathies. Mayo Clin Proc 1998;73:567–574.

Warner MA, Martin JT, Schroeder DR, et al. Lower-extremity motor neuropathy associated with surgery performed on patients in a lithotomy position. Anesthesiology 1994;81:6–12.

Warner MA, Warner DO, Harper CM, et al. Lower extremity neuropathies associated with the lithotomy position. Anesthesiology 2000;93:938–942.

Index

Note: Page numbers followed by f indicate figures; those followed by t indicate tables.

ISBN 0-443-06601-9